HANDBOOK OF DEPRESSION IN CHILDREN AND ADOLESCENTS

Handbook of Depression in Children and Adolescents

Edited by
John R. Z. Abela
Benjamin L. Hankin

THE GUILFORD PRESS
New York   London

© 2008 The Guilford Press
A Division of Guilford Publications, Inc.
72 Spring Street, New York, NY 10012
www.guilford.com

Printed in the United States of America

This book is printed on acid-free paper.

Last digit is print number: 9 8 7 6 5 4 3 2 1

The authors have checked with sources believed to be reliable in their efforts to provide information that is complete and generally in accord with the standards of practice that are accepted at the time of publication. However, in view of the possibility of human error or changes in medical sciences, neither the authors, nor the editor and publisher, nor any other party who has been involved in the preparation or publication of this work warrants that the information contained herein is in every respect accurate or complete, and they are not responsible for any errors or omissions or the results obtained from the use of such information. Readers are encouraged to confirm the information contained in this book with other sources.

Library of Congress Cataloging-in-Publication Data
Handbook of depression in children and adolescents / edited by John R. Z. Abela, Benjamin L. Hankin.
   p. ; cm.
  Includes bibliographical references and indexes.
  ISBN-13: 978-1-59385-582-6 (hardcover : alk. paper)
  ISBN-10: 1-59385-582-6 (hardcover : alk. paper)
  1. Depression in children. 2. Depression in adolescence. I. Abela, John R. Z.
II. Hankin, Benjamin L.
  [DNLM: 1. Depressive Disorder. 2. Adolescents. 3. Children. 4. Depression.
WM 171 H2368 2008]
  RJ506.D4H362 2008
  618.92′8527—dc22
                                       2007036573

To my parents, John and Kathleen Abela,
and my partner, Hubert Comtois.
Thank for your never-ending love, guidance, and support.
I owe where I am today, in large part, to you.

—John R. Z. Abela

To my parents, Lawrence and Lee Hankin,
and my wife, Michelle, and children, Noah and Jacob.
Your support, laughter, and love are invaluable
and make all things possible.

—Benjamin L. Hankin

About the Editors

John R. Z. Abela, PhD, is Associate Professor and William Dawson Scholar in the Departments of Psychology and Psychiatry at McGill University and Director of the Cognitive Behavior Therapy Clinic at Montreal Children's Hospital. A clinical psychologist, Dr. Abela is a two-time recipient of the Young Investigator Award from the National Alliance for Research on Schizophrenia and Depression, among many other awards. His research on cognitive and interpersonal vulnerability to depression in children, adolescents, and adults has also been funded by the National Institute of Mental Health, the Canadian Institutes of Health Research, the Canada Foundation for Innovation, the Social Sciences and Research Council of Canada, and the Canadian Psychiatric Research Foundation.

Benjamin L. Hankin, PhD, is Assistant Professor of Psychology at the University of South Carolina. Dr. Hankin is a developmental psychopathologist interested in vulnerability and stress models to depression. His research on depression has been funded by the National Institute of Mental Health, the National Science Foundation, the National Cancer Institute, the American Foundation for Suicide Prevention, and the Canadian Institutes of Health Research. He has served on the editorial boards of several journals, including *Journal of Abnormal Psychology, Journal of Consulting and Clinical Psychology, Journal of Abnormal Child Psychology,* and *Journal of Clinical Child and Adolescent Psychology,* and has received awards from the Society for Research in Psychopathology and the Association of Behavioral and Cognitive Therapies.

Contributors

Jamie L. Abaied, MA, Department of Psychology, University of Illinois at Urbana–Champaign, Champaign, Illinois

John R. Z. Abela, PhD, Department of Psychology, McGill University, Montreal, Quebec, Canada

Afroze Anjum, PsyD, Toronto District School Board, Toronto, Ontario, Canada

Shelli Avenevoli, PhD, Division of Pediatric Translational Research and Treatment Development, Department of Health and Human Services, National Institute of Mental Health, National Institutes of Health, Bethesda, Maryland

Theodore W. Bender, BS, Department of Psychology, Florida State University, Tallahassee, Florida

Steven M. Brunwasser, BA, Department of Psychology, University of Michigan, Ann Arbor, Michigan

Catherine Cheely, BS, Department of Psychology, Barnwell College, University of South Carolina, Columbia, South Carolina

C. Emily Durbin, PhD, Department of Psychology, Northwestern University, Evanston, Illinois

Thalia C. Eley, PhD, Social, Genetic, and Developmental Psychiatry Centre, Institute of Psychiatry, King's College, London, London, United Kingdom

Ilyan Ferrer, BA, Department of Psychology, McGill University, Montreal, Quebec, Canada

Melissa Fisher, MS, Department of Educational Psychology, University of Texas, Austin, Texas

Megan Flynn, MA, Department of Psychology, University of Illinois at Urbana–Champaign, Champaign, Illinois

Eric Fombonne, MD, Department of Psychiatry, Montreal Children's Hospital, McGill University, Montreal, Quebec, Canada

Derek R. Freres, MA, Annenberg School for Communication, University of Pennsylvania, Philadelphia, Pennsylvania

Jane E. Gillham, PhD, Department of Psychology, Swarthmore College, Swarthmore, Pennsylvania, and Department of Psychology, University of Pennsylvania, Philadelphia, Pennsylvania

Golda S. Ginsburg, PhD, Division of Child and Adolescent Psychiatry, Johns Hopkins University School of Medicine, Baltimore, Maryland

Sherryl H. Goodman, PhD, Department of Psychology, Emory University, Atlanta, Georgia

Michelle Greenberg, MS, Department of Educational Psychology, University of Texas, Austin, Texas

Benjamin L. Hankin, PhD, Department of Psychology, Barnwell College, University of South Carolina, Columbia, South Carolina

Jennifer Hargrave, PhD, Department of Educational Psychology, University of Texas, Austin, Texas

Kate L. Harkness, PhD, Department of Psychology, Queen's University, Kingston, Ontario, Canada

Jenny Herren, MS, Department of Educational Psychology, University of Texas, Austin, Texas

Brooke Hersh, MS, Department of Educational Psychology, University of Texas, Austin, Texas

Nora Hilmy, BA, Department of Psychology, McGill University, Montreal, Quebec, Canada

Thomas E. Joiner, Jr., PhD, Department of Psychology, Florida State University, Tallahassee, Florida

Ronald C. Kessler, PhD, Department of Health Care Policy, Harvard Medical School, Boston, Massachusetts

Erin Knight, BA, Section on Developmental Genetic Epidemiology, Mood and Anxiety Disorders Program, Department of Health and Human Services, National Institute of Mental Health, National Institutes of Health, Bethesda, Maryland

Jennifer Y. F. Lau, PhD, Mood and Anxiety Disorders Program, Department of Health and Human Services, National Institute of Mental Health, National Institutes of Health, Bethesda, Maryland

Margaret N. Lumley, PhD, Department of Psychology, Queen's University, Kingston, Ontario, Canada

Chad McWhinnie, BA, Department of Psychology, McGill University, Montreal, Quebec, Canada

Kathleen Ries Merikangas, PhD, Section on Developmental Genetic Epidemiology, Mood and Anxiety Disorders Program, Department of Health and Human Services, National Institute of Mental Health, National Institutes of Health, Bethesda, Maryland

Laura Mufson, PhD, Department of Psychiatry, Columbia University College of Physicians and Surgeons, and New York State Psychiatric Institute, New York, New York

Amélie Nantel-Vivier, BA, Department of Psychology, McGill University, Montreal, Quebec, Canada

Robert O. Pihl, PhD, Department of Psychology, McGill University, Montreal, Quebec, Canada

Tayyab Rashid, PhD, Positive Psychology Center, University of Pennsylvania, Philadelphia, Pennsylvania

Mark A. Reinecke, PhD, Division of Psychology, Feinberg School of Medicine, Northwestern University, Chicago, Illinois

Karen D. Rudolph, PhD, Department of Psychology, University of Illinois at Urbana–Champaign, Champaign, Illinois

Edward A. Selby, BS, BA, Department of Psychology, Florida State University, Tallahassee, Florida

Daphna M. Shafir, BA, Department of Psychology, Northwestern University, Evanston, Illinois

Susan H. Spence, PhD, Faculty of Health, Griffith University, Queensland, Australia

Kevin D. Stark, PhD, Department of Educational Psychology, University of Texas, Austin, Texas

Erin Tully, PhD, Department of Psychology, University of Minnesota, Minneapolis, Minnesota

Kimberly A. Van Orden, MS, Department of Psychology, Florida State University, Tallahassee, Florida

Emily Wetter, BA, Department of Psychology, Barnwell College, University of South Carolina, Columbia, South Carolina

Tracy K. Witte, MS, Department of Psychology, Florida State University, Tallahassee, Florida

Jami F. Young, PhD, Department of Psychiatry, Columbia University College of Physicians and Surgeons, and New York State Psychiatric Institute, New York, New York

Suzanne Zinck, MD, IWK Children's Health Centre/Maritime Psychiatry, Halifax, Nova Scotia, Canada

Contents

I. INTRODUCTION AND EPIDEMIOLOGY OF DEPRESSION

1. Depression in Children and Adolescents: Causes, Treatment, and Prevention   3
   John R. Z. Abela and Benjamin L. Hankin

2. Epidemiology of Depression in Children and Adolescents   6
   Shelli Avenevoli, Erin Knight, Ronald C. Kessler, and Kathleen Ries Merikangas

II. ETIOLOGY OF DEPRESSION

3. Cognitive Vulnerability to Depression in Children and Adolescents: A Developmental Psychopathology Perspective   35
   John R. Z. Abela and Benjamin L. Hankin

4. A Developmental Perspective on Interpersonal Theories of Youth Depression   79
   Karen D. Rudolph, Megan Flynn, and Jamie L. Abaied

5. Biological Vulnerability to Depression   103
   Amélie Nantel-Vivier and Robert O. Pihl

6. New Behavioral Genetic Approaches to Depression in Childhood and Adolescence   124
   Jennifer Y. F. Lau and Thalia C. Eley

7. Emotion Regulation and Risk for Depression   149
   C. Emily Durbin and Daphna M. Shafir

III. TREATMENT OF DEPRESSION

8. Cognitive-Behavioral Treatment of Depression during Childhood and Adolescence   179
   Mark A. Reinecke and Golda S. Ginsburg

9. Psychopharmacological Treatment of Depression   207
   in Children and Adolescents
   Eric Fombonne and Suzanne Zinck

10. Treatment of Childhood Depression: The ACTION Treatment Program   224
    Kevin D. Stark, Jennifer Hargrave, Brooke Hersh, Michelle Greenberg,
    Jenny Herren, and Melissa Fisher

11. Positive Psychotherapy for Young Adults and Children   250
    Tayyab Rashid and Afroze Anjum

12. Interpersonal Psychotherapy for Treatment and Prevention   288
    of Adolescent Depression
    Jami F. Young and Laura Mufson

IV. PREVENTION OF DEPRESSION

13. Preventing Depression in Early Adolescence: 309
    The Penn Resiliency Program
    Jane E. Gillham, Steven M. Brunwasser, and Derek R. Freres

14. Integrating Individual and Whole-School Change Approaches   333
    in the Prevention of Depression in Adolescents
    Susan H. Spence

15. Positive Youth Development Programs: An Alternative Approach   354
    to the Prevention of Depression in Children and Adolescents
    Chad McWhinnie, John R. Z. Abela, Nora Hilmy, and Ilyan Ferrer

V. SPECIAL POPULATIONS

16. Sex Differences in Child and Adolescent Depression: 377
    A Developmental Psychopathological Approach
    Benjamin L. Hankin, Emily Wetter, and Catherine Cheely

17. Children of Depressed Mothers: Implications for the Etiology,   415
    Treatment, and Prevention of Depression in Children and Adolescents
    Sherryl H. Goodman and Erin Tully

18. Suicidal Behavior in Youth   441
    Kimberly A. Van Orden, Tracy K. Witte, Edward A. Selby,
    Theodore W. Bender, and Thomas E. Joiner, Jr.

19. Child Abuse and Neglect and the Development of Depression   466
    in Children and Adolescents
    Kate L. Harkness and Margaret N. Lumley

Author Index   489

Subject Index   515

INTRODUCTION AND EPIDEMIOLOGY OF DEPRESSION

1 Depression in Children and Adolescents

Causes, Treatment, and Prevention

John R. Z. Abela and Benjamin L. Hankin

Children and adolescents are currently experiencing depression at an unprecedented rate. As prevalence rates of depression in Western cultures have soared to epidemic proportions, the average age of onset has rapidly decreased (Reich et al., 1987). Researchers have reported that by the age of 14, as many as 9% of youth have already experienced at least one episode of severe depression (Lewinsohn, Hops, Roberts, Seeley, & Andrews, 1993). Lifetime prevalence rates of major depressive disorder for adolescents between the ages of 15 and 18 are estimated to be approximately 14%, with an additional 11% reporting minor depression (for review, see Hammen & Rudolph, 2004). Even when diagnostic criteria are not met, subsyndromal depressive symptoms are indicative of impaired functioning and may lead to the later development of diagnosable disorders (Roberts, Lewinsohn, & Seeley, 1991). Early-onset depression is a chronic disorder with as many as 84% of those depressed as youths experiencing depressive episodes in adulthood (Harrington, Rutter, & Frombonne, 1996). Further, early-onset depression has been shown to be associated with a wide range of psychiatric and physical health problems in adulthood as well as impairment in multiple domains of functioning (e.g., Achenbach, Howell, McConaughy, & Stanger, 1995a, 1995b; Fleming, Boyle, & Offord, 1993; Kandel & Davies, 1986; Rao et al., 1995).

Until recent years, most of the research examining the etiology, treatment, and prevention of depression has been conducted using adult samples. This is unfortunate, given that results from studies examining models of depression in adults cannot be extended downward to children and adolescents. Rather, age-related differences in cognition, emotion, behavior, and physical development must be taken into account, and theories of etiology as well as the efficacy of treatment/prevention interventions must be examined using child, adolescent, and adult samples.

Substantial progress has been made in the past decade in understanding the etiology of depression in child and adolescent populations within a vulnerability–stress, developmental psychopathology framework from cognitive, interpersonal, biological, genetic, and emotion regulation perspectives. In addition, research on the etiology of depression in youth has begun to be translated into effective treatments for youth suffering from depressive disorders, as well as effective prevention programs for use with both unselected and high-risk samples of youth.

The goal of this edited book is to bring together some of the foremost experts who are conducting groundbreaking research examining the causes, treatment, and prevention of depression in children and adolescents, to summarize the theoretical and empirical literature that has accumulated on these topics in the past decade and to propose future directions for theory, research, and clinical practice. The two major unique and distinct aspects of this book are (1) its interdisciplinary approach to understanding the development of depression in youth within a vulnerability–stress, developmental psychopathological framework and (2) its attempt to bridge the gap between research on the etiology of depression and the various approaches to treatment and prevention.

Chapter 2 reviews recent literature on the epidemiology of depression in children and adolescence, touching on issues such as (1) the classification of depressive disorders, (2) developmental differences in the manifestation of depressive symptoms, (3) the prevalence/incidence of depressive disorders in youth, (4) gender differences in the prevalence rates of depression in youth, (5) socioeconomic, ethnic, and cultural differences in the prevalence rates of depression in youth, (5) the continuous versus categorical nature of depression, and (6) the developmental course and prognosis of childhood and adolescent depression.

Part II of the book presents contemporary theoretical models of the etiology and maintenance of depression in youth from a diverse array of theoretical perspectives (e.g., childhood adversity, cognitive, interpersonal, biological, genetics, and emotion regulation) Theories are organized within a vulnerability–stress, developmental psychopathology framework. Research examining the etiological components of such theoretical models in children, preadolescents, and adolescents is discussed. Emphasis is placed on the impact of developmental factors on the etiological chains proposed by the various models. Directions for future research are outlined.

Part III focuses on both individual and group treatments for depression in youth. Treatments representing a wide variety of theoretical orientations (cognitive, interpersonal, and biological) are included. Each chapter presents a step-by-step overview of the implementation of a particular intervention with children and adolescents. Attention is paid to drawing connections between the therapeutic techniques employed and the theoretical models on which the interventions are based. The available research examining both the efficacy of interventions and their mechanisms of action is summarized. Directions for future research are outlined.

Part IV focuses on the prevention of depression in youth. The theoretical framework underlying three specific empirically supported, cognitive-behavioral depression programs is described in detail. The techniques employed in such programs are presented in a step-by-step manner. The available research examining both the efficacy of the interventions and their mechanisms of action is summarized. The authors outline future directions for modification of their programs in order to increase their efficacy for use with both unselected samples of youth and at-risk populations.

Part V touches on issues presented in the previous four sections as they pertain to specific populations. The topics covered include (1) research pertaining to the epidemiology, etiology, treatment, and prevention of depression in children of depressed parents, (2) theoretical models of suicidality, as well as interventions for working with suicidal youth, and (3) cognitive, interpersonal, life stress, and biological models proposed specifically to clarify the emergence of gender differences in the prevalence of depression.

This book seeks to provide a critical analysis of the prevailing theories of vulnerability to depression in youth, as well as the treatment/prevention programs based on such theories. Because it represents one of the first attempts to place such theories and interventions within a developmental psychopathology framework, more questions are posed than answers given. At the same time, the book aims to serve as a springboard to the development of more holistic, developmentally sensitive models of the etiology, treatment, and prevention of depression in youth from a vulnerability–stress perspective.

REFERENCES

Achenbach, T. M., Howell, C. T., McConaughy, S. H., & Stanger, C. (1995a). Six-year predictors of problems in a national sample of children and youths: I. Cross-informant syndromes. *Journal of the American Academy of Child and Adolescent Psychiatry, 34,* 336–347.

Achenbach, T. M., Howell, C. T., McConaughy, S. H., & Stanger, C. (1995b). Six-year predictors of problems in a national sample of children and youths: II. Signs of disturbance. *Journal of the American Academy of Child and Adolescent Psychiatry, 34,* 488–498.

Fleming, J. E., Boyle, M. H., & Offord, D. R. (1993). The outcome of adolescent depression in the Ontario Child Health Study follow-up. *Journal of the American Academy of Child and Adolescent Psychiatry, 32,* 28–33.

Hammen, C., & Rudolph, K. D. (2003). Childhood mood disorders. In E. J. Mash & R. A. Barkley (Eds.), *Child psychopathology* (2nd ed., pp. 233–278). New York: Guilford Press.

Harrington, R., Rutter, M., & Frombonne, E. (1996). Developmental pathways in depression: Multiple meanings, antecedents, and endpoints. *Development and Psychopathology, 8,* 601–616.

Kandel, D. B., & Davies, M. (1986). Adult sequelae of adolescent depressive symptoms. *Archives of General Psychiatry, 43,* 255–262.

Lewinsohn, P. M., Hops, H., Roberts, R. E., Seeley, J. R., & Andrews, J. A. (1993). Adolescent psychopathology: I. Prevalence and incidence of depression and other DSM-III-R disorders in high school students. *Journal of Abnormal Psychology, 102,* 133–144.

Rao, U., Ryan, N. D., Birmaher, B., Dahl, R. E., Williamson, D. E., Kaufman, J., et al. (1995). Clinical outcome in adulthood. *Journal of the American Academy of Child and Adolescent Psychiatry, 34,* 566–578.

Reich, T., Van Eerdewegh, P., Rice, J., Mullaney, J., Klerman, G., & Endicott, J. (1987). The family transmission of primary depressive disorder. *Journal of Psychiatric Research, 21,* 613–624.

Roberts, R. E., Lewinsohn, P. M., & Seeley, J. R. (1991). Screening for adolescent depression: A comparison of depression scales. *Journal of the American Academy of Child and Adolescent Psychology, 30,* 58–66.

2 Epidemiology of Depression in Children and Adolescents

Shelli Avenevoli, Erin Knight, Ronald C. Kessler,
and Kathleen Ries Merikangas

This chapter provides an update on previous reviews of the epidemiological literature on childhood and adolescent unipolar depression (Kessler, Avenevoli, & Merikangas, 2001; Merikangas & Avenevoli, 2002). Less than two decades ago, information on the prevalence, course, and risk of depression among children and adolescents was based on studies with small, unrepresentative, or primarily clinical samples of youth or on retrospective accounts from studies of adults. Since that time, a number of community surveys have been carried out that studied the epidemiology of depression among youths. Moreover, child and adolescent psychiatric epidemiological research has progressed from descriptive to analytical aims (Earls, 1979). Prompted in part by a trend to integrate developmental issues (Costello, Foley, & Angold, 2006), several community studies have followed cohorts over time and have provided valuable information on changes in prevalence, trajectories of illness, and mechanisms of risk across child, adolescent, and early adult development. These studies are reviewed here, with an emphasis on findings regarding prevalence, comorbidity, developmental course, correlates, consequences, and treatment. Consistent with the available literature, the information presented focuses on major depression or collapsed indices of depressive disorders. When available, findings for dysthymia and minor depression are discussed; the epidemiology of bipolar disorder is not reviewed in this chapter.

METHODOLOGICAL ISSUES

Definition

Depression has been defined in a number of ways in the research literature (Angold, 1988; Compas, Ey, & Grant, 1993), including as a transient mood or affective state, a syndrome of related symptoms, and a clinical disorder defined by official nosologies (e.g.,

Diagnostic and Statistical Manual of Mental Disorders, fourth edition [DSM-IV; American Psychiatric Association, 1994], *International Classification of Diseases*, 10th edition [ICD; World Health Organization, 1993]). These conceptualizations represent different approaches to measurement and highlight two controversial issues in child and adolescent psychiatry. The first issue concerns the threshold at which clinically significant depression is defined among children and adolescents. Consistent with empirical evidence that the essential features of depression are similar in adults and adolescents (Angst, 1988; Roberts, Lewinsohn, & Seeley, 1995; Lewinsohn, Pettit, Joiner, & Seeley, 2003), the diagnostic criteria for all mood disorders are virtually identical for children and adults. The few exceptions in DSM-IV for major depression and dysthymia include irritable mood as a proxy for depressed mood, failure to make expected weight gains as a proxy for weight loss, and shorter required duration for dysthymia.

Despite similarities in the core symptoms of depression, however, there is evidence of age differences in symptom expression that may reflect developmental changes in cognitive, emotional, biological, and social competencies (Avenevoli & Steinberg, 2001; Cichetti & Toth 1998; Kovacs, Obrosky, & Sherrill, 2003; Weiss & Garber 2003). Findings consistently suggest that somatic complaints among youth with depressive disorders decrease with age, hypersomnia and reduced appetite (for girls) increase during adolescence, and suicide risk peaks during middle (girls) or late (boys) adolescence (Kashani, Rosenberg, & Reid, 1989; Kovacs & Gatsonis, 1989; Kovacs et al., 2003; Mitchell, McCauley, Burke, & Moss, 1988; Ryan et al., 1987; Weiss et al., 1992). In addition, a growing literature highlights the significance of syndromes (e.g., minor depression) that fall below diagnostic thresholds by number of symptoms or duration of episodes. The large proportion of children and adolescents with subthreshold depressive symptoms (Kessler & Walters, 1998; Angold, Costello, Farmer, Burns, & Erkanli, 1999) report as much or nearly as much functional impairment and seek treatment at the same or higher rates as adolescents with major depression (Angold, Costello, Farmer, Burns, & Erkanli, 1999; Gonzalez-Tejera et al., 2005). Thus, although child and adolescent studies collectively support the downward extension of adult criteria, insufficient attention to developmental differences may lead to the underidentification of clinically meaningful cases (Avenevoli & Steinberg, 2001; Weiss & Garber 2003). This may be particularly true among preadolescent children, owing to the fact that few studies have examined differences in syndrome expression between school-age children and adults (but see Luby, Heffelfinger, et al., 2003; Luby, Mrarotsky, et al., 2003, and Egger & Angold, 2006, for early work on nosology in preschool children).

A related controversy concerns whether depression ought to be considered on a continuum of severity or as a categorical disorder. The categorical approach is required for clinical decision, but a dimensional approach allows examination of the full severity gradient and makes it possible to study correlates of severity. The dimensional approach is also favored by some researchers because it typically yields greater statistical power in data analyses. However, the dimensional approach is often limited to assessment during recent time intervals (e.g., the past week), in contrast to categorical approaches that can be adapted to assess lifetime history. There are statistical methods to determine whether the implicit assumption of discrete latent categories (taxa) that distinguish cases and noncases can be rejected in analysis of dimensional symptom distributions (Kessler, 2002). Most research along these lines on adults and adolescents has failed to find strong evidence to support a categorical characterization of depression (Hankin, Fraley, Lahey, & Waldman, 2005; Kessler, Zhao, Blazer, & Swartz, 1997; Ruscio & Ruscio, 2000; Slade & Andrews, 2005); however, there is some evidence that depression, or specific subtypes, may be taxonic (Ambrosini, Bennett, Cleland, & Haslam, 2002; Beach & Amir, 2003; Solomon, Ruscio, Seeley, & Lewinsohn, 2006). Some recent commentators have called for additional empirical research to further examine the structure of child psychopathology (e.g., Lahey et al., 2004) and to systematically evaluate methodological factors (Solomon et al., 2006), whereas others have cautioned that there is no "right" approach and that categorical and dimensional approaches both have utility in different contexts and with different research questions (Rutter, 2003; Pickles & Angold, 2003).

As much of the psychiatric epidemiological literature is based on the categorical approach, most of the findings on prevalence, comorbidity, course, and outcomes presented in this chapter focus on depressive disorders as defined by DSM.

Assessment

Structured and semistructured diagnostic interviews have been developed to assess child and adolescent depressive disorders (e.g., Angold et al., 1995; Chambers et al., 1985). Diagnostic interviews employ rules for assessing syndromes in terms of frequency, duration, and impairment and stipulate procedures for defining dichotomous caseness based on current taxonomies. However, use of these interviews presents three important challenges in epidemiological research.

One challenge in using diagnostic interviews is that the ICD-10 and DSM-IV criteria do not provide clear guidelines regarding a number of required classification distinctions, such as "clinically significant" impairment and "marked" distress (Angold et al., 1995). Developers of diagnostic interviews have made their own decisions about operational definitions in an effort to increase the reliability of an assessment. These decisions, however, are not always applied consistently across research programs. As a result, fully structured respondent-based assessments are likely to yield more consistent data across raters, although the flexibility of semistructured interviews may yield higher validity.

A second challenge is that diagnostic interviews are typically administered to multiple respondents, including a parent, a teacher, and/or the child or adolescent. Although there is sufficient evidence to support the use of multiple informants (i.e., each offers a unique perspective; Achenbach, McConaughy, & Howell, 1987; Kraemer et al., 2003), there is little consensus on how best to integrate the often inconsistent information obtained from multiple informants to yield optimally valid diagnoses. This problem is especially acute in following youth over time, as the norm in the literature is not to interview children under the age of approximately 12 but to rely entirely on parent and/or teacher interviews, thus creating an inconsistency in data density when youth are followed from an earlier age into adolescence. Common approaches to resolving interrater discrepancies in reports include carrying out separate parallel analyses for each informant, combining diagnostic information using an "OR" rule (i.e., accepting positive reports from any informant) either at the diagnostic level or at the symptom level, or using an "AND" rule (i.e., requiring that all informants report the symptom or syndrome as present to qualify as a case). Another option is to integrate data across sources into clinical "best estimates."

A third challenge is that the reliability and validity of diagnostic interviews change with the age of the respondent. This is due to an increase in the reliability and validity of child reports with age, to the increased recognition of psychiatric symptoms by children and parents as children get older, and to the likelihood that symptoms themselves become clearer with age. These age-related changes increase the complexity of studies of change, as true change in symptoms can be confounded with age-related variation in instability due to unreliability and invalidity.

PREVALENCE

Prevalence Estimates of Depressive Disorders

Twenty-eight national and international studies employing community samples and standardized diagnostic criteria provide estimates of prevalence for major depression, dysthymia, and other depressive disorders (see Table 2.1). There is wide variation in prevalence estimates across these studies.

In general, prevalence estimates of depression in schoolchildren (approximately 7–12 years) are lower than those of depression in adolescents (approximately 13–18 years) and young adults (approximately 19–26 years). As evidenced in Table 2.1, point prevalence estimates for major depression range from less than 1% (Costello et al., 1996) to 2% (Kashani & Simonds, 1979) among school-age children and from about 1% (Fergusson, Horwood, & Lynskey, 1993) to 7% (Garrison et al., 1997) among adolescents. As would be expected, 6- and 12-month prevalence estimates were somewhat higher, with ranges from less than 1% (Anderson, Williams, McGee, & Silva, 1987; Costello et al., 1988) to almost 3% (Velez, Johnson, & Cohen, 1989) among preadolescents and from 2% (McGee et al., 1990; Velez et al., 1989) to 13% (Feehan, McGee, Raja, & Williams, 1994) among adolescents. In the two studies that assessed young adults, 12-month prevalence estimates were 8.2% (Pine, Cohen, Gurley, Brook, & Ma, 1998) and 16.8% (Newman, Moffit, Caspi, & Magdol, 1996).

Lifetime prevalence of major depression in children was reported in only one study (1.1% at age 9; Kashani et al., 1983). Six studies reported lifetime prevalence in adolescents, with estimates ranging from 4.0% (Whitaker et al., 1990) to 24.0% (Lewinsohn, Hops, Roberts, Seeley, & Andrews, 1993). Estimates for young adults were at the upper end of the adolescent range (Reinherz, Paradis, Giaconia, Stashwick, & Fitzmaurice, 2003). The only study based on a national probability sample of adolescents and young adults reported a 15% lifetime prevalence estimate (Kessler & Walters, 1998).

Estimates of prevalence for dysthymic disorder follow the same general pattern as for major depression, with prevalence estimates higher in adolescents than in children. Prevalence estimates of dysthymia among school-age children are similar to those of major depression (Costello et al., 1988; Costello, Mustillo, Erkanli, Keeler, & Angold, 2003). For adolescents and young adults, in comparison, prevalence estimates of dysthymia are typically lower than those of major depression (Feehan et al., 1994; Kim-Cohen et al., 2003; Lewinsohn et al., 1993; Newman et al., 1996; Verhulst, van der Ende, Ferdinand, & Kasius, 1997; Wittchen, Nelson, & Lachner, 1998). In contrast, prevalence estimates of subthreshold depressive disorders and syndromes, including minor depression and depression not otherwise specified (NOS), are generally higher than those of major depression across all age groups (Angold et al., 2002; Costello et al., 2003; Gonzalez-Tejera et al., 2005; Kashani et al., 1983; Lewinsohn, Shankman, Gau, & Klein, 2004).

Age and Sex Patterns of Prevalence

Retrospective studies of adults with depression suggest that first onset is most likely to occur in the age range between mid-to-late adolescence and young adulthood (Burke, Burke, Regier, & Rae, 1990; Kessler, McGonagle, Swartz, Blazer, & Nelson, 1993; Lewinsohn, Duncan, Stanton, & Hautzinger, 1986). In the only nationally representative general population sample to examine age of onset, approximately 25% of adults with major depression or dysthymia reported onset prior to young adulthood, and almost

TABLE 2.1. Prevalence Estimates of Depressive Disorders in Community Samples of Children and Adolescents

Authors	Location	Wave	n	Age (yr)	Dx criteria	Dx intvw[a,b]	Period[c]	MDE/D[d,e]	Other depression[f]
United States									
Angold et al. (2002)	North Carolina		920	9–17	DSM-IV	CAPA	3M	1.0%	0.3% (DY), 1.7% (mDep)
Bird et al. (1988)	Puerto Rico		386	4–16	DSM-III	DISC		5.9% (I)	
Canino et al. (2004)	Puerto Rico		1,886	4–17	DSM-IV	Spanish DISC	12M	3.6%, 3.0 (I)	0.6% (DY), 0.5% (DY;I)
Gonzalez-Tejera et al. (2005)			891	11–17				4.4%	5.3% (mDep)
Costello et al. (1988)	Pittsburgh		300	7–11	DSM-III	DISC	12M	0.4%	1.3% (DY)
Costello et al. (1996)	North Carolina	1	1,015	9, 11, 13	DSM-III-R	CAPA	3M	0.03%	0.1%(DY), 1.5% (NOS)
Costello et al. (2003)		FU to 16		9–16	DSM-IV			0.4%	0.3% (DY), 1.5% (NOS), 2.2% (Any)
Deykin, Levy, & Wells (1987)	Boston		424	16–19	DSM-III	DIS	LT	6.8%	
Garrison et al. (1997)	Southeastern United States	1 2	359	11–16 12–17	DSM-III	K-SADS	PT	7.0% 5.4%	2.6% (DY) 4.3% (DY)
Kashani & Simonds (1979)	Missouri		103	7–12	DSM-III		PT	1.9%	
Kashani et al. (1987a, 1987b)	Missouri		150	14–16	DSM-III	DICA	PT	4.7%	
Kashani et al. (1989)	Missouri		210	8, 12, 17	DSM-III	CAS	PT	1.5, 1.5, 5.7%	
Kessler & Walters (1998)	United States		1,769	15–24	DSM-III-R	CIDI	30D, 12M, LT	5.8% (30D) 12.4% (12M) 15.3% (LT)	2.1% (mDep, 30D) 7.1% (mDep, 12M) 9.9% (mDep, LT)

Study	Location	#	N	Age	Criteria	Instrument	Time	Prevalence	Other
Kilpatrick et al. (2003)	U.S. probability		4,023	12–17	DSM-IV	NWS	6M	M: 7.4%, F:13.9%	3.2% (DY, LT)
Lewinsohn et al. (1991)	Oregon	1	1,709	14–18	DSM-III-R	K-SADS-E	PT, LT	2.9% (PT), 20.4% (LT)	
Lewinsohn et al. (2004)									25.9% (sMDD, LT)
Lewinsohn et al. (1993)		2	1,507	15–19		LIFE	PT, LT	3.1% (PT), 24.0% (LT)	0.1% (DY, PT), 3.0% (DY,LT)
Lewinsohn, personal communication (2006)		3	941	24	DSM-IV		PT	2.4%	0.5% (DY)
		4	816				PT	4.1%	0.8% (DY)
Reinherz, Giaconia, Lefkowitz, Pakiz, & Frost (1993)	Northeastern United States	1	386	18	DSM-III-R	DIS	1M,	2.9% (1M),	
Giaconia et al. (1994)							6M, LT	6.0% (6M), 9.4% (LT)	
Reinherz, Giaconia, Carmela-Hauf, Wasserman, & Silverman (1999)		2	375	21			LT	10%	
Reinherz et al. (2003)		3	354	18–26	DSM-IV		LT	23.2%	
Shaffer, Fisher, Dulcan, & Davies (1996)	Atlanta, GA; New Haven, CT; New York; Puerto Rico		1,285	9–17	DSM-III-R	DISC	6M	5.6% (I), 7.1% (no I)	7.2% (Any, I), 8.8% (Any, no I)
Simonoff et al. (1997)	Virginia		2,762 twins	8–16	DSM-III-R	CAPA	3M	1.2% (I), 1.3% (no I)	
Velez et al. (1989)	New York State	1	776	1–10	DSM-III-R	No assessment	12M	2.5%	
		2	760	9–12		DISC		3.7%	
				13–18				2.5%	
		3	716	11–14				3.1%	
				15–20					
Pine et al. (1998)		4	716	17–26				M: 5.0%, F: 11.5%	
Whitaker et al. (1990)	New Jersey		356	13–18	DSM-III	Clinical Intrw	LT	4.0%	4.9% (DY)

(continued)

11

TABLE 2.1. (continued)

Authors	Location	Wave	n	Age (yr)	Dx criteria	Dx intvw[a,b]	Period[c]	MDE/D[d,e]	Other depression[f]
International									
Kashani et al. (1983)	Dunedin, New Zealand	B	189	9	DSM-III	K-SADS-E	PT, LT	1.8% (PT), 1.1% (LT)	2.5% (PT mDep), 9.7% (LT mDep)
Anderson et al. (1987)		1	792	11		DISC	12M	0.5%	1.8%* (Any)
McGee & Williams (1988)		2	762	13			PT	0.4%	1.6% (DY)
McGee et al. (1990)		3	943	15		DISC short	PT, 12M	1.2% (PT), 1.9% (12M)	1.1% (DY, 12M)
Feehan et al. (1994)		4	930	18	DSM-III-R	DIS	PT, 12M	3.4% (PT), 13.3% (12M)	3.2% (DY, 12M)
Newman et al. (1996)		5	961	21			12M	16.8%	3.0% (DY)
Kim-Cohen et al. (2003)		6	976	26	DSM-IV		12M	16.5%	0.8% (DY)
Canals, Marti-Henneberg, Fernandez-Ballert, & Marti-Henneberg (1995)	Spain	1	500	10–11		No assessment			
Canals, Domenech, Carbajo, & Blade (1997)		2	290	18 (FU)	DSM-III-R	SCAN	PT	2.4%	5.8% (DY), 0.7% (mDep)
Fergusson et al. (1993)	Christchurch, New Zealand	1	1,265	15	DSM-III-R	DISC	PT, 12M	0.7% (PT), 4.2% (12M)	0.4% (DY, PT)
Fergusson & Woodward (2002)		2–4	1,006	16–21	DSM-IV	CIDI	interval	33.5% (cumulative)	
Fleming, Offord, & Boyle (1989)	Ontario, Canada		2,852	6–16	DSM-III	SDI	6M	5.9%	

Study	Location	Design	N	Age	Criteria	Interview	Time	Prevalence	Other
Gau, Chong, Chen, & Cheng (2005)	Taiwan	3-year panel	1,070	7th 8th 9th grade	DSM-IV	Chinese KSADS-E	Unk	0.5% 2.5% 4.4%	0.2% (DY) 0.2% (DY) 0.6% (DY)
Goodyer & Cooper (1993)	Cambridgeshire, England		1,068 girls	11–16	DSM-III-R	DISC	PT, 12M	3.6% (PT), 6.0% (12M)	
Rutter, Tizard, & Whitmore (1970)	Isle of Wight		2,303	14–15	—	Clinical intvw	PT	1.5%	
Verhulst et al. (1997)	Netherlands		780	13–18	DSM-III-R	DISC	6M	3.6%	2.3% (DY)
Wittchen et al. (1998)	Munich, Germany		3,021	14–24	DSM-IV	CIDI	12M LT	3.6% (12M) 9.3% (LT)	2.9% (DY,12M) 3.0% (DY,LT)
Pezawas et al. (2003)			2,548	14–22			LT		2.6% (RBD/sRBD)
Yang, Soong, Kuo, Chang, & Chen (2004)	Taipei		178	12–16	DSM-IV	K-SADS	PT	3.7% (no I) 2.4% (I)	2.7% (DY, no I) 0.3% (DY,I)

[a] Diagnostic interview.

[b] Abbreviations of diagnostic interviews: CAS, Child Assessment Schedule; CAPA, Child and Adolescent Psychiatric Assessment; CIDI, Composite International Diagnostic Interview; DICA, Diagnostic Interview for Children and Adolescents; DIS, Diagnostic Interview Schedule; DISC, Diagnostic Interview Schedule for Children; K-SADS, Schedule for Affective Disorders and Schizophrenia for School-Age Children; NWS, National Women's Study, Major depression module; SCAN, Schedules for Clinical Assessment in Neuropsychiatry; SDI, Survey Diagnostic Instrument.

[c] Time period abbreviations: PT, point; 30D, 30 days; 1M, 1 month; 6M, 6 months; 12M, 12 months; LT, lifetime.

[d] Major depressive episode or disorder.

[e] Abbreviations: I, with impairment; no I, without impairment; M, males; F, females.

[f] Other depressive disorders abbreviations: Any, any depressive disorder; DY, dysthymia; mDep, minor depression; NOS, not otherwise specified; RBD, recurrent brief depression; sMDD, subthreshold major depression; sRBD, subthreshold recurrent brief depression.

50% by age 30 (see Figure 2.1). Longitudinal studies of treatment and community samples of children and adolescents suggest an earlier average age of onset between 11 and 14 years for major depression and dysthymia (Kovacs, Feinberg, Crouse-Novak, Paulauskas, & Finkelstein, 1984; Lewinsohn et al., 1993). In addition, prospective studies that follow the same children over time reveal a dramatic increase in the prevalence of major depressive episodes after age 11 and again after age 15, with a flattening of rates in young adulthood (ages 21–26) (McGee, Feehan, Williams, & Anderson, 1992; Newman et al., 1996; Kim-Cohen et al., 2003).

It has been well documented in national epidemiological studies that the prevalence of depression is nearly twice as high among adult females as among adult males in developing countries (Kessler et al., 1993). Among preadolescents, community studies report either no sex differences in depression (Fleming, Offord, & Boyle, 1989; Kashani et al., 1983; Velez et al., 1989) or somewhat higher prevalence among preadolescent boys than girls (Anderson et al., 1987; Costello et al., 1988; Angold, Costello, & Worthman, 1998). During adolescence and young adulthood, however, depression is more common among females than males (Cohen et al., 1993; Costello et al., 2003; Kessler & Walters, 1998; Lewinsohn et al., 1993; McGee et al., 1990; Reinherz, Giaconia, Lefkowitz, Pakiz, & Frost, 1993; Whitaker et al., 1990; Wittchen et al., 1998). Sex differences in depression are evident for both major depression and dysthymia; however, findings on sex differences in minor depression (Kessler & Walters 1998; Gonzalez-Tejera et al., 2005), recurrent brief depression (Pezawas et al., 2003), and depressive symptoms (Petersen, Sarigiani, & Kennedy, 1991) are mixed across studies.

The female preponderance of depression begins to emerge around the age of 13 (McGee et al., 1992; Nolen-Hoeksema & Girgus, 1994). In a longitudinal follow-up of a large birth cohort, the change in the sex ratio was attributable to an increase in the incidence of depression among females after age 11 and again between 15 and 18 (Hankin et al., 1998). Although depression increases among both males and females during the middle adolescent years, the incidence among females is far greater than among males (Hankin et al., 1998; Lewinsohn et al., 1993).

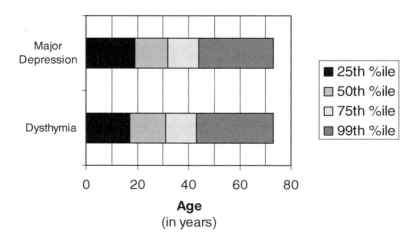

FIGURE 2.1. Age at onset of mood disorders in U.S. general population (*n* = 9,282). Data from Kessler, Berglund, Demler, Jin, and Walters (2005).

CONCURRENT AND LIFETIME COMORBIDITY

Community studies show a consistently high comorbidity of depression with other mental disorders among children and adolescents (Angold, Costello, & Erkanli, 1999; Merikangas & Angst, 1995; Nottelmann & Jensen, 1995) and suggest that these associations are not fully explained by biases, expectancies, overlapping taxonomies, and other methodological factors (Angold, Costello, & Erkanli, 1999) and that pure depression may be relatively rare among youth (Avenevoli, Stolar, Li, Dierker, & Merikangas, 2001; Lewinsohn, Rohde, & Seeley, 1998). Comorbidity has been associated with greater severity of depression and, in some cases, its co-occurring conditions, (e.g., anxiety; Last, Perrin, Hersen, & Kazdin, 1996), greater risk of suicide (Rohde, Lewinsohn, & Seeley, 1991), and greater functional impairment (Lewinsohn et al., 1998). In this chapter, findings on concurrent (defined here as comorbidity within the same year), lifetime, and sequential comorbidity (i.e., one disorder preceding the other in time) are reviewed separately. The first two are reviewed in this section, and sequential comorbidity is discussed in the context of the course of depression (heterotypic continuity) in the next section.

Evidence from community studies of children and adolescents reveal that depression is associated with a significantly elevated risk of anxiety, behavior, eating, and substance use disorders (e.g., Gotlib & Hammen, 1992; Lewinsohn et al., 1993; Simonoff et al., 1997). Depression and anxiety disorders are the most common concurrent conditions in youth, with median prevalence estimates of more than 39% anxiety among youth with depression and almost 17% depression among children and adolescents with anxiety disorders (median odds ratio = 8.2; see Angold, Costello, and Erkanli, 1999, for a list of studies and estimates). Major depression is significantly associated with most of the major subtypes of anxiety disorders, with the exception of obsessive–compulsive disorder, and shows particularly strong associations with overanxious and generalized anxiety disorders (Costello, Egger, & Angold, 2004; Lewinsohn, Zinbarg, Lewinsohn, & Sack, 1997). Estimates of comorbid associations between anxiety and depression appear to decrease as the time period of assessment increases (i.e., odds ratios are lower for associations assessed over a 12-month period, as compared with a 3-month period) and are lowest for lifetime associations, suggesting that the two disorders are more likely to occur at the same point in time than at different points in time (Lewinsohn et al., 1993, 1998).

Community samples also yield high estimates of concurrent comorbidity between depression and conduct disorder, with a median prevalence of 27.3% conduct disorder among youth with depression, 12.2% depression among youth with conduct disorder, and a median odds ratio of 6.6 (Angold, Costello, & Erkanli, 1999). Associations between depression and substance use disorders among children and adolescents are generally lower than associations between depression and anxiety and behavioral disorders for both concurrent (median odds ratio = 2.2) and lifetime (median odds ratio = 3.3) time periods (see Armstrong & Costello, 2002, for a list of studies and estimates). Although few studies have systematically examined sex differences in patterns of comorbidity, there is evidence to suggest that comorbidity between depression and anxiety is similar for females and males, but that comorbidity with substance use is greater among boys (Costello et al., 2003).

Findings on comorbidity between subthreshold depressive syndromes and anxiety or behavioral disorders are mixed and may be explained by differences in definitions of subthreshold depression. Whereas some studies report high past-year comorbidity (Gonzalez-Tejera et al., 2005), other studies show no significant comorbidity (Lewinsohn et al., 2004). However, patterns of concurrent comorbidity between recurrent brief depression and anxiety may be more distinct than those between major depression and anxiety. In contrast to the broad association between major depression and most anxiety subtypes, recurrent brief depression shows associations with select anxiety disorders (i.e., agoraphobia, specific phobia with complications) (Pezawas et al., 2003).

CONTINUITY/COURSE

Whereas many previous studies of persistence were based on retrospective reports of adult samples, a number of longitudinal community studies can now provide prospective estimates of the continuity of depression across childhood and adolescence and into adulthood. Findings of both homotypic and heterotypic continuity are reviewed here. In keeping with the traditional use of these terms in developmental psychopathology, *homotypic continuity* is defined as stability in the same or similar behavioral responses over time and *heterotypic continuity* is defined as stability of an underlying construct that is manifested differentially across time as a result of changing developmental capacities (e.g., Avenevoli & Steinberg, 2001; Kagan & Moss, 1962; Sroufe & Rutter, 1984).

Homotypic Continuity

There is a great deal of evidence supporting the homotypic continuity of depression during childhood and adolescence in clinical and community samples. Youth who have experienced major depressive episodes have a high risk of recurrence within a few years (Kovacs, 1996; Lewinsohn et al., 1993), with a cumulative probability of recurrence of 40% by 2 years and 70% by 5 years (Birmaher et al., 1996). Depression during childhood is associated with risk of depression during adolescence, even after controlling for comorbid disorders (Costello et al., 2003). Likewise, childhood-onset dysthymia is associated with a high risk of major depression in adolescence (Kovacs, 1996; Lewinsohn, Rohde, Seeley, & Hops, 1991). Although there are few community studies that have followed children under the age of 12 into adulthood, there is some evidence from studies of community and clinically referred youth that depression in childhood is predictive of depression in young adulthood (Geller, Zimerman, Williams, Bolhofner, & Craney, 2001; Kim-Cohen et al., 2003; Kovacs, 1996).

Prospective community studies also show that depression that begins in adolescence is associated with risk for recurrence in young adulthood (Bardone, Moffit, Caspi, Dickson, & Silva, 1996; Fergusson & Woodward, 2002; Lewinsohn, Rohde, Klein, & Seeley, 1999; Pine et al., 1998; Canals, Domenech-Llaberia, Fernandez-Ballart, & Marti-Henneberg, 2002; Kim-Cohen et al., 2003). Approximately 40–70% of depressed adolescents have a recurrence in adulthood, and depressed adolescents have two to seven times increased odds of recurrence in adulthood as compared with adolescents without depression (Rutter, Kim-Cohen, & Maughan, 2006). Although only an average of 9% of respondents from the Oregon Adolescent Depression Project who were depressed as adolescents met the criteria for the *Diagnostic and Statistical Manual of Mental Disorders*, third edition, revised (DSM-III-R), major depression in any given year as young adults (as compared with 3.7% among controls; Lewinsohn et al., 1999), more than half did so at some time in the 5-year follow-up period used in this study (Lewinsohn, Rohde, Seeley, Klein, & Gotlib, 2000). Other prospective studies have shown associations between subthreshold levels of depressive symptoms during adolescence and adult depression

(Bardone et al., 1996; Fergusson, Horwood, Ridder, & Beautrais, 2005; Garrison et al., 1997; Pine, Cohen, Cohen, & Brook, 1999).

In contrast to prospective studies of the continuity of childhood disorders, follow-back analyses using prospective studies are critical to examine the roots of adult depression. In the Dunedin cohort assessed at ages 11, 13, 15, 18, 21, and 26, 45% of those with a mood disorder at age 21 had a prior history of depression, as compared with 27% with a history of a different disorder and 28% with no psychiatric history (Newman et al., 1996). Those with depression at age 26 were 2.5 times more likely than those without depression at that age to have had depression in adolescence (i.e., at age 11 or 15). The proportion of adult depression cases that can be attributed to any juvenile disorder and/ or to depression, specifically, at age 11 or 15, was 23% and 6%, respectively (Kim-Cohen et al., 2003). These estimates are conservative, as no diagnostic data were available for the participants in this study prior to age 11 or between ages 12 and 14, and data at age 18 were not used in these analyses. Moreover, when subthreshold levels of depression are considered, estimates of continuity appear to be much higher (Canals et al., 2002).

It has been suggested repeatedly that "early-onset" depression is predictive of greater continuity of depression in adulthood. However, confusion about the operationalization of "early onset" has led to the inaccurate assumption that child-onset depression and adolescent-onset depression are equally continuous with depression in adulthood. There is evidence for heterogeneity of juvenile depression, with depression that has an onset prior to puberty appearing to follow a different course and to be etiologically distinct from depression that begins in adolescence. For example, in a clinical sample of youth with depression, Harrington and colleagues (Harrington, Fudge, Rutter, Pickles, & Hill, 1990) found that the continuity of major depression from childhood to adulthood was lower in those with prepubertal-onset versus postpubertal-onset depression. In a much larger clinical study, Weissman et al. (1999) reported that prepubertally depressed children were not at increased risk for depression in adulthood (as compared with children with anxiety and children without psychopathology). Two community studies also suggest that depression and internalizing symptoms show greater continuity from adolescence to adulthood than from childhood to adulthood (Pine et al., 1998; the difference was not statistically significant due to small group sizes, once the sample was stratified by age; Hofstra, Van der Ende, & Verhulst, 2000; a difference was found only among girls). These findings, together with evidence of increased heritability with age (Silberg et al 1999; Thapar & McGuffin, 1997) and differences in neurobiological correlates with age (Kaufman, Martin, King, & Charney, 2001), support the notion of heterogeneity of depression among youth. Caution in interpretation is warranted, however, given the limited number of studies that have evaluated the continuity of depression from childhood to adulthood. Additional research, particularly in community samples, is needed to examine the full course of prepubertal or child-onset depression in comparison to the course of post-pubertal or adolescent-onset depression.

Heterotypic Continuity

Evidence of discontinuity from the studies reviewed above may also suggest some underlying heterotypic continuity. Clinical, high-risk family, and community studies converge in suggesting that anxiety and depression share common etiological roots (Beidel & Turner, 1997; Thapar & McGuffin, 1997; Warner, Weissman, Mufson, & Wickramaratne, 1999) and that childhood anxiety is likely an early precursor to later depressive disorders (Costello et al., 2003; Rende, Warner, Wickramaratne, &

Weissman, 1999; Silberg, Rutter, & Eaves, 2001). Most subtypes of anxiety in adolescence show prospective continuity with major depression in adulthood, although findings on specific associations are somewhat mixed across studies (Bittner et al., 2004; Pine et al., 1998; Pine, Cohen, & Brook, 2001; Wittchen, Kessler, Pfister, & Lieb, 2000). Depressed adults are twice as likely as adults without depression to have had an anxiety disorder during adolescence (Kim-Cohen et al., 2003). Likewise, there appears to be continuity between depression during adolescence and anxiety (particularly Generalized Anxiety Disorder) in adulthood, as evidenced by both prospective and follow-back analyses (Kim-Cohen et al., 2003; Fergusson & Woodward, 2002). Generally, estimates of homotypic continuity of depression are greater than those for heterotypic continuity between anxiety and depression.

There is some suggestion that early conduct disorder is associated with depression in adulthood (Kim-Cohen et al., 2003), although the etiologic roots of conduct disorder and depression have not been extensively examined. Few studies have shown continuity between adolescent depression and adolescent or adult substance use or disorders, particularly after adjusting for other comorbid disorders (Costello et al., 2003; Fergusson & Woodward, 2002; Kim-Cohen et al., 2003).

CORRELATES

Socioeconomic Status, Race, Ethnicity, Culture

In studies of adults, depression has been associated with lower socioeconomic status (Kessler et al., 2003); in contrast, studies of children and adolescents yield less consistent findings. Whereas some studies report a lack of association between depressive disorders and socioeconomic status (Costello et al., 1988; Whitaker et al., 1990; Costello et al., 2003), others report a significant association, at least with the most impoverished groups (Bird et al., 1988; Costello et al., 1996; Reinherz, Giaconia, Pakiz, et al., 1993; Gilman, Kawachi, Fitzmaurice, & Buka, 2003). A large meta-analysis of 310 samples of children who completed the Children's Depression Inventory (CDI) found no association between depressive symptoms and socioeconomic status (Twenge & Nolen-Hoeksema, 2002).

The small sample size of ethnic minority youth in most community studies of children and adolescents diminishes the statistical power to test differences in the prevalence of disorders between specific subgroups. The few studies that have compared racial or ethnic groups yielded no differences in the prevalence of depressive disorders between European American and African American (Angold et al., 2002; Costello et al., 1988) or American Indian youth (Costello, Farmer, Angold, Burns, & Erkanli, 1997). Evidence for ethnic differences in depressive symptoms in children and adolescents is mixed, with some support for increased depressive symptoms among Hispanic, as compared with European American and African American youth (Twenge & Nolen-Hoeksema, 2002).

Family and Genetic Risk

Twin, family, and adoption studies all strongly suggest that familial factors are important determinants of depression (Sullivan, Neale, & Kendler, 2000). Children of depressed parents are approximately four times more likely to have an episode of major depression than children of normal controls and two times more likely to have depression than children of parents with other psychiatric disorders or medical conditions (Rice, Harold, & Thapar, 2002). This elevated risk increases with age (Beardslee, Keller, Lavori, Staley, &

Sacks, 1993; Weissman, Fendrich, Warner, & Wickramaratne, 1992; Weissman, Warner, Wickramaratne, Moreau, & Olfson, 1997), with an estimated cumulative probability for major depression of almost 70% by late adolescence (Hammen, Burge, Burney, & Adrian, 1990). Furthermore, parental concordance for mood disorders and a heavy familial loading for depression (e.g., a double dose of parent and grandparent depression) are associated with even greater risk of depression in offspring (Merikangas, Prusoff, & Weissman, 1988; Weissman et al., 2005). The effects of parental psychopathology may be due to genetic influences, environmental influences, or a combination. The difficulty in sorting out causal pathways is that parental psychopathology is often part of a complex cluster of risk factors that includes family violence, neglect, poor parenting, stress, and other types of childhood adversity (Kessler, Davis, & Kendler, 1997; Goodman & Gotlib, 1999).

Most twin studies suggest that there is moderate genetic influence for childhood depressive symptoms, with heritability estimates in the range of 30–80% (Eley & Plomin, 1997; Murray & Sines, 1996; Thapar & McGuffin 1994, 1997). In addition, heritability appears to increase from childhood to adolescence (Scourfield et al., 2003). Although there has been an extensive search for genes underlying both bipolar and unipolar depression through genetic linkage and association studies, there are still no genetic loci for depression that have been replicated in independent studies (Shih, Belmonte, & Zandi, 2004). The aggregate evidence from family and twin studies suggests that transmission of depression in families results from a complex combination of genetic and environmental factors (Levinson, 2006; Merikangas & Low, 2005; Sullivan, Prescott, & Kendler, 2002). The identification of the serotonin transporter (SERT) as a susceptibility gene that leads to depression only in the presence of acute life stress, by Caspi et al. (2003), has generated substantial focus on more complex modes of transmission of depression, particularly on the role of gene–environment interaction in the etiology of depression. However, reviews of the evidence from subsequent studies do not provide consistent support for the SERT locus as an important determinant of depression (Zammit & Owen, 2006).

Biological Factors

The major theories of the neurobiology of depression are based on dysregulation of the human stress system through activation of the hypothalamic–pituitary–adrenal (HPA) axis (Nestler et al., 2002). The preponderance of female depression has generated substantial research on the role of sex steroids in regulation of the HPA axis (Young & Altemus, 2004). Aside from stress reactivity, other biological systems that have been investigated in depression include sleep dysregulation, circadian rhythm disturbances, and impaired reward and motivational pathways (Shaffery, Hoffmann, & Armitage, 2003).

The hippocampus is the main feedback site for the adrenal glucocorticoids that turn off the stress response (McEwen, 1995). Recent neuroimaging studies have identified brain areas other than the hippocampus, such as the nucleus accumbens, amygdala, and specific hypothalamic nuclei that regulate motivation, eating, sleeping, circadian rhythm, pleasure, and response to stress (Nestler et al., 2002). As progress is made in identifying neural circuits *in vivo*, it is becoming increasingly possible to identify circuits involved in normal mood regulation that may be disturbed in depression. However, the molecular, cellular, and circuital bases of the complex behaviors underlying depression still remain obscure (Nestler et al., 2002). Future progress in understanding the neurobiological pathways of depression will require greater focus on developmental and sex differences in the manifestation of depression, as well as identification of genetic factors that confer vulnerability to depression.

Life Events/Stress

Exposure to stressful life events is one of the most widely studied risk factors for depressive disorder and symptoms. In both clinical and community samples, depressed children and adolescents report more stressful life events than youth without depression (e.g., Costello et al., 1988; Franko et al., 2004; Lewinsohn, Allen, & Seeley, 1999; Williamson, Ryan, Birmaher, Dahl, & Nelson, 1995). Although major life events such as parental death, serious illness, and sexual and physical abuse are linked with youth depression (Kendler, Kuhn, & Prescott, 2004; O'Sullivan, 2004; Roy, 1985; Williamson, Birmaher, Dahl, & Ryan, 2005), less traumatic events and hassles (e.g., changes in family, peer, and romantic relations, the transition from junior high to high school) are also related to increased depressive symptoms (Isakon & Jarvis, 1999; Monroe, Rohde, Seeley, & Lewinsohn, 1999; O'Sullivan, 2004). Adverse life events, like many other social correlates, however, appear to be nonspecific risk factors for depression. These events are also associated with increased risk for a number of other types of psychopathology (Kendler, Neale, Kessler, Heath, & Eaves, 1992; Kessler, Davis, & Kendler, 1997; Lewinsohn, Gotlib, & Seeley, 1997; Phillips, Hammen, Brennan, Najma, & Bor, 2005).

Studies have shown that stressful life events aggregate in families (McGuffin, Katz, & Bebbington, 1988), are heritable (Silberg et al., 1999), and mediate the association between parent and child depression (Hammen, Shih, & Brennan, 2004). Most likely, stressors are insufficient to contribute to depression without an underlying vulnerability to depression (Hankin & Abela, 2005). For example, during the past few years there has been a surge of studies that have focused on particular genetic markers, such as the serotonin receptor or the SERT that may interact with life events to induce the onset of depression (e.g., Caspi et al., 2003). However, the findings have been highly variable with respect to the nature and severity of the events—ranging from traumatic childhood events to unemployment—and to the definitions of depression—ranging from major depression to physical symptoms of depression (Zammit & Owen, 2006).

CONSEQUENCES

In addition to a risk for recurrence of depression, children and adolescents with depression are more likely to experience a number of negative outcomes across the lifespan. Although not specific to depression, the most common sequelea of depression in childhood and adolescence include impairment in school and work performance, in relationships with family and friends, and in cognitive functioning (Reinherz, Giaconia, R.M., Pakiz, et al., 1993; Kessler & Walters, 1998). Depression during adolescence is also associated with poor outcomes in adulthood, including increased stressful life events, loss of social support, low satisfaction in life roles, low income levels, low educational aspirations, early marriage, early parenthood, and low marital satisfaction (Franko et al., 2005; Gotlib, Lewinsohn, & Seeley, 1998; Rao et al., 1995). The adverse consequences of depression are more severe among youth with recurrent depressive disorders than among those with depressive symptoms alone (Wittchen et al., 1998). Depression may also be a risk factor for drug use and abuse and smoking (Franko et al., 2005; Schepis & Rao, 2005; Conway, Compton, Stinson, & Grant, 2006), although these associations may be explained by other comorbid disorders (Costello et al., 2003).

The most severe consequence of depression in adolescents is suicide. Forty-one percent of adolescents with depression in the Oregon Adolescent Depression Project reported suicidal ideation, and 21% of depressed youth in the National Comorbidity Survey (NCS) reported a suicide attempt (Kessler & Walters, 1998). Depression comorbid with substance abuse, anxiety disorders, and personality disorders may be more predictive of suicide and repeated suicide attempts than non-comorbid depression (Hoberman & Bergmann, 1992).

HELP SEEKING AND TREATMENT

The World Health Organization (WHO) Global Burden of Disease study concluded that unipolar depression is the leading disease causing disability among those ages 15–44 in the developed world (Murray & Lopez, 1996). With evidence that depression often has its roots in childhood and adolescence and shows continuity into adulthood, there is an increasing need to focus on early intervention to reduce the burden of this disease. However, studies consistently show that only a minority of depressed children or adolescents receive treatment before reaching adulthood.

Epidemiological studies of children and adolescents suggest that only about one-fourth to one-half of children with psychiatric disorders, including depression, have received some kind of mental health services (e.g., school, primary care, child welfare) within the same 3-, 6-, or 12-month period, and far fewer have received services directly from mental health care specialists (Angold et al., 2002; Canino et al., 2004; Costello et al., 1988; Kessler & Walters, 1998; Wu et al., 1999). African American youth appear to receive fewer health services than European American youth with the same mental health problems (Elster, Jarosik, Van Geest, & Fleming, 2003), although this disparity may be limited in some parts of the country to care from the specialty mental health sector (Angold et al., 2002). Other factors associated with service utilization include high global impairment, comorbidity, prior history of depression, suicide attempt, and impact of the child's problem on the family (Angold et al., 2002; Canino et al., 2004; Fergusson & Horwood, 2001; Lewinsohn et al., 1998; Wittchen et al., 1998). School services are the most common point of entry for children seeking services, although those who enter through the education sector are least likely to transition to specialty mental health services (Farmer, Burns, Phillips, Angold, & Costello, 2003).

Epidemiological studies of adults with depression that compare retrospectively reported ages of disorder onset with ages of first seeking professional treatment yield three consistent findings (Christiana et al., 2000; Kessler, Olfson, & Berglund, 1998; Olfson, Kessler, Berglund, & Lin, 1998). First, the majority of people with child- and adolescent-onset depression eventually obtain treatment. Second, delays in initial help seeking are pervasive and inversely related to age at onset. Third, the probability of obtaining treatment for depression has increased in recently studied cohorts, although delays are still quite common.

FUTURE DIRECTIONS

This chapter has reviewed findings from community studies of children and adolescents on the prevalence, comorbidity, continuity, correlates, consequences, and treatment of depression. Epidemiological research on depression has advanced significantly over the past two decades. Findings are now derived from community samples that minimize the biases associated with treatment samples and retrospective reporting. These studies suggest a high prevalence of depression during adolescence and young adulthood, significant comorbidity and impairment beginning in childhood, and low service utilization during early initial episodes of depression. Longitudinal follow-up of these community samples have yielded valuable information on the increasing rates of depression from childhood to adolescence, emerging sex differences in rates of depression, moderate stability of depression into adulthood, risk factors for depression, and prospective associations between childhood anxiety and adult depression (and vice versa).

Despite these advances, there are many areas ripe for future research. First, evaluations of continuity in long-term longitudinal studies are needed to inform both the nosology and measurement of depression. In terms of nosology, data that show the adult outcomes of children with subthreshold depressive syndromes and disorders would be useful in resolving current uncertainties about the prognostic significance of these symptoms and the threshold levels at which to define clinically meaningful depression. In addition, evaluations of developmental patterns in symptom expression from early childhood to adulthood would be helpful in further defining meaningful depressive syndromes. Regarding measurement, data showing the extent to which discrepant information from different reporters (parents, teachers, children) predict the subsequent emergence of clear adult disorders could help resolve the current uncertainties about how to combine information into classifications of child and adolescent disorders.

Second, evaluations of the course of depression from childhood to adulthood are needed to identify sources of the heterogeneity of depression and to identify multiple pathways to depression across development. Current evidence suggests that depression that varies by age of onset and patterns of comorbidity may indicate divergent pathways to adult health and depression. In terms of age of onset, studies are needed to evaluate the heterogeneity of juvenile-onset depression by examining the course and predictive significance of child-, or prepubertal-, onset depression in comparison to that of adolescent-onset depression. Likewise, more thorough evaluations of patterns of comorbidity (e.g., evaluations of epiphenomenal comorbidity and a focus on comorbid disorders that share etiological links) over time and at different points in development are needed to determine whether specific comorbid disorders represent distinct subtypes of depression. Special attention to relationships between childhood anxiety and adolescent and adult depression and between conduct disorder and depression is warranted. Fortunately, these questions may be addressed by exploiting data from existing prospective studies and by continuing to follow existing cohorts into adulthood.

Third, much more research is needed to identify etiological factors associated with the onset and recurrence of depression. Although it is well known that a number of cognitive, biological, family, and environmental factors are associated with depression, it is necessary to move beyond simplistic models of associations in order to advance our understanding of the stages of depressive disorders. Studies are needed to examine the predictive significance of known correlates and the interplay between these factors across time. The transition to adolescence stands out as a particularly important period for research on the over-time unfolding of depression and other problems of internalization. Studies that span developmental transitions may be further enriched by evaluating developmentally salient biological, cognitive, and social factors in relation to the increasing incidence of depression and the emergence of sex differences during adolescence. These goals will require large studies with sufficient power to evaluate complex models. As the tools available to neuroscientists and geneticists become more sophisticated, it will be possible to elucidate the biological mechanisms underlying depression and to develop more comprehensive theories of etiology.

Future studies on the course and etiology of depression have important implications for informing the timing and targets of intervention efforts and for identifying factors that are amenable to change in prevention and treatment programs. Data on the predictors of the unfolding, progression, and resolution of child and adolescent depression in adulthood may help to refine our ability to predict which youngsters are at risk of serious adult disorders and which factors may be modulated to minimize depressive outcomes. Further evidence on the course of depression across developmental transitions may also pinpoint sensitive periods for preventive and treatment efforts. The feasibility of mounting targeted early outreach and intervention programs to decrease child suffering and adult psychopathology hinges centrally on our ability to improve accuracy in determining the targets and timing for these efforts.

REFERENCES

Achenbach, T. M., McConaughy, S. H., & Howell, C. T. (1987). Child/adolescent behavioral and emotional problems: Implications of cross-informant correlations for situational specificity. *Psychological Bulletin, 101,* 213–232.

Ambrosini, P., Bennett, D., Cleland, C. M., & Haslam, N. (2002). Taxonicity of adolescent melancholia: A categorical or dimensional construct? *Journal of Psychiatric Research, 36,* 247–256.

American Psychiatric Association. (1994). *Diagnostic and statistical manual of mental disorders* (4th ed.). Washington, DC: Author.

Anderson, J. C., Williams, S., McGee, R., & Silva, P. A. (1987). DSM-III disorders in preadolescent children: Prevalence in a large sample from the general population. *Archives of General Psychiatry, 44,* 69–76.

Angold, A. (1988). Childhood and adolescent depression: I. Epidemiological and aetiological aspects. *British Journal of Psychiatry, 152,* 601–617.

Angold, A., Costello, E. J., & Erkanli, A. (1999). Comorbidity. *Journal of Child Psychology and Psychiatry and Allied Disciplines, 40,* 57–87.

Angold, A., Costello, E. J., Farmer, E. M., Burns, B. J., & Erkanli, A. (1999). Impaired but undiagnosed. *Journal of the American Academy of Child and Adolescent Psychiatry, 38,* 129–137.

Angold, A., Costello, E. J., & Worthman, C. M. (1998). Puberty and depression: The roles of age, pubertal status, and pubertal timing. *Psychological Medicine, 28,* 51–61.

Angold, A., Erkanli, A., Farmer, E., Fairbank, J. A., Burns, B. J., Keeler, G., et al. (2002). Psychiatric disorder, impairment, and service use in rural African American and white youth. *Archives of General Psychiatry, 59,* 893–901.

Angold, A., Prendergast, M., Cox, A., Harrington, R., Simonoff, E., & Rutter, M. (1995). The Child and Adolescent Psychiatric Assessment (CAPA). *Psychological Medicine, 25,* 739–753.

Angst, J. (1988). Clinical course of affective disorders. In T. Helagson & R. J. Daly (Eds.), *Illness: Prediction of course and outcome* (pp. 1–48). Berlin: Springer-Verlag.

Armstrong, T. D., & Costello, E. J. (2002). Community studies on adolescent substance use, abuse, or dependence and psychiatric comorbidity. *Journal of Consulting and Clinical Psychology, 70,* 1224–1239.

Avenevoli, S., & Steinberg, L. (2001). The continuity of depression across the adolescent transition. In H. Reese & R. Kail (Eds.), *Advances in child development and behavior* (pp. 139–173). San Diego: Academic Press.

Avenevoli, S., Stolar, M., Li, J., Dierker, L., & Merikangas, K. R. (2001). Comorbidity of depression in children and adolescents: Models and evidence from a prospective high-risk family study. *Biological Psychiatry, 49,* 1071–1081.

Bardone, A. M., Moffit, T., Caspi, A., Dickson, N., & Silva, P. A. (1996). Adult mental health and social outcomes of adolescent girls with depression and conduct disorder. *Development and Psychopathology, 8,* 811–829.

Beach, S. R. H., & Amir, N. (2003). Is depression taxonic, dimensional, or both? *Journal of Abnormal Psychology, 112,* 228–236.

Beardslee, W. R., Keller, M. B., Lavori, P. W., Staley, J. E., & Sacks, N. (1993). The impact of parental affective disorders on depression in offspring: A longitudinal follow-up in a nonreferred sample. *Journal of the American Academy of Child and Adolescent Psychiatry, 32,* 723–730.

Beidel, D. C., & Turner, S. M. (1997). At risk for anxiety: I. Psychopathology in the offspring of anxious parents. *Journal of the American Academy of Child and Adolescent Psychiatry, 36,* 918–924.

Bird, H. R., Canino, G., Rubio-Stipec, M., Gould, M. S., Ribera, J., Sesman, M., et al. (1988). Estimates of the prevalence of childhood maladjustment in a community survey in Puerto Rico: The use of combined measures. *Archives of General Psychiatry, 45,* 1120–1126.

Birmaher, B., Ryan, N. D., Williamson, D. E., Brent, D. A., Kaufman, J., Dahl, R. E., et al. (1996). Childhood and adolescent depression: A review of the past 10 years: Part I. *Journal of the American Academy of Child and Adolescent Psychiatry, 35,* 1427–1439.

Bittner, A., Goodwin, R. D., Wittchen, H.-U., Beesdo, K., Hofler, M., & Lieb, R. (2004). What characteristics of primary anxiety disorders predict subsequent major depressive disorder? *Journal of Clinical Psychiatry, 65,* 618–626.

Burke, K. C., Burke, J. D., Regier, D. A., & Rae, D. S. (1990). Age at onset of selected mental disorders in five community populations. *Archives of General Psychiatry, 47,* 511–518.

Canals, J., Domenech, E., Carbajo, G., & Blade, J. (1997). Prevalence of DSM-III-R and ICD-10 psychiatric disorders in a Spanish population of 18-year-olds. *Acta Psychiatrica Scandinavica, 96,* 287–294.

Canals, J., Domenech-Llaberia, E., Fernandez-Ballart, J., & Marti-Henneberg, C. (2002). Predictors of depression at eighteen: A 7 year follow-up in a Spanish nonclinical population. *European Child and Adolescent Psychiatry, 11,* 226–233.

Canals, J., Marti-Henneberg, C., Fernandez-Ballart, J., & Domenech, E. (1995). A longitudinal study of depression in an urban Spanish pubertal population. *European Child and Adolescent Psychiatry, 4,* 102–111.

Canino, G., Shrout, P. E., Rubio-Stipec, M., Bird, H. R., Bravo, M., Ramirez, R., et al. (2004). The DSM-IV rates of child and adolescent disorders in Puerto Rico: Prevalence, correlates, service use, and effects of impairment. *Archives of General Psychiatry, 61,* 85–93.

Caspi, A., Sugden, K., Moffitt, T. E., Taylor, A., Craig, I. W., Harrington, H. L., et al. (2003). Influence of life stress on depression: Moderation by a polymorphism in the 5-HTT gene. *Science, 301,* 386–389.

Chambers, W. J., Puig-Antich, J., Hirsch, M., Paez, P., Ambrosini, P. J., Tabrizi, M. A., et al. (1985). The assessment of affective disorders in children and adolescents by semi-structured interview: Test–retest reliability of the Schedule for Affective Disorders and Schizophrenia for School-age Children, Present Episode Version. *Archives of General Psychiatry, 42,* 696–702.

Christiana, J. M., Gilman, S. E., Guardino, M., Kessler, R. C., Mickelson, K., Morselli, P. L., et al. (2000). Duration between onset and time of obtaining initial treatment among people with anxiety and mood disorders: An international survey of members of mental health patient advocate groups. *Psychological Medicine, 30,* 693–703.

Cicchetti, D., & Toth, S. L. (1998). The development of depression in children and adolescents. *American Psychologist, 53,* 221–241.

Cohen, P., Cohen, J., Kasen, S., Velez, C. N., Hartmark, C., Johnson, J., et al. (1993). An epidemiological study of disorders in late childhood and adolescence: I. Age and gender-specific prevalence. *Journal of Child Psychology and Psychiatry and Allied Disciplines, 34,* 851–867.

Compas, B. E., Ey, S., & Grant, K. E. (1993). Taxonomy, assessment, and diagnosis of depression during adolescence. *Psychological Bulletin, 114,* 323–344.

Conway, K. P., Compton, W., Stinson, F. S., & Grant, B. F. (2006). Lifetime comorbidity of DSM-IV mood and anxiety disorders and specific drug use disorders: Results from the national epidemiologic survey on alcohol and related conditions. *Journal of Clinical Psychiatry, 67,* 247–257.

Costello, E. J., Angold, A., Burns, B. J., Stangl, D. K., Tweed, D. L., Erkanli, A., et al. (1996). The

Great Smoky Mountains Study of Youths: Goals, design, methods, and the prevalence of DSM-III-R disorders. *Archives of General Psychiatry, 53,* 1129–1136.

Costello, E. J., Costello, A. J., Edelbrock, C., Burns, B. J., Dulcan, M. K., Brent, D. A., et al. (1988). Psychiatric disorders in pediatric primary care: Prevalence and risk factors. *Archives of General Psychiatry, 45,* 1107–1116.

Costello, E. J., Egger, H. L., & Angold, A. (2004). The developmental epidemiology of anxiety disorders. In T. Ollendick & J. March (Eds.), *Phobic and anxiety disorders in children and adolescents: A clinician's guide to effective psychosocial and pharmacological interventions* (pp. 61–91). New York: Oxford University Press.

Costello, E. J., Farmer, E., Angold, A., Burns, B., & Erkanli, A. (1997). Psychiatric disorders among American Indian and white youth in Appalachia: The Great Smoky Mountains Study. *American Journal of Public Health, 87,* 827–832.

Costello, E. J., Foley, D. L., & Angold, A. (2006). 10-year research update review: The epidemiology of child and adolescent psychiatric disorders: II. Developmental epidemiology. *Journal of the American Academy of Child and Adolescent Psychiatry, 45,* 8–25.

Costello, E. J., Mustillo, S., Erkanli, A., Keeler, G., & Angold, A. (2003). Prevalence and development of psychiatric disorders in childhood and adolescence. *Archives of General Psychiatry, 60,* 837–844.

Deykin, E. Y., Levy, J. C., & Wells, V. (1987). Adolescent depression, alcohol and drug abuse. *American Journal of Public Health, 77,* 178–182.

Earls, F. (1979). Epidemiology and child psychiatry: Historical and conceptual development. *Comprehensive Psychiatry, 20,* 256–269.

Egger, H. L., & Angold, A. (2006). Common emotional and behavioral disorders in preschool children: Presentation, nosology, and epidemiology. *Journal of Child Psychology and Psychiatry, 47,* 313–337.

Eley, T. C., & Plomin, R. (1997). Genetic analyses of emotionality. *Current Opinion in Neurobiology, 7,* 279–284.

Elster, A., Jarosik, J., VanGeest, J., & Fleming, M. (2003). Racial and ethnic disparities in health care for adolescents: A systematic review of the literature. *Archives of Pediatric and Adolescent Medicine, 157,* 867–874.

Farmer, E. M., Burns, B. J., Phillips, S. D., Angold, A., & Costello, E. J. (2003). Pathways into and through mental health services for children and adolescents. *Psychiatric Services, 54,* 60–66.

Feehan, M., McGee, R., Raja, S. N., & Williams, S. M. (1994). DSM-III-R disorders in New Zealand 18-year-olds. *Australian and New Zealand Journal of Psychiatry, 28,* 87–99.

Fergusson, D. M., & Horwood, L. J. (2001). The Christchurch Health and Development Study: Review of findings on child and adolescent mental health. *Australian and New Zealand Journal of Psychiatry, 35,* 287–296.

Fergusson, D. M., Horwood, L. J., & Lynskey, M. T. (1993). Prevalence and comorbidity of DSM-III-R diagnoses in a birth cohort of 15-year-olds. *Journal of the American Academy of Child and Adolescent Psychiatry, 32,* 1127–1134.

Fergusson, D. M., Horwood, L. J., Ridder, E. M., & Beautrais, A. L. (2005). Subthreshold depression in adolescence and mental health outcomes in adulthood. *Archives of General Psychiatry, 62,* 66–72.

Fergusson, D. M., & Woodward, L. J. (2002). Mental health, educational, and social role outcomes of adolescents with depression. *Archives of General Psychiatry, 59,* 225–231.

Fleming, J. E., Offord, D. R., & Boyle, M. H. (1989). Prevalence of childhood and adolescent depression in the community—Ontario Child Health Study. *British Journal of Psychiatry, 155,* 647–654.

Franko, D. L., Striegel-Moore, R. H., Bean, J., Tamer, R., Kraemer, H. C., Dohm, F. A., et al. (2005). Psychosocial and health consequences of adolescent depression in black and white young adult women. *Health Psychology, 24,* 586–593.

Franko, D. L., Striegel-Moore, R. H., Brown, K. M., Barton, B. A., McMahon, R. P., Schreiber, G. B., et al. (2004). Expanding our understanding of the relationship between negative life events and depressive symptoms in black and white adolescent girls. *Psychological Medicine, 34,* 1319–1330.

Garrison, C. Z., Waller, J. L., Cuffe, S. P., McKeown, R. E., Addy, C. L., & Jackson, K. L. (1997). Incidence of major depressive disorder and dysthymia in young adolescents. *Journal of the American Academy of Child and Adolescent Psychiatry, 36,* 458–465.

Gau, S. S., Chong, M. Y., Chen, T. H., & Cheng, A. T. (2005). A 3-year panel study of mental disorders among adolescents in Taiwan. *American Journal of Psychiatry, 162,* 1344–1350.

Geller, B., Zimerman, B., Williams, M., Bolhofner, K., & Craney, J. (2001). Bipolar disorder at prospective follow-up of adults who had prepubertal major depressive disorder. *American Journal of Psychiatry, 158,* 125–127.

Giaconia, R. M., Reinherz, H. Z., Silverman, A. B., Pakiz, B., Frost, A. K., & Cohen, E. (1994). Ages of onset of psychiatric disorders in a community population of older adolescents. *Journal of the American Academy of Child and Adolescent Psychiatry, 33,* 706–717.

Gilman, S. E., Kawachi, I., Fitzmaurice, G. M., & Buka, L. (2003). Socio-economic status, family disruption and residential stability in childhood: Relation to onset, recurrence and remission of major depression. *Psychological Medicine, 33,* 1341–1355.

Gonzalez-Tejera, G., Canino, G., Ramirez, R., Chavez, L., Shrout, P., Bird, H., et al. (2005). Examining minor depression and major depression in adolescents. *Journal of Child Psychology and Psychiatry, 46,* 888–899.

Goodman, S. H., & Gotlib, I. H. (1999). Risk for psychopathology in the children of depressed mothers: A developmental model for understanding mechanisms of transmission. *Psychological Review, 106,* 458–490.

Goodyer, I., & Cooper, P. (1993). A community study of depression in adolescent girls: II. The clinical features of identified disorder. *British Journal of Psychiatry, 163,* 374–380.

Gotlib, I. H., & Hammen, C. L. (1992). *Psychological aspects of depression: Toward a cognitive-interpersonal integration.* Chichester, UK: Wiley.

Gotlib, I. H., Lewinsohn, P. M., & Seeley, J. R. (1998). Consequences of depression during adolescence: Marital status and marital functioning in early adulthood. *Journal of Abnormal Psychology, 107,* 686–690.

Hammen, C., Burge, D., Burney, E., & Adrian, C. (1990). Longitudinal study of diagnosis in children of women with unipolar and bipolar affective disorder. *Archives of General Psychiatry, 47,* 1112–1117.

Hammen, C., Shih, J. H., & Brennan, P. A. (2004). Intergenerational transmission of depression: Test of an interpersonal stress model in a community sample. *Journal of Consulting and Clinical Psychology, 72,* 511–522.

Hankin, B. L., & Abela, J. R. Z. (Eds.). (2005). *Development of psychopathology: A vulnerability-stress perspective.* Thousand Oaks, CA: Sage.

Hankin, B. L., Abramson, L. Y., Moffitt, T. E., Silva, P. A., McGee, R., & Angell, K. E. (1998). Development of depression from preadolescence to young adulthood: Emerging gender differences in a 10-year longitudinal study. *Journal of Abnormal Psychology, 107,* 128–140.

Hankin, B. L., Fraley, R. C., Lahey, B. B., & Waldman, I. D. (2005). Is depression best viewed as a continuum or discrete category? A taxometric analysis of childhood and adolescent depression in a population based sample. *Journal of Abnormal Psychiatry, 114,* 96–110.

Harrington, R., Fudge, H., Rutter, M., Pickles, A., & Hill, J. (1990). Adult outcomes of childhood and adolescent depression: I. Psychiatric status. *Archives of General Psychiatry, 47,* 465–473.

Hoberman, H. M., & Bergmann, P. E. (1992). Suicidal behavior in adolescence. *Current Opinion in Psychiatry, 5,* 508–517.

Hofstra, M. B., Van der Ende, J., & Verhulst, F. C. (2000). Continuity and change of psychopathology from childhood into adulthood: A 14-year follow-up study. *Journal of the American Academy of Child and Adolescent Psychiatry, 39,* 850–858.

Isakson, K., & Jarvis, P. (1999). The adjustment of adolescents during the transition into high school: A short term longitudinal study. *Journal of Youth and Adolescence, 28,* 1–26.

Kagan, J., & Moss, H. A. (1962). *Birth to maturity.* New York: Wiley.

Kashani, J., Beck, N., Hoeper, E., Fallahi, M. A., Corcoran, C. M., McAllister, J. A., et al. (1987). Psychiatric disorders in a community sample of adolescents. *American Journal of Psychiatry, 144*, 584–589.

Kashani, J. H., Carlson, G. A., Beck, N. C., Hoeper, E. W., Corcoran, C. M., McAllister, J. A., et al. (1987). Depression, depressive symptoms, and depressed mood among a community sample of adolescents. *American Journal of Psychiatry, 144*, 931–934.

Kashani, J. H., McGee, R. O., Clarkson, S. E., Anderson, J. C., Walton, L. A., Williams, S., et al. (1983). Depression in a sample of 9-year-old children. *Archives of General Psychiatry, 40*, 1217–1223.

Kashani, J. H., Rosenberg, T. K., & Reid, J. C. (1989). Developmental perspectives in child and adolescent depressive symptoms in a community sample. *American Journal of Psychiatry, 146*, 871–875.

Kashani, J. H., & Simonds, J. F. (1979). The incidence of depression in children. *American Journal of Psychiatry, 136*, 1203–1205.

Kaufman, J., Martin, A., King, R. A., & Charney, D. (2001). Are child-, adolescent-, and adult-onset depression one in the same disorder? *Biological Psychiatry, 49*, 980–1001.

Kendler, K. S., Kuhn, J. W., & Prescott, C. A. (2004). Childhood sexual abuse, stressful life events and risk for major depression in women. *Psychological Medicine, 34*, 1475–1482.

Kendler, K. S., Neale, M. C., Kessler, R. C., Heath, A. C., & Eaves, L. J. (1992). A population-based twin study of major depression in women: The impact of varying definitions of illness. *Archives of General Psychiatry, 49*, 257–266.

Kessler, R. C. (2002). The categorical versus dimensional assessment controversy in the sociology of mental illness. *Journal of Health and Social Behavior, 43*, 171–188.

Kessler, R. C., Avenevoli, S., & Merikangas, K. R. (2001). Mood disorders in children and adolescents: An epidemiological perspective. *Biological Psychiatry, 49*, 1002–1014.

Kessler, R. C., Berglund, P., Demler, O., Jin, R., Koretz, D., Merikangas, K. R., et al. (2003). The epidemiology of major depressive disorder: Results from the National Comorbidity Survey Replication (NCS-R). *Journal of the American Medical Association, 289*, 3095–3105.

Kessler, R. C., Berglund, P., Demler, O., Jin, R., & Walters, E. (2005). Lifetime prevalence and age-of-onset distributions of DSM-IV disorders in the National Comorbidity Survey Replication. *Archives of General Psychiatry, 62*, 593–602.

Kessler, R. C., Davis, C. G., & Kendler, K. S. (1997). Childhood adversity and adult psychiatric disorder in the U.S. National Comorbidity Survey. *Psychological Medicine, 27*, 1101–1119.

Kessler, R., McGonagle, K., Swartz, M., Blazer, D., & Nelson, C. (1993). Sex and depression in the National Comorbidity Survey: I. Lifetime prevalence, chronicity and recurrence. *Journal of Affective Disorders, 29*, 85–96.

Kessler, R. C., Olfson, M., & Berglund, P. A. (1998). Patterns and predictors of treatment contact after first onset of psychiatric disorders. *American Journal of Psychiatry, 155*, 62–69.

Kessler, R. C., & Walters, E. E. (1998). Epidemiology of DSM-III-R major depression and minor depression among adolescents and young adults in the National Comorbidity Survey. *Depression and Anxiety, 7*, 3–14.

Kessler, R. C., Zhao, S., Blazer, D. B., & Swartz, M. (1997). Prevalence, correlates, and course of minor depression and major depression in the National Comorbidity Survey. *Journal of Affective Disorders, 45*, 19–30.

Kilpatrick, D. G., Ruggiero, K. J., Acierno, R., Saunders, B. E., Resnick, H. S., & Best, C. L. (2003). Violence and risk of PTSD, major depression, substance abuse/dependence, and comorbidity: Results from the national survey of adolescents. *Journal of Consulting and Clinical Psychology, 71*, 692–700.

Kim-Cohen, J., Caspi, A., Moffit, T. E., Harrington, H. L., Milne, B. J., & Poulton, R. (2003). Prior juvenile diagnoses in adults with mental disorder: Developmental follow-back of a prospective-longitudinal cohort. *Archives of General Psychiatry, 60*, 709–717.

Kovacs, M. (1996). The course of childhood-onset depressive disorders. *Psychiatric Annals, 26*, 326–330.

Kovacs, M., Feinberg, T. L., Crouse-Novak, M. A., Paulauskas, S. L., & Finkelstein, R. (1984). Depressive disorders in childhood: I. A longitudinal prospective study of characteristics and recovery. *Archives of General Psychiatry, 41,* 229–237.

Kovacs, M., & Gatsonis, C. (1989). Stability and change in childhood-onset depressive disorders: Longitudinal course as a diagnostic validator. In L. E. Robbins & J. E. Barrett (Eds.), *the validity of psychiatric diagnoses* (pp. 57–75). New York: Raven Press.

Kovacs, M., Obrosky, D. S., & Sherrill, J. (2003). Developmental changes in the phenomenology of depression in girls compared to boys from childhood onward. *Journal of Affective Disorders, 74,* 33–48.

Kraemer, H. C., Measelle, J. R., Ablow, J. C., Essex, M. J., Boyce, W. T., & Kupfer, D. J. (2003). A new approach to integrating data from multiple informants in psychiatric assessment and research: Mixing and matching contexts and perspectives. *American Journal of Psychiatry, 160,* 1566–1577.

Lahey, B. B., Applegate, B., Waldman, I. D., Loft, J. D., Hankin, B. L., & Rick, J. (2004). The structure of child and adolescent psychopathology: Generating new hypotheses. *Journal of Abnormal Psychology, 113,* 358–385.

Last, C. G., Perrin, S., Hersen, M., & Kazdin, A. (1996). A prospective study of childhood anxiety disorders. *Journal of the American Academy of Child and Adolescent Psychiatry, 35,* 1502–1510.

Levinson, D. F. (2006). The genetics of depression: A review. *Biological Psychiatry, 60,* 84–92.

Lewinsohn, P. M., Allen, N. B., & Seeley, J. R. (1999). First onset versus recurrence of depression: Differential processes of psychosocial risk. *Journal of Abnormal Psychology, 108,* 483–489.

Lewinsohn, P. M., Duncan, E. M., Stanton, A. K., & Hautzinger, M. (1986). Age at first onset for nonbipolar depression. *Journal of Abnormal Psychology, 95,* 378–383.

Lewinsohn, P. M., Gotlib, I. H., & Seeley, J. R. (1997). Depression-related psychosocial variables: Are they specific to depression in adolescents? *Journal of Abnormal Psychology, 106,* 365–375.

Lewinsohn, P. M., Hops, H., Roberts, R. E., Seeley, J. R., & Andrews, J. A. (1993). Adolescent psychopathology: I. Prevalence and incidence of depression and other DSM-III-R disorders in high school students. *Journal of Abnormal Psychology, 102,* 133–144.

Lewinsohn, P. M., Pettit, J. W., Joiner, T. E., & Seeley, J. R. (2003). The symptomatic expression of major depressive disorder in adolescents and young adults. *Journal of Abnormal Psychology, 112,* 244–252.

Lewinsohn, P. M., Rohde, P., Klein, D. N., & Seeley, J. R. (1999). Natural course of adolescent major depressive disorder: I. Continuity into young adulthood. *Journal of the American Academy of Child and Adolescent Psychiatry, 38,* 56–63.

Lewinsohn, P. M., Rohde, P., & Seeley, J. R. (1998). Major depressive disorder in older adolescents: Prevalence, risk factors, and clinical implications. *Clinical Psychology Review, 18,* 765–794.

Lewinsohn, P. M., Rohde, P., Seeley, J. R., & Hops, H. (1991). Comorbidity of unipolar depression: I. Major depression with dysthymia. *Journal of Abnormal Psychology, 100,* 205–213.

Lewinsohn, P. M., Rhode, P., Seeley, J. R., Klein, D. N., & Gotlib, I. H. (2000). Natural course of adolescent major depressive disorder in a community sample: Predictors of recurrence in young adults. *American Journal of Psychiatry, 157,* 1584–1591.

Lewinsohn, P. M., Shankman, S. A., Gau, J. M., & Klein, D. N. (2004). The prevalence and comorbidity of subthreshold psychiatric conditions. *Psychological Medicine, 34,* 613–622.

Lewinsohn, P. M., Zinbarg, J., Lewinsohn, M., & Sack, W. (1997). Lifetime comorbidity among anxiety disorders and between anxiety disorders and other mental disorders in adolescents. *Journal of Anxiety Disorders, 11,* 377–394.

Luby, J., Heffelfinger, A., Mrakotsky, C., Brown, K., Hessler, M., Wallis, J., et al. (2003). The clinical picture of depression in preschool children. *Journal of the American Academy of Child and Adolescent Psychiatry, 42,* 340–348.

Luby, J., Mrakotsky, C., Heffelfinger, A., Brown, K., Hessler, M., & Spitznagel, E. (2003). Modification of DSM-IV criteria for depressed preschool children. *American Journal of Psychiatry, 160,* 1169–1172.

McEwen, B. S., & Sapolsky, R. M. (1995). Stress and cognitive function. *Current Opinion in Neurobiology, 5,* 205–216.

McGee, R., Feehan, M., Williams, S., & Anderson, J. (1992). DSM-III disorders from age 11 to age 15 years. *Journal of the American Academy of Child and Adolescent Psychiatry, 31,* 50–59.

McGee, R., Feehan, M., Williams, S., Partridge, F., Silva, P. A., & Kelly, J. (1990). DSM-III disorders in a large sample of adolescents. *Journal of the American Academy of Child and Adolescent Psychiatry, 29,* 611–619.

McGee, R., & Williams, S. (1988). A longitudinal study of depression in nine-year-old children. *Journal of the American Academy of Child and Adolescent Psychiatry, 27,* 342–348.

McGuffin, P., Katz, R., & Bebbington, P. (1988). The Camberwell Collaborative Depression Study: III. Depression and adversity in the relatives of depressed probands. *British Journal of Psychiatry, 152,* 775–782.

Merikangas, K. R., & Angst, J. (1995). The challenge of depressive disorders in adolescence. In R. Michael (Ed.), *Psychosocial disturbances in young people: Challenges for prevention* (pp. 131–165). New York: Cambridge University Press.

Merikangas, K. R., & Avenevoli, S. (2002). Epidemiology of mood and anxiety disorders in children and adolescents. In M. T. Tsuang & M. Tohen (Eds.), *Textbook in psychiatric epidemiology* (pp. 657–704). New York: Wiley-Liss.

Merikangas, K. R., & Low, N. C. (2005). Genetic epidemiology of anxiety disorders. *Handbook of Experimental Pharmacology, 169,* 163–179.

Merikangas, K. R., Prusoff, B. A., & Weissman, M. M. (1988). Parental concordance for affective disorders: Psychopathology in offspring. *Journal of Affective Disorders, 15,* 279–290.

Mitchell, J., McCauley, E., Burke, P. M., & Moss, S. J. (1988). Phenomenology of depression in children and adolescents. *Journal of the American Academy of Child and Adolescent Psychiatry, 27,* 12–20

Monroe, S. M., Rohde, P., Seeley, J. R., & Lewinsohn, P. M. (1999). Life events and depression in adolescence: Relationship loss as a prospective risk factor for first onset of major depressive disorder. *Journal of Abnormal Psychology, 108,* 606–614.

Murray, C. J. L., & Lopez, A. D. (Eds.). (1996). *The global burden of disease: A comprehensive assessment of mortality and disability from diseases, injuries, and risk factors in 1990 and projected to 2020.* Cambridge, MA: Harvard University Press.

Murray, K. T., & Sines, J. O. (1996). Parsing the genetic and nongenetic variance in children's depressive behavior. *Journal of Affective Disorders, 38,* 23–34.

Nestler, E. J., Barrot, M., DiLeone, R. J., Eisch, A. J., Gold, S. J., & Monteggia, L. M. (2002). Neurobiology of depression. *Neuron, 34,* 13–25.

Newman, D. L., Moffitt, T. E., Caspi, A., & Magdol, L. (1996). Psychiatric disorder in a birth cohort of young adults: Prevalence, comorbidity, clinical significance, and new case incidence from ages 11–21. *Journal of Consulting and Clinical Psychology, 64,* 552–562.

Nolen-Hoeksema, S., & Girgus, J. S. (1994). The emergence of gender differences in depression during adolescence. *Psychological Bulletin, 115,* 424–443.

Nottelmann, E. D., & Jensen, P. S. (1995). Comorbidity of disorders in children and adolescents. In T. H. Ollendick & R. J. Prinz (Eds.), *Advances in clinical child psychology* (Vol. 17, pp. 109–155). New York: Plenum Press.

Olfson, M., Kessler, R. C., Berglund, P. A., & Lin, E. (1998). Psychiatric disorder onset and first treatment contact in the United States and Ontario. *American Journal of Psychiatry, 155,* 1415–1422.

O'Sullivan, C. (2004). The psychosocial determinants of depression: A lifespan perspective. *Journal of Nervous Mental Disorders, 192,* 585–594.

Petersen, A. C., Sarigiani, P. A., & Kennedy, R. E. (1991). Adolescent depression: Why more girls? *Journal of Youth and Adolescence, 20,* 247–271.

Pezawas, L., Wittchen, H.-U., Pfister, H., Angst, J., Lieb, R., & Kasper, S. (2003). Recurrent brief depressive disorder reinvestigated: A community sample of adolescents and young adults. *Psychological Medicine, 33,* 407–418.

Phillips, N. K., Hammen, C. L., Brennan, P. A., Najman, J. M., & Bor, W. (2005). Early adversity and the prospective prediction of depressive and anxiety disorders in adolescents. *Journal of Abnormal Child Psychology, 33,* 13–24.

Pickles, A., & Angold, A. (2003). Natural categories or fundamental dimensions: On carving nature at the joints and rearticulation of psychopathology. *Development and Psychopathology, 15,* 529–551.

Pine, D. S., Cohen, E., Cohen, P., & Brook, J. (1999). Adolescent depressive symptoms as predictors of adult depression: Moodiness or mood disorder? *American Journal of Psychiatry, 156,* 133–135.

Pine, D. S., Cohen, P., & Brook, J. (2001). Adolescent fears as predictors of depression. *Biological Psychiatry, 50,* 721–724.

Pine, D. S., Cohen, P., Gurley, D., Brook, J., & Ma, Y. (1998). The risk for early adulthood anxiety and depressive disorders in adolescents with anxiety and depressive disorders. *Archives of General Psychiatry, 55,* 56–64.

Rao, U., Ryan, N. D., Birmaher, B., Dahl, R. E., Williamson, D. E., Kaufman, J., et al (1995). Unipolar depression in adolescents: Clinical outcome in adulthood. *Journal of the American Academy of Child and Adolescent Psychiatry, 34,* 566–578.

Reinherz, H. Z., Giaconia, R. M., Carmola-Hauf, A. M., Wasserman, M. S., & Silverman, A. B. (1999). Major depression in the transition to adulthood: Risks and impairments. *Journal of Abnormal Psychology, 108,* 500–510.

Reinherz, H. Z., Giaconia, R. M., Lefkowitz, E. S., Pakiz, B., & Frost, A. (1993). Prevalence of psychiatric disorders in a community population of older adolescents. *Journal of the American Academy of Child and Adolescent Psychiatry, 32,* 369–377.

Reinherz, H. Z., Giaconia, R. M., Pakiz, B., Silverman, A. B., Frost, A. K., & Lefkowitz, E. S. (1993). Psychosocial risks for major depression in late adolescence: A longitudinal community study. *Journal of the American Academy of Child and Adolescent Psychiatry, 32,* 1155–1163.

Reinherz, H. Z., Paradis, A. D., Giaconia, R. M., Stashwick, C. K., & Fitzmaurice, G. (2003). Childhood and adolescent predictors of major depression in the transition to adulthood. *American Journal of Psychiatry, 160,* 2141–2147.

Rende, R., Warner, V., Wickramaratne, P., & Weissman, M. M. (1999). Sibling aggregation for psychiatric disorders in offspring at high and low risk for depression: 10-year follow-up. *Psychological Medicine, 29,* 1291–1298.

Rice, F., Harold, G., & Thapar, A. (2002). The genetic aetiology of childhood depression: A review. *Journal of Child Psychology and Psychiatry, 43,* 65–79.

Roberts, R. E., Lewinsohn, P. M., & Seeley, J. R. (1995). Symptoms of DSM-III-R major depression in adolescence: Evidence from an epidemiological survey. *Journal of the American Academy of Child and Adolescent Psychiatry, 34,* 1608–1617.

Rohde, P., Lewinsohn, P. M., & Seeley, J. R. (1991). Comorbidity of unipolar depression: II. Comorbidity with other mental disorders in adolescents and adults. *Journal of Abnormal Psychology, 100,* 214–222.

Roy, A. (1985). Early parental separation and adult depression. *Archives of General Psychiatry, 42,* 987–991.

Ruscio, J., & Ruscio, A. M. (2000). Informing the continuity controversy: A taxometric analysis of depression. *Journal of Abnormal Psychology, 109,* 473–487.

Rutter, M. (2003). Categories, dimensions, and the mental health of children and adolescents. *Annals of the New York Academy of Science, 1008,* 11–21.

Rutter, M., Kim-Cohen, J., & Maughan, B. (2006). Continuities and discontinuities in psychopathology between childhood and adult life. *Journal of Child Psychology and Psychiatry, 47,* 276–295.

Rutter, M., Tizard, J., & Whitmore, K. (1970). *Education, health, and behavior.* New York: Longman.

Ryan, N. D., Puig-Antich, J., Ambrosini, P., Rabinovich, H., Robinson, D., Nelson, B., et al. (1987). The clinical picture of major depression in children and adolescents. *Archives of General Psychiatry, 44,* 854–861.

Schepis, T. S., & Rao, U. (2005). Epidemiology and etiology of adolescent smoking. *Current Opinion in Pediatrics, 17,* 607–612.

Scourfield, J., Rice, F., Thapar, A., Harold, G. T., Martin, N., & McGuffin, P. (2003). Depressive symptoms in children and adolescents: Changing aetiological influences with development. *Journal of Child Psychology and Psychiatry, 44,* 968–976.

Shaffer, D., Fisher, P., Dulcan, M. K., & Davies, M. (1996). The NIMH Diagnostic Interview Schedule for Children Version 2.3 (DISC-2.3): Description, acceptability, prevalence rates, and performance in the MECA study. *Journal of the American Academy of Child and Adolescent Psychiatry, 35,* 865–877.

Shaffery, J., Hoffmann, R., & Armitage, R. (2003). The neurobiology of depression: Perspectives from animal and human sleep studies. *Neuroscientist, 9*(1), 82–98.

Shih, R. A., Belmonte, P. L., & Zandi, P. P. (2004). A review of the evidence from family, twin, and adoption studies for a genetic contribution to adult psychiatric disorders. *International Review of Psychiatry, 16,* 260–283.

Silberg, J., Pickles, A., Rutter, M., Hewitt, J., Simonoff, E., Maes, H., et al (1999). The influence of genetic factors and life stress on depression among adolescent girls. *Archives of General Psychiatry, 56,* 225–232.

Silberg, J. L., Rutter, M., & Eaves, L. (2001). Genetic and environmental influences on the temporal association between earlier anxiety and later depression in girls. *Biological Psychiatry, 49,* 1040–1049.

Simonoff, E., Pickles, A., Meyer, J., Silberg, J. L., Maes, H. H., Loeber, R., et al. (1997). The Virginia twin study of adolescent behavioral development: Influences of age, sex, and impairment on rates of disorders. *Archives of General Psychiatry, 47,* 487–496.

Slade, T., & Andrews, G. (2005). Latent structure of depression in a community sample: A taxometric analysis. *Psychological Medicine, 35,* 489–497.

Solomon, A., Ruscio, J., Seeley, J. R., & Lewinsohn, P. M. (2006). A taxometric investigation of unipolar depression in a large community sample. *Psychological Medicine, 15,* 1–13.

Sroufe, A., & Rutter, M. (1984). The domain of developmental psychopathology. *Child Development, 55,* 17–29.

Sullivan, P. F., Neale, M. C., & Kendler, K. S. (2000). Genetic epidemiology of major depression: Review and meta-analysis. *American Journal of Psychiatry, 157,* 1552–1562.

Sullivan, P. F., Prescott, C. A., & Kendler, K. S. (2002). The subtypes of major depression in a twin registry. *Journal of Affective Disorders, 68,* 273–284.

Thapar, A., & McGuffin, P. (1994). A twin study of depressive symptoms in childhood. *British Journal of Psychiatry, 165,* 259–265.

Thapar, A., & McGuffin, P. (1997). Anxiety and depressive symptoms in childhood: A genetic study of comorbidity. *Journal of Child Psychology and Psychiatry and Allied Disciplines, 38,* 651–656.

Twenge, J. M., & Nolen-Hoeksema, S. (2002). Age, gender, race, socioeconomic status, and birth cohort differences on the Children's Depression Inventory: A meta-analysis. *Journal of Abnormal Psychology, 111*(4), 578–588.

Velez, C., Johnson, J., & Cohen, P. (1989). A longitudinal analysis of selected risk factors for childhood psychopathology. *Journal of the American Academy of Child and Adolescent Psychiatry, 28,* 861–864.

Verhulst, F. C., van der Ende, J., Ferdinand, R. F., & Kasius, M. C. (1997). The prevalence of DSM-III-R diagnoses in a national sample of Dutch adolescents. *Archives of General Psychiatry, 54,* 329–336.

Warner, V., Weissman, M. M., Mufson, L., & Wickramaratne, P. J. (1999). Grandparents, parents, and grandchildren at high risk for depression: A three-generation study. *Journal of the American Academy of Child and Adolescent Psychiatry, 38,* 289–296.

Weiss, B., & Garber, J. (2003). Developmental differences in the phenomenology of depression. *Development and Psychopathology, 15,* 403–430.

Weiss, B., Weisz, J. R., Politano, M., Carey, M., Nelson, W. M., & Finch, A. J. (1992). Relations among self-reported depressive symptoms in clinic-referred children versus adolescents. *Journal of Abnormal Psychology, 101,* 391–397.

Weissman, M. M., Fendrich, M., Warner, V., & Wickramaratne, P. (1992). Incidence of psychiatric disorder in offspring at high and low risk for depression. *Journal of the American Academy of Child and Adolescent Psychiatry, 31,* 640–648.

Weissman, M. M., Warner, V., Wickramaratne, P., Moreau, D., & Olfson, M. (1997). Offspring of depressed parents: Ten years later. *Archives of General Psychiatry, 54,* 932–940.

Weissman, M. M., Wickramaratne, P., Nomura, Y., Warner, V., Verdeli, H., Pilowsky, D. J., et al. (2005). Families at high and low risk for depression: A 3-generation study. *Archives of General Psychiatry, 6,* 29–36.

Weissman, M. M., Wolk, S., Wickramaratne, P., Goldstein, R. B., Adams, P., Greenwald, S., et al. (1999). Children with pre-pubertal onset major depressive disorder and anxiety grown up. *Archives of General Psychiatry, 56,* 794–801.

Whitaker, A., Johnson, J., Shaffer, D., Rapoport, J. L., Kalikow, K., Walsh, B. T., et al. (1990). Uncommon troubles in young people: Prevalence estimates of selected psychiatric disorders in a nonreferred population. *Archives of General Psychiatry, 47,* 487–496.

Williamson, D. E., Birmaher, B., Dahl, R. E., & Ryan, N. D. (2005). Stressful life events in anxious and depressed children. *Journal of Child and Adolescent Psychopharmacology, 15,* 571–580.

Williamson, D. E., Ryan, N. D., Birmaher, B., Dahl, R. E., & Nelson, B. (1995). A case-control family history study of depression in adolescents. *Journal of the American Academy of Child and Adolescent Psychiatry, 34,* 1596–1607.

Wittchen, H.-U., Kessler, R. C., Pfister, H., & Lieb, M. (2000). Why do people with anxiety disorders become depressed? A prospective-longitudinal community study. *Acta Psychiatrica Scandinavica, 102*(Suppl.), 14–23.

Wittchen, H.-U., Nelson, C. B., & Lachner, G. (1998). Prevalence of mental disorders and psychosocial impairments in adolescents and young adults. *Psychological Medicine, 28,* 109–126.

World Health Organization. (1993). *ICD-10 classification of mental and behavioural disorders.* Geneva: Author.

Wu, P., Hoven, C. W., Bird, H. R., Moore, R. E., Cohen, P., Alegria, M., et al. (1999). Depressive and disruptive disorders and mental health utilization in children and adolescents. *Journal of the American Academy of Child and Adolescent Psychiatry, 38,* 1081–1090.

Yang, H. J., Soong, W. T., Kuo, P. H., Chang, H. L., & Chen, W. J. (2004). Using the CES-D in a two-phase survey for depressive disorders among nonreferred adolescents in Taipei: A stratum-specific likelihood ratio analysis. *Journal of Affective Disorders, 82,* 419–430.

Young, E. A., & Altemus, M. (2004). Puberty, ovarian steroids, and stress. *Annals of the New York Academy of Science, 1021,* 124–133.

Zammit, S., & Owen, M. J. (2006). Stressful life events, 5-HTT genotype and risk of depression. *British Journal of Psychiatry, 188,* 199–201.

II ETIOLOGY OF DEPRESSION

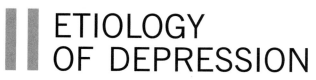

3 Cognitive Vulnerability to Depression in Children and Adolescents

A Developmental Psychopathology Perspective

John R. Z. Abela and Benjamin L. Hankin

Ever since their introduction in the late 1960s, cognitive theories of vulnerability to depression have generated a vast amount of empirical attention (Abramson et al., 2002; Clark & Beck, 1999; Nolen-Hoeksema & Corte, 2004; Zuroff, Santor, & Mongrain, 2004). Initial research testing these theories focused on examining either the cross-sectional association between vulnerability factors and depressive symptoms or the main effect of vulnerability factors on change in depressive symptoms over time. Critical reviews of the literature, however, argued that such early studies provided an inadequate examination of the cognitive theories as they failed to examine the theories' central hypothesis, that cognitively vulnerable individuals are more likely than other individuals to experience increases in depressive symptoms only in the face of negative events; in the absence of such events, cognitively vulnerable individuals are no more likely than others to exhibit depression (Abramson, Alloy, & Metalsky, 1988; Alloy, Hartlage, & Abramson, 1988). In response to such critiques, the field saw a major shift in methodologies used to test cognitive theories and prospective diathesis–stress designs became the gold standard.

During the 1980s and 1990s, as diathesis–stress studies began to rapidly accumulate in the literature, a striking trend began to emerge. More specifically, the vast majority of studies testing the cognitive theories were using adult samples, with relatively few examining the applicability of these theories to youth. Such a trend would be understandable if depression was a disorder that is rare in children and adolescents. Results from studies examining the prevalence of depression in youth, however, indicate that depressive disorders are relatively common, with up to 9% of youth experiencing at least one major depressive episode by the age of 14 (Lewinsohn, Rohde, Seeley, & Fischer, 1993). Further, results from epidemiological studies indicate that adolescence is a critical period for understanding depression, as it is during this time that the majority of individuals who develop depression experience their first clinically significant episode and that the sex difference in depression rates emerges (Hankin et al., 1998). Thus, examining the applicability of cognitive vulnerability theories to youth at different developmental stages is essential in order to gain a deep understanding of the mechanisms and processes underlying the onset, maintenance, and recurrence of this disorder.

In recent years, the field has seen a rapid growth in prospective studies testing cognitive theories of vulnerability to depression in child and adolescent samples. For example, of the 48 prospective studies that we review in this chapter, 38 have been conducted within the past 6 years. This increased attention to examining these theories in youth is due, in part, to increased awareness of the high prevalence, chronic course, and debilitating nature of childhood and adolescent depression (Shwartz, Gladstone, & Kaslow, 1998). This is also due, in part, to the seminal work of pioneering developmental psychopathologists who have highlighted the importance of examining cognitive vulnerability theories within a developmental framework (Garber, 2000; Hammen, 1992). We begin by discussing the central tenets of cognitive theories of vulnerability to depression. We next present a comprehensive review of prospective research examining four of the predominant cognitive models of depression: (1) the hopelessness theory (Abramson, Metalsky, & Alloy, 1989; Abramson, Seligman, & Teasdale, 1978), (2) Beck's (1967) cognitive theory, (3) response styles theory (Nolen-Hoeksema, 1991), and (4) theories of personality predispositions to depression (Beck, 1983; Blatt & Zuroff, 1992). In the remaining sections, we highlight several areas that should be priorities for research on cognitive vulnerability to depression in youth, including (1) new conceptual approaches to understanding the relationships between cognitive vulnerability factors, (2) developmental issues, and (3) methodological and statistical issues that may enhance tests of the cognitive theories.

COGNITIVE VULNERABILITY TO DEPRESSION: THEORY AND EVIDENCE

Cognitive theories of depression are primarily concerned with the relationship between human mental activity and the experience of depressive symptoms and episodes (Ingram, Miranda, & Segal, 1998). Cognition is thought to encompass the mental processes of perceiving, recognizing, conceiving, judging, and reasoning. According to cognitive theorists, these cognitive variables have significant causal implications for the onset, maintenance, and remission of depression.

Cognitive theories of depression define vulnerability as an internal and stable feature of an individual that predisposes him or her to develop depression following the occurrence of negative events (Ingram et al., 1998). It is important to emphasize that cognitive models are fundamentally diathesis–stress models in that they posit that depression is produced by the *interaction* between an individual's cognitive vulnerability and certain environmental conditions that serve to trigger this diathesis into operation (Ingram et al., 1998). Evidence suggests that under ordinary conditions, persons thought to be vulnerable to depression are indistinguishable from the general population. Only when confronted with certain stressors do differences between vulnerable and nonvulnerable individuals emerge (Ingram et al., 1998; Ingram & Luxton, 2005; Monroe & Simons, 1991). For individuals who possess cognitive vulnerability factors, the occurrence of a negative event triggers a pattern of negatively biased, self-referent information processing that initiates a downward spiral into depression. Nonvulnerable individuals react with an appropriate level of distress and depressive affect to the event but do not spiral into depression.

Cognitive theories of vulnerability to depression are essentially titration models (Abramson, Alloy, & Metalsky, 1995, p. 118). In other words, such theories posit that cognitive vulnerability is best conceptualized along a continuum, with some individuals exhibiting higher levels of cognitive vulnerability than others. Similarly, negative events are best conceptualized along a continuum, with some negative events being more negative than others. According to such a perspective, the higher the level of cognitive vulnerability an individual possesses, the less stressful the negative event must be to trigger the onset of depressive symptoms/episodes. Conversely, even youth possessing average or low levels of cognitive vulnerability may be at risk for developing depression following the occurrence of extreme stressors.

Within a titration framework, depression is also viewed as existing along a continuum of severity, ranging from subclinical depressive mood reactions to enduring clinically significant depressive episodes (Abramson et al., 1988; Alloy et al., 1988; see Hankin, Fraley, Lahey, & Waldman, 2005, for evidence that depression among youth exists on a continuum). Severity of depression is hypothesized to vary as a function of (1) the severity of cognitive vulnerability factors, (2) the severity of negative events, and (3) the content (e.g., situation-specific versus generalized) of the thought processes that ensue following the occurrence of stressors. Thus, cognitive diatheses can serve as vulnerability factors to either subclinical depressive mood reactions or clinically significant depressive episodes, depending on the severity of stressors encountered and the generality of the depressogenic thought processes triggered by such stressors. As cognitive theories state that a less severe analogue to clinical depression exists when stressors and vulnerability factors are not extreme and depressogenic thought processes are event-specific, researchers have examined such theories from multiple perspectives, ranging from predicting depressive mood reactions following the occurrence of stressful events (e.g., Abela, 2002; Abela & Seligman, 2000) to predicting the development of clinically significant depressive episodes in high-risk populations (e.g., Alloy et al., 2006; Hammen, Adrian, & Hiroto, 1988).

Although a multitude of vulnerability factors have been posited by cognitive theorists, we focus our review on the following vulnerability factors, as they have been studied the most extensively across child, early adolescent, and adolescent populations: (1) depressogenic inferential styles about causes, consequences, and the self (Abramson et al., 1978, 1989), (2) dysfunctional attitudes (Beck, 1967), (3) the tendency to ruminate in response to depressed mood (Nolen-Hoeksema, 1991), and (4) personality predispositions to depression (Beck, 1983; Blatt & Zuroff, 1992). In addition, we focus our review on prospective studies, as they provide the most powerful tests of theories of cognitive vulnerability.

Hopelessness Theory

The hopelessness theory is a cognitive diathesis–stress theory that posits a series of contributory causes that interact with one another to culminate in the proximal sufficient cause of a specific subtype of depression: hopelessness depression (Abramson et al., 1989). The theory postulates three distinct depressogenic inferential styles that serve as distal contributory causes of hopelessness depression: (1) the tendency to attribute negative events to global and stable causes, (2) the tendency to perceive negative events as having many disastrous consequences, and (3) the tendency to view the self as flawed or deficient following negative events. Each depressogenic inferential style predisposes individuals to the development of hopelessness depression by increasing the likelihood that they will make depressogenic inferences following negative events. Making such inferences increases the likelihood that hopelessness will develop. Hopelessness is defined as the expectation that negative events will occur and that positive events will not occur, coupled with the expectation that one can do nothing to change this. Once hopelessness develops, hopelessness depression is inevitable, as the hopelessness theory views hopelessness as the proximal sufficient cause of hopelessness depression.

Most of the research testing the diathesis–stress component of the hopelessness theory in children and adolescents has examined the question of whether youth who possess a depressogenic attributional style are more likely than other youth to experience increases in depressive symptoms following negative events. As illustrated in Table 3.1, several studies have provided full support for the attributional vulnerability hypothesis in youth (e.g., Abela, Parkinson, Stollow, & Starrs, in press; Dixon & Ahrens, 1992; Hankin, Abramson, & Siler, 2001; Hankin & Roesch, 2005; Hilsman & Garber, 1995; Joiner, 2000; Panak & Garber, 1992; Prinstein & Aikins, 2004; Southall & Roberts, 2002). Yet other studies have provided only partial support (Abela, 2001, 2002; Abela & Seligman, 2000; Brozina & Abela, 2006; Conley, Haines, Hilt, & Metalsky, 2001; Gibb & Alloy, 2006; Lewinsohn, Joiner, & Rohde, 2001; Nolen-Hoeksema, Girgus, & Seligman, 1986, 1992; Robinson, Garber, & Hilsman, 1995) or no support (Abela & Sarin, 2002; Bennett & Bates, 1995; Hammen et al., 1988; Spence, Sheffield, & Donovan, 2002) for this hypothesis. Fewer studies have examined the question of whether depressogenic inferential styles about consequences and the self serve as vulnerability factors to depression in youth. The results from those that have are mixed with studies providing full (Hankin & Roesch, 2005), partial (Abela, 2001, 2002; Abela & Seligman, 2000), or no support (Abela & Sarin, 2002) for this component of the hopelessness theory.

Beck's Cognitive Theory

Similar to hopelessness theory, Beck's cognitive theory is a diathesis–stress theory that posits a series of contributory causes that interact with one another to culminate in depression (Beck, 1967, 1983). Central to Beck's theory is the construct of schema. Beck defines schema as stored bodies of knowledge (i.e., mental representations of the self and prior experience) that are relatively enduring characteristics of a person's cognitive organization. When an individual is confronted with a situation, the schema most relevant to the situation is activated. Schema activation subsequently influences how the person perceives, encodes, and retrieves information regarding the situation.

Beck (1967, 1983) proposes that certain individuals possess depressogenic schema that confer vulnerability to depression. Beck hypothesizes that depressogenic schema are typically organized as sets of dysfunctional attitudes such as "I am nothing if a person I love doesn't like me" or "If I fail at my work than I am a failure as a person." Such schema are activated following the occurrence of negative events. Once activated, depressogenic schema trigger a pattern of negatively biased, self-referent information processing characterized by negative errors in thinking (e.g., negatively skewed interpretations of negative life events such as overgeneralization and catastrophizing). Negative errors in thinking increase the likelihood that an individual will develop the negative cognitive triad. Beck defines the negative cognitive triad as containing three distinct

TABLE 3.1. Summary of Prospective Studies Testing the Hopelessness Theory

Study	Sample type	Follow-up	Depression measure	Results	Sample size
Abela (2001)	3rd and 7th graders	1.5 months	CDI	DIS-causes × stress predicted increases in depressive symptoms in 7th graders but not 3rd graders.	382
				DIS-consequences × stress predicted increases in depressive symptoms in 3rd and 7th graders.	
				DIS-self × stress predicted increases in depressive symptoms in 3rd and 7th grade girls, not boys.	
Abela (2002)	12th graders	0.25–2 months	MAACL	DIS-causes, DIS-consequences, and DIS-self predicted enduring, but not immediate, depressive mood responses to a negative event.	136
Abela & McGirr (2007)	6- to 14-year-olds with an affectively ill parent	12 months, multiwave	CDI	Weakest link interacted with fluctuations in hassles to predict fluctuations in depressive symptoms.	140
Abela, McGirr, & Skitch (2007)	3rd and 7th graders	1.5 months, multiwave	CDI	Weakest link interacted with fluctuations in hassles to predict fluctuations in depressive symptoms.	382
Abela, Parkinson, Stolow, & Starrs (in press)	9th graders	1.5 months	CDI	DIS-causes × stress predicted increases in depressive symptoms.	319
Abela & Payne (2003)	3rd and 7th graders	1.5 months	CDI	Weakest link × stress predicted increases in depressive symptoms in 3rd graders and 7th grade boys with low, but not high, self-esteem.	314
Abela & Sarin (2002)	7th graders	2.5 months	CDI	DIS-causes × stress, DIS-consequences × stress, DIS-Self × Stress did not predict change in depressive symptoms.	79
				Weakest link × stress predicted increases in depressive symptoms.	
Abela & Seligman (2000)	12th graders	0.25–2 months	MAACL	DIS-causes, DIS-consequences, and DIS-self predicted immediate, but not enduring, depressive mood responses to a negative event.	77
Abela, Skitch, Adams, & Hankin (2006)	6- to 14-year-olds with an affectively ill parent	12 months, multiwave	CDI	Weakest link interacted with fluctuations in parental depressive symptoms to predict fluctuations in children's depressive symptoms.	140
Bennett & Bates (1995)	11- to 13-year-olds	6 months	CDI	DIS-causes × stress did not predict change in depressive symptoms.	95

(continued)

TABLE 3.1. *(continued)*

Study	Sample type	Follow-up	Depression measure	Results	Sample size
Brozina & Abela (2006)	3rd to 6th graders	1.5 months	CDI	DIS-causes × stress, DIS-consequences × stress, and DIS-self × stress predicted increases in depressive symptoms in children possessing low, but not high, initial levels of symptoms.	480
Conley et al. (2001)	5- to 10-year-olds	0.5–1 months	CDI	DIS-causes × stress predicted increases in depressive symptoms in 5- to 7-year-olds with low self-esteem, but not in 8- to 10-year-olds.	147
Dixon & Ahrens (1992)	9- to 12-year-olds at summer camp	1 month	CDI	DIS-causes × stress predicted increases in depressive symptoms.	84
Gibb & Alloy (2006)	4th and 5th graders	6 months	CDI	DIS-causes × stress predicted increases in depressive symptoms in 5th but not 4th graders.	415
Hammen et al. (1988)	8- to 16-year-olds with either affectively ill, medically ill, or control parents	6 months	K-SADS	DIS-causes × stress did not predict onset of depressive disorder.	79
Hankin & Roesch (2005)	6th to 10th graders	4 months; multiwave	CDI	DIS-causes × stress, DIS-consequences × stress, and DIS-self × stress predicted trajectories of depressive symptoms.	320
Hankin, Abramson, & Siler (2001)	9th to 12th graders	1.25 months	BDI, HDSQ-R	DIS-causes × stress predicted increases in depressive symptoms.	270
Hilsman & Garber (1995)	5th to 6th graders	0.2 months	CES-DC	DIS-causes × stress predicted enduring but not immediate depressive symptoms in children possessing low, but not high, competence and perceptions of control.	439
Joiner (2000)	9- to 17-year-old mixed clinical sample	2 months	CDI	DIS-causes × stress predicted increases in depressive symptoms.	34
Lewinsohn, Joiner, & Rohde (2001)	9th to 12th graders	12 months	K-SADS	DIS-causes interacted with low stress to predict onset of depressive episode.	1,507
Nolen-Hoeksema et al. (1986)	3rd to 5th graders	12 months	CDI	DIS-causes × stress predicted increases in depressive symptoms in two out of four follow-up assessments.	168

(continued)

TABLE 3.1. *(continued)*

Study	Sample type	Follow-up	Depression measure	Results	Sample size
Nolen-Hoeksema et al. (1992)	3rd to 8th graders	60 months	CDI	DIS-causes × stress predicted increases in depressive symptoms in 5th to 8th graders but not 3rd or 4th graders.	336
Panak & Garber (1992)	3rd to 5th graders	12 months	CDI DACL	DIS-causes × stress predicted increases in depressive symptoms.	521
Prinstein & Aikins (2004)	15- to 17-year-olds	17 months	CDI	DIS-causes × stress predicted increases in depressive symptoms.	158
Robinson, Garber, & Hilsman (1995)	12-year-olds	4–5 months	CDI	DIS-causes × stress predicted increases in depressive symptoms among youth with low, not high, self-esteem.	371
Southall & Roberts (2002)	9th to 12th graders	3.5 months	CDI	DIS-causes × stress predicted increases in depressive symptoms.	115
Spence, Sheffield, & Donovan (2002)	11- to 13-year-olds	12 months	BDI	DIS-causes × stress did not predict depressive symptoms.	773

Note. CDI, Children's Depression Inventory; DIS-causes, depressogenic inferential style about causes (attributional style); DIS-consequences, depressogenic inferential style about consequences; DIS-self, depressogenic inferential style about the self; weakest link, an individual's most depressogenic inferential style; MAACL, Multiple Adjective Affect Checklist; K-SADS, Kiddie Schedule for Affective Disorders; BDI, Beck Depression Inventory; HDSQ-R, Hopelessness Depressive Symptoms Questionnaire, Revised; CES-DC, Center for Epidemiologic Studies Depression Scale for Children; DACL, Depressive Adjective Checklist.

depressogenic cognitive patterns: negative views of the self (e.g., the belief that one is deficient, inadequate, or unworthy), negative views of the world (e.g., construing life experiences in terms of themes of defeat or disparagement), and negative views of the future (e.g., the expectation that one's difficulties will persist in the future and there is nothing one can do to change this). As Beck views the negative cognitive triad as a proximal, sufficient cause of depression, once an individual develops the negative cognitive triad, he or she will develop depressive symptoms.

To our knowledge, four prospective studies have examined the diathesis–stress component of Beck's cognitive theory in adolescent samples, and one has done so in a child sample (see Table 3.2). Although some of these studies have provided full support for the cognitive vulnerability hypothesis of Beck's theory (Hankin, Lakdawalla, Lee, Grace, & Roesch, 2004; Lewinsohn et al., 2001), others have provided only partial support (Abela & D'Alessandro, 2002; Abela & Skitch, 2007; Abela & Sullivan, 2003).

Response Styles Theory

The response styles theory posits that the way in which individuals respond to their symptoms of depression determines both the severity and duration of symptoms (Nolen-Hoeksema, 1991). Two such responses are proposed: rumination and distraction. Nolen-Hoeksema argues that individuals who engage in ruminative responses are likely to expe-

TABLE 3.2. Summary of Prospective Studies Testing Beck's Cognitive Theory

Study	Sample type	Follow-up	Depression measure	Results	Sample size
Abela & D'Alessandro (2002)	12th graders	0.25–2 months	MAACL	Dysfunctional attitudes × stress predicted immediate, but not enduring, depressive mood response to a negative event.	136
Abela & Skitch (2007)	6- to 14-year-olds with an affectively ill parent	12 months; multiwave	CDI	Dysfunctional attitudes interacted with fluctuations in hassles to predict fluctuations in depressive symptoms among youth with low, but not high, self-esteem.	140
Abela & Sullivan (2003)	7th graders	1.5 months	CDI	Dysfunctional attitudes × stress predicted increases in depressive symptoms among youth with high, but not low, social support and self-esteem.	184
Hankin, Lakdawalla, Lee, Grace, & Roesch (2004)	6th to 10th graders	4 months; multiwave	CDI	Dysfunctional sttitudes × stress predicted trajectories of depressive symptoms.	320
Lewinsohn, Joiner, & Rhode (2001)	9th to 12th graders	12 months	K-SADS	Dysfunctional attitudes × stress predicted onset of depressive disorder episodes.	1,507

Note. MAACL, Multiple Adjective Affect Checklist; CDI, Children's Depression Inventory; K-SADS, Kiddie Schedule for Affective Disorders.

rience increased severity and duration of symptoms, whereas those who engage in distracting responses are likely to experience relief. The response styles theory was originally proposed to explain the finding that prevalence rates of depression are higher among women than men. Nolen-Hoeksema proposed that this difference could be accounted for, at least in part, by the differential response styles of the sexes. More specifically, she hypothesized that women are more likely to ruminate in response to depressed mood whereas men are more likely to distract.

To our knowledge, seven prospective studies have examined the vulnerability hypothesis of the response styles theory in youth (see Table 3.3). Results from these studies have consistently been supportive of the hypothesis that rumination is associated with greater severity of depressive symptoms over time (Abela, Aydin, & Auerbach, 2007; Abela, Brozina, & Haigh, 2002; Abela, Parkinson, et al., in press; Broderick & Korteland, 2004; Driscoll & Kistner, 2007; Hankin, Lakdawalla, et al., 2004; Schwartz & Koenig, 1996). Support for the hypothesis that girls exhibit greater rumination than boys, however, is mixed, with the majority of studies using child and early adolescent samples failing to obtain the hypothesized sex difference (Abela, Aydin, et al., 2007; Abela et al., 2002; Abela, Vanderbilt, & Rochon, 2004; Broderick & Korteland, 2004; for an exception, see Ziegert & Kistner, 2002) and studies using middle to late adolescent samples obtaining the hypothesized sex difference (Abela, Parkinson, et al., in press; Schwartz & Koenig, 1996). To date, no studies have obtained support for the hypothesis that boys are more likely than girls to engage in distraction in response to depressed mood.

TABLE 3.3. Summary of Prospective Studies Testing the Response Styles Theory

Study	Sample type	Follow-up	Depression measure	Results	n
Abela, Aydin, & Auerbach (2007)	6- to 14-year-olds with an affectively ill parent	1.5 months	CDI	Rumination predicted increases in depressive symptoms. Distraction predicted decreases in depressive symptoms. Rumination to distraction ratio scores predicted increases in depressive symptoms above and beyond rumination and distraction. No sex difference in rumination or distraction.	140
Abela, Brozina, & Haigh (2002)	3rd and 7th graders	1.5 months	CDI	Rumination predicted increases in depressive symptoms. Distraction not associated with change in depressive symptoms. No sex difference in rumination or distraction.	314
Abela, Parkinson, Stolow, & Starrs (in press)	9th graders	1.5 months	CDI	Rumination predicted increases in depressive symptoms. Girls exhibited higher levels of rumination than boys.	319
Broderick & Korteland (2004)	4th to 6th graders	36 months	CDI	Rumination associated with higher levels of depressive symptoms at follow-up, but did not control for initial depressive symptoms. No sex difference in rumination.	79
Driscoll & Kistner (2006)	2nd to 7th graders	8 months	CDI	Rumination × stress predicted increases in depressive symptoms. Distraction × stress predicted increases in depressive symptoms (i.e., low distraction × high stress). 6th- and 7th-grade girls exhibited higher levels of rumination than 6th- and 7th-grade boys during the initial, but not follow-up, assessment. No sex difference in rumination among 2nd to 5th graders at either assessment. No sex difference in distraction.	202
Hankin, Lakdawalla, Lee, Grace, & Roesch (2004)	6th to 10th graders	4 months; multiwave	CDI	Rumination predicted trajectories of depressive symptoms.	320
Schwartz & Koenig (1996)	9th to 12th graders	1.5 months	CDI	Rumination predicted increases in depressive symptoms. Distraction not associated with change in depressive symptoms. Girls exhibited higher levels of rumination than boys. No sex difference in distraction.	397

Note. CDI, Children's Depression Inventory.

Personality Predispositions to Depression

Researchers from diverse theoretical orientations have proposed that certain personality traits serve as vulnerability factors to depression (Beck, 1983; Blatt & Zuroff, 1992). Although differences in conceptualizations exist, each theory proposes a personality predisposition focused on interpersonal issues and another focused on achievement issues. Psychodynamic theorists label these personality predispositions as *dependency* and *self-criticism* (Blatt & Zuroff, 1992), whereas cognitive theorists label them as *sociotropy* and *autonomy* (Beck, 1983). Individuals high in dependency/sociotropy are concerned with interpersonal issues; they need the approval of others to maintain a sense of well-being. Dependent/sociotropic individuals are hypothesized to be at risk for developing depression when they perceive disruptions in their relationships with others, interpersonal loss, and/or social rejection. Individuals high in self-criticism/autonomy, however, are concerned with achievement issues; they need to meet their own and/or others' standards to maintain a sense of well-being. Self-critical individuals are hypothesized to be at risk for developing depression when they perceive that they are not meeting such standards. The specific vulnerability hypothesis posits that individuals who possess personality predispositions are at risk for developing depression only following the occurrence of negative events congruent with their personality vulnerabilities. More specifically, it is hypothesized that dependent/sociotropic individuals are at risk for developing depression following negative interpersonal events, whereas self-critical/autonomous individuals are at risk for developing depression following negative achievement events.

Support for the vulnerability hypothesis of theories of personality predispositions to depression in youth has been mixed (see Table 3.4). With respect to self-criticism, five studies have found self-criticism to confer vulnerability to depression in youth (Abela, Sakellaropoulo, & Taxel, 2007; Abela & Taylor, 2003; Adams, Abela, Auerbach, & Skitch, 2007; Shahar & Priel, 2003; Shahar, Blatt, Zuroff, Kuperminc, & Leadbeater, 2004) and two have not (Little & Garber, 2000, 2004). With respect to dependency, four studies have found dependency to confer vulnerability to depression in youth (Adams et al., 2007; Little & Garber, 2000, 2004, 2005) and four have not (Abela, Sakellaropoulo, & Taxel, 2007; Abela & Taylor, 2003; Shahar & Priel, 2003; Shahar et al., 2004). Among the studies that have examined the specific vulnerability hypothesis, specificity (Abela, Sakellaropoulo, & Taxel, 2007; Abela & Taylor, 2003, seventh graders; Little & Garber, 2000, 2004), reverse specificity (Shahar & Priel, 2003), and nonspecificity (Abela & Taylor, 2003, third graders) have all been observed.

Empirical Status of Theories of Cognitive Vulnerability to Depression in Youth

There are several main points to emphasize based on our brief review of the literature. First, it is clear that the preponderance of evidence supports the hypothesis that cognitive vulnerability factors interact with negative events to predict increases in depressive symptoms in both children and adolescents—although the pattern of findings does not always conform exactly to what was originally proposed by the theories (e.g., reverse specificity for specific vulnerability hypothesis).

Second, the extant corpus of evidence supporting/contradicting theories of cognitive vulnerability to depression in child and adolescent samples parallels that found in adult samples (see Hankin & Abela, 2005, for a review and elaboration on this point). On bal-

TABLE 3.4. Summary of Prospective Studies Testing Theories of Personality Predispositions to Depression

Study	Sample type	Follow-up	Depression measure	Results	n
Abela, Sakellaropoulo, & Taxel (2007)	7th graders	1.5 months	CDI	Self-criticism interacted with negative achievement, but not interpersonal, events to predict increases in depressive symptoms.	79
				Dependency did not predict change in depressive symptoms.	
Abela & Taylor (2003)	3rd and 7th graders	2.5 months	CDI	Self-criticism interacted with negative achievement, but not interpersonal, events to predict increases in depressive symptoms in 7th-grade boys, but not girls, with low, but not high, self-esteem.	303
				Self-criticism interacted with both negative achievement and negative interpersonal events to predict increases in depressive symptoms in 3rd-graders with low, but not high, self-esteem.	
				Dependency did not predict change in depressive symptoms.	
Adams et al. (2007)	7- to 14-year-olds with an affectively ill parent	2 months; multiwave experience sampling	CDI	Self-criticism interacted with fluctuations in hassles to predict fluctuations in depressive symptoms.	56
				Dependency interacted with fluctuations in hassles to predict fluctuations in depressive symptoms.	
Hammen & Goodman-Brown (1990)	8- to 16-year-olds with either affectively ill, medically ill, or control parents	6 months	CDI	Children exhibited increases in depressive symptoms following the occurrence of negative events congruent with their personality predisposition (achievement or interpersonal).	64
				The authors did not test the specific vulnerability hypothesis separately in the achievement and interpersonal domains.	
Little & Garber (2000)	5th to 6th graders	3 months	CDI	Connectedness interacted with negative interpersonal, but not achievement, events to predict increases in depressive symptoms in boys.	486
				Connectedness predicted increases in depressive symptoms regardless of negative interpersonal or achievement events in girls.	
				Neediness predicted increases in depressive symptoms in both boys and girls regardless of negative interpersonal or achievement events	
				Neither self-criticism nor individualistic achievement orientation predicted change in depressive symptoms	

(continued)

TABLE 3.4. *(continued)*

Study	Sample type	Follow-up	Depression measure	Results	*n*
Little & Garber (2004)	8th graders	12 months	CDI	Neediness and connectedness interacted with negative peer, but not academic, events to predict increases in depressive symptoms in girls but not boys.	129
				Neither self-criticism nor individualistic achievement orientation predicted change in depressive symptoms.	
Little & Garber (2005)	6th graders with an affectively ill parent	12 months	CDI CDI-PR CDRS-R	Neediness and connectedness predicted increases in depressive symptoms through the mediating role of dependent interpersonal negative events, but not dependent noninterpersonal negative events or independent negative events.	185
Shahar et al. (2004)	6th to 7th graders	12 months	BDI	Self-criticism predicted increases in depressive symptoms in girls, but not boys, regardless of negative events.	460
				Dependency did not predict change in depressive symptoms.	
Shahar & Priel (2003)	9th graders	4 months	CES-DC	Self-criticism interacted with negative interpersonal, but not achievement, events to predict increases in depressive symptoms.	603
				Dependency predicted increases in depressive symptoms regardless of negative interpersonal or achievement events.	

Note. CDI, Children's Depression Inventory; CDI-PR, Child Depression Inventory; CDRS-R, Children's Depression Rating Scale—Revised; BDI, Beck Depression Inventory; CES-DC, Center for Epidemiologic Studies Depression Scale for Children.

ance, there exist proportionally as many studies with adults, as there do with children and adolescents that support the cognitive theories of depression.

Third, the majority of studies testing theories of cognitive vulnerability to depression in youth have done so within the framework of the hopelessness theory, focusing particularly on the theory's attributional vulnerability hypothesis. Far fewer studies have investigated the vulnerability hypothesis of other cognitive theories. This stands in stark contrast to tests of theories of cognitive vulnerability to depression in adults wherein there is a far greater balance in research examining the various theories. As a result, there is still comparatively less knowledge about cognitive vulnerability to depression in youth than in adults, and most of this knowledge is based on attributional style as a vulnerability factor.

Fourth, the various independent tests of cognitive diathesis–stress theories in child, adolescent, and adult samples yield what appears, at least on the surface, to be a picture of mixed support, based on the use of traditional significance testing criteria (e.g., $p <$ 0.05; Cohen 1994) as the foundation for determining whether a study supports or refutes cognitive theories. This "counting the significance stars" approach (Meehl, 1978), however, such as we have implicitly used in this chapter, may incorrectly lead one to conclude that there is evidence to refute cognitive theories (in regard to adults, as well as youth) when overall the evidence supports them. Such an approach may also drive one to search for moderators to account for the "equivocal" evidence base when such a search is not needed. In contrast to counting how many studies have been supportive based on simple tests of significance, quantitative reviews, such as meta-analyses, can aggregate across the many individual studies, with varying samples sizes, methods, and designs, to provide a more accurate picture of the state of the field. We are aware of one such quantitative review (Lakdawalla & Hankin, 2007), and it provides relatively strong support for the hypothesis that cognitive vulnerability factors interact with negative events to predict increases in depressive symptoms in both children and adolescents.

Finally, there are likely meaningful developmental patterns in how cognitive vulnerability factors transact with negative events over time to influence the development of depression, yet it is not entirely clear how various developmental factors (e.g., biological, cognitive, and emotional development, changes in parental and peer relationships, etc.) affect this process despite some theorizing on the issue (e.g., Abela & Sarin, 2002; Cole & Turner, 1993; Gibb & Coles, 2005; Hankin & Abela, 2005; Hankin & Abramson, 2001; Ingram, 2001). A necessary, and helpful, start toward understanding how development influences both cognitive vulnerability factors and their interaction with negative events is derived from the fact that, based on the research conducted to date, the effect size for the interaction between cognitive vulnerability factors and negative life events is in the small range for preadolescent children and in the medium range for adolescents (Lakdawalla & Hankin, 2007). This change in effect size following the transition into adolescence could be due to multiple causes, including the strengthening of cognitive vulnerability factors, increases in the frequency and/or objective intensity of negative events, negative changes in interpersonal relationships that previously served as protective factors (i.e., parent–child relationship), preexisting cognitive vulnerability factors interacting synergistically with normative changes in cognitive development (i.e., increases in self-consciousness and egocentrism), and/or the use of measures of cognitive vulnerability that are not appropriate for use with younger children. At this point, the reason for this change is not entirely clear.

In sum, there is still a need for research examining theories of cognitive vulnerability to depression in children and adolescents. In the sections that follow, we highlight several areas that should be priorities for research examining the cognitive theories in youth, including (1) new conceptual approaches towards understanding the relationships between various cognitive vulnerability factors, (2) developmental issues, and (3) methodological and statistical issues that may enhance tests of the cognitive theories.

CONCEPTUALIZING THE RELATIONSHIPS BETWEEN THE VARIOUS COGNITIVE VULNERABILITY FACTORS

Despite the etiology of depression being widely acknowledged as multifactorial in nature (e.g., Gotlib & Hammen, 2002; Hankin & Abela, 2005; Ingram & Price, 2001), relatively little research has considered possible relationships between the many risk, vulnerability, and protective factors proposed *across* the various cognitive theories of depression. It is unlikely that each cognitive vulnerability theory is presenting a distinct etiological pathway leading to the development of depression that is unaffected by the various contributory causes of depression proposed by alternative theories. Consequently, the richest examination of such theories will ultimately involve the integration of the various distinct risk, vulnerability, and protective factors proposed by empirically supported theories.

To date, three approaches to conceptualizing the relationships between various cognitive vulnerability factors have been proposed: (1) the multiplicative approach, (2) the additive approach, and (3) the weakest link approach.

The Multiplicative Approach

Most research to date that has attempted to take an integrative approach has conceptualized the relationships between the multiple vulnerability factors being examined (i.e., usually two) using a *multiplicative approach*. Such an approach posits that the vulnerability factors will interact synergistically to potentiate the stress–depression relationship such that the greatest increases in depressive symptoms following increases in stress will be observed in individuals possessing both vulnerability factors. For example, high levels of self-esteem buffer youth who possess cognitive vulnerability factors such as depressogenic inferential styles (Abela & Payne, 2003; Conley et al., 2001; Robinson et al., 1995; Southall & Roberts, 2002), dysfunctional attitudes (Abela & Skitch, 2007), and self-criticism (Abela & Taylor, 2003) against experiencing increases in depressive symptoms following negative events.

Although a multiplicative approach has proven useful in examining the integration of any given *two* models of vulnerability to depression, such an approach becomes more cumbersome, both theoretically and methodologically, when attempting to integrate a wider range of models. As the pool of vulnerability factors increases, the precision of the hypotheses becomes so exact that only those possessing the complete "depressogenic profile" are hypothesized to show increases in depressive symptoms following the occurrence of stressors.

The Additive Approach

A second approach to conceptualizing the relationships between multiple vulnerability factors is an *additive approach*. Such an approach assumes that an individual's degree of vulnerability to depression depends on the ultimate *balance* between his or her vulnerability, protective, and risk factors. Vulnerability factors exhibit a cumulative effect, with the presence of each additional vulnerability factor leading to a greater degree of vulnerability. Conversely, protective factors exhibit a cumulative effect, with the presence of each additional protective factor leading to a lesser degree of vulnerability. This approach assumes that the factors work independently of one another, as shown by the factor analytic evidence just reviewed. For example, the additive approach would predict that a person with a depressogenic attributional style, a high propensity to ruminate, and low self-esteem (three vulnerabilities) is more vulnerable to depression than a person with a depressogenic attributional style, a high propensity to ruminate, and average self-esteem (two vulnerabilities). Furthermore, because of the counterbalancing effects of protective factors, such an approach would predict that a person with a depressogenic attributional style, an average propensity to engage in rumination, and average self-esteem (one vulnerability) is as vulnerable to depression as an individual with a depressogenic attributional style, a high propensity to ruminate, and high self-esteem (two vulnerabilities + one protective factor).

Several studies examining the hopelessness theory of depression in adult samples have taken an additive approach to conceptualizing the relationships between depressogenic inferential styles about the self, consequences, and causes. In doing so, researchers have assumed that the more depressogenic inferential styles an individual possesses, the more negative his or her overall cognitive style. Results from such studies have generally been supportive of the hopelessness theory (Alloy, Abramson, Hogan, Whitehouse, Rose, et al., 2000; Alloy et al., 2006; Hankin, Abramson, Miller, & Haeffel, 2004). At the same time, no study, to our knowledge, has demonstrated that additive composite scores predict increases in depressive symptoms following negative events *above and beyond* the three individual vulnerability–stress interactions featured in the hopelessness theory. Demonstration of such a unique effect is necessary to show that the sum of an individual's scores on measures of inferential styles provides information about his or her degree of vulnerability to depression above and beyond what would be known by looking at each of his or her inferential styles separately. Studies examining the vulnerability hypothesis of the hopelessness theory in youth using an additive approach have yielded less supportive findings than those obtained in adult studies, with additive composite scores not being a significant moderator of the association between increases in depressive symptoms following the occurrence of negative events (Abela & Payne, 2003; Abela & Sarin, 2002).

Recent work examining the vulnerability hypothesis of the response styles theory in youth has also begun to take an additive approach to conceptualizing the relationships between the various response styles proposed in the theory. More specifically, measures assessing ruminative and distracting response styles typically ask participants to rate the frequency with which they utilize various behaviors or coping strategies in response to depressed mood. Research with youth has found ruminative responses to be either not associated (Abela, Aydin, et al., 2007; Abela et al., 2002, seventh graders; Abela, Vanderbilt, & Rochon, 2004, seventh graders; Ziegert & Kistner, 2002) or positively associated (e.g., Abela et al., 2002, third graders; Abela, Vanderbilt, & Rochon, 2004, third graders) with distracting responses on such measures, suggesting that many youth may not exhibit a consistent response style but, rather, may utilize multiple responses to depression whose opposing effects counterbalance each other. Abela, Aydin, et al. (2007) proposed that when examining the response styles theory, researchers should utilize composite scores that take into account both the likelihood that a given individual will engage in ruminative responses to depressed mood (a vulnerability factor) and the likelihood that he or she will engage in distractive responses (a protective factor). Using a sample of 140 children, between the ages of 6 and 14, of affectively ill parents, Abela, Aydin, et al. (2007) reported that rumination scores, distraction scores, and additive composite scores were all significant predictors of change in depressive symptoms over time. At the same time, additive composite scores predicted change in depressive symptoms over time above and beyond both rumination and distraction scores.

The Weakest Link Approach

A third approach to conceptualizing the relationships between multiple vulnerability factors is a *weakest link approach* (Abela & Sarin, 2002). This approach posits that when multiple vulnerability factors predict depression through a *similar mediating pathway* (e.g., negative cognitive style, dysfunctional attitudes, and self-criticism/dependency each increase the likelihood an individual will engage in negative thinking following negative events and thus develop depression), then an individual's most depressogenic vulnerability is the best marker of his or her true propensity for developing depression. Thus, when considering similar vulnerabilities, this approach predicts that an individual is as vulnerable to depression as his or her most depressogenic vulnerability makes him or her.

The weakest link approach (Abela & Sarin, 2002) was originally developed within the framework of the hopelessness theory of depression. Within the framework of this theory, the weakest link hypothesis posits that an individual is as cognitively vulnerable to hopelessness depression as his or her most depressogenic inferential style makes him or her. Abela and Sarin argue that their hypothesis follows from the hopelessness theory's logic that depressogenic inferences about negative events, irrespective of whether they are about the self, consequences, or causes, increase the likelihood of developing hopelessness (and consequently hopelessness depression). In an initial test of this hypothesis in a sample of seventh-grade students, Abela and Sarin reported that the participants' "weakest links" interacted with subsequently occurring negative events to predict increases in depressive symptoms. In contrast, none of the three individual depressogenic inferential styles on their own interacted with negative events to predict such increases. Finally, the interaction between weakest link scores and negative events exhibited a unique effect above and beyond each of the three individual diathesis–stress interactions featured in the hopelessness theory. Similar findings have been reported in subsequent studies utilizing child and early adolescent samples (Abela & McGirr, 2007; Abela, McGirr, & Skitch, 2007; Abela & Payne, 2003; Abela, Skitch, Adams, & Hankin, 2006).

Abela and Sarin (2002) have noted that the weakest link hypothesis may have particularly important implications for research examining the vulnerability hypothesis of the hopelessness theory in youth. More specifically, research examining the hopelessness theory in adult samples has not found depressogenic inferential styles about causes, consequences, and the self to be empirically distinguishable (Abela, 2002; Abela & Seligman, 2000; Hankin, Carter, Lakdawalla, Abela, & Adams, 2007; Metalsky & Joiner, 1992), whereas research examining the vulnerability hypothesis of the hopelessness theory in children has (Abela, 2001; Abela & Sarin, 2002). Furthermore, studies using child and early adolescent samples have reported that a large proportion (e.g., > 20%) of youth in their samples would be classified as extremely pessimistic (1 SD above sample mean score) on one inferential style but extremely optimistic on at least one other (1 SD below sample mean score; Abela & Payne, 2003; Abela & Sarin, 2002). Given that a significant proportion of children exhibit a range in their thinking styles, a weakest link approach may be particularly warranted in order to provide an adequate test of the diathesis–stress component of the hopelessness theory in children.

It is possible that a weakest link approach can prove beneficial in examining the relationships between cognitive vulnerability factors on a broader level. In a preliminary study examining this possibility, Abela and Scheffler (2007) had children (ages 7–15) complete measures assessing depressive symptoms, four cognitive vulnerability factors (e.g., rumination, self-criticism, low self-esteem, and negative cognitive style), and four interpersonal vulnerability factors (e.g., low social support, negative attachment cognitions, dependency, and excessive reassurance seeking). The children were subsequently given handheld personal computers that were programmed to signal them to complete measures assessing depressive symptoms and negative events once a week, at a randomly selected time, for 6 weeks. With respect to cognitive vulnerability factors, a depressogenic weakest link was associated with increases in depressive symptoms following negative events. In contrast, additive composite scores were not associated with such increases. Interestingly, with respect to interpersonal vulnerability factors, both depressogenic weakest link and additive composite scores were associated with increases in depressive symptoms following negative events. Furthermore, both scores exhibited unique effects. Such a pattern of findings suggests that the best approach to take when integrating multiple vulnerability factors may vary according to the type of vulnerability factor examined. In addition, such results indicate that it is possible that multiple types of integrative relationships are present for certain types of vulnerability factors.

DEVELOPMENTAL CONSIDERATIONS

The Emergence and Consolidation of Cognitive Vulnerability Factors

Cognitive vulnerability factors to depression, by definition and theory, are believed to reflect stable individual differences, certainly by adulthood. However, both the age at which such vulnerability factors emerge and the extent to which they represent trait-like risk processes in youth remain unknown. It is vital to answer these questions, because understanding when and how vulnerability factors emerge as stable risks to depression is (1) essential for a fuller theoretical understanding of the development of and continuity/ change in vulnerability factors to depression and (2) can potentially advance knowledge about when to implement optimal, developmentally sensitive interventions for depression. Understanding how cognitive vulnerability factors to depression emerge and stabilize may also shed light on the pattern of depression rates observed in children, early adolescents, and adolescents, especially if different *processes* lead to depression at different developmental stages. More specifically, it is possible that the processes described by theories of cognitive vulnerability come into play only in later developmental stages, shortly before depression rates begin to increase. Alternatively, cognitive vulnerability factors may exist and operate earlier, yet remain relatively latent until the increase in stressors that occurs during the transition from early to middle adolescence causes them to be more chronically active. Presently, both hypotheses (and, of course, the combination of these two possibilities) are viable. The discussion that follows conveys what is known theoretically and empirically about developmental influences related to cognitive vulnerability to depression.

Early Research: Theory and Evidence

There has been great debate in the literature as to the developmental stage at which cognitive vulnerability factors emerge (Garber, 2000; Gibb & Coles, 2005; Hammen & Rudolph, 2003; Hankin & Abela, 2005). Several researchers (e.g., Cole & Turner, 1993) have hypothesized that cognitive vulnerability factors do not begin to moderate the relationship between stress and depression until the transition from middle childhood to early adolescence; these theorists connect the emergence of such vulnerability factors to the influence of increasing levels of experience and cognitive processing capacities. For example, from the perspective of Beck's (1967, 1983) cognitive theory, researchers have hypothesized that schema do not become consolidated until adolescence, or even early adulthood, after repeated learning experiences have reinforced them (Hammen & Zuppan, 1984; Young, 1999). From the perspective of the hopelessness theory (Abramson et al., 1989), researchers have hypothesized that a depressogenic attributional style emerges as a vulnerability factor only during the transition from childhood to adolescence, when children acquire the ability to engage in abstract reasoning and formal operational thought (Nolen-Hoeksema et al., 1992; Turner & Cole, 1994).

In explaining the mechanisms underlying such a developmental hypothesis, researchers have drawn from a wide variety of findings in the cognitive development literature— particularly those pertaining to middle childhood. For example, during middle childhood, children develop a more stable and less concrete sense of self (Rholes, Blackwell,

Jordan, & Walters, 1980). Their self-views become increasingly differentiated (Abela & Véronneau-McArdle, 2002) as they shift their focus from concrete, behavioral characteristics in early childhood, to trait-like characteristics in middle childhood, to more abstract psychological constructs during adolescence (Harter, 1986, 1990). During this developmental period, children also become less here-and-now oriented (Shirk, 1988) and more likely to integrate past experience into working knowledge in a manner that informs interpretations and predictions (Rholes et al., 1980). Although very young children have a rudimentary understanding of causality (e.g., Oakes, 1994), it is not until middle childhood that their use of stable personality traits to explain behavior increases dramatically (Corrigan, 1995). Finally, some researchers have suggested that young children do not have the cognitive capacity to develop hopelessness because they have difficulty conceptualizing the sequencing of events as well as the length of time between events (Kaslow, Adamson, & Collins, 2000). Consequently, such researchers have hypothesized that it is only in the transition from middle childhood to early adolescence when a future time orientation and the ability to assess probabilities emerge that hopelessness can develop (Kaslow et al., 2000). Yet, contrary to this hypothesis, Kazdin, French, Unis, Esveldt-Dawson, and Sherick (1983) found that hopelessness in younger children was associated with depressive symptoms, and this finding appears to contradict the hypothesis that a future orientation is necessary for hopelessness to operate. This example of a discrepancy between theory and evidence illustrates that more work is needed to address this and other related hypotheses seeking to integrate work in basic cognitive development with the emergence and consolidation of cognitive risk factors.

In addition, the developmental hypothesis that cognitive vulnerability emerges during the transition from middle childhood to early adolescence is largely based on early research examining the attributional vulnerability hypothesis of the hopelessness theory in youth. Results from three studies, in particular, provide the most compelling support for this hypothesis. In a 1-year longitudinal study of 8-to 11-year-old children, Nolen-Hoeksema et al. (1986) found that attributional style interacted with negative events to predict increases in depression in two out of four follow-up assessments. In a 5-year longitudinal study of third-grade schoolchildren, Nolen-Hoeksema et al. (1992) found that the interaction between a depressogenic attributional style and negative events predicted increases in depressive symptoms in early adolescence (sixth to eighth grades) but not in middle childhood (third to fifth grades). Finally, in a cross-sectional study of fourth-, sixth-, and eighth-grade schoolchildren, Turner and Cole (1994) found that a depressogenic attributional style interacted with negative events to predict higher levels of depressive symptoms in eighth-grade children but not in fourth- or sixth-grade children.

When interpreting the results of these three studies, it is important to note two issues. First, support for this development hypothesis is based on the practice of null hypothesis significance testing (e.g., a significant attributional style × stress interaction found in two of four analyses; Nolen-Hoeksema et al., 1986), and as argued earlier, this practice may not be effective or contribute to a progressive and cumulative scientific knowledge base (cf. Meehl, 1978). Second, attributional style was assessed in these studies using the Children's Attributional Style Questionnaire (CASQ; Seligman et al., 1984), a measure that is limited by its poor internal reliability (alpha range = .4–.6; Hankin & Abramson, 2002; Thompson, Kaslow, Weiss, & Nolen-Hoeksema, 1998). Subsequent research examining a wider range of cognitive vulnerability factors (e.g., depressogenic inferential styles about the self and consequences, a ruminative response style, dysfunctional attitudes, and self-criticism) and using improved measures of cognitive vulnerability, including more developmentally sensitive measures of attributional style (Conley et al., 2001), has yielded a pattern of findings that is contradictory to this developmental hypothesis. For example, as seen in Table 3.1, several studies support the cognitive vulnerability–stress hypothesis in third-grade schoolchildren and children between the ages of 6 and 14 (prior to the age when this effect should be observed, if Cole's developmental hypothesis were correct), whereas other studies failed to support the cognitive vulnerability–stress hypothesis in adolescence (after the age when the developmental hypothesis states that this interaction should be found).

Although the pattern of results obtained in research examining theories of cognitive vulnerability to depression in youth suggests that such theories may be equally applicable to children, early adolescents, and adolescents, it is likely that much change occurs with respect to cognitive vulnerability factors throughout childhood and adolescence. More specifically, it is likely that the accumulation of experience and increased cognitive processing abilities leads to both (1) greater stabilization and consolidation of specific cognitive vulnerability factors and (2) greater interrelatedness among different cognitive vulnerability factors.

Stabilization of Cognitive Vulnerabilities into Trait-Like Risk Factors

We have adapted and applied conceptual and empirical approaches from research on basic personality development in order to advance knowledge on how and when cognitive vulnerability factors emerge and stabilize (e.g., Caspi, Roberts, & Shiner, 2005; Fraley & Roberts, 2005), including examination of rank-order stability and mean-level changes in vulnerabilities over time. Different processes can explain how vulnerability factors to depression maintain rank-order, or test–retest, stability over time. As seen in Figure 3.1, these include (1) a trait-like model (top panel), (2) a contextual/autoregressive model (middle panel), and (3) a combined trait/contextual model (bottom panel). Trait models predict that the empirical test–retest correlations will be invariant (ignoring statistical fluctuations in measurement precision) as the length of the test–retest interval increases, because a stable psychological variable (i.e., a trait vulnerability) organizes the manifestation of depression vulnerability over time. In contrast, contextual models predict that the magnitude of the test–retest correlations for depression vulnerability will decrease monotonically as the size of the interval increases (i.e., an autoregressive simplex pattern; Kenny & Zautra, 2001), because there is no enduring trait vulnerability in the model contributing to stability over time.

In order to test these different organizing conceptual models rigorously, it is essential that multiple waves of data be used. The two time point study (e.g., Burns & Seligman, 1989, in adults; Voelz, Walker, Petit, Joiner, & Wagner, 2003, in youth) typically used to examine the stability of cognitive vulnerability factors is inadequate for doing so, as it is the pattern of test–retest correlations over time, not the strength of any given test–retest correlation, that indicates whether the vulnerability factor is organized in a trait, contextual, or combined manner (Fraley & Roberts, 2005). With multiwave data, structural equation modeling (SEM) can be used to examine the pattern of test–retest correlations over multiple follow-ups to determine whether a trait-like or autoregressive contextual model best explains the rank-order stability of data over time. Moreover, longitudinal analyses can evaluate whether mean levels of stability change significantly over time for participants.

On the basis of this personality framework, Hankin, Fraley, and Abela (2005) recently provided the first examination of the *processes underlying the stability of cognitive vulnerability*, in any age group, using data from a 35-day diary study with late ado-

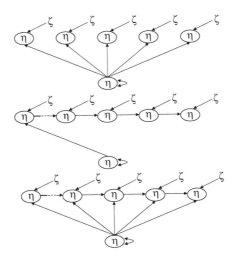

FIGURE 3.1. Processes explaining how vulnerability factors to depression maintain rank-order, or test–retest, stability over time: (1) a trait-like model (top panel), (2) a contextual/autoregressive model (middle panel), and (3) a combined trait/contextual model (bottom panel).

lescents ($n = 210$). Participants completed daily ratings of the inferences they made for the most negative event experienced every day for a month, based on the hopelessness theory. With respect to mean-level stability, cognitive vulnerability scores did not change on average over the 35 days. With respect to rank-order stability, cognitive vulnerability (negative cognitive style) was moderately stable over time (average test–retest $r = .38$, $SD = .08$, range = .56–.15). Using SEM, the pattern of this test–retest stability was best explained by a trait-like model. The contextual/autoregressive model provided a poor fit to the test–retest data, and the combined trait and contextual model fit as well as the trait model alone.

In addition, research with younger adolescents (grades 6–10; $n = 280$; Hankin, 2005) found that both depressogenic inferential styles and dysfunctional attitudes exhibited moderate mean-level stability over time, and this stability was explained best by a trait-like model. The adolescents' average levels of cognitive vulnerabilities (both depressogenic inferential styles and dysfunctional attitudes) were stable and did not significantly change over time. Moderate rank-order stability was observed: The mean correlation across the four waves of data for depressogenic inferential styles was .61 ($SD = .12$; range = .44–.74) and .29 ($SD = .15$; range = .08–.43) for dysfunctional attitudes. Using SEM, a trait model fit the cognitive vulnerability data over the four waves best for the sample as a whole, whereas an autoregressive model fit these data poorly. Finally, the youths' grades were examined to determine whether grade, as a rough index of developmental level, influenced the fit of these models, given the possibility that cognitive vulnerability factors may evolve into a more stable, trait-like vulnerability as a function of increasing grade. Consistent with this hypothesis, the trait model fit *both* the older (ninth and tenth graders) and younger (sixth to eighth graders) youth well. At the same time, the contextual model also fit *moderately* well in the younger, but not older, grades. These results provide initial evidence that cognitive vulnerability factors appear to have stabilized into a relatively stable, trait-like pattern, at least by sixth grade, although there is likely some continued change (i.e., greater stabilization) throughout early adolescence.

Developmental Changes in the Interrelation among Cognitive Vulnerability Factors

Another conceptual and analytic approach for understanding the emergence and stabilization of cognitive vulnerability factors is to examine the degree to which such factors interrelate with one another over time. Although various forms of cognitive vulnerability (e.g., depressogenic inferential styles, dysfunctional attitudes, rumination, self-criticism, etc.) may emerge and stabilize along a similar time course, their degree of interrelatedness may change as a function of development. For example, cognitive vulnerability factors may be relatively independent of one another early in development (Abela & Sarin, 2002). As development progresses, however, these vulnerability factors may become increasingly more interrelated and consolidated. Such a pattern of increasing interrelatedness would be consistent with research on temperament and personality development, in which many narrow, lower-order factors are observed early in development and the standard Big-5 factors are obtained in middle adolescence through adulthood (e.g., Caspi & Shiner, 2006; Rothbart & Bates, 2006).

The results from factor analytic studies suggest that cognitive vulnerability factors are more distinct in children than in adolescents and young adults (e.g., Adams, Abela, & Hankin, 2007; Hankin, Carter, et al., 2007; Joiner & Rudd, 1996). It appears that the various cognitive vulnerability factors may initially be relatively independent of one another but then become more interrelated during the transition from childhood to adolescence. As multiple vulnerability factors coalesce into a consolidated *set* of moderately intercorrelated cognitive vulnerabilities, youths' degree of vulnerability to depression may heighten. Interestingly, this contamination process may occur at about the same time that many researchers (Nolen-Hoeksema et al., 1992; Turner & Cole, 1994) have hypothesized that cognitive vulnerability to depression in youth first emerges.

Given that cognitive vulnerability factors become more interrelated with one another with age, different approaches to conceptualizing the relationship between multiple cognitive vulnerability factors may be optimal for youth at different developmental stages. When youths' cognitive vulnerability factors are still relatively distinct, knowledge of any particular factor may convey minimal information about the overall degree of vulnerability to depression. At this stage of development, a weakest link approach may be the most appropriate approach, as a child's most depressogenic vulnerability factor is likely be the best indicator of his or her propensity to engage in depressogenic thinking following stressors (Abela & Sarin, 2002). As cognitive vulnerability factors become increasingly interrelated over time, however, knowledge of a child's level with respect to any given vulnerability factor provides information about his or her levels with respect to other vulnerability factors. At this point in development, an additive approach may become more appropriate than a weakest link approach, as the presence of multiple vulnerabilities may become an equally, if not more, important indicator of both the likelihood that he or she engages in depressogenic thought processes and the degree of negativity and generality of such processes.

Developmental Changes in Levels of Cognitive Vulnerability

An alternative way in which theories of cognitive vulnerability could shed light on the pattern of depression rates across development is if levels of the vulnerability and risk factors featured in such theories vary as a function of development. In other words, although similar processes may be related to the onset of depression in both children and adolescents, differing levels of causal variables (e.g., vulnerability factors and stressors) may account for differing rates of depression in these age groups. For example, youth, especially girls, begin to encounter more stressors starting at about age 13 (Hankin & Abramson, 2001), so the increase in overall levels of stress, combined with cognitive vulnerabilities, could explain, at least in part, the rise in depression rates observed during adolescence. Few studies have prospectively followed groups of youth over time, monitoring changes in levels of cognitive vulnerability, so it is unclear whether cognitive vulnerability factors increase during the transition from childhood to early adolescence.

It is important to note that research examining changes in levels of cognitive vulnerability factors over time must consider not only the possibility that increases in levels of specific vulnerability factors contribute to increased depression rates, but also that a *lack of decreases* in levels of certain vulnerability factors may also contribute to increased depression rates. We have found a cross-sectional association between age and dependency (Abela & Taylor, 2003) and reassurance seeking (e.g., Abela, Hankin, et al., 2005; Abela, Zuroff, Ho, Adams, & Hankin, 2006), with younger children reporting higher levels of such variables than older children. It is possible that elevated levels of such cognitive-interpersonal variables are both normative and adaptive in younger children, and consequently elevated levels of such factors begin to confer vulnerability to depression only during the transition from childhood to early adolescence when they are expected to become developmentally atypical. As normative base rates of dependency and reassurance seeking decrease, the interpersonal behaviors associated with them may be viewed as developmentally atypical and, consequently, elicit more negative responses from others (e.g., parents, peers, etc.). Providing indirect support for such a hypothesis, although elevated levels of dependency have been found to serve as a vulnerability factor to depressive symptoms in both adolescents and adults (see Zuroff et al., 2004), dependency has not been consistently found to confer vulnerability to depression in children (e.g., Abela, Sakellaropoulo, & Taxel, 2007; Abela & Taylor, 2003). Furthermore, although elevated levels of dependency have been found to be associated with impairment in social functioning in adolescents and adults (e.g., see Zuroff et al., 2004), elevated levels of dependency have been found to be positively associated with social functioning in children (Fichman, Koestner, & Zuroff, 1996).

The Developmental Origins of Cognitive Vulnerability

The developmental origins of cognitive vulnerabilities to depression have received far less attention than the diathesis–stress hypothesis of cognitive theories. Although a detailed discussion of this topic is beyond the scope of this chapter, we provide a brief overview of theories and topics that have generated the most theoretical debate and empirical research (for more detailed discussions, see Blatt & Homann, 1992; Garber & Flynn, 1998; Haines, Metalsky, Cardamone, & Joiner, 1999; see also special issues of *Cognitive Therapy and Research*, edited by Ingram, 2001, 2003a, 2003b).

Some researchers have hypothesized that experiencing a sustained episode of depression may lead to the development of cognitive vulnerability factors that persist even after the depressive episode itself remits. According to this perspective, a youth's initial depressive episode may be caused by factors other than cognitive vulnerability (e.g., a youth's coping abilities are overwhelmed following the experiencing of a severe stressor). However, as a result of experiencing such an episode, he or she becomes cognitively vulnerable to the recurrence of depression. Nolen-Hoeksema and colleagues (1992) outline several pathways through which the experience of a depressive episode may lead to the development of cognitive vulnerability factors in youth. For example, depressed children often exhibit deficits in both academic performance and peer relations (Nolen-Hoeksema et al., 1986, 1992). Such deficits may lead these children to believe that they have low abilities and cannot control important outcomes in their lives. In addition, depression may facilitate access to negative memories and thoughts, owing to the priming effects of mood on cognition (Blaney, 1986; Bower, 1981). If such negative cognitions persist over an extended period of time, particularly when a child's self-view and styles of thinking are still developing, they may have a strong influence on the ultimate content of the belief systems and cognitive styles the child develops and maintains even after the episode of depression remits. Finally, research suggests that youth exhibiting depressive symptoms may generate stress (Hankin, Mermelstein, & Roesch, 2007; Rudolph & Hammen, 1999). Such youth may consequently act in ways that reinforce the development of cognitive vulnerability factors. For example, a depressed child deficient in social skills, who consequently encounters rejection, may learn to expect such rejection. Subsequent behavior, such as withdrawing from social activity, may lead to an increase in social rejection and consequently reinforce the negativity of developing cognitive styles (Ingram, 2001). Some studies have provided support for the hypothesized relationship between the experience of elevated levels of depressive symptoms and the subsequent development of cognitive vulnerability factors in youth (e.g., Gibb et al., 2006; Nolen-Hoeksema et al., 1986, 1992), whereas other longitudinal studies (e.g., Lewinsohn, Steinmetz, Larson, & Franklin, 1981; Rohde, Lewinsohn, & Seeley, 1994) have failed to obtain support for such a relationship.

Other researchers have hypothesized that certain types of negative life events may play a significant role in the development of cognitive vulnerability factors. More specifically, such researchers have proposed that (1) repeated exposure to negative events that occur in multiple and likely interacting domains (i.e., family conflict, divorce, poverty) and (2) chronic and/or major traumatic negative life events lead to the development of personal themes of derogation and unworthiness (Janoff-Bulman, 1992; Rose & Abramson, 1992). Such themes are posited, in turn, to become deeply ingrained in self-structures, consequently conferring vulnerability to subsequent episodes of depression. Consistent with this hypothesis, Garber and Flynn (1998) found that mothers' reports of the negative life events experienced by their children over the previous year predicted increases in depressogenic attributional style a year later. Further, in a prospective study of fifth and sixth graders, Rudolph, Kurlowsky, and Conley (2001) found that numerous facets of family disturbance (i.e., divorce, abandonment, parental death, or severe, recurrent, and inadequately resolved interparental conflict) and recent stress led to concurrent and subsequent deficits in perceptions of control and increased levels of helplessness.

Within the framework of the hopelessness theory of depression, Rose and Abramson (1992) have hypothesized that maltreatment, whether it is physical, emotional or sexual, is a specific type of negative life event that is particularly likely to lead to the development of depressogenic inferential styles. Following the experience of maltreatment events, youth attempt to understand the causes, meaning, and consequences of such events. In the case of an isolated experience of maltreatment, a child is not necessarily likely to make depressogenic inferences, as he or she is apt to interpret the event in a way that allows him or her to maintain hope ("My mom/dad was in a bad mood that day"). When such events become chronic (recurrent across time) and pervasive (recurrent across situations), however, a child is especially likely to begin to make depressogenic inferences about the maltreatment. The repetition of such depressogenic inferences following maltreatment consequently leads to the formation of a more general depressogenic inferential style. Rose and Abramson (1992) suggest that when a child is emotionally maltreated, he or she may be particularly likely to develop depressogenic inferential styles, as the child is directly provided with the negative cognitions from the abuser that ultimately form his or her depressogenic inferential styles. Several studies have supported this hypothesis in adults (e.g., Gibb et al., 2001; Feiring, Taska, & Lewis 1998; Hankin, 2005; Rose, Abramson, Hodulik, Halberstadt, & Leff, 1994) and children (Gibb et al., 2006; Gibb & Abela, in press; Gibb & Alloy, 2006). Moreover, a history of childhood emotional, but not physical or sexual, maltreatment predicted depressive symptoms and episodes in adults, and this relationship was mediated by depressogenic inferential styles (Gibb et al., 2001; Hankin, 2005).

Some researchers have connected the development of cognitive vulnerability factors to maladaptive parenting practices. Within a cognitive-developmental framework, parenting consists of patterns of behaviors that convey information to the child, which may be internalized and subsequently contribute to the formation of beliefs about the self and the world (Bruce et al., 2006). Parenting that is characterized by high levels of warmth, acceptance, autonomy promotion, consistency, and positive reinforcement is likely to contribute to the development of positive views of the self and the world, whereas parenting that is characterized by high levels of criticism, rejection, control, and inconsistency is likely to contribute to the formation of negative views of the self and the world (Ainsworth, 1979; Beck, 1967; Blatt & Homann, 1992; Bowlby, 1969, 1980; Young, 1999). Several cross-sectional studies have provided support for the hypothesized link between maladaptive parenting practices and cognitive vulnerability factors. For example, within the framework of Beck's cognitive theory of depression, high levels of parental criticism, indifference, and control and low levels of parental acceptance and care have been found to be associated with higher levels of dysfunctional attitudes and cognitive distortions in youth (Alloy et al., 2001; Bruce et al., 2006; Garber & Flynn, 2001; Liu, 2003). Similarly, high levels of parental rejection, inconsistency, and restrictiveness and low levels of parental care, acceptance, and autonomy promotion have been found to be associated with a negative self-concept in youth (Bruce et al., 2006; Jaenicke et al., 1987; Liu, 2003). Finally, within the framework of the hopelessness theory of depression, high levels of parental criticism and control and low levels of parental care and acceptance have been found to be associated with a depressogenic attributional style in youth (Alloy et al., 2001; Bruce et al., 2006; Garber & Flynn, 2001; Jaenicke et al., 1987). In one of the few prospective studies to examine the hypothesized association between maladaptive parenting practices and cognitive vulnerability factors, Koestner, Zuroff, and Powers (1991) reported that maternal reports of parenting behaviors reflecting high rejection and restrictiveness when children were age 5 prospectively predicted elevated levels of self-criticism when youth were age 12—even after controlling for mothers' reports of their children's early temperament.

Other researchers have proposed that children may acquire cognitive vulnerability factors through modeling processes. It is thought that children learn to make causal inferences by observing their parents' inferential styles concerning the parents' own behavior. For example, Seligman et al. (1984) found that children's inferential style about the causes of negative events correlated with those of their mothers, but not their fathers. Yet others have failed to replicate these findings concerning the relationship between child and parental inferential styles (e.g., Garber & Flynn, 2001; Kaslow, Rehm, Pollack, & Siegel, 1988).

A variation on the modeling hypothesis is that rather than modeling their parents' inferential styles, children model the inferential feedback communicated to them about events in their own lives. Most studies have tested this hypothesis by examining whether parents' typical inferential communications to their children are associated with their children's inferential styles. For example, Garber and Flynn (2001) reported that although mothers' and children's attributional styles were not significantly associated, mothers' and children's attributions regarding the same child-focused events were. Several other studies have obtained similarly strong support for this variant on the modeling hypothesis (e.g., Alloy et al., 2001; Dweck, Davidson, Nelson, & Enna, 1978; Fincham & Cain, 1986; Garber & Flynn, 2001; Turk & Bry, 1992; for an exception, see Gibb et al., 2006).

Finally, normative changes in cognitive development during the transition from middle childhood may play a role in either the development or the exacerbation of cognitive vulnerability factors. Elkind (1967, 1978) hypothesized that normative increases in self-consciousness and egocentrism during early adolescence contribute to increases in depression rates in this age group. Early adolescents maintain the false belief that others are as concerned about their thoughts and behaviors as they are. One consequence of adolescents' belief in an "imaginary audience" is heightened concern about what others think about them. Elkind has suggested that adolescents who are critical of themselves will anticipate a critical audience and, consequently, will be at risk for depression. Expanding on this hypothesis, Garber, Weiss, and Shanley (1993) posited that the relationship between adolescent cognitions (i.e., self-consciousness and egocentrism) and depressive symptoms is mediated by depressogenic cognitive styles. In line with this hypothesis, Garber and colleagues reported a significant relation between adolescent cognitions and both depressive symptoms and cognitive vulnerability factors (e.g., depressogenic attributional style, dysfunctional attitudes, negative automatic thoughts, helplessness expectancies, and negative outcome expectancies). Garber and colleagues hypothesized that self-consciousness and egocentrism may make adolescents particularly vulnerable to developing cognitive vulnerability factors, and consequently depression, if they experience stressors that impinge on their personal areas of specific concern (e.g., Hammen, 1990). That is, the interaction of normative adolescent cognitions with stressors that are common during this developmental stage (e.g., academic, social, and physical changes) may contribute to increased depression during adolescence through the mediating role of depressogenic cognitive styles.

METHODOLOGICAL CONSIDERATIONS IN THE STUDY OF COGNITIVE VULNERABILITY TO DEPRESSION IN YOUTH

In the past few years there has been a surge in literature examining possible methodological reasons for inconsistencies in the findings of studies examining theories of cognitive vulnerability to depression in children, adolescents, and adults (for reviews, see Gibb & Coles, 2005, and Hankin & Abela, 2005). We briefly discuss some of these reasons, as more methodologically rigorous research is likely to lead to greater consistency in findings in the examination of cognitive vulnerability to depression at all stages of development.

Nomothetic Versus Idiographic Approaches to Analysis

In recent years, researchers have increasingly turned to examining theories of cognitive vulnerability to depression in youth using multiwave longitudinal designs. The use of such designs has opened many new avenues of inquiry, including the examination of the vulnerability–stress hypothesis of cognitive theories using idiographic as opposed to nomothetic approaches to analysis, as well as the examination of processes that explain how cognitive vulnerabilities maintain rank-order, or test–retest, stability over time.

In the typical study examining the diathesis–stress component of cognitive theories of vulnerability to depression (e.g., Abela & Sullivan, 2003; Hankin et al., 2001; Lewinsohn et al., 2001), vulnerability factors and depressive symptoms are assessed at Time 1. Depressive symptoms and the occurrence of negative events are assessed at Time 2 (e.g., 6 months later). Analyses are then conducted to examine whether the vulnerability factors interact with the occurrence of negative events to predict increases in depressive symptoms. Implicit within such a design is the reliance on a nomothetic (between-subject) approach to operationalizing high levels of stress. Within a nomothetic framework, an individual is considered to be experiencing a high level of stress when his or her level of stress is high in comparison to the sample's average level of stress. Thus, when testing the diathesis–stress component of cognitive theories utilizing a nomothetic approach, researchers are examining whether individuals who possess high levels of vulnerability are more likely than other individuals to experience increases in depressive symptoms when their levels of stress are higher than the sample's average level of stress. Although such an approach sounds plausible on the surface, it is likely to lead to inaccurate predictions at the level of individual study participants.

Consider the following example. Scores on a measure assessing the frequency of negative events over a 6-week interval range from 0 to 60, with a mean of 30 and a standard deviation of 10. Participant 1 and participant 2 both have high levels of cognitive vulnerability at Time 1. Participant 1 is coming out of a stressful period of her life. Although her score on the life event measure at Time 2 is 40, this score is considerably lower than the score she would have received had she completed the life events measure at Time 1. In fact, this score is the lowest she would have obtained over the past 12 months. Participant 2, however, has experienced several negative events in the past 6 weeks, causing him to receive a score of 25 on the life events measure. This score is considerably higher than the score he would have received had he completed the life events measure at Time 1. In fact, this score is the highest he would have obtained over the past 12 months.

Cognitive theories of vulnerability to depression would predict that participant 1 is not likely to exhibit increases in depressive symptoms during the course of the study, as the frequency of negative events in her life in the past 6 weeks has been low in comparison to the frequency of negative events she experienced in the 42 weeks prior to participating in the study. In contrast, cognitive theories of vulnerability to depression would predict that participant 2 is likely to exhibit increases in depressive symptoms during the course of the study, given that the frequency of negative events in his life in the past 6 weeks is high in comparison to the frequency with which he experienced negative events in the 42 weeks prior to participating in the study.

A nomothetic approach to operationalizing high levels of stress, however, would predict the exact opposite. More specifically, such an approach would predict that participant 1 is likely to show increases in depressive symptoms between Time 1 and Time 2 because her level of stress is higher than the sample's average level of stress. In contrast, such an approach would predict that participant 2 is not likely to experience increases in depressive symptoms between Time 1 and Time 2 as his level of stress is lower than that of the sample's average level of stress. Thus, when utilizing a nomothetic approach, important contextual information is likely to be lost, leading to inaccurate predictions at the level of individual participants.

Several researchers have recently proposed that the use of an idiographic (within-subject), as opposed to a nomothetic, approach to operationalizing high levels of stress is likely to lead to a more powerful examination of the diathesis–stress component of cognitive theories of vulnerability to depression (Abela, Aydin, & Auerbach, 2006; Abela & Skitch, 2007; Abela, Skitch, Adams, & Hankin, 2006; Abela, Webb, Ho, Wagner, & Adams, 2006; Abela, Zuroff, Ho, Adams, & Hankin, 2006). From an idiographic perspective, an individual is considered to be experiencing a high level of stress when he or she is experiencing a level of stress that is higher than his or her own average level of stress. In considering our previous example, an idiographic approach would predict that participant 1 is not likely to show increases in depressive symptoms between Time 1 and Time 2, because the frequency of negative events she experienced in the past 6 weeks is lower than the preceding 42 weeks, whereas participant 2 is likely to show increases in depressive symptoms, as the frequency of negative events he experienced in the past 6 weeks is higher than in the preceding 42 weeks. Thus, an idiographic approach retains contextual information that is likely to lead to more accurate predictions at the level of individual participants.

The most powerful examination of cognitive vulnerability–stress theories requires the use of a multiwave longitudinal design in which stress and depression are assessed at multiple time points. The use of such a design allows researchers to examine the relationship between fluctuations in stress and fluctuations in depressive symptoms over time in individuals possessing varying levels of vulnerability. As can be seen in the upper panel of Figure 3.2, for an individual who possesses high vulnerability, cognitive theories would predict that stress and depressive symptoms should covary to a significant degree over time, with such individuals reporting higher levels of the depressive symptoms when they are experiencing high stress than when experiencing low stress. In contrast, as can be seen in the middle panel of Figure 3.2, for an individual who possesses low levels of vulnerability, cognitive theories would predict that although levels of stress are likely to fluctuate over time, levels of depressive symptoms should stay relatively low and stable. Thus, as illustrated in the bottom panel of Figure 3.2, when an idiographic approach is taken, vulnerability theories posit that stress and depressive symptoms will covary to a greater degree in individuals who possess high vulnerability than in individuals who possess low vulnerability. To date, studies have obtained consistent support for the diathesis–stress component of such theories in both children (Abela & McGirr, 2007; Abela, McGirr, et al., 2007; Abela & Skitch, 2007; Abela, Skitch, Adams, & Hankin, 2006; Abela, Zuroff, Ho, Adams, & Hankin, 2006) and adults (Abela, Aydin, et al., 2006; Abela, Webb, Ho, Wagner, & Adams, 2006) when using an idiographic, as opposed to a nomothetic, approach.

Research has only recently begun to examine the diathesis–stress component of cognitive vulnerability theories of depression using an idiographic approach to analysis. At the same time, nomothetic and idiographic approaches may be integrated. For example, Abela, Foa, and McWhinnie (2007) simultaneously examined the between- versus within-subject effects of both stress and hopelessness on depressive symptoms from a multiwave (nine waves of data collection) longitudinal study of 140 children (ages 6–14) of affectively ill parents over a 1-year interval. Results suggest that as individuals' average stress levels increase, the strength of the association between fluctuations in negative cognitions and fluctuations in depressive symptoms becomes stronger. This suggests a possible explanation for changes in the epidemiology of depression in adolescence. Mean levels of stress increase during the transitions from early to middle adolescence and from middle to late adolescence (Hankin & Abramson, 2001), so the association between neg-

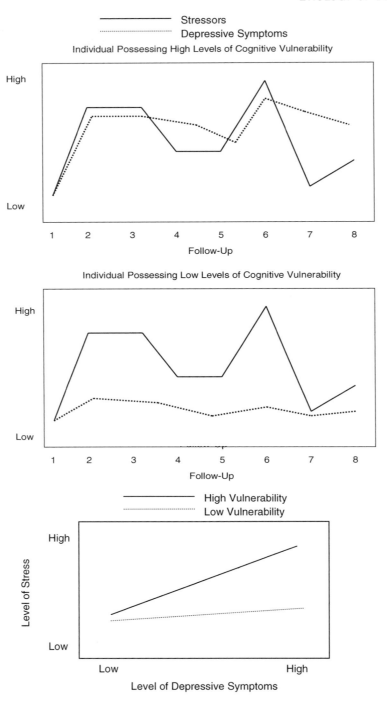

FIGURE 3.2. Hypothesized relationship between stress and depressive symptoms for individuals possessing high (top panel) and low (middle panel) levels of cognitive vulnerability. Hypothesized slope of the relationship between levels of stress and depressive symptoms for individuals possessing high and low levels of cognitive vulnerability (bottom panel).

ative cognitions and depressive outcomes may be potentiated, particularly for girls, who begin to experience higher average stress levels during the transition from early to middle adolescence than boys.

Priming of Cognitive Vulnerability Factors

Several cognitive theorists have argued that cognitive vulnerability factors are typically latent and must be activated by negative mood states and/or the occurrence of stressors in order to be assessed accurately (Beck, 1967; Persons & Miranda, 1992; Riskind & Rholes, 1984; Teasdale, 1983). Therefore, studies that do not activate or prime cognitive vulnerability factors before assessing them are likely to inadequately assess the true propensity of participants' depressogenic thinking, and as a result, may be less likely to yield results that are supportive of cognitive theories. Using various information-processing tasks and paradigms drawn from basic cognitive psychological research , a large body of research, using adult samples, has accumulated in recent years, providing support for this priming hypothesis (e.g., Gotlib et al., 2004; Gotlib, Krasnoperova, Yue, & Joormann, 2004; Joormann & Gotlib, 2007; Johnson, Joormann, & Gotlib, 2007; for review see Scher, Ingram, & Segal, 2005). In addition, prospective studies using adult samples have demonstrated that primed assessments of cognitive vulnerability factors, such as depressogenic inferential styles, predict increases in depressive symptoms following negative events above and beyond those predicted by unprimed assessments of such factors (Abela & Brozina, 2004; Abela, Brozina, & Seligman, 2004). Far fewer studies have examined the priming hypothesis in youth. Of those conducted, however, results have been consistently supportive (e.g., Joormann, Talbot, & Gotlib, 2007; Taylor & Ingram, 1999; Timbremont & Braet, 2004a, 2004b).

To our knowledge, no prospective studies examining theories of cognitive vulnerability to depression in youth have utilized priming procedures when assessing cognitive vulnerability factors. Thus, we cannot be certain that youths' true propensities for depressogenic thinking in such studies were accurately assessed. Future research is likely to benefit from incorporating priming techniques into its assessment procedures in order to increase the accuracy of its assessments of cognitive vulnerability factors.

Specific Vulnerability

Several theories of vulnerability to depression have proposed that certain individuals possess cognitive vulnerability only in specific content domains. Consequently, such individuals are vulnerable to developing depression only following the occurrence of domain-congruent stressors. For example, as outlined earlier, the specific vulnerability hypotheses of both Beck's (1983) and Blatt and Zuroff's (1992) theories of personality predispositions to depression posit that individuals possessing high levels of self-criticism/autonomy are vulnerable to depression following negative achievement, but not interpersonal, events, whereas individuals possessing high levels of dependency/sociotropy are vulnerable to depression following negative interpersonal, but not achievement, events. Similarly, the hopelessness theory posits that certain individuals possess depressogenic inferential styles in only the achievement or interpersonal domains and thus are vulnerable only to domain-congruent stressors (Abramson et al., 1995).

Research with adult samples has generally been supportive of the specific vulnerability hypotheses of both theories of personality predispositions to depression (for reviews, see Clark & Beck, 1999, and Zuroff et al., 2004) and the hopelessness theory (Abela,

2002; Metalsky, Halberstadt, & Abramson, 1987; for exception see Abela & Seligman, 2000). Research with child and adolescent populations, however, has yielded more mixed results, with some studies reporting specificity (Abela & Sakellaropoulo, & Taxel, 2007; Abela & Taylor, 2003; Hammen & Goodman-Brown, 1990; Little & Garber, 2002, 2004), other studies reporting nonspecificity (Abela & Taylor, 2003, third graders), and others reporting reverse specificity (Shahar & Priel, 2003).

Although not enough research has yet accumulated to allow us to determine the mechanisms underlying such discrepant patterns of support, we outline possible explanations that may prove beneficial for future exploration. One possible explanation is that young children's self-concepts may not yet be differentiated enough for them to exhibit specific vulnerability (Abela & Taylor, 2003). In other words, in young children, interpersonal and achievement events may impinge on the same or similar self-aspects. As the complexity of children's self-concepts increases during middle childhood (e.g., Abela & Véronneau-McArdle, 2002), youth may increasingly perceive different domains of their lives (e.g., interpersonal and achievement events) as relevant to different self-aspects and consequently begin to exhibit specific vulnerability. Consistent with this explanation, research has demonstrated that whereas high levels of self-criticism predicts increases in depressive symptoms following both negative achievement and negative interpersonal events in third-grade schoolchildren, high levels of self-criticism predict increases in depressive symptoms following negative achievement, but not interpersonal, events in seventh-grade schoolchildren (Abela, Sakellaropoulo, & Taxel, 2007; Abela & Taylor, 2003).

A second possible explanation is that dependency/sociotropy and self-criticism/autonomy are multidimensional constructs (Little & Garber, 2002), with some dimensions being maladaptive and others being adaptive. Among the currently used measures of these constructs, different measures may tap into different dimensions (e.g., adaptive versus maladaptive). This could account for, in part, the differences between studies obtaining greater support for theories of personality predispositions in youth in the achievement (Abela, Sakellaropoulo, & Taxel, 2007; Abela & Taylor, 2003; Shahar & Priel, 2003) versus the interpersonal domain (Little & Garber, 2002, 2004, 2005). Studies supporting theories of personality predispositions in the achievement, but not interpersonal, domain may have used measures tapping into the maladaptive components of self-criticism/autonomy, but the adaptive components of dependency/sociotropy, and vice versa for the interpersonal domain. It is important to note that different dimensions of these constructs may be adaptive or maladaptive at different developmental stages.

Finally, younger children may not perceive the world as divided into the same domains as do adults. This could mean that the specific vulnerability hypotheses derived from research with adult populations would not extend downward to youth. In line with this possibility, whereas research with adult samples has typically found the Dysfunctional Attitudes Scale to break down into belief clusters (e.g., factors) centering on themes of sociotropy and autonomy (Cane, Olinger, Gotlib, & Kuiper, 1986; Oliver & Baumgart, 1985; Rude & Burnham, 1993), research with youth has found the Children's Dysfunctional Attitudes Scale to break down into belief clusters centering on themes of self-critical perfectionism and personal standards perfectionism (McWhinnie, Abela, & Knauper, in press). Interestingly, items loading onto both factors contain both interpersonal and achievement themes. Similarly, in a study examining the factor structure of the Hassles Scale for Children in a sample of third- through sixth-grade schoolchildren, Abela, Brozina, and McWhinnie (2004) reported that hassles broke down into home-related hassles and school-related hassles, rather than achievement and interpersonal hassles. Thus, it is possible that both personality predispositions to depression themselves and the negative events they interact with break down into different content domains in youth than in adults. Consequently, a more developmentally sensitive approach to examining specific vulnerability may be needed.

It is important to note that such constructs may also break down differently as a function of both developmental stage (e.g., childhood, early and late adolescence) and sex (e.g., see Abela & Taylor, 2003; Little & Garber, 2000; Shahar & Priel, 2003). In their elaborated cognitive vulnerability–transactional stress model of depression, Hankin and Abramson (2001) posit that there may be age- and development-related changes in the motivational strivings in individuals' primary domain of cognitive vulnerability. For example, preadolescent children's vulnerabilities may center on themes of family cohesion or academic success, whereas adolescent girls may focus on themes of physical appearance/body image, and middle age adults may think more about potential declines in physical health.

FUTURE DIRECTIONS

As the discussion in this chapter has illustrated, there is now fairly convincing evidence demonstrating that various cognitive vulnerability factors, interact with negative events to predict increases in depressive symptoms in both children and adolescents. Although more research is needed in order to understand the parameters of this cognitive vulnerability–stress process in explaining the onset, maintenance, remission, and recurrence of depression in youth, it seems safe to conclude that cognitive factors, particularly in interaction with negative events, play an important etiological role in the development of youth depression. In this final section, we focus on potentially important future directions for research aimed at advancing knowledge about the role of cognition in the ontogeny of depression in youth.

First, there is an urgent need for enhanced research investigating the developmental aspects of cognitive theories of vulnerability to depression. Such research may examine many issues. For example, as outlined earlier, research is needed examining both the emergence and consolidation of cognitive vulnerability factors. Prospective research is also needed examining the developmental processes that contribute to the formation of cognitive vulnerability factors. There must also be greater attention given to understanding whether distinct cognitive models are needed to understand the development of depression at different ages or whether a general cognitive theory, with slight modifications that take into account normative developmental changes, is applicable across the lifespan. Some have suggested fairly distinct models of depression for children versus adolescents and adults (e.g., Cole & Turner's [1993] mediation-moderation model). At the same time, some of the evidence reviewed in this chapter implies that potentially similar cognitive factors and processes are relevant for predicting depressive symptoms in children, adolescents, and adults. We believe that recent theoretical/conceptual, methodological, and statistical advances in the field, as described in this chapter, can better enable future research to evaluate this and related issues and to ascertain whether distinct cognitive models are needed to understand depression at different ages or whether a universal cognitive theory can successfully be applied to understanding the etiology of depression across development.

Second, there is a need to integrate cognitive vulnerability factors with other theoretically interesting and empirically supported vulnerability factors, especially neural, genetic, social/interpersonal, and emotional influences. Some exciting theoretical work integrating these previously disparate etiological factors has begun (e.g., Abramson et al., 2002; Davidson, 2004; Gotlib, Joormann, Minor, & Cooney, 2006; Hankin & Abramson, 2001; Nelson, Leibenluft, McClure, & Pine, 2005), and some intriguing empirical research has recently been initiated. For example, a recent neuroimaging study combining information-processing tasks and affective stimuli found that depressed adults revealed reduced activity in the frontotemporal and limbic areas in response to happy words, as compared with controls, whereas for sad words they showed greater activation, as compared with controls in the inferior parietal region but less activity in superior temporal gyrus and cerebellum (Canli et al., 2004). There may be developmental differences in the extent to which various neural areas are engaged in the processing of affective stimuli, socially relevant events, and thus how these neural circuits may instantiate some cognitive vulnerability processes (e.g., memory or attention biases). Consistent with this possibility, adolescents have been found to exhibit greater neural activity in the anterior cingulate for remembered angry faces and greater activity in the right temporal pole when viewing remembered fearful faces, as compared with adults (Nelson et al., 2003; see also Pine et al., 2001). Other research has connected emotionality and temperament with cognitive vulnerabilities. In a 4-year longitudinal study, 3-year-old children's low levels of positive emotionality predicted various measures of cognitive vulnerability—specifically, negative attributional style and depressogenic schema—when they were at age 7 (Hayden, Klein, Durbin, & Olino, 2006). This finding supports Hankin and Abramson's (2001) model, in which it was hypothesized that temperament, especially negative and positive emotionality, distally predicts depression, in part, through stress generation processes (Hammen, 1991) and the development of cognitive vulnerability factors. Consistent with this hypothesis, results from a four-wave prospective study showed that adolescents with low positive emotionality and those with high negative emotionality experienced greater levels of depressive symptoms and encountered more negative events over time (Hankin, 2006). Moreover, the interaction of cognitive vulnerability factors with these negative events partially accounted for the association between negative emotionality and later depression (Hankin, 2006). Cognitive and genetic influences on depression can be integrated as well. Of particular interest, a recent behavioral genetic study reported evidence that a negative attributional style is also moderately heritable (Lau, Rijsdijk, & Eley, 2006), as predicted by Hankin and Abramson (2001). Other research has used molecular genetic techniques to study functional genetic polymorphisms (e.g., the serotonin transporter, 5-HTT) and found that particular alleles (e.g., one or two copies of the short allele form of 5-HTT), interacting with negative events, predict depression (e.g., Caspi et al., 2003; Eley et al., 2004; see Moffitt, 2005, for a review). These exciting results raise the hypothesis that cognitive vulnerability factors may operate as an endophenotype (an intermediate trait; Gottesman & Gould, 2003) between latent genetic risk for depression and the behavioral phenotype of depressive disorder. Longitudinal research aimed at examining genetic risks in combination with cognitive vulnerability factors and negative events could test this hypothesis, as well as the potential for a genetic–cognitive integrated account of the development of depression. It would also be informative and exciting to conduct neuroimaging studies with youth who are genotyped while they are completing affective and information processing tasks aimed at assessing cognitive vulnerability factors (see Pezawas et al., 2005, for an example). Such research could begin to elucidate the interplay of genetic, neural, affective, and cognitive risks in the ontogeny of depression in children and adolescents. In sum, we look forward to the new advances in knowledge based on the potential for transdisciplinary research that seeks to coherently integrate cognitive vulnerability factors with other depression risk and vulnerability factors.

Third, cognitive vulnerability theories should continue to be applied in the quest to understand the "big facts" of depression, such as the dramatic rise in rates of depression starting in middle adolescence, the emergence of the sex difference in depression starting in early adolescence, and the strong continuity and recurrence of depression. For example, Hankin and Abramson's (2001) elaborated cognitive vulnerability–transactional stress theory of depression contains particular hypotheses, based in part on cognitive factors and processes, that can be tested to better understand the emergence of the sex difference and the overall rise in depression. In addition, other researchers have begun to examine how cognitive factors can help explain the course of depression: Negative life events have been found to predict first onsets of depression, whereas cognitive vulnerability factors, such as dysfunctional attitudes, are more strongly associated with recurrence of depression in adolescents (Lewinsohn, Allen, Seeley, & Gotlib, 1999).

Fourth, the greater part of research that has been conducted to date with youth examining cognitive theories of depression has assumed that negative events are independent of preexisting diatheses as well as independent of baseline depression levels. The diathesis–stress interaction has been overwhelmingly interpreted as a linear interaction: Negative events interact with the diathesis and the disorder follows. This underlying assumption of independence between the diathesis and environmental stressors has, for the most part, remained unquestioned, with researchers implicitly assuming that there is a random distribution of negative events across the population that determines who will develop depression and who will remain symptom free. Equally, baseline levels of depression have been consistently viewed as confounds of tests of the etiological chain and have therefore been tightly controlled for in selecting populations for study. Recent research, however, initially with adults (Hammen, 1991) and more recently with youth (Little & Garber, 2005; Rudolph et al., 2000; Shih, Abela, & Starrs, 2007), using semistructured clinical interviews aimed at differentiating between dependent and independent negative events, suggests that these assumptions may be incorrect and that stressful events are far from independent of these elements at least for some subsets of individuals. For example, using a sample of sixth-grade children of affectively ill parents, Little and Garber (2005) reported that neediness and connectedness predicted increases in depressive symptoms over a 1-year follow-up interval through the mediating role of dependent interpersonal negative events, but not dependent noninterpersonal negative events or independent negative events. Similarly, using a sample of 6- to 14-year-olds of affectively ill parents, Shih and colleagues reported that a depressogenic attributional style, self-criticism, and rumination all prospectively predicted the occurrence of dependent, but not independent, negative events over a 1-year follow-up interval even after controlling for initial levels of both parent and child depressive symptoms. Such findings suggest that youth who possess cognitive vulnerability factors may be in a double bind. In other words, not only do they possess cognitive factors that make them more likely than other youth to develop depressive symptoms following the occurrence of stressors, but they also play a role in creating the stressors that interact with their vulnerabilities. Future research is likely to benefit from examining cognitive diathesis–stress theories from a transactional perspective (see, e.g., Hankin & Abramson, 2001) in order to better understand both the cognitive and interpersonal processes underlying the onset of depression in youth. Such research is also likely to benefit from examining the impact of age and sex on such processes, given that preliminary research in this area has uncovered both age and sex differences (Rudolph et al., 2000; Rudolph & Hammen, 1999; Shih et al., 2007).

Finally, the comorbidity of depression with other emotional and behavioral problems and disorders is a well-known fact of psychopathology (e.g., Angold, Costello, &

Erkanli, 1999). Consequently, cognitive vulnerability factors need to be examined as depression-specific or disorder-general factors. Surprisingly little research has examined whether cognitive vulnerability factors, such as those discussed in this chapter, either alone or in interaction with negative events, specifically predict the development of depressive symptoms. Providing preliminary support for the specificity of such factors, Hankin and Abramson (2002) found that depressogenic inferential styles predicted depressive symptoms, but not externalizing problems, in a sample of adolescents. Similarly, in a four-wave longitudinal study of adolescents, Hankin, Lakdawalla, et al. (2004) found that both depressogenic inferential styles and dysfunctional attitudes interacted with negative events to predict trajectories of depressive symptoms more strongly than anxiety symptoms but not externalizing problems. Several other past studies have also found that the cognitive vulnerability factors discussed in this chapter are more specifically associated with depression than with other comorbid problems (e.g., Gladstone, Kaslow, Seeley, & Lewinsohn, 1997; Lewinsohn, Zinbarg, Seeley, Lewinsohn, & Sack, 1997; Robinson et al., 1995; Quiggle, Garber, Panak, & Dodge, 1992; Weiss, Susser, & Catron, 1998). Moreover, evidence has accumulated suggesting a sequential unfolding of comorbid patterns with depression such that anxiety typically precedes depression and earlier externalizing behaviors tend to predict later depressive symptoms (see Hankin & Abela, 2005, for a review). How do cognitive factors help to explain this typical developmental sequence of comorbidity between depression and other internalizing and externalizing problems? For example, the cognitive content specificity hypothesis suggests that depression is associated with negative cognitions involving loss and past failures, whereas anxiety is associated with cognitions involving harm and threat, and anger is associated with thoughts of unfairness. Do children with anxiety problems and thoughts centered on harm and threat become depressed adolescents with negative cognitions concerning loss and failure (cf. the helplessness–hopelessness model; Alloy, Kelly, Mineka, & Clements, 1990)? Solid theory and evidence seeking to understand the developmental unfolding of comorbidity patterns over time from a cognitive perspective are lacking, but they hold promise for enhancing etiological models and potentially identifying at-risk youth who may benefit from early prevention efforts.

In conclusion, the surge of interest in recent years in examining cognitive models of vulnerability to depression in children and adolescents has led to the accumulation of a substantial body of literature supporting the applicability of such theories to youth. At the same time, research has only just begun to examine many questions crucial to understanding the impact of development on the cognitive theories. For example, there remains much to be discovered about the processes through which cognitive vulnerability factors develop, how the latent structure and organization of cognitive vulnerability factors change as a function of development, and how cognitive diathesis–stress theories can provide insight into changes in the epidemiology of depression over the course of development—particularly with respect to the transition from early to late adolescence. The questions raised in this chapter and the theoretical and methodological innovations discussed are intended to serve as guides for theorists and researchers interested in expanding this important area of research. As literature examining these and other related questions accumulates, a stronger developmental psychopathology perspective on the etiology, maintenance, and recurrence of depression will emerge. Such an increased understanding from a developmental perspective will ultimately contribute to the most important goal of our field—the development of empirically supported treatment approaches for use with children and adolescents suffering from depression, as well as the creation of effective depression prevention programs for those at risk.

REFERENCES

Abela, J. R. Z. (2001). The hopelessness theory of depression: A test of the diathesis–stress and causal mediation components in third and seventh grade children. *Journal of Abnormal Child Psychology, 29,* 241–254.

Abela, J. R. Z. (2002). Depressive mood reactions to failure in the achievement domain: A test of the integration of the hopelessness and self-esteem theories of depression. *Cognitive Therapy and Research, 26,* 531–552.

Abela, J. R. Z., Aydin, C., & Auerbach, R. P. (2006). Operationalizing the "vulnerability" and "stress" components of the hopelessness theory of depression: A multi-wave longitudinal study. *Behaviour Research and Therapy, 44,* 1565–1583.

Abela, J. R. Z., Aydin, C., & Auerbach, R. P. (2007). Responses to depression in children: Reconceptualizing the relation among response styles. *Journal of Abnormal Child Psychology, 35,* 913–927.

Abela, J. R. Z., & Brozina, K. (2004). The use of negative events to prime cognitive vulnerabilities to depression. *Cognitive Therapy and Research, 28,* 209–227.

Abela, J. R. Z., Brozina, K., & Haigh, E. P. (2002). An examination of the response styles theory of depression in third and seventh grade children: A short-term longitudinal study. *Journal of Abnormal Child Psychology, 30,* 513–525.

Abela, J. R. Z., Brozina, K., & McWhinnie, C. M. (2004). *The assessment of domain specific hassles in children and adolescents.* Paper presented at the World Congress of Behavioural and Cognitive Therapies, Kobe, Japan.

Abela, J. R. Z., Brozina, K., & Seligman, M. E. P. (2004). A test of the integration of the activation hypothesis and the diathesis–stress component of the hopelessness theory of depression. *British Journal of Clinical Psychology, 43,* 111–128.

Abela, J. R. Z., & D'Alessandro, D. U. (2002). Beck's cognitive theory of depression: A test of the diathesis–stress and causal mediation components. *British Journal of Clinical Psychology, 41,* 111–128.

Abela, J. R. Z., Foa, C., & McWhinnie, C. M. (2007). *The between- versus within-subject effects of negative life events and hopelessness on depressive symptoms in children of affectively ill parents.* Manuscript submitted for publication.

Abela, J. R. Z., Hankin, B. L., Haigh, E. A. P., Vinokuroff, T., Trayhern, L., & Adams, P. (2005). Interpersonal vulnerability to depression in high-risk children: The role of insecure attachment and reassurance seeking. *Journal of Clinical Child and Adolescent Psychology, 34,* 182–192.

Abela, J. R. Z., & McGirr, A. (2007). Operationalizing "cognitive vulnerability" and "stress" from the perspective of the hopelessness theory: A multi-wave longitudinal study of children of affectively ill parents. *British Journal of Clinical Psychology, 46.*

Abela, J. R. Z., McGirr, A., & Skitch, S. A. (2007). Depressogenic inferential styles, negative events, and depressive symptoms in youth: An attempt to reconcile past inconsistent findings. *Behaviour Research and Therapy, 45,* 2397–2406.

Abela, J. R. Z., Parkinson, C., Stolow, D., & Starrs, C. (in press). A test of the integration of the hopelessness and response styles theories of depression in middle adolescence. *Journal of Clinical Child and Adolescent Psychology.*

Abela, J. R. Z., & Payne, A. V. L. (2003). A test of the integration of the hopelessness and self-esteem theories of depression in schoolchildren. *Cognitive Therapy and Research, 27,* 519–535.

Abela, J. R. Z., Sakellaropoulo, M., & Taxel, E. (2007). Integrating two subtypes of depression: Psychodynamic theory and its relation to hopelessness depression in schoolchildren. *Journal of Early Adolescence, 27,* 363–385.

Abela, J. R. Z., & Sarin, S. (2002). Cognitive vulnerability to hopelessness depression: A chain is only as strong as its weakest link. *Cognitive Therapy and Research, 26,* 811–829.

Abela, J. R. Z., & Scheffler, P. (2007). *A diathesis–stress test of additive and "weakest link" of cognitive and interpersonal vulnerabilities in high risk children.* Manuscript submitted for publication.

Abela, J. R. Z., & Seligman, M. E. P. (2000). The hopelessness theory of depression: A test of the diathesis–stress component in the interpersonal and achievement domains. *Cognitive Therapy and Research, 24,* 361–378.

Abela, J. R. Z., & Skitch, S. A. (2007). Dysfunctional attitudes as a cognitive vulnerability factor for depression in children of affectively ill parents: A multi-wave longitudinal study. *Behaviour Research and Therapy, 45,* 1127–1140.

Abela, J. R. Z., Skitch, S. A., Adams, P., & Hankin, B. L. (2006). The timing of parent and child depression: A hopelessness theory perspective. *Journal of Clinical Child and Adolescent Psychology, 35,* 253–263.

Abela, J. R. Z., & Sullivan, C. (2003). A test of Beck's cognitive diathesis–stress theory of depression in early adolescents. *Journal of Early Adolescence, 23,* 384–404.

Abela, J. R. Z., & Taylor, G. (2003). Specific vulnerability to depressive mood reactions in children: The moderating role of self-esteem. *Journal of Clinical Child and Adolescents Psychology, 32,* 408–418.

Abela, J. R. Z., Vanderbilt, E., & Rochon, A. (2004). A test of the integration of the response styles and social support theories of depression in third and seventh grade children. *Journal of Social and Clinical Psychology, 5,* 653–674.

Abela, J. R. Z., & Véronneau-McArdle, M. (2002). The relationship between self-complexity and depressive symptoms in third and seventh grade children: A short-term longitudinal study. *Journal of Abnormal Child Psychology, 30,* 155–166.

Abela, J. R. Z., Webb, C. A., Ho, M., Wagner, C., & Adams, P. (2006). The role of self-criticism, dependency, and hassles in the course of depressive illness: A multi-wave longitudinal study of vulnerability and resiliency. *Personality and Social Psychology Bulletin, 32,* 328–338.

Abela, J. R. Z., Zuroff, D. C., Ho, R., Adams, P., & Hankin, B. L. (2006). Excessive reassurance seeking, hassles, and depressive symptoms in children of affectively ill parents: A multi-wave longitudinal study. *Journal of Abnormal Child Psychology, 34,* 171–187.

Abramson, L. Y., Alloy, L. B., Hankin, B. L., Haeffel, J. G., MacCoon, D. G., & Gibb, B. E. (2002). Cognitive vulnerability–stress models of depression in a self-regulatory and psychobiological context. In I. H. Gotlib & C. L. Hammen (Eds.), *Handbook of depression* (pp. 268–294). New York: Guilford Press.

Abramson, L. Y., Alloy, L. B., & Metalsky, G. I. (1988). The cognitive diathesis–stress theories of depression: Toward an adequate evaluation of the theories' validities. In L. B. Alloy (Ed.), *Cognitive processes in depression* (pp. 3–30). New York: Guilford Press.

Abramson, L. Y., Alloy, L. B., & Metalsky, G. I. (1995). Hopelessness depression. In G. M. Buchanan & M. E. P. Seligman (Eds.), *Explanatory style* (pp. 113–134). Hillsdale, NJ: Erlbaum.

Abramson, L. Y., Metalsky, G. I., & Alloy, L. B. (1989). Hopelessness depression: A theory-based subtype of depression. *Psychological Review, 96,* 358–372.

Abramson, L. Y., Seligman, M. E. P., & Teasdale, J. (1978). Learned helplessness in humans: Critique and reformulation. *Journal of Abnormal Psychology, 87,* 49–74.

Adams, P., Abela, J. R. Z., Auerbach, R. P., & Skitch, S. A. (2007). *Self-criticism, dependency, and stress reactivity: An experience sampling approach to testing Blatt and Zuroff's (1992) theory of personality predispositions to depression in high-risk youth.* Manuscript submitted for publication.

Adams, P., Abela, J. R. Z., & Hankin, B. L. (2007). Factorial categorization of depression related constructs in children and early adolescents. *Journal of Cognitive Psychotherapy, 21,* 123–139.

Ainsworth, M. D. S. (1979). Infant–mother attachment. *American Psychologist, 34,* 932–937.

Alloy, L. B., Abramson, L. Y., Hogan, M. E., Whitehouse, W. G., Rose, D. T., Robinson, M. S., et al. (2000). The Temple–Wisconsin Cognitive Vulnerability to Depression Project: Lifetime history of Axis-I psychopathology in individuals at high and low cognitive risk for depression. *Journal of Abnormal Psychology, 109,* 403–418.

Alloy, L. B., Abramson, L. Y., Tashman, N. A., Berrebbi, D. S., Hogan, M. E., Whitehouse, W. G., et al. (2001). Developmental origins of cognitive vulnerability to depression: Parenting, cognitive, and inferential feedback styles of the parents of individuals at high and low cognitive risk for depression. *Cognitive Therapy and Research, 25*, 397–423.

Alloy, L. B., Abramson, L. Y., Whitehouse, W. G., Hogan, M. E., Panzarella, C., & Rose, D. T. (2006). Prospective incidence of first onsets and recurrences of depression in individuals at high and low cognitive risk for depression. *Journal of Abnormal Psychology, 115*, 145–156.

Alloy, L. B., Hartlage, S., & Abramson, L. Y. (1988). Testing the cognitive diathesis–stress theories of depression: Issues of research design, conceptualization, and assessment. In L. B. Alloy (Ed.), *Cognitive processes in depression* (pp. 31–73). New York: Guilford Press.

Alloy, L. B., Kelly, K. A., Mineka, S., & Clements, C. M. (1990). Comorbidity of anxiety and depressive disorders: A helplessness–hopelessness perspective. In J. D. Maser & C. R. Cloninger (Eds.), *Comorbidity of mood and anxiety disorders* (pp. 499–543). Washington, DC: American Psychiatric Press.

Angold, A., Costello, E. J., & Erkanli, A. (1999). Comorbidity. *Journal of Child Psychology and Psychiatry, 40*, 57–87.

Beck, A. T. (1967). *Depression: Clinical, experimental, and theoretical aspects.* New York: Harper & Row.

Beck, A. T. (1983). Cognitive therapy of depression: New perspectives. In P. J. Clayton & J. E. Barrett (Eds.), *Treatment of depression: Old controversies and new approaches* (pp. 256–284). New York: Raven Press.

Bennett, D. S., & Bates, J. E. (1995). Prospective models of depressive symptoms in early adolescence: Attributional style, stress, and support. *Journal of Early Adolescence, 15*, 299–315.

Blaney, P. H. (1986). Affect and memory: A review. *Psychological Bulletin, 99*, 229–246.

Blatt, S. J., & Homann, E. (1992). Parent–child interaction in the etiology of dependent and self-critical depression. *Clinical Psychology Review, 12*, 47–91.

Blatt, S. J., & Zuroff, D. C. (1992). Interpersonal relatedness and self-definition: Two prototypes for depression. *Clinical Psychology Review, 12*, 527–562.

Bower, G. H. (1981). Mood and memory. *American Psychologist, 36*, 129–148.

Bowlby, J. (1969). *Attachment and loss: Vol. 1. Attachment.* New York: Basic Books.

Bowlby, J. (1980). *Attachment and loss: Vol. 3. Loss: Sadness and depression.* New York: Basic Books.

Broderick, P. C., & Korteland, C. (2004). A prospective study of rumination and depression in early adolescence. *Clinical Child Psychology and Psychiatry, 9*, 383–394.

Brozina, K., & Abela, J. R. Z. (2006). Symptoms of hopelessness depression and anxiety in children: Specificity of the hopelessness theory. *Journal of Clinical Child and Adolescent Psychology, 35*, 515–527.

Bruce, A. E., Cole, D. A., Dallaire, D. H., Jacquez, F. M., Pineda, A. Q., & LaGrange, B. (2006). Relation of parenting and negative life events to cognitive diatheses for depression in children. *Journal of Abnormal Child Psychology, 34*, 321–333.

Burns, M. O., & Seligman, M. E. P. (1989). Explanatory style across the life span: Evidence for stability over 52 years. *Journal of Personality and Social Psychology, 56*, 471–477.

Cane, D. B., Olinger, L. J., Gotlib, I. H., & Kuiper, N. A. (1986). Factor structure of the Dysfunctional Attitudes Scale in a student population. *Journal of Clinical Psychology, 42*, 307–309.

Canli, T., Sivers, H., Thomason, M. E., Whitfield-Gabrieli, S., Gabrieli, J. D. E., & Gotlib, I. H. (2004). Brain activation to emotional words in depressed vs. healthy subjects. *Neuroreport: For Rapid Communication of Neuroscience Research, 15*, 2585–2588.

Caspi, A., Roberts, B. W., & Shiner, R. L. (2005). Personality development: Stability and change. *Annual Review of Psychology, 56*, 453–484.

Caspi, A., & Shiner, R. L. (2006). Personality development. In W. Damon, R. M. Lerner, & N. Eisenberg (Eds.), *Handbook of child psychology: Vol. 3. Social, emotional, and personality development* (6th ed., pp. 300–365). New York: Wiley.

Caspi, A., Sugden, K., Moffit, T. E., Taylor, A., Craig, I. W., & Harrington, H. (2003). Influence of life stress on depression: Moderation by a polymorphism in the 5-HTT gene. *Science, 301,* 386–389.

Clark, D. A., & Beck, A. T. (1999). *Scientific foundations of cognitive theory and therapy of depression.* New York: Wiley.

Cohen, J. (1994). The earth is round (*p* < .05). *American Psychologist, 49,* 997–1003.

Cole, D. A., & Turner, J. E., Jr. (1993). Models of cognitive mediation and moderation in child depression. *Journal of Abnormal Psychology, 102,* 271–281.

Conley, C. S., Haines, B. A., Hilt, L. M., & Metalsky, G. I. (2001). The children's attributional style interview: Developmental tests of cognitive diathesis–stress theories of depression. *Journal of Abnormal Child Psychology, 29,* 445–463.

Corrigan, R. (1995). How infants and young children understand the causes of negative events. In N. Eiseberg (Ed.), *Social development* (pp. 1–26). Thousand Oaks, CA: Sage.

Davidson, R. (2004). Affective style: Causes and consequences. In J. T. Cacioppo & G. T. Berntson (Eds.), *Essays in social neuroscience* (pp. 77–91). Cambridge, MA: MIT Press.

Dixon, J. F., & Ahrens, A. H. (1992). Stress and attributional styles as predictors of self-reported depression in children. *Cognitive Therapy and Research, 16,* 623–634.

Driscoll, K., & Kistner, J. (2007). *Response styles theory: A longitudinal test of the diathesis–stress model in children.* Manuscript submitted for publication.

Dweck, C. S., Davidson, W., Nelson, S., & Enna, B. (1978). Sex differences in learned helplessness: II. The contingencies of evaluative feedback in the classroom, and III. An experimental analysis. *Developmental Psychology, 14,* 268–276.

Eley, T. C., Sugden, K., Corsico, A., Gregory, A. M., Sham, P., McGuffin, P., et al. (2004). Gene–environment interaction analysis of serotonin system markers with adolescent depression. *Molecular Psychiatry, 9,* 908–915.

Elkind, D. (1967). Egocentrism in adolescence. *Child Development, 38,* 1025–1034.

Elkind, D. (1978). Understanding the young adolescent. *Adolescence, 49,* 127–134.

Feiring, C., Taska, L., & Lewis, M. (1998). The role of shame and attributional style in children's and adolescents' adaptation to sexual abuse. *Childhood Maltreatment, 3,* 129–142.

Fichman, L., Koestner, R., & Zuroff, D. C. (1996). Dependency, self-criticism, and perceptions of inferiority at summer camp: I'm even worse than you think. *Journal of Youth and Adolescence, 25,* 113–126.

Fincham, F. D., & Cain, K. M. (1986). Learned helplessness in humans: A developmental analysis. *Developmental Review, 6,* 301–333.

Fraley, C., & Roberts, B. W. (2005). Patterns of continuity: A dynamic model for conceptualizing the stability of individual differences in psychological constructs across the lifecourse. *Psychological Review, 112,* 60–74.

Garber, J. (2000). Development and depression. In A. J. Sameroff, M. Lewis, & S. M. Miller (Eds.), *Handbook of developmental psychopathology* (pp. 467–490). New York: Kluwer.

Garber, J., & Flynn, C. (1998). Origins of the depressive cognitive style. In D. Routh & R. J. DeRebeis (Eds.), *The science of clinical psychology: Evidence of a century's progress* (pp. 53–93). Washington, DC: American Psychological Association.

Garber, J., & Flynn, C. (2001). Predictors of depressive cognitions in young adolescents. *Cognitive Therapy and Research, 25,* 353–376.

Garber, J., Weiss, B., & Shanley, N. (1993). Cognitions, depressive symptoms, and development in adolescents. *Journal of Abnormal Psychology, 102,* 47–57.

Gibb, B. E., & Abela, J. R. Z. (in press). Emotional abuse, verbal victimization, and the development of children's negative inferential styles and depressive symptoms. *Cognitive Therapy and Research.*

Gibb, B. E., & Alloy, L. B. (2006). A prospective test of the hopelessness theory of depression in children. *Journal of Clinical Child and Adolescent Psychology, 35,* 264–274.

Gibb, B. E., Alloy, L. B., Abramson, L. Y., Rose, D. T., Whitehouse, W. G., Donovan, P., et al. (2001). History of childhood maltreatment, negative cognitive styles, and episodes of depression in adulthood. *Cognitive Therapy and Research, 25,* 425–446.

Gibb, B. E., Alloy, L. B., Walshaw, P. D., Comer, J. S., Shen, G. H. C., & Villari, A. G. (2006). Predictors of attributional style change in children. *Journal of Abnormal Child Psychology, 34,* 425–439.

Gibb, B. E., & Coles, M. (2005). Cognitive vulnerability–stress models of psychopathology: A developmental perspective. In B. L. Hankin & J. R. Z. Abela (Eds.), *Development of psychopathology: A vulnerability–stress perspective* (pp. 104–135). Thousand Oaks, CA: Sage.

Gladstone, T. R. G., Kaslow, N. J., Seeley, J. R., & Lewinsohn, P. M. (1997). Sex differences, attributional style, and depressive symptoms among adolescents. *Journal of Abnormal Child Psychology, 25,* 297–305.

Gotlib, I. H., & Hammen, C. L. (Eds.). (2002). *Handbook of depression.* New York: Guilford Press.

Gotlib, I. H., Joormann, J., Minor, K. L., & Cooney, R. E. (2006). Cognitive and biological functioning in children at risk for depression. In T. Canli (Ed.), *Biology of personality and individual differences* (pp. 353–382). New York: Guilford Press.

Gotlib, I. H., Kasch, K. L., Traill, S., Joormann, J., Arnow, B. A., & Johnson, S. L. (2004). Coherence and specificity of information-processing biases in depression and social phobia. *Journal of Abnormal Psychology, 113,* 386–398.

Gotlib, I. H., Krasnoperova, E., Yue, D. N., & Joormann, J. (2004). Attentional biases for negative interpersonal stimuli in clinical depression. *Journal of Abnormal Psychology, 113,* 127–135.

Gottesman, H., & Gould, T. D. (2003). The endophenotype concept in psychiatry: Etymology and strategic intentions. *American Journal of Psychiatry, 160,* 636–645.

Haines, B. A., Metalsky, G. I., Cardamone, A. L., & Joiner, T. (1999). Interpersonal and cognitive pathways into the origins of attributional style: A developmental perspective. In T. Joiner & J. C. Coyne (Eds.), *The interactional nature of depression* (pp. 65–92). Washington, DC: American Psychological Association.

Hammen, C. (1990). Self-schemas and vulnerability to specific life stress in children at risk for depression. *Cognitive Therapy and Research, 14,* 215–227.

Hammen, C. (1991). The generation of stress in the course of unipolar depression. *Journal of Abnormal Psychology, 100,* 555–561.

Hammen, C. L. (1992). Cognitive, life stress, and interpersonal approaches to a developmental psychopathology model of depression. *Development and Psychopathology, 4,* 189–206.

Hammen, C. L., Adrian, C., & Hiroto, D. (1988). A longitudinal test of the attributional vulnerability model of depression in children at risk for depression. *British Journal of Clinical Psychology, 27,* 37–46.

Hammen, C., & Goodman-Brown, T. (1990). Self-schemas and vulnerability to specific life stress in children at risk for depression. *Cognitive Therapy and Research, 14,* 215–227

Hammen, C., & Rudolph, K. D. (2003). Childhood mood disorders. In E. J. Mash & R. A. Barkley (Eds.), *Child psychopathology* (2nd ed., pp. 233–278). New York: Guilford Press.

Hammen, C., & Zupan, B. A. (1984). Self-schemas, depression, and the processing of personal information in children. *Journal of Experimental Child Psychology, 37,* 598–608.

Hankin, B. L. (2005). Childhood maltreatment and psychopathology: Prospective tests of attachment, cognitive vulnerability, and stress as mediating processes. *Cognitive Therapy and Research, 29,* 645–671.

Hankin, B. L. (2006). *Temperament as vulnerability to depression in youth: A multi-wave analysis of mediating mechanisms.* Manuscript in preparation.

Hankin, B. L., & Abela, J. R. Z. (2005). Depression from childhood through adolescence and adulthood: A developmental vulnerability–stress perspective. In B. L. Hankin & J. R. Z. Abela (Eds.), *Development of psychopathology: A vulnerability–stress perspective* (pp. 245–288). Thousand Oaks, CA: Sage.

Hankin, B. L., & Abramson, L. Y. (2001). Development of sex differences in depression: An elaborated cognitive vulnerability–transactional stress theory. *Psychological Bulletin, 127,* 773–796.

Hankin, B. L., & Abramson, L. Y. (2002). Measuring cognitive vulnerability to depression in adolescence: Reliability, validity, and gender differences. *Journal of Child and Adolescent Clinical Psychology, 31,* 491–504.

Hankin, B. L., Abramson, L. Y., Miller, N., & Haeffel, G. (2004). Cognitive vulnerability–stress theories of depression: Examining affective specificity in the prediction of depression versus anxiety in three prospective studies. *Cognitive Therapy and Research, 28,* 309–345.

Hankin, B. L., Abramson, L. Y., Moffitt, T. E., Silva, P. A., McGee, R., & Angell, K. A. (1998). Development of depression from preadolescence to young adulthood: Emerging gender differences in a 10 year longitudinal study. *Journal of Abnormal Psychology, 107,* 128–141.

Hankin, B. L., Abramson, L. Y., & Siler, M. (2001). A prospective test of the hopelessness theory of depression in adolescence. *Cognitive Therapy and Research, 25,* 607–632.

Hankin, B. L., Carter, I., Lakdawalla, Z., Abela, J. R. Z., & Adams, P. (2007). Are neuroticism, cognitive vulnerability and self-esteem overlapping or distinct risks for depression? Evidence from exploratory and confirmatory factor analyses. *Journal of Social and Clinical Psychology, 26,* 29–63.

Hankin, B. L., Fraley, R. C., & Abela, J. R. Z. (2005). Daily depression and cognitions about stress: Evidence for a trait-like depressogenic cognitive style and the prediction of depressive symptoms trajectories in a prospective daily diary study. *Journal of Personality and Social Psychology, 88,* 673–685.

Hankin, B. L., Fraley, R. C., Lahey, B. B., & Waldman, I. (2005). Is youth depressive disorder best viewed as a continuum or discrete category? A taxometric analysis of childhood and adolescent depression in a population-based sample. *Journal of Abnormal Psychology, 114,* 96–110.

Hankin, B. L., Lakdawalla, Z., Lee, A., Grace, D., & Roesch, L. (2004, November). Cognitive vulnerabilities for emotional distress in adolescence: Disentangling the comorbidity of depression and anxiety in a multi-wave prospective study. In B. L. Hankin & J. R. Z. Abela (co-chairs), *Depression and anxiety: Issues of specificity and comorbidity.* Symposium conducted at the 38th annual meeting of the Association for Advancement of Behavior Therapy, New Orleans.

Hankin, B. L., Mermelstein, R., & Roesch, L. (2007). Sex differences in adolescent depression: Stress exposure and reactivity models. *Child Development, 78,* 279–295.

Hankin, B. L., & Roesch, L. (2005, April). Cognitive vulnerabilities to depression and stress: General and specific predictors of psychopathology in youth. In B. L. Hankin (Chair), *Methodological advances in the study of vulnerability to depression in youth.* Symposium conducted at the annual meeting of the Society for Research in Child Development, Atlanta, GA.

Harter, S. (1986). Processes underlying the construction, maintenance, and enhancement of the self-concept in children. In J. Suis & A. Greenwald (Eds.), *Psychological perspectives on the self* (Vol. 3, pp. 137–181). Hillsdale, NJ: Erlbaum.

Harter, S. (1990). Causes, correlates, and the functional role of global self-worth: A life-span perspective. In R. J. Sternberg & J. Kolligan, Jr. (Eds.), *Competence considered* (pp. 67–97). New Haven: Yale University Press.

Hayden, E. P., Klein, D. N., Durbin, C. E., & Olino, T. M. (2006). Positive emotionality at age 3 predicts cognitive styles in 7-year-old children. *Development and Psychopathology, 18,* 409–423.

Hilsman, R., & Garber, J. (1995). A test of the cognitive diathesis–stress model of depression in children: Academic stressors, attributional style, perceived competence, and control. *Journal of Personality and Social Psychology, 69,* 370–380.

Ingram, R. E. (2001). Developing perspectives on the cognitive-developmental origins of depression: Back is the future. *Cognitive Therapy and Research, 25,* 497–504.

Ingram, R. E. (2003a). Twenty-five years of inquiry and insight. *Cognitive Therapy and Research, 27,* 1–17.

Ingram, R. E. (2003b). Origins of cognitive vulnerability to depression. *Cognitive Therapy and Research, 27,* 77–88.

Ingram, R. E., & Luxton, D. D. (2005). Vulnerability–stress models. In B. L. Hankin & J. R. Z. Abela (Eds.), *Development of psychopathology: A vulnerability–stress perspective* (pp. 32–46). Thousand Oaks, CA: Sage.

Ingram, R. E., Miranda, J., & Segal, Z. V. (1998). *Cognitive vulnerability to depression*. New York. Guilford Press.

Ingram, R. E., & Price, J. M. (2001). *Vulnerability to psychopathology*. New York: Guilford Press.

Jaenicke, C., Hammen, C., Zupan, B., Hiroto, D., Gordon, D., Adrian, C., et al. (1987). Cognitive vulnerability in children at risk for depression. *Journal of Abnormal Child Psychology, 15,* 559–572.

Janoff-Bulman, R. (1992). *Shattered assumptions: Towards a new psychology of trauma*. New York: Free Press.

Johnson, S., Joormann, J., & Gotlib, I. H. (2007). Information processing biases as predictors of symptomatic improvement and diagnostic recovery from major depression. *Emotion, 7,* 201–206.

Joiner, T. E., Jr. (2000). A test of the hopelessness theory of depression in youth psychiatric inpatients. *Journal of Clinical Child Psychology, 29,* 167–176.

Joiner, T. E., Jr., & Rudd, M. D. (1996). Toward a categorization of depression-related psychological constructs. *Cognitive Therapy and Research, 20,* 51–68.

Joormann, J., & Gotlib, I. H. (2007). Selective attention to emotional faces following recovery from depression. *Journal of Abnormal Psychology, 116,* 80–85.

Joormann, J., Talbot, L., & Gotlib, I. H. (2007). Biased processing of emotional information in girls at risk for depression. *Journal of Abnormal Psychology, 116,* 135–143.

Kaslow, N. J., Adamson, L. B., & Collins, M. H. (2000). A developmental psychopathology perspective on the cognitive components of child and adolescent depression. In A. J. Sameroff, M. Lewis, & S. M. Miller (Eds.), *Handbook of developmental psychopathology* (pp. 491–510). New York: Kluwer.

Kaslow, N. J., Rehm, L. P., Pollack, S. L., & Siegel, A. W. (1988). Attributional style and self-control behavior in depressed and nondepressed children and their parents. *Journal of Abnormal Child Psychology, 16,* 163–175.

Kazdin, A. E., French, N. H., Unis, A. S., Esveldt-Dawson, K., & Sherick, R. B. (1983). Hopelessness, depression, and suicidal intent among psychiatrically disturbed inpatient children. *Journal of Consulting and Clinical Psychology, 51,* 504–510.

Kenny, D. A., & Zautra, A. (2001). Trait–state models for longitudinal data. In L. M. Collins & A. G. Sayer (Eds.), *New methods for the analysis of change*. Washington, DC: American Psychological Association.

Koestner, R., Zuroff, D. C., & Powers, T. A. (1991). Family origins of adolescent self-criticism and its continuity into adulthood. *Journal of Abnormal Psychology, 100,* 191–197.

Lakdawalla, Z., & Hankin, B. L. (2007). Cognitive theories of depression in children and adolescents: A conceptual and quantitative review. *Clinical Child and Family Psychology Review, 10,* 1–24.

Lau, J. Y. F., Rijsdijk, F., & Eley, T. C. (2006). I think, therefore I am: A twin study of attributional style in adolescents. *Journal of Child Psychology and Psychiatry, 47,* 696–703.

Lewinsohn, P. M., Allen, N. B., Seeley, J. R., & Gotlib, I. H. (1999). First onset versus recurrence of depression: Differential processes of psychosocial risk. *Journal of Abnormal Psychology, 108,* 483–489.

Lewinsohn, P. M., Joiner, T. E., & Rohde, P. (2001). Evaluation of cognitive diathesis–stress models in predicting major depressive disorder in adolescents. *Journal of Abnormal Psychology, 110,* 203–215.

Lewinsohn, P., Rohde, P., Seeley, J., & Fischer, S. (1993). Age-cohort changes in the lifetime occurrence of depression and other mental disorders, *Journal of Abnormal Psychology, 102,* 110–120.

Lewinsohn, P. M., Steinmetz, J. L., Larson, D. W., & Franklin, J. (1981). Depression-related cognitions: Antecedent or consequence? *Journal of Abnormal Psychology, 90,* 213–219.

Lewinsohn, P. M., Zinbarg, R., Seeley, J. R., Lewinsohn, M., & Sack, W. H. (1997). Lifetime comorbidity among anxiety disorders and between anxiety disorders and other mental disorders in adolescents. *Journal of Anxiety Disorders, 11,* 377–394.

Little, S. A., & Garber, J. (2000). Interpersonal and achievement orientations and specific stressors predicting depressive and aggressive symptoms in children. *Cognitive Therapy and Research*, *24*, 651–670.

Little, S. A., & Garber, J. (2004). Interpersonal and achievement orientations and specific stressors predict depressive and aggressive symptoms. *Journal of Adolescent Research*, *19*, 63–84.

Little, S. A., & Garber, J. (2005). The role of social stressors and interpersonal orientation in explaining the longitudinal relation between externalizing and depressive symptoms. *Journal of Abnormal Psychology*, *114*, 432–443.

Liu, Y. (2003). The mediators between parenting and adolescent depressive symptoms: Dysfunctional attitudes and self-worth. *International Journal of Psychology*, *38*, 91–100.

McWhinnie, C., Abela, J. R. Z., & Knauper, B. (in press). Assessing dysfunctional attitudes in children: The development and validation of the Children's Dysfunctional Attitudes Scale—Revised. *British Journal of Clinical Psychology*.

Meehl, P. E. (1978). Theoretical risks and tabular asterisks: Sir Karl, Sir Ronald, and the slow progress of soft psychology. *Journal of Consulting and Clinical Psychology*, *46*, 806–834.

Metalsky, G. I., Halberstadt, L. J., & Abramson, L. Y. (1987). Vulnerability to depressive mood reactions: Toward a more powerful test of the diathesis–stress and causal mediation components of the reformulated theory of depression. *Journal of Personality and Social Psychology*, *52*, 386–393.

Metalsky, G. I., & Joiner, T. E., Jr. (1992). Vulnerability to depressive symptomatology: A prospective test of the diathesis–stress and causal mediation components of the hopelessness theory of depression. *Journal of Personality and Social Psychology*, *63*, 667–675.

Moffitt, T. E. (2005). The new look of behavioral genetics in developmental psychopathology: Gene–environment interplay in antisocial behaviors. *Psychological Bulletin*, *131*, 533–554.

Monroe, S. M., & Simons, A. D. (1991). Diathesis–stress theories in the context of life stress research: Implications for the depressive disorders. *Psychological Bulletin*, *110*, 406–425.

Nelson, E. E., Leibenluft, E., McClure, E., & Pine, D. S. (2005). The social re-orientation of adolescence: A neuroscience perspective on the process and its relation to psychopathology. *Psychological Medicine*, *35*, 163–174.

Nelson, E. E., McClure, E. B., Monk, C. S., Zarahn, E., Leibenluft, E., Pine, D. S., et al. (2003). Developmental differences in neuronal engagement during implicit encoding of emotional faces: An event-related fMRI study. *Journal of Child Psychology and Psychiatry*, *44*, 1015–1024.

Nolen-Hoeksema, S. (1991). Responses to depression and their effects on the duration of depressive episodes. *Journal of Abnormal Psychology*, *100*, 569–582.

Nolen-Hoeksema, S., & Corte, C. (2004). Gender and self-regulation. In R. F. Baumeister & K. D. Vohs (Eds.), *Handbook of self-regulation: Research, theory, and applications* (pp. 411–421). New York: Guilford Press.

Nolen-Hoeksema, S., Girgus, J. S., & Seligman, M. E. P. (1986). Learned helplessness in children: A longitudinal study of depression, achievement, and attributional style. *Journal of Personality and Social Psychology*, *51*, 435–442.

Nolen-Hoeksema, S., Girgus, J. S., & Seligman, M. E. P. (1992). Predictors and consequences of childhood depressive symptoms: A five-year longitudinal study. *Journal of Abnormal Psychology*, *101*, 405–422.

Oakes, L. M. (1994). Development of infants' use of continuity cues in their perceptions of causality. *Developmental Psychology*, *30*, 869–879.

Oliver, J. M., & Baumgart, E. P. (1985). The Dysfunctional Attitudes Scale: Psychometric properties and relation to depression in an unselected adult population. *Cognitive Therapy and Research*, *9*, 161–167.

Panak, W. F., & Garber, J. (1992). Role of aggression, rejection, and attributions in the prediction of depression in children. *Development and Psychopathology*, *4*, 145–165.

Persons, J. B., & Miranda, J. (1992). Cognitive theories of vulnerability to depression: Reconciling negative evidence. *Cognitive Therapy and Research*, *16*, 485–502.

Pezawas, L., Meyer-Lindberg, A., Drabant, E. M., Verchinski, B. A., Munoz, K. E., Kolachana, B. S., et al. (2005). 5-HTTLPR polymorphism impacts human cingulated-amygdala interactions: A genetic susceptibility mechanism for depression. *Nature Neuroscience, 8*, 828–834.

Pine, D. S., Grun, J., Zarahn, E., Fyer, A., Koda, V., Li, W., et al. (2001). Corticol brain regions engaged by masked emotional faces in adolescents and adults: An fMRI study. *Emotion, 1*, 137–147.

Prinstein, M. J., & Aikins, J. W. (2004). Cognitive moderators of the longitudinal association between peer rejection and adolescent depressive symptoms. *Journal of Abnormal Child Psychology, 32*, 147–158.

Quiggle, N. L., Garber, J., Panak, W. F., & Dodge, K. A. (1992). Social information processing in aggressive and depressed children. *Child Development, 63*, 1305–1320.

Riskind, J. H., & Rholes, W. S. (1984). Cognitive accessibility and the capacity of cognitions to predict future depression: A theoretical note. *Cognitive Therapy and Research, 8*, 1–12.

Rholes, W. S., Blackwell, J., Jordan, C., & Walters, C. (1980). A developmental study of learned helplessness. *Developmental Psychology, 16*, 616–624.

Robinson, N. S., Garber, J., & Hilsman, R. (1995). Cognitions and stress: Direct and moderating effects on depressive versus externalizing symptoms during the junior high school transition. *Journal of Abnormal Psychology, 104*, 453–463.

Rohde, P., Lewinsohn, P. M., & Seeley, J. R. (1994). Are adolescents changed by an episode of major depression? *Journal of the American Academy of Child and Adolescent Psychiatry, 33*, 1289–1298.

Rose, D. T., & Abramson, L. Y. (1992). Developmental predictors of depressive cognitive style: Research and theory. In D. Cicchetti & S. L. Toth (Eds.), *Rochester symposium on developmental psychopathology* (Vol. 4, pp. 323–349). Hillsdale, NJ: Erlbaum.

Rose, D. T., Abramson, L. Y., Hodulik, C. J., Halberstadt, L., & Leff, G. (1994). Heterogeneity of cognitive style among depressed inpatients. *Journal of Abnormal Psychology, 103*, 419–429.

Rothbart, M. K., & Bates, J. E. (2006). Temperament. In W. Damon, R. M. Lerner, & N. Eisenberg (Eds.), *Handbook of child psychology: Vol. 3. Social, emotional, and personality development* (6th ed., pp. 99–166). New York: Wiley.

Rude, S. S., & Burnham, B. L. (1993). Do interpersonal and achievement vulnerabilities interact with congruent life events to predict depression? Comparison of DEQ, DAS, and combined scale. *Cognitive Therapy and Research, 17*, 531–548.

Rudolph, K. D., & Hammen, C. (1999). Age and gender as determinants of stress exposure, generation, and reactions in youngsters: A transactional perspective. *Child Development, 70*, 660–677.

Rudolph, K. D., Hammen, C., Burge, D., Lindberg, N., Herzberg, D., & Daley, S. E. (2000). Toward an interpersonal life-stress model of depression: The developmental context of stress generation. *Development and Psychopathology, 12*, 215–234.

Rudolph, K. D., Kurlakowsky, K. D., & Conley, C. S. (2001). Developmental and social-contextual origins of depressive control-related beliefs and behavior. *Cognitive Therapy and Research, 25*, 447–475.

Scher, C. D., Ingram, R. E., & Segal, Z. V. (2005). Cognitive reactivity and vulnerability: Empirical evaluation of construct activation and cognitive diatheses in unipolar depression. *Clinical Psychology Review, 25*, 487–510.

Seligman, M. E. P., Peterson, C., Kaslow, N. J., Tenenbaum, R. L., Alloy, L. B., & Abramson, L. Y. (1984). Attributional style and depressive symptoms among children. *Journal of Abnormal Psychology, 93*, 235–241.

Shahar, G., Blatt, S. J., Zuroff, D. C., Kuperminc, G., & Leadbeater, B. J. (2004). Reciprocal relations between depressive symptoms and self-criticism (but not dependency) among early adolescent girls (but not boys). *Cognitive Therapy and Research, 28*, 85–103.

Shahar, G., & Priel, B. (2003). Active vulnerability, adolescent distress, and the mediating/suppressing role of life events. *Personality and Individual Differences, 35*, 199–218.

Shih, J., Abela, J. R. Z., & Starrs, C. (2007). *Cognitive and interpersonal predictors of stress gener-ation in children*. Manuscript submitted for publication.

Shirk, S. R. (1988). Causal reasoning and children's comprehension of therapeutic interpretations. In S. R. Shirk (Ed.), *Cognitive development and child psychotherapy* (pp. 53–89). New York: Plenum Press.

Shwartz, J. A. J., Gladstone, T. R. G., & Kaslow, N. (1998). Depressive disorders. In T. H. Ollendick & M. Hersen (Eds.), *Handbook of child psychopathology* (3rd ed., pp. 269–289). New York: Plenum Press.

Shwartz, J. A. J., & Koenig, L. J. (1996). Response styles and negative affect among adolescents. *Cognitive Therapy and Research, 20,* 13–36.

Southall, D., & Roberts, J. E. (2002). Attributional style and self-esteem in vulnerability to adoles-cent depressive symptoms following life stress: A 14-week prospective study. *Cognitive Ther-apy and Research, 26,* 563–579.

Spence, S. H., Sheffield, J., & Donovan, C. (2002). Problem–solving orientation and attributional style: Moderators of the impact of negative life events on the development of depressives in adolescence? *Journal of Clinical Child Psychology, 31,* 219–229.

Taylor, L., & Ingram, R. E. (1999). Cognitive reactivity and depressotypic information processing in children of depressed mothers. *Journal of Abnormal Psychology, 108,* 202–210.

Teasdale, J. D. (1983). Negative thinking in depression: Cause, effect, or reciprocal relationship? *Advances in Behavior Research and Therapy, 5,* 3–25.

Thompson, M., Kaslow, N. J., Weiss, B., & Nolen-Hoeksema, S. (1998). Children's Attributional Style Questionnaire—Revised: Psychometric examination. *Psychological Assessment, 10,* 166–170.

Timbremont, B., & Braet, C. (2004a). Cognitive vulnerability in remitted depressed children and adolescents. *Behaviour Research and Therapy, 42,* 423–437.

Timbremont, B., & Braet, C. (2004b). Selective information-processing in depressed children and adolescents: Is there a difference in processing of self-referent and other-referent information? *Behaviour Change, 22,* 143–155.

Turk, E., & Bry, B. (1992). Adolescents' and parents' explanatory styles and parents' causal expla-nations about their adolescents. *Cognitive Therapy and Research, 16,* 349–357.

Turner, J. E., & Cole, D. A. (1994). Developmental differences in cognitive diatheses for child depression. *Journal of Abnormal Child Psychology, 22*(1), 15–32.

Voelz, Z. R., Walker, R. L., Petit, J. W., Joiner, T. E., Jr., & Wagner, K. D. (2003). Depressogenic attributional style: Evidence of trait-like nature in youth psychiatric inpatients. *Personality and Individual Differences, 37,* 1129–1140.

Weiss, B., Susser, K., & Catron, T. (1998). Common and specific features of childhood psychopath-ology. *Journal of Abnormal Psychology, 107,* 118–128.

Young, J. E. (1999). *Cognitive therapy for personality disorders: A schema-focused approach* (3rd ed.). Sarasota, FL: Professional Resource Press.

Ziegert, D., & Kistner, J. (2002). Response styles theory: Downward extension to children. *Journal of Clinical Child and Adolescent Psychology, 31*(3), 325–334.

Zuroff, D. C., Santor, D. A., & Mongrain, M. (2004). Dependency, self-criticism, and maladjust-ment. In J. S. Auerbach, K. J. Levy, & C. E. Schaffer (Eds.), *Relatedness, self-definition and mental representation: Essays in honor of Sidney J. Blatt* (pp. 75–90). London: Brunner-Routledge.

4 A Developmental Perspective on Interpersonal Theories of Youth Depression

Karen D. Rudolph, Megan Flynn, and Jamie L. Abaied

Youth depression is, in many ways, a disorder that occurs within an interpersonal context. Depressed youth experience significant disruptions in many aspects of their relationships. They view themselves and are viewed by others as having considerable impairment in their social skills. They often encounter rejection and conflict in their relationships. Consequently, most contemporary theories of depression incorporate the role of interpersonal factors. In this chapter we present a model that delineates the interpersonal antecedents, correlates, and consequences of youth depression (see Figure 4.1). According to this model, *early family disruption* (e.g., insecure parent–child attachment, parental depression) interferes with the development of adaptive interpersonal behaviors and fosters maladaptive interpersonal behaviors. These *social-behavioral deficits* cause youth to generate *disturbances in their relationships*, which heighten risk for subsequent depression. Depressive symptoms further undermine interpersonal functioning, leading to the perpetuation or exacerbation of depression and risk for recurrence.

The model also incorporates a number of factors that may moderate the extent to which social-behavioral deficits and relationship disturbances heighten risk for depression, as well as the extent to which depression interferes with interpersonal functioning (see Figure 4.1). Possible moderating variables to be discussed include (1) *personality characteristics and social-cognitive style* (e.g., interpersonal dependency or sociotropy, need for approval, attributional style); (2) *gender* and *gender-linked characteristics* of youth (e.g., interpersonal orientation, social goals), which are hypothesized to create greater sensitivity to interpersonal problems in girls than in boys; and (3) normative *developmental transitions* (e.g., physical, psychological, and social changes associated with the transition to adolescence).

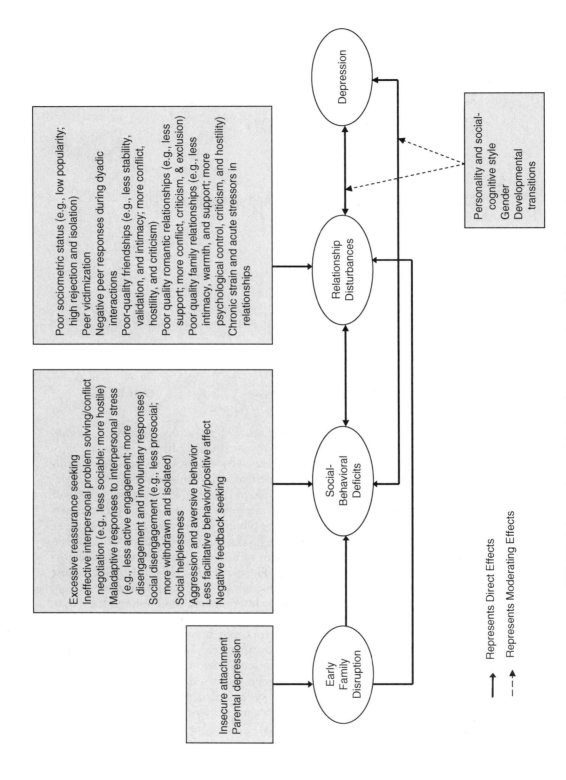

FIGURE 4.1. Developmentally based interpersonal model of youth depression.

INTERPERSONAL THEORIES OF DEPRESSION: TAKING A DEVELOPMENTAL PERSPECTIVE

Interpersonal theories of depression propose that characteristics and behaviors of depressed and depression-prone individuals disrupt social relationships by evoking negative responses from others (Coyne, 1976; Gotlib & Hammen, 1992; Joiner, 2002; Joiner, Coyne, & Blalock, 1999) and generating interpersonal stress and conflict (Hammen, 1992; Rudolph et al., 2000). It is theorized that depressed individuals induce negative affect in those with whom they interact, which causes people to avoid or reject them. Further, according to the theory, a "depressive social process" (Coyne, 1976, p.187) emerges within social networks in which depressed individuals cannot be avoided. Specifically, depressed individuals deny the encouragement and reassurance initially provided by others, thereby maintaining their depression and the negative impact they have on those around them. As depressed individuals observe inconsistencies between others' reassurance and behavior, they increase their expression of symptoms, thereby eliciting further negative affect and creating interpersonal difficulties. Interpersonal difficulties serve to perpetuate or exacerbate symptoms and promote the future recurrence of depression. This cycle may be particularly problematic for youth, who have less flexibility in their social environments and interact regularly with the same people (e.g., families, schoolmates).

Traditional interpersonal theories of depression provide a useful foundation on which to build an interpersonal model of youth depression. However, these theories originated in efforts to understand adult depression and therefore neglect to consider the developmental context of interpersonal dysfunction and depression. Efforts to understand the interpersonal antecedents and consequences of depression in youth would therefore benefit from the application of a developmental psychopathology perspective on disorders. This perspective emphasizes the intersection between normative and atypical development and the continuous unfolding of transactions between youth and their environments over time (Cicchetti, 1993; Lewis, 1990). The model presented in this chapter integrates these developmental emphases in several ways. First, the model proposes that normative intrapersonal and social changes associated with the transition to adolescence enhance interpersonal vulnerability and intensify the link between interpersonal dysfunction and depression. Second, the model proposes that disruptions in early family experiences associated with insecure attachment and parental depression undermine the normative development of interpersonal competencies, contributing to interpersonal vulnerability to depression (i.e., social-behavioral deficits and relationship disturbances). Third, the model proposes that early-onset symptoms interrupt normative developmental trajectories, resulting in long-term adverse interpersonal consequences of depression. More broadly, the model highlights how depressed youth both *react* and *contribute* to disturbances in their relationships.

SOCIAL-BEHAVIORAL DEFICITS OF DEPRESSED YOUTH

Research consistently reveals that depressed youth display *social-behavioral deficits* across a range of interpersonal contexts, including peer, romantic, and family relationships. Depressed youth describe themselves as less socially competent (e.g., less able to resolve conflict or to provide effective emotional support to peers, less able to make friends) than do their nondepressed peers (Hammen, Shih, & Brennan, 2004; Rudolph & Clark, 2001; Rudolph, Hammen, & Burge, 1997). Consistent with early interpersonal models of depression (Coyne, 1976), depressed youth report that they engage in excessive reassurance seeking (i.e., repeatedly seeking assurance about their self-worth) with close relationship partners (Prinstein, Borelli, Cheah, Simon, & Aikins, 2005; for a review, see Joiner, Metalsky, Katz, & Beach, 1999).

Depressed youth also demonstrate ineffective interpersonal problem-solving skills and maladaptive responses to interpersonal stress. For example, when asked how they typically respond or how they would respond to social dilemmas, depressed youth endorse fewer sociable and assertive responses and more hostile responses than do nondepressed youth (Quiggle, Garber, Panak, & Dodge, 1992; Rudolph, Hammen, & Burge, 1994). In the context of interpersonal stressors (e.g., problems with friends or family), depressed youth report that they engage in lower levels of active, problem-focused, and engagement coping (e.g., problem solving, positive thinking; Connor-Smith, Compas, Wadsworth, Thomsen, & Saltzman, 2000) and higher levels of disengagement coping (e.g., avoidance, denial; Steele, Forehand, & Armistead, 1997) and involuntary responses to stress (e.g., rumination, emotional arousal, inaction; Jaser et al., 2005).

Although the self-perceptions of depressed youth may, in part, reflect negatively biased estimates of their interpersonal competence (Brendgen, Vitaro, Turgeon, & Poulin, 2002; McGrath & Repetti, 2002; Rudolph & Clark, 2001), reports by significant others (e.g., parents, teachers, peers) and direct observations of depressed youth in both natural and laboratory settings corroborate the presence of social-behavioral deficits. According to teachers, depressed youth demonstrate lower levels of prosocial behavior and higher levels of aggression and withdrawal than do nondepressed youth (Bell-Dolan, Reaven, & Peterson, 1993; Rudolph & Clark, 2001). Observations of depressed youth interacting on the playground reveal similar interpersonal profiles; depressed youth are more likely than nondepressed youth to play alone and to engage in aggressive and aversive behaviors when interacting with peers (Altmann & Gotlib, 1988). Supporting depressed youths' own reports of deficits in interpersonal problem solving and maladaptive responses to interpersonal stress, observations of dyadic interactions reveal that depressed youth show poorer conflict negotiation skills and heightened emotion dysregulation when faced with a social challenge (Rudolph et al., 1994). Consistent with these observations, teachers describe depressed youth as more helpless (e.g., showing a lack of initiative and persistence) in challenging social situations than nondepressed youth (Nolen-Hoeksema, Girgus, & Seligman, 1992; Rudolph, Kurlakowsky, & Conley, 2001). In romantic relationships, both depressed adolescent women and their partners perceive these women as less interpersonally competent than do their nondepressed counterparts (Daley & Hammen, 2002).

Observations of depressed youth during family interactions also find a range of maladaptive interpersonal behaviors. For example, when interacting with parents, depressed youth are more likely than nondepressed youth to show ineffective problem solving, less behavior that facilitates the ongoing exchange (e.g., affirmations, positive affect directed toward others; Sheeber & Sorensen, 1998), more solitary behavior, and fewer positive reactions to others, suggesting an overall deficit in positive interpersonal behavior with parents (Messer & Gross, 1995). Depressed youth also show less autonomous assertion than nondepressed youth during parent–child interactions (Kobak & Ferenz-Gillies, 1995).

RELATIONSHIP DISTURBANCES IN DEPRESSED YOUTH

Given the range of social-behavioral deficits manifested by depressed youth, it is not surprising that their relationships are compromised. With regard to peer relationships, depression is linked to self-, parent, teacher, and peer reports of poor sociometric status (i.e., low popularity, high rejection and isolation) and exposure to peer victimization (Cole, 1990; Crick & Grotpeter, 1996; Nolan, Flynn, & Garber, 2003; Rudolph & Clark, 2001; Rudolph et al., 1994). Observations of depressed youth confirm that they encounter negative reactions from peers. For example, observers report that peers show more negative responses to depressed than nondepressed youth during structured dyadic interactions; moreover, the interaction partners of depressed youth evaluate them more negatively than the partners of nondepressed youth (Baker, Milich, & Manolis, 1996; Connolly, Geller, Marton, & Kutcher, 1992; Rudolph et al., 1994).

Significantly less research examines the close friendships of depressed youth. However, it has been suggested that interpersonal negativity may be intensified during interactions between depressed individuals and intimate partners, as compared with their interactions in the general peer group (Joiner, 2002). Indeed, self-reports and interviews with depressed youth and their parents suggest that depression is concurrently associated with less stable friendships and poorer friendship quality (e.g., lower levels of validation, intimacy, and conflict resolution; higher levels of conflict, hostility, and perceived criticism; Borelli & Prinstein, 2006; Goodyer, Wright, & Altham, 1990; La Greca & Harrison, 2005; Prinstein et al., 2005; Puig-Antich et al. 1993; Windle, 1994). Interestingly, less consistent findings emerge when friend reports of friendship quality are used. For example, one study revealed no differences in the friend-reported friendship quality of depressed and nondepressed youth (Brendgen et al., 2002). In another study, the friends of depressed female adolescents reported that they provided *more* emotional support in their friendships than did the friends of nondepressed adolescents (Daley & Hammen, 2002). The discrepancy between youth and friend reports of friendship quality may be due to several factors, including a negative perceptual bias in depressed youth or an inability for depressed youth to accept initial offers of support, perhaps leading to withdrawal of support and dissolution of the friendship over time. Research also links depression with problematic romantic relationships. For example, adolescents with higher levels of depressive symptoms report more negative qualities (e.g., conflict, criticism, and exclusion) in their romantic relationships (La Greca & Harrison, 2005). According to both adolescent women with depressive symptoms and their romantic partners, these women receive less emotional support from their partners than do nondepressed women (Daley & Hammen, 2002).

A considerable data base also reveals significant disturbance in the family relationships of depressed youth. Research based on youth perceptions consistently links depression with several types of dysfunction, including decreased intimacy and satisfaction in parent–child relationships (Herman-Stahl & Petersen, 1999), lower levels of parental acceptance and higher levels of parental psychological control (Garber, Robinson, & Valentiner, 1997; Rudolph et al., 1997), and higher levels of maternal criticism (Frye & Garber, 2005). Depressed youth also describe their families as less cohesive and adaptable, less open to emotional expressiveness, more hostile and rejecting, more conflictual and disorganized, and less likely to engage in pleasant activities (Hops, Lewinsohn, Andrews, & Roberts, 1990; Sheeber & Sorensen, 1998). Once again, other sources of information confirm that self-reports of family relationship difficulties are, at least in part, accurate appraisals of reality. For example, parents of depressed youth describe more impairment (e.g., less warmth and more hostility) in the mother–child relationship relative to the parents of nondepressed youth (Puig-Antich et al., 1993). Moreover, research on expressed emotion reveals higher levels of criticism and emotional over-involvement in the parents' descriptions about depressed children than about non-depressed children (Asarnow, Tompson, Woo, & Cantwell, 2001; Goodman, Adamson, Riniti, & Cole, 1994).

Observations of family interactions provide similar evidence of disruption in parent–child relationships. For instance, the mothers of depressed youth are more dominant in parent–child interactions (Kobak, Sudler, & Gamble, 1991) and show less support, validation, and positive behavior (e.g., smiling, approving) toward their children (Messer & Gross, 1995; Sheeber & Sorensen, 1998) than the mothers of nondepressed children. In family-wide interactions, mothers of depressed youth direct more negative attention toward their children than do the mothers of nondepressed youth (Dadds, Sanders, Morrison, & Rebgetz, 1992). Although depressed youth report higher levels of family conflict, observations of parent–child interactions do not always reveal overtly hostile or conflictual behavior (Sheeber & Sorensen, 1998).

Consistent with research examining specific types of impairment in close relationships, life stress research paints a general picture of interpersonal disruption and conflict in the lives of depressed youth. For example, extensive interviews of depressed youth and their parents reveal that these youth experience heightened chronic strain (e.g., more isolation and negativity, less reciprocity) and acute life stress (e.g., arguments, termination of relationships) in their peer, romantic, and family relationships (Daley & Hammen, 2002; Rudolph et al., 2000).

It is likely that the social-behavioral deficits of depressed youth explain, in part, their involvement in negative and stressful relationships. However, other processes (e.g., peer group selection and peer group influence) may also increase the likelihood that depressed youth experience relationship disturbances. For example, depressed youth may have more limited options for friends owing to their inadequate social skills, or may be attracted to peers or romantic partners with depression or other types of disorders owing to homophily effects (Hogue & Steinberg, 1995) or assortative mating. Indeed, female adolescents with depressive symptoms tend to pair themselves with romantic partners who have heightened levels of personality disorder symptoms (Daley & Hammen, 2002). As a result, depressed youth may become friends or romantic partners with socially unskilled peers, resulting in poorer quality relationships. Peer group selection effects also may result from depressed youths' tendency to engage in negative feedback seeking. Specifically, research demonstrates that depressed youth are more likely than nondepressed youth to seek out and prefer negative evaluations from peers (Cassidy, Aikins, & Chernoff, 2003; Joiner, Katz, & Lew, 1997). Finally, relationship disturbances may arise from the "contagion" effects of depressive symptoms and associated deficits, resulting in the spread of impairment among friends (Hogue & Steinberg, 1995; Stevens & Prinstein, 2005). This contagion effect may cause the deterioration of relationships over time.

TRANSACTIONS BETWEEN INTERPERSONAL DYSFUNCTION AND DEPRESSION

Despite ample evidence that depressed youth show social-behavioral deficits and disturbances in their relationships, much of the research to date involves concurrent designs

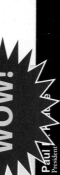
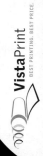

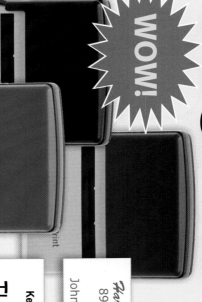
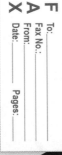

that fail to examine the transactional aspect of interpersonal models. Moreover, little theoretical elaboration has been provided concerning the processes that account for the reciprocal linkages between interpersonal dysfunction and depression. In the following sections, we propose several explanations for why interpersonal dysfunction may serve as a risk factor for depression, and why depression may contribute to declines in interpersonal functioning. We also present supportive empirical evidence for this bidirectional partnership.

Interpersonal Dysfunction as a Risk Factor for Depression

There are several pathways through which interpersonal dysfunction (i.e., social-behavioral deficits and relationship disturbances) may influence the onset, persistence, or recurrence of depression. First, interpersonal dysfunction may contribute to maladaptive social-cognitive processes and negative self-evaluation. For example, according to Cole's competence-based model of depression (Cole, Martin, & Powers, 1997; Cole, Martin, Powers, & Truglio, 1996), children internalize negative competence-related feedback from significant others in the form of negative self-perceptions, which heighten the risk for future depression. Youth who consistently experience interpersonal dysfunction, as reflected in their own social-behavioral deficits or disturbances in their relationships, may develop negative beliefs about their own competence and worth in relationships (e.g., Caldwell, Rudolph, Troop-Gordon, & Kim, 2004; Egan & Perry, 1998), may internalize blame for these difficulties (Graham & Juvonen, 1998), and may feel helpless about their ability to improve their relationships (Rudolph et al., 2001). These negative self-views and perceived loss of control over their social worlds may then precipitate negative affect, feelings of worthlessness or hopelessness, and other symptoms of depression (Abramson et al., 2002). Second, chronic interpersonal dysfunction may interfere with the development of effective self-regulation abilities. Youth exposed to significant relationship disturbances may lack adequate opportunities to learn adaptive ways of managing their emotions or may become sensitized to challenging social situations. Difficulties with self-regulation may increase the likelihood that youth become overwhelmed by negative emotions, thereby heightening their risk for depression (Garber, Braafladt, & Zeman, 1991). Third, exposure to interpersonal dysfunction may disrupt the biological systems underlying stress responses (Suomi, 1991). This sensitivity of the stress–response system may then heighten reactivity to future problems in relationships, creating a risk for depression. Finally, interpersonal dysfunction may diminish the positive reinforcement and support that youth typically receive from their relationship partners (Joiner, 2002), thereby precipitating or maintaining depression (Lewinsohn, 1974).

Some prospective longitudinal research supports the idea that interpersonal dysfunction serves as a risk factor for depression. Social-behavioral deficits, such as excessive reassurance seeking, social withdrawal, and negative feedback seeking, predict subsequent depression in youth (Boivin, Hymel, & Bukowski, 1995; Borelli & Prinstein, 2006; Prinstein et al., 2005). Research also links relationship disturbances, such as peer rejection (Nolan et al., 2003; Panak & Garber, 1992) and termination of romantic relationships (Monroe, Rohde, Seeley, & Lewinsohn, 1999), with subsequent depression. Similarly, disturbances in family relationships contribute to youth depression over time. For instance, youths' perceptions of diminished parental (Lewinsohn et al., 1994; Stice, Ragan, & Randall, 2004) and family-wide (Davies & Windle, 1997) support and intimacy, and multi-informant reports (self, parent, observations) of less supportive and more conflictual parent–child relationships (Sheeber, Hops, Alpert, Davis, & Andrews,

1997), predict future depressive symptoms. More broadly, research from a life stress perspective reveals that youth exposed to stressful events within their relationships experience more depression over time (Hankin, Mermelstein, & Roesch, 2007).

Interpersonal Dysfunction as a Consequence of Depression

Despite the transactional emphasis of interpersonal models of depression (Coyne, 1976; Joiner, 2002) and more general developmental psychopathology models of depression (Cicchetti & Toth, 1998; Hammen, 1992; Hankin & Abramson, 2001; Rudolph, Hammen, & Daley, 2006), most of the research in this area focuses on the interpersonal *antecedents* of depression. Far less is known about the interpersonal *consequences* of depression. Especially lacking is prospective longitudinal research examining how depression influences subsequent interpersonal functioning. Depressive symptoms and associated impairment may have both short-term and long-term adverse interpersonal consequences. Specific symptoms and features of depressed youth may interfere with the expression of competent interpersonal behavior and promote maladaptive interpersonal behavior, thereby resulting in proximal relationship disturbances. Moreover, depression may leave an interpersonal "scar" (Rohde, Lewinsohn, & Seeley, 1990) that lasts well beyond the acute episode, interfering with the development of subsequent interpersonal competencies and causing long-term disturbances in relationships.

Short-Term Social-Behavioral Deficits and Relationship Disturbances

In the short term, specific symptoms and associated characteristics of depressed youth may undermine their ability to function adaptively in social situations and may compromise their relationships. For example, depressive symptoms and behaviors such as fatigue, lack of motivation, social withdrawal, and anhedonia may cause depressed youth to disengage from their social environments, leading to isolation from peers, poor quality friendships and romantic relationships, or alienation from family members. Moreover, irritability and difficulties with emotion regulation in depressed youth may foster aversive social interactions, thus eliciting peer rejection or creating conflict within the family. Symptoms of depression such as self-doubt and feelings of worthlessness may lead youth to engage in excessive efforts to seek reassurance from significant others; if these efforts fail to pacify the depressed youth, significant others may eventually react with annoyance and anger or may withdraw from the youth, which can lead to stress in relationships (Joiner, Metalsky, et al., 1999; Potthoff, Holahan, & Joiner, 1995). Depressive symptoms also lead to a negative focus on the self (Cole, Martin, Peeke, Seroczynski, & Hoffman, 1998; Pomerantz & Rudolph, 2003) and a tendency to engage in more negative statements during conversations with friends (Segrin & Flora, 1998). Excessive negative self-focus may make interactions with depressed youth unpleasant and frustrating and may therefore alienate relationship partners.

Research supports the idea that specific behaviors of depressed youth interfere with the expression of adaptive interpersonal competencies. For example, one study revealed that depressed inpatient youth engage in less social activity and show less affect-related expression than do nondepressed youth (Kazdin, Esveldt-Dawson, Sherick, & Colbus, 1985). Moreover, observations of depressed youth during structured laboratory interactions reveal that they show heightened emotion dysregulation and evoke negative responses from their partners even when interacting with *unfamiliar* peers (Connolly et al., 1992; Rudolph et al., 1994), suggesting that depressive symptoms and behaviors interfere with interpersonal interactions during the formation of new relationships. Consistent with these observations, interviews with depressed youth and their parents suggest that these youth experience more self-generated interpersonal stress, or stress to which they contribute, than do nondepressed youth (Rudolph et al., 2000). Thus, depressed youth, in part, seem to create aversive interpersonal encounters and relationship disturbances.

Long-Term Social-Behavioral Deficits and Relationship Disturbances

Traditional interpersonal models of depression focus in large part on the proximal social-behavioral deficits and relationship disturbances created by depressive symptoms. However, equally important are the potential long-term interpersonal consequences of depression. Early-onset depressive symptoms may interfere with the achievement of key developmental tasks within relationships; thus, youth with a history of depression may fail to acquire the critical skills necessary to develop and maintain high-quality relationships.

Despite the importance of understanding the long-term interpersonal impact of depression, little is known about how depression influences subsequent relationship well-being. Some prospective longitudinal research does support the idea that depression contributes to social-behavioral deficits and relationship disturbances over relatively short periods. For instance, depressive symptoms in youth predict heightened social helplessness (Nolen-Hoeksema et al., 1992), negative feedback seeking (Borelli & Prinstein, 2006), peer rejection (Little & Garber, 1995), instability of friendships (Prinstein et al., 2005), poorer self-reported (but not friend-reported) friendship quality (Prinstein et al., 2005), and the generation of romantic relationship stress (Hankin et al., 2007) over the course of 3 months to 12 months, although some research does not support links between depression and subsequent social difficulties (e.g., Brendgen et al., 2002; Cole et al., 1996). Little research examines the longer-term interpersonal consequences of depression, although one study revealed that depression predicts declines in perceived peer support in girls over the course of 2 years (Stice et al., 2004). More broadly, adolescent depression predicts considerable psychosocial maladjustment associated with the transition to adulthood, including disturbances in romantic relationships (e.g., Gotlib, Lewinsohn, & Seeley, 1998; Rao, Hammen, & Daley, 1999). Several studies suggest that depressive symptoms do not predict long-term declines in family relationships (Hankin et al., 2007; Rao et al., 1999; Sheeber et al., 1997; Stice et al., 2004).

DEVELOPMENTAL ORIGINS OF INTERPERSONAL VULNERABILITY: HOW DOES EARLY FAMILY DISRUPTION CONTRIBUTE TO SOCIAL-BEHAVIORAL DEFICITS AND RELATIONSHIP DISTURBANCES?

Collectively, the aforementioned findings illustrate the importance of interpersonal models that emphasize the ongoing transactions between depressed youth and their interpersonal environments over time. However, interpersonal theories of depression and the supportive empirical evidence provide little insight into how the social-behavioral deficits and relationship disturbances characteristic of depression-prone youth develop. Creating a comprehensive, developmentally sensitive interpersonal model of depression requires a consideration of how individual differences in interpersonal vulnerability (i.e., social-behavioral deficits and relationship disturbances) emerge. In particular, we consider the role of early family disruption (see Figure 4.1). Although a variety of forms of early family disruption (e.g., parental psychopathology, maltreatment, maladaptive parent socialization) likely contribute to the development of interpersonal vulnerability to depression, we focus for two reasons on insecure parent–child attachment and parental depression. First, other types of interpersonal adversity are highlighted in another chapter in this book (see Harkness & Lumley, Chapter 19, this volume). Second, considerable theory and research implicate insecure parent–child attachment and parental depression as early precursors of youth depression—we suggest that interpersonal vulnerability serves as a key explanatory mechanism underlying this link.

Attachment and Interpersonal Vulnerability

Attachment theory (Bowlby, 1969) emphasizes the role of early interactions with caregivers (e.g., responsiveness, emotional support) in the emergence of relatively stable attachment orientations and internal working models of the self (as worthy or unworthy of love and nurturance) and others (as responsive and trustworthy or unresponsive and untrustworthy) (Ainsworth, Blehar, Waters, & Wall, 1978; Main, Kaplan, & Cassidy, 1985). These internal working models are believed to influence youths' developing interpersonal competencies and relationships. Youth who form insecure attachments are presumed to develop maladaptive conceptions of self and others in relationships and accompanying interpersonal dysfunction. Although insecure attachment may be viewed as a type of relationship disturbance, and thus a proximal antecedent of depression, we conceptualize insecure attachment as a distal developmental foundation for relationships that is translated into more proximal forms of interpersonal vulnerability later in life.

Consistent with this conceptualization, youth with insecure attachment show specific social-behavioral deficits and relationship disturbances that are linked to depression. With regard to social-behavioral deficits, an insecure attachment orientation interferes with the development of socially competent behavior and effective emotion regulation. Insecurely attached youth show a tendency to seek less positive feedback than securely attached youth (Cassidy, Ziv, Mehta, & Feeney, 2003). Insecurely attached adolescents report lower levels of interpersonal competence with peers, including less assertiveness (Kobak & Sceery, 1988) and more submissiveness (Irons & Gilbert, 2005) in social situations, although observations suggest that insecurely attached preschoolers display heightened aggression against peers (Troy & Sroufe, 1987). Insecurely attached infants engage in more self-directed (e.g., self-soothing, distraction) than parent-directed emotion regulation strategies when experiencing distress (Diener, Mangelsdorf, McHale, & Frosch, 2002). Moreover, insecurely attached infants demonstrate increasing levels of negative emotionality into toddlerhood (Kochanska, 2001). During adolescence, insecurely attached youth report that they engage in less support seeking (Shirk, Gudmundsen, & Burwell, 2005) and more maladaptive avoidant responses to stress (Howard & Medway, 2004). Moreover, peers describe insecurely attached adolescents as less ego-resilient than securely attached adolescents (Kobak & Sceery, 1988). Insecurely attached youth also show a variety of relationship disturbances that are linked to depression. For example, these youth are more likely than secure youth to be targets of peer victimization (Troy & Sroufe, 1987) and to develop lower-quality friendships (Lieberman, Doyle, & Markiewicz, 1999; Youngblade & Belsky, 1992).

In sum, research supports the idea that a history of insecure caregiver–child attachment predicts the emergence of social-behavioral deficits and relationship disturbances that heighten vulnerability to depression. Insecurely attached youth have difficulty forming and maintaining adaptive relationships, perhaps because of their negative emotionality, maladaptive responses to interpersonal stress, and tendency to seek out negative feedback from others. Thus, these youth may create aversive social environments over time, which then reinforce maladaptive internal working models of the self and others and heighten their risk for depression.

Parental Depression and Interpersonal Vulnerability

Another key risk factor for youth depression is a child's being raised by a depressed parent (for a review, see Goodman & Gotlib, 1999; see also Goodman & Tully, Chapter 17, this volume). Heightened risk for depression in the offspring of depressed parents is likely mediated in part by social-behavioral deficits and relationship disturbances. Depressed mothers are more hostile and critical, more withdrawn, and less positive with their children than are nondepressed mothers (Lovejoy, Graczyk, O'Hare, & Neuman, 2000). In their review, Goodman and Gotlib (1999) propose that because depressed mothers are preoccupied with negative cognitions, affect, and behavior, and their parent–child interactions are marked by discord, depressed mothers prove to be poor social partners for their children, often leaving their offspring with their socioemotional needs unmet. This lack of social support, in combination with high levels of stress in the families of depressed mothers, prevent youth from developing adequate social skills (Goodman & Gotlib, 1999), potentially leading to social-behavioral deficits that heighten their risk for depression. Maternal depression also is linked to dysfunctional socialization of coping (Abaied & Rudolph, 2007) and to atypical development of neural circuits guiding emotion regulation and expression (Dawson et al., 2003). Both psychological and physiological processes may therefore underlie the development of emotion regulation deficits and maladaptive responses to stress that create a vulnerability to depression. Beyond depressive symptoms, heightened interpersonal stress experienced by depressed mothers has adverse effects on parenting quality, which in turn predicts relationship disturbances in youth (e.g., low peer acceptance, poorer-quality friendships, and the generation of interpersonal stress; Hammen et al., 2004).

In sum, parental depression contributes to youths' interpersonal vulnerability to depression by compromising their acquisition of social competencies and effective emotion regulation strategies. These social-behavioral deficits may heighten both the generation of, and reactivity to, relationship disturbances in the offspring of depressed parents. It also is possible that depressed parents contribute a genetic liability to interpersonal vulnerability through the transmission of personality characteristics that foster interpersonal dysfunction, a possibility that awaits further exploration.

VULNERABILITY–STRESS PERSPECTIVES IN AN INTERPERSONAL CONTEXT

Consistent with vulnerability–stress perspectives on youth depression (Hankin & Abela, 2005), youth may differ in the extent to which interpersonal dysfunction heightens their risk for depression or in the extent to which depression undermines interpersonal functioning. Consideration of vulnerability–stress perspectives therefore highlights the interface between interpersonal models and other perspectives on youth depression. Here we briefly discuss three possible moderators of the link between interpersonal dysfunction and depression: (1) personality and social-cognitive style; (2) gender and gender-linked processes, and (3) developmental transitions, particularly the transition to adolescence. Most of the research in this area focuses on moderation of the association between relationship disturbances and depression. However, it also is feasible that these moderators influence the association between social-behavioral deficits and depression (see Figure 4.1).

Personality and Social-Cognitive Style

Vulnerability–stress models propose a number of personality and social-cognitive characteristics that intensify depressive responses to stress (Hankin & Abela, 2005). Although much of the work in this area does not focus specifically on interpersonal dysfunction, some theory and research distinguishes between interpersonal and noninterpersonal types of vulnerability and stress. Psychodynamic and cognitive vulnerability–stress models of depression similarly propose that a personality style characterized by a tendency to base one's self-worth on success or approval in relationships, called "interpersonal dependency" (Blatt & Homann, 1992) or "sociotropy" (Clark, Steer, Beck, & Ross, 1995), heightens depressive responses to interpersonal stress. Consistent with these theories, some research supports the idea that youth who endorse high levels of sociotropy or dependency are more likely to become depressed in the face of interpersonal dysfunction than those who endorse low levels (e.g., Abela, McIntyre-Smith, & Dechef, 2003; Fichman, Koestner, & Zuroff, 1997; Little & Garber, 2005), although other research does not support this view (Abela & Taylor, 2003).

More generally, research demonstrates that a number of personality and social-cognitive characteristics, such as a heightened need for approval (Rudolph, Caldwell, & Conley, 2005), insecure attachment cognitions (Abela et al., 2005; Hammen et al., 1995), an investment in peer status and a negative attributional style (Prinstein & Aikins, 2004), and an anxious behavioral style (Gazelle & Rudolph, 2004) interact with social-behavioral deficits (e.g., excessive reassurance seeking) and relationship disturbances (e.g., peer rejection, victimization, and exclusion; stressful interpersonal life events) to predict depression. Together, this research points to the importance of considering why some individuals are more susceptible to depression in the face of interpersonal dysfunction than others. Little research has investigated individual differences in the influence of depression on subsequent interpersonal behavior and relationships, but one might imagine that certain personality or social-cognitive styles would increase the likelihood that depressive symptoms are expressed in ways that cause social-behavioral deficits and relationship disturbances. Future research needs to examine this possibility.

Gender and Gender-Linked Processes

Contemporary theories of depression emphasize the role of gender-linked interpersonal processes in the onset and course of depression (Hankin & Abramson, 2001; Nolen-Hoeksema, 2002; Rudolph, 2002). In particular, theory and research suggest that, in comparison to males, females are more likely to rely on relationships as a source of self-definition, show heightened interpersonal dependency, emphasize relationship-oriented goals, and have concerns about social evaluation (for a review, see Rose & Rudolph, 2006). Moreover, girls are more likely than boys to respond to interpersonal stress in ways that exacerbate depressive symptoms, such as ruminating about their problems (for a review, see Rose & Rudolph, 2006). This type of interpersonal orientation and response style likely amplifies girls' depressive responses to interpersonal dysfunction.

As discussed earlier, research suggests that certain female-linked interpersonal orientation styles (e.g., a tendency toward dependency and sociotropy) interact with interpersonal dysfunction to predict depression. Little research has examined the moderating role of other gender-linked characteristics, such as goal orientation or social-evaluative concerns. However, direct investigations of sex differences in stress reactivity generally support the idea that relationship disturbances are linked more strongly to depression in girls than in boys (e.g., Ge, Lorenz, Conger, Elder, & Simons, 1994; Hankin et al., 2007; Rudolph, 2002; Rudolph & Hammen, 1999; cf. La Greca & Harrison, 2005). Moreover, research suggests that poor friendship quality and peer rejection predict depressive symptoms over time in girls but not in boys, specifically in girls with high levels of reassurance seeking (for friendship quality; Prinstein et al., 2005), highly reactive temperaments (for peer rejection; Brendgen, Wanner, Morin, & Vitaro, 2005), negative attributional styles (for peer rejection; Prinstein & Aikins, 2004), and a high investment in peer status (for peer rejection; Prinstein & Aikins, 2004). In the family, lower perceptions of parental support predict subsequent depressive symptoms in girls but not in boys (Slavin & Rainer, 1990), although this sex difference may be limited to *self-perceptions* of diminished family support (Sheeber et al., 1997).

Depression may also have more negative interpersonal *consequences* for girls than for boys. Girls' friendships are characterized by a greater exchange of emotional provisions such as validation, affection, and nurturance than those of boys. Moreover, girls are more likely than boys to engage in intimate self-disclosure with their close friends (for a review, see Rose & Rudolph, 2006). Thus, developing and maintaining relationships may place larger emotional demands on girls than on boys. Depressive symptoms such as a lack of motivation and anhedonia may interfere with girls' ability to engage in relationship-building and relationship-maintaining behaviors. In support of this idea, one study revealed that depressive symptoms during third grade predicted a decline in the number of reciprocal friendships and poorer friendship quality in girls, but not in boys, 3 years later, suggesting that early-onset symptoms may exert long-term negative effects on girls' friendships (Rudolph, Ladd, & Dinella, 2007). Moreover, depression-linked social-behavioral deficits (e.g., excessive reassurance seeking) may be met with more negative reactions in female than in male friendships because girls expect friends to accept their offers of support and reassurance. Consistent with this idea, one study revealed that reassurance seeking predicted poorer friendship quality over time in girls but not in boys, although gender did not moderate the influence of depressive symptoms on subsequent friendship quality (Prinstein et al., 2005). More research is needed to examine whether certain aspects of interpersonal behavior and relationships are more adversely affected by depression in girls than in boys.

Developmental Transitions

Developmental transitions may constitute sensitive periods for the activation of depression-linked interpersonal processes, particularly in girls (Rudolph et al., 2006). Normative challenges and disruptions that occur during transitions may intensify youths' interpersonal vulnerability to depression and may exacerbate the interpersonal consequences of depression. In particular, understanding developmental influences on the interpersonal context of depression is critical during the transition to adolescence. Rates of depression rise sharply during adolescence, especially in girls (Hankin et al., 1998). Moreover, the transition to adolescence is marked by a variety of social challenges produced by major maturational changes (e.g., the onset of puberty) and social-contextual changes (e.g., the transition to middle school). During this time, the peer group takes on a more powerful role as a context of socialization as youth begin to rely more on their friends for intimacy and support (Brown, Dolcini, & Leventhal, 1997). At the same time, peer networks may be disrupted as a result of alienation from familiar peers and the formation of new relationships that co-occur with school transitions (Simmons, Burgeson, Carlton-Ford, & Blyth, 1987). Moreover, youth become increasingly involved in platonic heterosexual relationships and romantic relationships that present new challenges and stressors (Leaper & Anderson, 1997). Significant changes also occur in family relationships during this time, including increased parent–child conflict (for a review, see Laursen, 1996). Along with these varied interpersonal disruptions, adolescents are faced with the challenges of negotiating the physical, psychological, and social changes accompanying puberty.

Normative interpersonal challenges associated with the adolescent transition may both directly increase risk for depression and may moderate the influence of nonnormative interpersonal dysfunction. These processes may be particularly salient in adolescent girls, given the intensification of sex differences in interpersonal orientation and response style discussed earlier, as well as the intensification of sex differences in the nature of relationships (e.g., increased stress and conflict) during adolescence (for a review, see Rose & Rudolph, 2006). Moreover, depression may have more adverse interpersonal consequences during adolescence than during preadolescence. That is, socialbehavioral deficits and relationship disturbances resulting from depression may become particularly impairing when youth, especially girls, are required to negotiate the more complex, emotionally charged, and stressful relationships that evolve during adolescence.

Research supports the idea that heightened interpersonal challenges explain, in part, the emergence of sex differences in depression during adolescence. For example, relative to adolescent boys, adolescent girls face more stress within their own friendships (Rudolph, 2002), peer relationships (Hankin et al., 2007), and family relationships (Hankin et al., 2007), and report more stressors experienced by their friends (Gore, Aseltine, & Colton, 1993). This exposure to stress helps to account for sex differences in depression. Moreover, heightened peer stress partially accounts for the association between early pubertal timing and depression in girls (Conley & Rudolph, 2007), suggesting that the physical manifestations of puberty may be translated into stressful interpersonal contexts that increase risk for depression in adolescent girls. Adolescent girls (particularly those with a preoccupied relational style) who are involved in romantic relationships also are at higher risk for subsequent depression in comparison to their nondating peers (Davila, Steinberg, Kachadourian, Cobb, & Fincham, 2004), indicating the stressful nature of these emerging relationships.

Few studies have examined age differences in the interpersonal antecedents of depression. Some limited research suggests that relationship disturbances contribute to depression more strongly in older than in younger youth (e.g., Cole et al., 1996). Focusing on physical maturation rather than age, other research indicates that pubertal development and relationship disturbances interact in their contribution to depression. For instance, early pubertal timing predicts subsequent depression in girls who experience high levels of stress in their peer relationships but not in those who experience low levels of peer stress (Conley & Rudolph, 2006). Moreover, heterosexual romantic involvement is especially likely to predict depressive symptoms in adolescent girls who are more advanced in their pubertal development (Hayward & Sanborn, 2002). Early maturing girls may be particularly sensitive to interpersonal stress because they experience various interpersonal challenges (e.g., the onset of dating) earlier than their age-mates, perhaps before they are psychologically prepared to deal with these challenges.

Overall, therefore, a developmentally based interpersonal model has significant promise for explaining why girls are especially vulnerable to increases in depression during adolescence. Research has not directly investigated whether depression has different interpersonal consequences across development. Once again, we might hypothesize that the adverse effects of depression would be heightened during the adolescent period. This stage likely taxes youths' interpersonal resources and capacities owing to the many changes they need to negotiate. However, as discussed earlier, it is possible that depression occurring early in life leaves a permanent interpersonal "scar" (Rohde et al., 1990), such that social-behavioral deficits stemming from early-onset depression interfere with emerging relationships during the adolescent transition even in the absence of concurrent depression.

SUMMARY OF A DEVELOPMENTALLY BASED INTERPERSONAL MODEL OF DEPRESSION

To summarize the proposed developmentally based interpersonal model of youth depression (see Figure 4.1), early family disruption (e.g., insecure attachment or parental depression) interferes with the development of social competencies, leading to a range of social-behavioral deficits. This intergenerational transmission of interpersonal impairment likely occurs as a function of direct modeling of parental social behavior, explicit and implicit parental socialization of maladaptive responses to stress, genetic liability to emotion dysregulation and associated social-behavioral deficits, and the internalization of maladaptive conceptions of self and others. Social-behavioral deficits, in turn, cause youth to create disturbances in their relationships (e.g., isolation, conflict, poor quality relationships) and to select into maladaptive relationships. Early disruption due to insecure parent–child attachment and parental depression may also be directly expressed as ongoing difficulties within the family. These relationship disturbances create a vulnerability to depression, particularly in youth with personality and social-cognitive styles that intensify their adverse reactions to interpersonal stress. Interpersonal vulnerability to depression is amplified during the transition to adolescence, particularly in girls, owing to the simultaneous challenges faced by youth (e.g., negotiating the physical, psychological, and social changes of puberty; the growing complexity of relationships; the emergence of romantic relationships) and the intensification of gender-linked interpersonal characteristics and experiences that heighten girls' risk. Depression, in turn, compromises youths' short-term interpersonal functioning and long-term social development, setting them on a trajectory toward recurrent or chronic depression.

FUTURE DIRECTIONS

Considerable progress has been made in understanding the interpersonal context of youth depression. Moreover, recent prospective longitudinal research has begun to provide a more careful evaluation of the interpersonal antecedents and, to a lesser extent, consequences of youth depression. To further advance both theory and research in this area, future work would benefit from a developmentally informed approach that places interpersonal theories of depression into a developmental context. Here we propose four critical areas that warrant attention: (1) expanding on the early origins of interpersonal vulnerability, (2) elucidating the developmental processes underlying the reciprocal link between interpersonal dysfunction and depression, (3) understanding developmental changes in interpersonal vulnerability, and (4) identifying developmentally relevant moderators of the association between interpersonal dysfunction and depression.

Expanding on the Early Origins of Interpersonal Vulnerability

Although preliminary research sheds some light on how early family disruption associated with insecure attachment and parental depression contributes to the emergence of interpersonal vulnerability to depression, much remains to be learned about the origins of depression-linked social-behavioral deficits and relationship disturbances. Moreover, such research needs to be integrated more comprehensively into interpersonal models of depression. In particular, theory and empirical research must address whether particular types of family disruption contribute to particular aspects of interpersonal vulnerability (e.g., excessive reassurance seeking, negative feedback seeking, maladaptive responses to interpersonal stress), and whether the contribution of family disruption differs according to the stage of development during which it occurs. More in-depth investigations are also needed to identify forms of early disruption other than insecure attachment relationships and parental depression (e.g., family conflict, maltreatment) that contribute to interpersonal vulnerability to depression.

Elucidating the Developmental Processes Linking Interpersonal Dysfunction and Depression

Advancing current interpersonal models of depression requires an understanding of the processes through which interpersonal dysfunction confers risk for depression. In this chapter, we proposed several possible pathways, including the internalization of relationship disturbances in the form of negative beliefs about one's worth, competence, and control; compromised self-regulatory abilities; and dysfunctional biological responses to stress. Although little empirical attention has been paid to this issue, some research points to possible mechanisms. For example, one study revealed that rumination partially accounted for the concurrent association between diminished perceived social support and depression (Abela, Vanderbilt, & Rochon, 2004). In another study, negative self-evaluation mediated the longitudinal association between interpersonal stress and subsequent depressive symptoms (Groot & Rudolph, 2007). These studies suggest that relationship disturbances set in motion a negative, ruminative self-focus that increases vulnerability to depression. Research is needed to examine directly other possible pathways underlying the adverse influence of interpersonal dysfunction on depression.

Moreover, significantly more research is needed to understand the short- and long-term interpersonal consequences of depression. Specifically, we need to expand our knowledge about how depressed youth create interpersonal dysfunction, both during the course of a depressive episode and over time. Do specific types of symptoms (e.g., fatigue and anhedonia versus self-doubt versus irritability) lead to particular types of interpersonal dysfunction (e.g., social disengagement versus excessive reassurance seeking versus interpersonal conflict)? Are there particular critical periods during which depression interferes with the maturation of interpersonal competencies, setting youth on a long-term trajectory of interpersonal dysfunction? Delineating these pathways can inform dynamic interpersonal theories that consider youth as active participants in the construction and shaping of their social worlds, as well as provide information about potential targets of intervention with depressed youth.

Understanding Developmental Changes in the Interpersonal Antecedents and Consequences of Depression

Much remains to be learned about how depression-linked interpersonal dysfunction changes across development. Very little research has examined age or maturation differences in the interpersonal antecedents or consequences of depression. However, some research, discussed earlier, does identify the transition to adolescence as a sensitive period during which heightened interpersonal dysfunction accounts for higher rates of depression, particularly in girls. Moreover, the transition through puberty (particularly when it is early relative to one's peers) appears to intensify depressive responses to relationship disturbances in girls. Clearly, it is essential to both theory and intervention to understand more about the extent to which interpersonal processes underlying the onset and course of depression change across development.

Identifying Developmentally Relevant Moderators of the Interpersonal Dysfunction–Depression Association

Research supports the idea that youth with certain personality and social-cognitive styles are more vulnerable than others to the adverse emotional effects of interpersonal dysfunction. Interpersonal perspectives on depression would benefit from continued integrative efforts aimed at understanding the vulnerability–stress interactions underlying the onset and course of depression, with a focus on those that are relevant at particular stages of development. Other promising candidates include genetic and biological vulnerabilities that heighten youths' depressive responses to social challenges. For instance, recent research reveals that genetic liability interacts with stressful life experiences to predict adolescent depression (Eley et al., 2004), but follow-ups of these findings need to examine the specific liability underlying depressive responses to interpersonal stress. Moreover, despite significant attention to the potential role of neuroendocrine dysregulation and structural and functional brain abnormalities in depression (for a review, see Kaufman, Martin, King, & Charney, 2001), research has not investigated directly how these abnormalities interact with youths' exposure to relationship disturbances to predict depression. One recent study did reveal that a reduced posterior right hemisphere bias in emotion processing was associated with depressive symptoms in youth exposed to high, but not low, levels of peer stress, suggesting that hemispheric asymmetries may create a vulnerability to interpersonal stress (Flynn & Rudolph, 2007). Even less attention has been devoted to examining whether depression undermines interpersonal functioning more strongly in some youth than in others. Further investigation of characteristics and experiences that moderate the association between interpersonal dysfunction and depression is critical for understanding the long-term developmental trajectories of depressed youth and for identifying at-risk youth.

ACKNOWLEDGMENTS

Preparation of this chapter was supported in part by National Institute of Mental Health Grant MH068444 awarded to Karen D. Rudolph. We thank Cathy Koerber for her assistance in preparation of this chapter.

REFERENCES

Abaied, J., & Rudolph, K. D. (2007). *Maternal socialization of coping during early adolescence.* Manuscript submitted for publication.

Abela, J. J. R., Hankin, B. L., Haigh, E. A. P., Adams, P., Vinokuroff, T., & Trayhern, L. (2005). Interpersonal vulnerability to depression in high-risk children: The role of insecure attachment and reassurance seeking. *Journal of Clinical Child and Adolescent Psychology, 34,* 182–192.

Abela, J. R. Z., McIntyre-Smith, A., & Dechef, M. L. E. (2003). Personality predispositions to depression: A test of the specific vulnerability and symptom specificity hypotheses. *Journal of Social and Clinical Psychology, 22,* 493–514.

Abela, J. R. Z., & Taylor, G. (2003). Specific vulnerability to depressive mood reactions in school-children: The moderating role of self-esteem. *Journal of Clinical Child and Adolescent Psychology, 32,* 408–418.

Abela, J. R. Z., Vanderbilt, E., & Rochon, A. (2004). A test of the integration of the response styles and social support theories of depression in third and seventh grade children. *Journal of Social and Clinical Psychology, 23,* 653–674.

Abramson, L. Y., Alloy, L. B., Hankin, B. L., Haeffell, G. J., MacCoon, D. G., & Gibb, B. E. (2002). Cognitive vulnerability–stress models of depression in a self-regulatory and psychobiological context. In I. H. Gotlib & C. L. Hammen (Eds.), *Handbook of depression* (pp. 268–294). New York: Guilford Press.

Ainsworth, M. D., Blehar, M., Waters, E., & Wall, S. (1978). *Patterns of attachment: A psychological study of the Strange Situation.* Hillsdale, NJ: Erlbaum.

Altmann, E. O., & Gotlib, I. H. (1988). The social behavior of depressed children: An observational study. *Journal of Abnormal Child Psychology, 16,* 29–44.

Asarnow, J. R., Tompson, M. C., Woo, S., & Cantwell, D. P. (2001). Is expressed emotion a specific risk factor for depression or a nonspecific correlate of psychopathology? *Journal of Abnormal Child Psychology, 29,* 573–583.

Baker, M., Milich, R., & Manolis, M. (1996). Peer interactions of dysphoric adolescents. *Journal of Abnormal Child Psychology, 24,* 241–255.

Bell-Dolan, D. J., Reaven, N. M., & Peterson, L. (1993). Depression and social functioning: A multidimensional study of the linkages. *Journal of Clinical Child Psychology, 22,* 306–315.

Blatt, S. J., & Homann, E. (1992). Parent–child interaction in the etiology of dependent and self-critical depression. *Clinical Psychology Review, 12,* 47–91.

Boivin, M., Hymel, S., & Bukowski, W. M. (1995). The roles of social withdrawal, peer rejection, and victimization by peers in predicting loneliness and depressed mood in childhood. *Development and Psychopathology, 7,* 765–785.

Borelli, J. L., & Prinstein, M. J. (2006). Reciprocal, longitudinal associations among adolescents' negative feedback-seeking, depressive symptoms, and peer relations. *Journal of Abnormal Child Psychology, 34,* 159–169.

Bowlby, J. (1969). *Attachment and loss: Vol. I. Attachment.* New York: Basic Books.

Brendgen, M., Vitaro, F., Turgeon, L., & Poulin, F. (2002). Assessing aggressive and depressed children's social relations with classmates and friends: A matter of perspective. *Journal of Abnormal Child Psychology, 30,* 609–624.

Brendgen, M., Wanner, B., Morin, A. J. S., & Vitaro, F. (2005). Relations with parents and peers, temperament, and trajectories of depressed mood during early adolescence. *Journal of Abnormal Child Psychology, 33,* 579–594.

Brown, B. B., Dolcini, M. N., & Leventhal, A. (1997). Transformations in peer relationships at adolescence: Implications for health-related behavior. In J. Schulenberg, J. L. Maggs, & K. Hurrelmann (Eds.), *Health risks and developmental transitions during adolescence* (pp. 161–189). New York: Cambridge University Press.

Caldwell, M. S., Rudolph, K. D., Troop-Gordon, W., & Kim, D. (2004). Reciprocal influences among relational self-views, social disengagement, and peer stress during early adolescence. *Child Development, 75,* 1140–1154.

Cassidy, J., Aikins, J. W., & Chernoff, J. J. (2003). Children's peer selection: Experimental examination and the role of self-perceptions. *Developmental Psychology, 39,* 495–508.

Cassidy, J., Ziv, Y., Mehta, T. G., & Feeney, B. C. (2003). Feedback seeking in children and adolescents: Associations with self-perceptions, attachment representations, and depression. *Child Development, 74,* 612–628.

Cicchetti, D. (1993). Developmental psychopathology: Reactions, reflections, projections. *Developmental Review, 13,* 471–502.

Cicchetti, D., & Toth, S. L. (1998). The development of depression in children and adolescents. *American Psychologist, 53,* 221–241.

Clark, D. A., Steer, R. A., Beck, A. T., & Ross, L. (1995). Psychometric characteristics of revised sociotropy and autonomy scales in college students. *Behavior Research and Therapy, 33,* 325–334.

Cole, D. A. (1990). The relation of social and academic competence to depressive symptoms in childhood. *Journal of Abnormal Psychology, 99,* 422–429.

Cole, D. A., Martin, J. M., Peeke, L. G., Seroczynski, A. D., & Hoffman, K. (1998). Are cognitive errors of underestimation predictive or reflective of depressive symptoms in children: A longitudinal study. *Journal of Abnormal Psychology, 107,* 481–496.

Cole, D. A., Martin, J. M., & Powers, B. (1997). A competency-based model of child depression: A longitudinal study of peer, parent, teacher, and self-evaluations. *Journal of Child Psychology and Psychiatry and Allied Disciplines, 38,* 505–514.

Cole, D. A., Martin, J. M., Powers, B., & Truglio, R. (1996). Modeling causal relations between academic and social competence and depression: A multitrait–multimethod longitudinal study of children. *Journal of Abnormal Psychology, 105,* 258–270.

Conley, C. S., & Rudolph, K. D. (2006). *Sex differences in depression: The interactive role of pubertal development and peer stress.* Manuscript submitted for publication.

Conley, C. S., & Rudolph, K. D. (2007). *The role of peer stress in mediating links between pubertal development and depression in adolescence.* Manuscript in preparation.

Connolly, J., Geller, S., Marton, P., & Kutcher, S. (1992). Peer responses to social interaction with depressed adolescents. *Journal of Clinical Child Psychology, 21,* 365–370.

Connor-Smith, J. K., Compas, B. E., Wadsworth, M. E., Thomsen, A. H., & Saltzman, H. (2000). Responses to stress in adolescence: Measurement of coping and involuntary stress responses. *Journal of Consulting and Clinical Psychology, 68,* 976–992.

Coyne, J. C. (1976). Depression and the response of others. *Journal of Abnormal Psychology, 85,* 186–193.

Crick, N. R., & Grotpeter, J. K. (1996). Children's treatment by peers: Victims of relational and overt aggression. *Development and Psychopathology, 8,* 367–380.

Dadds, M. R., Sanders, M. R., Morrison, M., & Rebgetz, M. (1992). Childhood depression and conduct disorder: II. An analysis of family interaction patterns in the home. *Journal of Abnormal Psychology, 101,* 505–513.

Daley, S. E., & Hammen, C. (2002). Depressive symptoms and close relationships during the transition to adulthood: Perspectives from dysphoric women, their best friends, and their romantic partners. *Journal of Consulting and Clinical Psychology, 70,* 129–141.

Davies, P. T., & Windle, M. (1997). Gender-specific pathways between maternal depressive symptoms, family discord, and adolescent adjustment. *Developmental Psychology, 33,* 657–668.

Davila, J., Steinberg, S. J., Kachadourian, L., Cobb, R., & Fincham, F. (2004). Romantic involvement and depressive symptoms in early and late adolescence: The role of a preoccupied relational style. *Personal Relationships, 11,* 161–178.

Dawson, G., Ashman, S. B., Panagiotides, H., Hessl, D., Self, J., Yamada, E., et al. (2003). Preschool outcomes of children of depressed mothers: Role of maternal behavior, contextual risk, and children's brain activity. *Child Development, 74,* 1158–1175.

Diener, M. L., Mangelsdorf, S. C., McHale, J. L., & Frosch, C. A. (2002). Infants' behavioral strategies for emotion regulation with fathers and mothers: Associations with emotional expressions and attachment quality. *Infancy, 3,* 153–174.

Egan, S. K., & Perry, D. G. (1998). Does low self-regard invite victimization? *Developmental Psychology, 34,* 299–309.

Eley, T. C., Sugden, K., Corsico, A., Gregory, A. M., Sham, P., McGuffin, P., et al. (2004). Gene–environment interaction analysis of serotonin system markers with adolescent depression. *Molecular Psychiatry, 9,* 908–918.

Fichman, L., Koestner, R., & Zuroff, D. C. (1997). Dependency and distress at summer camp. *Journal of Youth and Adolescence, 26,* 217–232.

Flynn, M., & Rudolph, K. D. (2007). Perceptual asymmetry and youths' responses to stress: Understanding vulnerability to depression. *Cognition and Emotion, 21,* 773–788.

Frye, A. A., & Garber, J. (2005). The relations among maternal depression, maternal criticism, and adolescents' externalizing and internalizing symptoms. *Journal of Abnormal Child Psychology, 33,* 1–11.

Garber, J., Braafladt, N., & Zeman, J. (1991). The regulation of sad affect: An information-processing perspective. In J. Garber & K. A. Dodge (Eds.), *The development of emotion regulation and dysregulation* (pp. 208–240). New York: Cambridge University Press.

Garber, J., Robinson, N. S., & Valentiner, D. (1997). The relation between parenting and adolescent depression: Self-worth as a mediator. *Journal of Adolescent Research, 12,* 12–33.

Gazelle, H., & Rudolph, K. D. (2004). Moving toward and away from the world: Social approach and avoidance trajectories in anxious solitary youth. *Child Development, 75,* 829–849.

Ge, X., Lorenz, F. O., Conger, R. D., Elder, G. G., & Simons, R. L. (1994). Trajectories of stressful life events and depressive symptoms during adolescence. *Developmental Psychology, 30,* 467–483.

Goodman, S. H., Adamson, L. B., Riniti, J., & Cole, S. (1994). Mother's expressed attitudes: Associations with maternal depression and children's self-esteem and psychopathology. *Journal of the American Academy of Child and Adolescent Psychiatry, 33,* 1265–1274.

Goodman, S. H., & Gotlib, I. H. (1999). Risk for psychopathology in the children of depressed mothers: A developmental model for understanding mechanisms of transmission. *Psychological Review, 106,* 458–490.

Goodyer, I. M., Wright, C., & Altham, P. M. E. (1990). The friendships and recent life events of anxious and depressed school-age children. *British Journal of Psychiatry, 156,* 689–698.

Gore, S., Aseltine, R. H., & Colton, M. E. (1993). Gender, social-relational involvement, and depression. *Journal of Research on Adolescence, 3,* 101–125.

Gotlib, I. H., & Hammen, C. (1992). *Psychological aspects of depression: Toward a cognitive-interpersonal integration.* London: Wiley.

Gotlib, I., Lewinsohn, P., & Seeley, J. (1998). Consequences of depression during adolescence: Marital status and marital functioning in early adulthood. *Journal of Abnormal Psychology, 107,* 686–690.

Graham, S., & Juvonen, J. (1998). Self-blame and peer victimization in middle school: An attributional analysis. *Developmental Psychology, 34,* 538–587.

Groot, A., & Rudolph, K. D. (2007). *Why does anxiety lead to depression? The mediating role of interpersonal stress and negative self-focus.* Manuscript in preparation.

Hammen, C. (1992). Cognitive, life stress, and interpersonal approaches to a developmental psychopathology model of depression. *Development and Psychopathology, 4,* 191–208.

Hammen, C., Burge, D., Daley, S. E., Davila, J., Paley, B., & Rudolph, K. D. (1995). Interpersonal attachment cognitions and prediction of symptomatic responses to interpersonal stress. *Journal of Abnormal Psychology, 104,* 436–443.

Hammen, C., Shih, J. H., & Brennan, P. A. (2004). Intergenerational transmission of depression: Test of an interpersonal stress model in a community sample. *Journal of Consulting and Clinical Psychology, 72,* 511–522.

Hankin, B. L., & Abela, J. R. Z. (2005). *Development of psychopathology: A vulnerability–stress perspective.* London: Sage.

Hankin, B. L., & Abramson, L. Y. (2001). Development of gender differences in depression: An elaborated cognitive vulnerability–transactional stress theory. *Psychological Bulletin, 127,* 773–796.

Hankin, B. L., Abramson, L. Y., Moffitt, T. E., Silva, P. A., McGee, R., & Angell, K. E. (1998). Development of depression from preadolescence to young adulthood: Emerging gender differences in a 10-year longitudinal study. *Journal of Abnormal Psychology, 107,* 128–140.

Hankin, B. L., Mermelstein, R., & Roesch, L. (2007). Sex differences in adolescent depression: Stress exposure and reactivity models in interpersonal and achievement contextual domains. *Child Development, 78,* 279–295.

Hayward, C., & Sanborn, K. (2002). Puberty and the emergence of gender differences in psychopathology. *Journal of Adolescent Health, 30,* 49–58.

Herman-Stahl, M., & Petersen, A. C. (1999). Depressive symptoms during adolescence: Direct and stress-buffering effects of coping, control beliefs, and family relationships. *Journal of Applied Developmental Psychology, 20,* 45–62.

Hogue, A., & Steinberg, L. (1995). Homophily of internalized distress in adolescent peer groups. *Developmental Psychology, 31,* 897–906.

Hops, H., Lewinsohn, P. M., Andrews, J. A., & Roberts, R. E. (1990). Psychosocial correlates of depressive symptomatology among high school students. *Journal of Clinical Child Psychology, 3,* 211–220.

Howard, M. S., & Medway, F. J. (2004). Adolescents' attachment and coping with stress. *Psychology in the Schools, 41,* 391–402.

Irons, C., & Gilbert, P. (2005). Evolved mechanisms in adolescent anxiety and depression symptoms: The role of the attachment and social rank systems. *Journal of Adolescence, 28,* 325–341.

Jaser, S. S., Langrock, A. M., Keller, G., Merchant, M. J., Benson, M. A., Reeslund, K., et al. (2005). Coping with the stress of parental depression: II. Adolescent and parent reports of coping and adjustment. *Journal of Clinical Child and Adolescent Psychology, 34,* 193–205.

Joiner, T. E. (2002). Depression in its interpersonal context. In I. H. Gotlib & C. L. Hammen (Eds.), *Handbook of depression* (pp. 295–313). New York: Guilford Press.

Joiner, T. E., Coyne, J. C., & Blalock, J. (1999). On the interpersonal nature of depression: Overview and synthesis. In T. E. Joiner & J. C. Coyne (Eds.), *The interactional nature of depression* (pp. 3–19). Washington, DC: American Psychological Association.

Joiner, T. E., Katz, J., & Lew, A. S. (1997). Self-verification and depression among youth psychiatric inpatients. *Journal of Abnormal Psychology, 106,* 608–618.

Joiner, T. E., Metalsky, G. I., Katz, J., & Beach, S. R. H. (1999). Depression and excessive reassurance-seeking. *Psychological Inquiry, 10,* 269–278.

Kaufman, J., Martin, A., King, R. A., & Charney, D. (2001). Are child-, adolescent-, and adult-onset depression one and the same disorder? *Biological Psychiatry, 49,* 980–1001.

Kazdin, A. E., Esveldt-Dawson, K., Sherick, R. B., & Colbus, D. (1985). Assessment of overt behavior and childhood depression among psychiatrically disturbed children. *Journal of Consulting and Clinical Psychology, 53,* 201–210.

Kobak, R. R., & Ferenz-Gillies, R. (1995). Emotion regulation and depressive symptoms during adolescence: A functionalist perspective. *Development and Psychopathology, 7,* 183–192.

Kobak, R. R., & Sceery, A. (1988). Attachment in late adolescence: Working models, affect regulation, and representations of self and others. *Child Development, 59,* 135–146.

Kobak, R. R., Sudler, N., & Gamble, W. (1991). Attachment and depressive symptoms during adolescence: A developmental pathways analysis. *Development and Psychopathology, 3,* 461–474.

Kochanska, G. (2001). Emotional development in children with different attachment histories: The first three years. *Child Development, 72,* 474–490.

La Greca, A. M., & Harrison, H. M. (2005). Adolescent peer relations, friendships, and romantic relationships: Do they predict social anxiety and depression? *Journal of Clinical Child and Adolescent Psychology, 34,* 49–61.

Laursen, B. (1996). Closeness and conflict in adolescent peer relationships: Interdependence with friends and romantic partners. In W. M. Bukowski & A. F. Newcomb (Eds.), *The company they keep: Friendship in childhood and adolescence. Cambridge studies in social and emotional development* (pp. 186–210). New York: Cambridge University Press.

Leaper, C., & Anderson, K. J. (1997). Gender development and heterosexual romantic relationships during adolescence. In S. Shulman & W. A. Collins (Eds.), *Romantic relationships in adolescence: Developmental perspectives. New directions for child development, No. 78* (pp. 85–103). San Francisco: Jossey-Bass.

Lewinsohn, P. M. (1974). A behavioral approach to depression. In R. Friedman & M. Katz (Eds.), *The psychology of depression: Contemporary theory and research* (pp. 157–185). Washington, DC: Winston-Wiley.

Lewinsohn, P. M., Roberts, R. E., Seeley, J. R., Rohde, P., Gotlib, I. H., & Hops, H. (1994). Adolescent psychopathology: II. Psychosocial risk factors for depression. *Journal of Abnormal Psychology, 103,* 302–315.

Lewis, M. (1990). Models of developmental psychopathology. In M. Lewis & S. M. Miller (Eds.), *Handbook of developmental psychopathology* (pp. 15–27). New York: Plenum Press.

Lieberman, M., Doyle, A., & Markiewicz, D. (1999). Developmental patterns in security of attachment to mother and father in late childhood and early adolescence: Associations with peer relations. *Child Development, 70,* 202–213.

Little, S. A., & Garber, J. (1995). Aggression, depression, and stressful life events predicting peer rejection in children. *Development and Psychopathology, 7,* 845–856.

Little, S. A., & Garber, J. (2005). The role of social stressors and interpersonal orientation in explaining the longitudinal relation between externalizing and depressive symptoms. *Journal of Abnormal Psychology, 114,* 432–443.

Lovejoy, C. M., Graczyk, P. A., O'Hare, E., & Neuman, G. (2000). Maternal depression and parenting behavior: A meta-analytic review. *Clinical Psychology Review, 20,* 561–592.

Main, M., Kaplan, N., & Cassidy, J. (1985). Security in infancy, childhood, and adulthood: A move to the level of representation. In I. Bretherton & E. Waters (Eds.), *Growing points in attachment theory and research. Monographs of the Society for Research in Child Development, 50,* 66–104.

McGrath, E. P., & Repetti, R. L. (2002). A longitudinal study of children's depressive symptoms, self-perceptions, and cognitive distortions about the self. *Journal of Abnormal Psychology, 111,* 77–87.

Messer, S. C., & Gross, A. M. (1995). Childhood depression and family interaction: A naturalistic observation study. *Journal of Clinical Child Psychology, 24,* 77–88.

Monroe, S. M., Rohde, P., Seeley, J. R., & Lewinsohn, P. M. (1999). Life events and depression in adolescence: Relationship loss as a prospective risk factor for first onset of major depressive disorder. *Journal of Abnormal Psychology, 108,* 606–614.

Nolan, S. A., Flynn, C., & Garber, J. (2003). Prospective relations between rejection and depression in young adolescents. *Journal of Personality and Social Psychology, 85,* 745–755.

Nolen-Hoeksema, S. (2002). Gender differences in depression. In I. H. Gotlib & C. L. Hammen (Eds.), *Handbook of depression* (pp. 492–509). New York: Guilford Press.

Nolen-Hoeksema, S., Girgus, J. S., & Seligman, M. E. P. (1992). Predictors and consequences of childhood depressive symptoms: A 5-year longitudinal study. *Journal of Abnormal Psychology, 101,* 405–422.

Panak, W. F., & Garber, J. (1992). Role of aggression, rejection, and attributions in the prediction of depression in children. *Development and Psychopathology, 4,* 145–165.

Pomerantz, E. M., & Rudolph, K. D. (2003). What ensues from emotional distress? Implications for competence estimation. *Child Development, 74,* 329–345.

Potthoff, J. G., Holahan, C. J., & Joiner, T. E. (1995). Reassurance seeking, stress generation, and depressive symptoms: An integrative model. *Journal of Personality and Social Psychology, 68,* 664–670.

Prinstein, M. J., & Aikins, J. W. (2004). Cognitive moderators of the longitudinal association between peer rejection and adolescent depressive symptoms. *Journal of Abnormal Child Psychology, 32*, 147–158.

Prinstein, M. J., Borelli, J. L., Cheah, C. S. L., Simon, V. A., & Aikins, J. W. (2005). Adolescent girls' interpersonal vulnerability to depressive symptoms: A longitudinal examination of reassurance-seeking and peer relationships. *Journal of Abnormal Psychology, 114*, 676–688.

Puig-Antich, J., Kaufman, J., Ryan, N. D., Williamson, D. E., Dahl, R. E., Lukens, E., et al. (1993). The psychosocial functioning and family environment of depressed adolescents. *Journal of the American Academy of Child and Adolescent Psychiatry, 32*, 244–253.

Quiggle, N. L., Garber, J., Panak, W. F., & Dodge, K. A. (1992). Social information processing in aggressive and depressed children. *Child Development, 63*, 1305–1320.

Rao, U., Hammen, C., & Daley, S. (1999). Continuity of depression during the transition to adulthood: A 5-year longitudinal study of young women. *Journal of the American Academy of Child and Adolescent Psychiatry, 38*, 908–915.

Rohde, P., Lewinsohn, P. M., & Seeley, J. R. (1990). Are people changed by the experience of having an episode of depression? A further test of the scar hypothesis. *Journal of Abnormal Psychology, 99*, 264–271.

Rose, A., & Rudolph, K. D. (2006). A review of sex differences in peer relationship processes: Potential trade-offs for the emotional and behavioral development of girls and boys. *Psychological Bulletin, 132*, 98–131.

Rudolph, K. D. (2002). Gender differences in emotional responses to interpersonal stress during adolescence. *Journal of Adolescent Health, 30*, 3–13.

Rudolph, K. D., Caldwell, M. S., & Conley, C. S. (2005). Need for approval and children's well-being. *Child Development, 76*, 309–323.

Rudolph, K. D., & Clark, A. G. (2001). Conceptions of relationships in children with depressive and aggressive symptoms: Social-cognitive distortion or reality? *Journal of Abnormal Child Psychology, 29*, 41–56.

Rudolph, K. D., & Hammen, C. (1999). Age and gender as determinants of stress exposure, generation, and reactions in youngsters: A transactional perspective. *Child Development, 70*, 660–677.

Rudolph, K. D., Hammen, C., & Burge, D. (1994). Interpersonal functioning and depressive symptoms in childhood: Addressing the issues of specificity and comorbidity. *Journal of Abnormal Child Psychology, 22*, 355–371.

Rudolph, K. D., Hammen, C., & Burge, D. (1997). A cognitive-interpersonal approach to depressive symptoms in preadolescent children. *Journal of Abnormal Child Psychology, 25*, 33–45.

Rudolph, K. D., Hammen, C., Burge, D., Lindberg, N., Herzberg, D. S., & Daley, S. E. (2000). Toward an interpersonal life-stress model of depression: The developmental context of stress generation. *Development and Psychopathology, 12*, 215–234.

Rudolph, K. D., Hammen, C., & Daley, S. E. (2006). Mood disorders. In D. A. Wolfe & E. J. Mash (Eds.), *Behavioral and emotional disorders in adolescents: Nature, assessment, and treatment* (pp. 300–342). New York: Guilford Press.

Rudolph, K. D., Kurlakowsky, K. D., & Conley, C. S. (2001). Developmental and social-contextual origins of depressive control-related beliefs and behavior. *Cognitive Therapy and Research, 25*, 447–475.

Rudolph, K. D., Ladd, G., & Dinella, L. (2007). Gender differences in the interpersonal consequences of early-onset depressive symptoms. *Merrill–Palmer Quarterly, 53*, 461–488.

Segrin, C., & Flora, J. (1998). Depression and verbal behavior in conversations with friends and strangers. *Journal of Language and Social Psychology, 17*, 492–503.

Sheeber, L., Hops, H., Alpert, A., Davis, B., & Andrews, J. A. (1997). Family support and conflict: Prospective relations to adolescent depression. *Journal of Abnormal Child Psychology, 25*, 333–344.

Sheeber, L., & Sorensen, E. (1998). Family relationships of depressed adolescents: A multimethod assessment. *Journal of Clinical Child Psychology, 27*, 268–277.

Shirk, S. R., Gudmundsen, G. R., & Burwell, R. A. (2005). Links among attachment-related cognitions and adolescent depressive symptoms. *Journal of Clinical Child and Adolescent Psychology, 34,* 172–181.

Simmons, R. G., Burgeson, R., Carlton-Ford, S., & Blyth, D. A. (1987). The impact of cumulative change in early adolescence. *Child Development, 58,* 1220–1234.

Slavin, L. A., & Rainer, K. L. (1990). Gender differences in emotional support and depressive symptoms among adolescents: A prospective analysis. *American Journal of Community Psychology, 18,* 407–421.

Steele, R. G., Forehand, R., & Armistead, L. (1997). The role of family processes and coping strategies in the relationship between parental chronic illness and childhood internalizing problems. *Journal of Abnormal Child Psychology, 25,* 83–94.

Stevens, E. A., & Prinstein, M. J. (2005). Peer contagion of depressogenic attributional styles among adolescents: A longitudinal study. *Journal of Abnormal Child Psychology, 33,* 25–37.

Stice, E., Ragan, J., & Randall, P. (2004). Prospective relations between social support and depression: Differential direction of effects for parent and peer support? *Journal of Abnormal Psychology, 113,* 155–159.

Suomi, S. J. (1991). Adolescent depression and depressive symptoms: Insights from longitudinal studies with rhesus monkeys. *Journal of Youth and Adolescence, 20,* 273–287.

Troy, M., & Sroufe, L. A. (1987). Victimization among preschoolers: Role of attachment history. *American Academy of Child and Adolescent Psychiatry, 26,* 166–172.

Windle, M. (1994). A study of friendship characteristics and problem behaviors among middle adolescents. *Child Development, 65,* 1764–1777.

Youngblade, L. M., & Belsky, J. (1992). Parent–child antecedents of 5-year-olds' close friendships: A longitudinal analysis. *Developmental Psychology, 28,* 700–713.

5 Biological Vulnerability to Depression

Amélie Nantel-Vivier and Robert O. Pihl

D*epression is a biological disease.* This bold, non-nuanced statement, initially provocative when confronted by the current cognitive zeitgeist, is neither new nor should it be particularly provocative. Historically, Hippocrates, in his humoral theory, saw depression as arising from an excess of black bile, a precursor to our common association of darkness with negative mood. Burton, in *The Anatomy of Melancholy*, written during Shakespeare's time, similarly saw the disorder as physiological. However, in addition to biological or medical treatments such as bloodletting, psychosocial interventions, including discussions with friends and interactive board games, were recommended.

Over the last 100 years, biological explanations waned as the importance of early developmental experiences, real and imagined, driven by psychoanalytic theorists, began to alter the perception of etiology. The putative physical basis for the disorder was hence lost for a time underneath the analytic couch. Interestingly, the introduction and widespread use of convulsive therapies for depression occurred concomitantly. This incongruence continues to some extent today between cognitive etiological theories and the still prevalent electrical convulsive therapy and the widespread growth and use of antidepressant medications. What this apparent incongruence reflects, however, is that it is becoming increasingly recognized that the etiology of the vast majority of mental disorders, including depression, can be best captured through a vulnerability–stress perspective. Putative biological, psychological, and environmental etiological mechanisms of depression and other mental disorders are therefore not mutually exclusive, but are rather intrinsically linked, interactive, and complementary.

Advances in the field of neurosciences over the last two decades have helped identify some of the neurobiological vulnerabilities of the diathesis–stress etiological chain associated with depression, vulnerabilities that are the focus of this chapter. A look at the literature on the etiology of depression quickly reveals that the vast majority of neurobiological studies have focused on adult clinical populations. However, faced with the increasing prevalence of depression and its progressively earlier onset, researchers are focusing more and more on the factors that render individuals vulnerable to depression. Increasing attention is therefore being paid to the biological correlates of pediatric depressive illness, with the hope of developing a closer understanding of the etiological roots of the disorder and creating better preventative tools.

Recent developments in brain-imaging techniques have allowed for the emergence of empirical investigations of brain differences between clinically depressed children and adolescents and healthy or psychiatric controls. This chapter offers an overview of the literature, describing the structural and functional brain anomalies associated with pediatric depression, as well as neurochemical correlates, and comparing available findings with those from adult populations. Empirical findings regarding the neurobiological etiology of depression must, however, be reflected upon in the context of important methodological and conceptual considerations, as well as current knowledge of normative neurobiological functioning and development. A brief description of these issues is therefore presented first.

METHODOLOGICAL AND CONCEPTUAL ISSUES

The assumption underlying research on the neurobiological bases of depression is that a significant causal relationship between depression and biological vulnerabilities exists and can be uncovered. Such assumption, however, proves to be a highly complex conceptual and empirical challenge. Until very recently, only "imprecise" technologies were available for studying the relationship between neurobiological functioning and mental states. Pharmacology, for example, has been the traditional route for developing biological explanations of depression and other psychopathologies. However, inferences regarding specific biochemical pathways involved in mental disorders based on treatment responses to medications have often been overnarrow, logically flawed, and consequently erroneous, as the vast majority of psychotropic drugs affect numerous neurochemical systems through complex interactive pathways. Techniques allowing for the supplementation or depletion of amino acid precursors have permitted the manipulation of levels of neurotransmitters, such as serotonin, in experimental participants and patients (Young, Smith, Pihl, & Ervin, 1985). Experimental manipulation of neurotransmitter levels through supplementation or depletion of amino acid precursors represents an important step toward establishing causal links between neurochemical states and psychiatric symptoms, although the specificity of the neurochemical changes associated with amino acid manipulation remains an issue.

Great excitement has been generated in the field of neurosciences by the ever evolving imaging techniques, which provide increasingly detailed descriptions of brain structure and functioning. Nuclear magnetic resonance imaging (MRI) uses a magnetic field to measure atoms and produces a detailed structural picture of the brain and its different areas. A blood oxygenation signal (functional magnetic resonance imaging; fMRI) can then be used to assess brain activity, as fluctuations in oxygenated blood flow signal fluctuations in the activity level of different brain areas. Positron emission tomography (PET) and single photon emission computed tomography (SPECT) are also informative, but more invasive, as they require the use of radioactive substances. Finally, diffusion tension imaging is an MRI procedure that specifically allows the investigation of white matter anomalies.

Despite the increasing precision and decreasing invasiveness of brain imaging techniques, the establishment of causal relationships between biological anomalies and mental disorders remains somewhat limited. To establish the psychophysiological underpinnings of mental states requires that no delay separates the recording of physiology and the occurrence of the mental states. However, as mental states are subjective, they are by definition impossible to objectively measure, leaving uncertainty as to their correspondence with any type of brain structure or activity (Schall, 2004). Furthermore, the typical research design used to investigate neurobiological correlates of mental disorders generally consists of identifying hormonal, neurochemical, brain structural, or functional anomalies through comparisons of patients suffering from a specific disorder of interest with healthy controls or patients suffering from other psychiatric illnesses. An important flaw in this design is that significant group differences in brain function or activity, and significant correlations between group membership and neurotransmitter metabolites or hormone levels, cannot be taken as direct evidence of causation of illness by biological forces. Rather, group differences and correlations could be caused by other factors associated with depression and other mental illnesses rather than by the illness per se, such as its treatment, concomitant illicit drug use, and the stress associated with the illness. In other words, when comparing patients with healthy controls or patients suffering from another mental illness, it is unclear whether we are measuring causal factors making an etiological contribution to the illness, or, conversely, consequences or associated factors of the illness. Such uncertainty may obscure our quest for neurobiological roots of depression and other mental disorders. This is why it is particularly crucial to focus on pediatric populations. By studying individuals at risk for developing depression (e.g., children of depressed parents) or individuals who can be considered to be very early in the course of their depressive illness (e.g., recently diagnosed children or adolescents who have yet to receive treatment), we significantly decrease the likelihood of the occurrence of confounding factors and can therefore more clearly investigate causative neurobiological forces by getting closer to their etiological roots.

In addition, although highly exciting and innovative, the use of imaging technologies remains somewhat limited with pediatric populations (Thompson & Nelson, 2001). For example, because PET imaging requires that participants be injected with a radioactive substance, it is understandably restricted to use in childhood clinical populations who have a medical vulnerability justifying the use of this type of scan. MRI and fMRI procedures are more promising for use with pediatric populations, as they do not require the injection of radioactive substances and are therefore much less invasive. However, because they require that participants lie still and refrain from moving within the enclosed, and often terrifying to some, scanner for quite extended periods of time, their use with very young participants is difficult. Moreover, there is still a certain level of uncertainty regarding the way in which children's physiology and physical build may affect scan results and the ensuing data. For example, children's heart and respiratory rates are approximately twice those of adults, which may impact blood flow and the blood-oxygen-level-dependent (BOLD) signal obtained from fMRI scans (Kotsoni, Byrd, & Casey, 2006). Furthermore, children's smaller head circumference, shorter neck, and narrower shoulders can affect placement within the scanner and, consequently, the subsequent signal. Adaptation of methodologies and equipment generally used with adult populations to specifically serve pediatric populations is therefore crucial (Kotsoni et al., 2006).

Finally, the greatest hurdle in the search for the neurobiological causes of depression and other mental disorders appears to be one of definition rather than of technology or methodology. *Depression*, like many psychopathological terms, is a big fat word. Its current obese condition is exemplified in the debate over the distinctiveness, or lack thereof, of depression and the rampant comorbidity that accompanies a diagnosis of depression. The consequence of this portly state is an inherent difficulty in determining where to aim the growing arsenal of technologically sophisticated biological measures. Psychopathologies are laden with noise, replete with debate, and lacking in specificity. This issue is exemplified by Andreasen (1999), who, in proposing a model for schizophrenia, wrote, "At present the most important problem in schizophrenia research is not finding the gene or localizing it in the brain and understanding its neural circuits. Our most important problem is identifying the correct target at which to aim our powerful new scientific weapons. Our most pressing problem is at the clinical level: defining what schizophrenia is" (p. 781). Similar statements can and should be repeatedly made concerning depression. Our diagnostic criteria and ensuing categories represent the way in which mental health specialists have carved out the frontiers of psychopathology. They are therefore a social construction, a construction not necessarily corresponding to any one biological phenomenon. The current system does not acknowledge the reality of comorbidity, presenting each disorder as a separate category. Comorbidity is, however, the rule rather than the exception in psychopathology. The most obvious example is the association between depression and anxiety. Studies have found high rates of comorbidity between depression and, for example, social anxiety, and have found the co-occurrence of both disorders in adolescence and early adulthood to be associated with a more severe later course of illness in adulthood (Stein et al., 2001). Disentangling the neurobiological etiological factors contributing to depression and other disorders constitutes an important step toward developing a taxonomy of mental illness that takes into consideration biological etiology rather than solely behavioral symptoms, perhaps yielding more homogeneous diagnostic categories that will be more amenable to targeted, specific, and effective treatments.

However, in spite of the methodological and conceptual limitations described above, great strides have been made toward identifying neurobiological correlates of adult and pediatric depressive illness. These exciting findings are reviewed, following a brief description of normative neurodevelopment and functioning.

NORMATIVE NEURODEVELOPMENT AND FUNCTIONING

From the onset of conception, the human brain goes through crucial formative and maturational processes, starting with neuron formation and migration. Such processes, described in Figure 5.1, adapted from Andreasen (1999), are importantly guided by genetic influences. As shown by Giedd (2004), using data from the National Institute of Mental Health (NIMH) longitudinal pediatric brain study, the brains of 6-year-old children are generally 90% of their adult size. Whole-brain volume is therefore determined quite early on in development. However, despite the relatively little change in whole-brain volume occurring beyond age 6, great change occurs in brain regional volumes over the course of childhood and adolescence.

One of these changes is increased myelination. White matter volumes have been shown to increase linearly throughout childhood and adolescence, at a similar rate across the four lobes (frontal, parietal, temporal, occipital; Giedd, 2004). Gray matter volumes, on the other hand, have been shown to follow an inverted U-shape developmental pattern, with significant decreases generally observed after age 12 (Casey, Giedd, & Thomas,

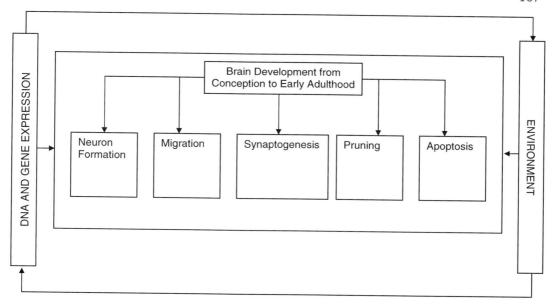

FIGURE 5.1. Developmental processes. Adapted from Andreasen (1999). Copyright 1999 by the American Medical Association. All rights reserved. Adapted by permission.

2000; Giedd, 2004). This decrease in gray matter volume during adolescence is a reflection of synaptic pruning, whereby unused connections are deleted (Giedd, 2004). Pruning is only one of the maturational processes taking place within the brain, accompanied by synaptogenesis and apoptosis, all dependent on activity and experience (see Figure 5.1).

Interestingly, one of the latest brain areas to exhibit the gray matter maturational pruning process described above is the dorsolateral prefrontal cortex (DLPC). The frontal lobes have been identified as the seat of executive cognitive functioning, generally understood to refer to the "ability to plan, initiate, and maintain or alter goal-directed behaviors" (Pihl, Vant, & Assaad, 2003). Through connections with other brain regions, the prefrontal cortex is part of an important circuitry that underlies the emergence of contextually appropriate affective and behavioural responses (Miller & Cohen, 2001). This process has been referred to as "affect-guided planning and anticipation" (Davidson, Pizzagalli, Nitschke, & Putnam, 2002, p. 548), where potentially rewarding responses will be undertaken and potentially harmful responses will be inhibited. Davidson and colleagues (2002) proposed that the anticipation of positive outcomes and approach behaviors may be subserved by the left prefrontal cortex, and inhibition and withdrawal tend be subserved by the right prefrontal cortex.

Connections of the prefrontal cortex with limbic structures, such as the amygdala and the hippocampus, appear to be crucial to affect-guided responding (Carlson, 2001). The primary role of the amygdala consists of promoting vigilance and attention to novel and/or affectively salient stimuli, whereas the hippocampus plays a key role in contextual memory and conditioning (Davidson et al., 2002). Both the amygdala and the hippocampus are central to the stress response (Davidson et al., 2002), constituting intricate components of the limbic–hypothalamic–pituitary–adrenocortical (LHPA) system (Gunnar & Vazquez, 2006). Given perceptions of stress, activating connections from limbic structures to the hypothalamus, a group of nuclei located at the base of the brain (Carlson,

2001), promote the secretion of corticotropin-releasing factor (CRF), which in turn triggers synthesis and release of adrenocorticotropin (ACTH) by the pituitary. ACTH then
stimulates synthesis and release of glucocorticoids by the adrenal cortex (Nestler et al.,
2002; Gunnar & Vazquez, 2006). Reciprocal feedback connections, consisting of
neuronal signaling and gene expression modulation, are intrinsic to the LHPA axis (Gunnar & Vazquez, 2006). For example, glucocorticoids first bind to mineralocorticoid
receptors, which play a permissive role and prepare individuals to react appropriately to
stressors. However, as the rate of glucocorticoid secretion increases, negative feedback,
for example, is achieved through binding of glucocorticoids to glucocorticoid receptors of
the hypothalamus, anterior pituitary, and the hippocampus, leading to a dampening of
the stress response (Gunnar & Vazquez, 2006; Nestler et al., 2002). High chronic levels
of glucocorticoids have been suggested to lead to hippocampal damage in the form of
reduced dendritic branching and glutamatergic dendritic spines, as well as reduced gene-
sis of granule cell neurons (Nestler et al., 2002). A vicious cycle may thus operate, as
decreased LHPA axis inhibition due to hippocampal damage would lead to increasing
glucocorticoid levels, which in turn may lead to further hippocampal damage (Nestler et
al., 2002). This pattern may explain why an inverse U-shape relationship is often
observed between stress response and functioning (Gunnar & Vazquez, 2006).

The prefrontal cortex, amygdala, and hippocampus, together with other brain
regions, are intrinsically linked and are crucial to our ability to appropriately respond to
our environment. Table 5.1, adapted from reviews by Davidson and colleagues (2002)
and Nestler and colleagues (2002), presents a list of the major brain regions that have
been associated with adult and pediatric depressive illness, as well as a summary of their
proposed functions and significance to the disorder.

STRUCTURAL IMAGING FINDINGS

Neuroimaging research on the brain correlates of depression in adult populations has
revealed significant structural anomalies between patients and controls. Although very
few studies have found support for differences in whole-brain volumes between patients
and healthy controls (Strakowski, Adler, & DelBello, 2002), anomalies have been noted

TABLE 5.1. Summary of Brain Regions Associated with Pediatric and Adult Depression

Brain region	Function	Significance in depression
Frontal lobes • Dorsolateral prefrontal cortex (DLPC) • Dorsomedial prefrontal cortex (DMPC) • Ventrolateral prefrontal cortex (VLPC) • Orbital prefrontal cortex • Subgenual prefrontal cortex • Insula	Executive functioning • Goal-directed behaviors • Affect-guided planning	Contribution to: • Cognitive impairments • Depressogenic cognitions • Anomalies in reward and punishment anticipation • Suicidality
Midline and medial temporal structures • Cingulate • Amygdala • Hippocampus • Caudate nucleus • Putamen • Thalamus	• Emotional memory • Contextual memory • Stress response • Regulation of drives	Contribution to: • Anhedonia • Anxiety • Vegetative symptoms

in regional volumes (Nestler et al., 2002). Reduction of frontal lobe volumes has been found, particularly of the subgenual prefrontal cortex (Drevets et al., 1997), as well as reduction of the greater right than left asymmetry, a finding associated with symptom severity (Beyer & Krishnan, 2002; Strakowski et al., 2002). Bilateral volume reductions, decreased cortical thickness, and decreased neuronal size and density have also been noted in the orbital region (Lai, Payne, Byrum, Steffens, & Krishnan, 2000; Rajkowska et al., 1999).

In one of the first structural imaging studies of depressed children and adolescents, Steingard and colleagues (Steingard et al., 1996) found evidence of a significant decrease in frontal lobe volumes and a significant increase in ventricular volumes in depressed pediatric inpatients as compared with nondepressed psychiatric controls, a pattern consistent with results from adult studies. Significantly smaller whole brain volumes and frontal lobe white matter volumes, but greater frontal lobe gray matter volumes, were also found in depressed adolescents as compared with healthy age-matched controls (Steingard et al., 2002). Botterton and colleagues (Botteron, Raichle, Drevrets, Heath, & Todd, 2002), in turn, reported that the left, but not the right, subgenual prefrontal cortex in young women presenting with a history of adolescent-onset major depressive disorder (MDD) was 19% smaller than that in controls. The extent of the reduction of the subgenual prefrontal cortex in these young women was similar to reductions found in a group of older women with major depression (Botteron et al., 2002). Lyoo and colleagues (Lyoo, Lee, Jung, Noam, & Renshaw, 2002), using a large sample of children with psychiatric disorders including bipolar disorder, MDD, schizophrenia, conduct disorder, and attention-deficit/hyperactivity disorder, investigated the presence of frontal white matter hyperintensities. White matter hyperintensities are indicative of increased water density. They are believed to contribute to cognitive impairment and have been studied in relation to a number of psychiatric disorders, generally in adult patients (Lyoo et al., 2002). Studies focusing on adult depression have shown that although the etiological role of white matter hyperintensities is unclear, their incidence is increased in depressed patients and they have been associated with decreased response to pharmacological interventions (Iosifescu et al. 2006). Results by Lyoo and colleagues (2002) indicated that the frontal lobes of children with major depressive disorder presented significantly greater white matter hyperintensities than those of controls. This was, however, also true of children with bipolar disorder, conduct disorder, and attention-deficit/hyperactivity disorder, so that frontal white matter hyperintensities could not be described as specific to early-onset depression.

Evidence for volumetric anomalies in brain regions other than the frontal cortex has been somewhat mixed (Beyer & Krishnan, 2002). Adult studies have provided partial support for decreased temporal cortical volumes (Strakowski et al., 2002). Because of their contribution to mood modulation and the processing of emotional stimuli, midline and medial temporal structures, such as the hippocampus, amygdala, and basal ganglia, have been the objects of a number of structural imaging studies of depression. Decreased hippocampal volume has been noted (Davidson et al., 2002; Strakowski et al., 2002), together with conflicting evidence concerning volumetric anomalies of the amygdala (Davidson et al., 2002). Finally, partial support has also been provided for an association between depression and decreased volume of the basal ganglia, specifically, the caudate nucleus and putamen (Beyer & Krishnan, 2002; Strakowski et al., 2002).

Rosso and colleagues (Rosso et al., 2005) found evidence for significant bilateral decrease in amygdala volumes in depressed children and adolescents as compared with healthy controls, but comparisons revealed no significant differences in hippocampal volumes. The decrease in amygdala volume was of approximately 12%. No significant association, however, emerged between amygdala volume reduction and depression severity, illness duration, and age of onset. MacMillan and colleagues (MacMillan et al., 2003) reported that medication-naive pediatric patients with MDD showed a bilateral increase in amygdala volume and a bilateral decrease in hippocampal volume, as compared with healthy controls. These differences, however, became nonsignificant after age and intracranial volume were controlled. When amygdala:hippocampal volume ratios were investigated, it was shown that bilateral amygdala:hippocampal volume ratios were significantly greater in depressed pediatric patients than in controls. Furthermore, greater left amygdala:hippocampal volume ratios were significantly positively associated with anxiety severity, but not with depression severity or illness duration. The authors thus concluded that increased amygdala:hippocampal volume ratios may be more indicative of comorbid anxiety than depression itself in pediatric major depression. MacMaster and Kusumakar (2004b) noted a significant decrease in left hippocampal volumes in medication-naive adolescents suffering from MDD. No significant relationship was found between depression severity and decreased hippocampal volume, but left hippocampal volume was significantly positively correlated with illness duration and negatively associated with age of onset. Decreased hippocampal volumes were more prominent in male patients. Amygdala volumes were, however, not investigated. Finally, an additional study by MacMaster and Kusumakar (2004a) found that although age was positively associated with pituitary volume in healthy controls, no such relationship was observed in depressed adolescent patients. Moreover, depressed adolescents exhibited 25% greater pituitary volumes than healthy controls, which the authors suggested may be associated with dysregulation of the LHPA axis.

FUNCTIONAL IMAGING FINDINGS

Functional imaging studies focusing on adult clinical populations have repeatedly found evidence for hypometabolism of the dorsolateral and dorsomedial prefrontal cortex of depressed patients, particularly in the left hemisphere (Davidson et al., 2002; Drevets, 2000; Liotti & Mayberg, 2001), whereas increased activity in the subgenual prefrontal cortex, as well as the bilateral posterior orbital cortex, left ventrolateral prefrontal cortex, and anterior insula has been noted (Drevets, 2000). Adult depressed patients have also been found to exhibit decreased hippocampal activity (Davidson et al., 2002; Strakowski et al., 2002), whereas increases in amygdala activity have been noted (Davidson et al., 2002).

Relatively less is known concerning the brain functional correlates of pediatric depressive illness, with very few studies having applied the most recent functional imaging technologies to pediatric populations. A recent investigation by Killgore and colleagues (Killgore & Yurgelun-Todd, 2006), focusing on the association between healthy adolescents' depressed mood scores and brain functional activity as measured by fMRI, found that higher depressed mood scores were associated with increased activity in the medial orbitofrontal and rostral anterior cingulate gyri while participants were shown fearful faces. This finding, however, may be representative of "normative" sadness rather than depression, as the range of depressed mood scores observed for the sample was below the clinical range. Thomas and colleagues (Thomas et al., 2001) similarly investigated brain functional correlates of exposure to fearful faces, this time using a clinical sample of children with anxiety or depressive disorders. Results indicated that although children diagnosed with an anxiety disorder showed an increased amygdala response to the presentation of fearful faces, as compared with healthy children, the amygdala response of depressed children to the same fearful stimuli was blunted (Thomas et al., 2001). Bonte and colleagues (Bonte et al., 2001; Bonte, 1999), using SPECT imaging, identified cerebral blood flow anomalies in depressed children and adolescents. In one study, two subgroups of depressed children were identified; the first characterized primarily by decreased activity of the occipital region, and a second group characterized primarily by frontal functional anomalies. In addition, Kowatch and colleagues (Kowatch et al., 1999), also using SPECT imaging, compared the regional blood flow of depressed adolescents and healthy controls. Results showed decreased blood flow in the left parietal lobe, anterior thalamus, and the right caudate nucleus of depressed adolescents, whereas increased activity was noted for the mesial temporal cortex, the right superior anterior temporal lobe, and the left inferior lateral temporal lobe. Tutus and colleagues (Tutus, Kibar, Sofuoglu, Basturk, & Gönül, 1998), using SPET technology, investigated differences in cortical activity between depressed adolescents and healthy controls under two conditions, using a repeated measure design for the clinical group. Patients were scanned twice, first when undergoing no pharmacological treatment, and second once depressive symptoms had receded. Results indicated significantly decreased activity of the left anterofrontal and left temporal cortical areas in nonmedicated depressed adolescents. However, no significant differences were noted at the second scan, once symptoms had subsided, suggesting that pharmacological treatment may have contributed to the normalization of brain activity in these patients.

Brain imaging research in both adult and child clinical populations have therefore found somewhat consistent evidence for prefrontal, temporal, and limbic anomalies in depressed patients. The equivocal nature of some of these empirical findings may be partly explained by the heterogeneity of the disorder. It is possible that certain subtypes of depression are associated with certain brain anomalies and not others (Davidson et al., 2002). For example, increased amygdala, orbital cortex, and thalamic activity, together with decreased activity of the prefrontal cortex and volumetric anomalies of the basal ganglia, have been noted to be more frequent in adult patients with a positive family history of major depression (Drevets, 2000). Similarly, Nolan and colleagues (2002), when comparing depressed pediatric patients with no family history of depression, depressed pediatric patients with a positive family history of depression, and healthy controls, found that patients with no family history of major depression had larger left prefrontal volumes than patients with a positive family history and healthy controls, and that the latter two groups did not significantly differ from each other in terms of prefrontal volumes. Moreover, sulcal and ventricular enlargement have been shown to be more pronounced in individuals presenting with a late-onset form of major depression (Drevets, 2000). Identifying depression subtypes based on age of onset and neurobiological characteristics may provide us with more etiologically consistent and uniform diagnostic categories.

NEUROCHEMICAL CONTRIBUTIONS

Neurotransmitters

Neurochemical explanations of adult-onset depressive disorder have largely focused on the monoamine neurotransmitter systems. Greatest attention has been given to serotonin, with the latest generation of antidepressants, the selective serotonin reuptake inhibitors

(SSRIs), showing significant effectiveness in reducing symptoms (Stockmeier, 2003). In addition, experimental manipulation of tryptophan, a serotonergic dietary precursor, has been shown to impact symptom recurrence in approximately 50–60% of remitted patients formerly treated with SSRI antidepressant medication (Van der Does, 2001). Performing a reanalysis of individual data from six separate tryptophan depletion studies, Booij and colleagues (Booij et al., 2002) identified history of recurrent depressive episodes, suicidal thoughts and behaviors, past treatment with SSRIs, and female gender to be predictive of individual differences in the mood response to tryptophan depletion, with illness chronicity being the strongest predictor of a lowered mood response. Research has also shown that lowered mood resulting from tryptophan depletion tends to be stronger in remitted patients with a positive family history of psychiatric disorders than in patients with no such history (Leyton et al., 2000). Furthermore, tryptophan depletion has been shown to decrease mood in healthy males with a positive family history of affective disorders (Benkelfat, Ellenbogen, Dean, Palmour, & Young, 1994). Low serotonergic metabolites in the cerebrospinal fluids of depressed patients with a history of suicide attempts have also been found, as well as decreased neuroendocrine response to serotonin stimuli and anomalies in serotonergic receptor binding sites (Stockmeier, 2003). It is important to note, however, that norepinephrine receptor and transporter anomalies, as well as decreased levels of GABA, have also been reported, indicating that serotonin most likely acts in conjunction with other neurotransmitter systems in contribution to the neurochemical basis of depression (Stockmeier, 2003).

As with other facets of neurobiological correlates of depressive illness, the contribution of serotonin and other neurochemicals to early-onset depression has received much less attention than has been given to its adult-onset counterpart. The involvement of such systems is therefore less clear, with serotonergic challenge studies in children and adolescents having yielded mixed findings. Evidence of increased, decreased, or no different hormonal response in depressed children and adolescents, as compared with healthy controls, has been found (Ryan et al., 1992; Hardan et al., 1999; Ghaziuddin et al., 2000)

Nevertheless, prescription rates of SSRIs have been dramatically rising since the 1990s, particularly in the preschool-age group (Andersen & Navalta, 2004). SSRIs, however, do not appear to be as effective in treating depression in children and adolescents as they are in adults, perhaps reflecting the more severe nature of early-onset depressive illness, or a deleterious effect of SSRI administration on the clinical course (Andersen & Navalta, 2004). There is relatively little evidence concerning the potential effects of antidepressant use on the developing brain. It has been established that the development of the monoamine systems, including the serotonergic system, follows an inverted U-shape pattern, with overproduction of neural connections in childhood followed by pruning of up to 40% of connections over the course of adolescence (Andersen & Navalta, 2004). Because the monoamines play a trophic role (Andersen & Navalta, 2004), altering levels of these neurotransmitters may impact the selection process occurring during pruning, and this effect may be observable only when the targeted systems reach maturity, long after treatment has been terminated.

Other neurochemicals that have been the focus of neurobiological investigations of pediatric depressive illness include choline/creatine, choline/N-acetylaspartate, and glutamate. Because choline, creatine, N-acetylaspartate, and glutamate play an important role in neuronal signaling, their levels are believed to be indicative of brain metabolism and may thus be informative for studies of neuropsychiatric disorders. Levels of these chemicals have been shown to be altered in depressed adult populations and tend to normalize with antidepressant pharmacological treatment (Steingard et al., 2000). Steingard and colleagues

(2000) found evidence of altered chemistry of the orbitofrontal cortex in depressed adolescents. As compared with healthy controls, depressed adolescents showed increased choline:creatine and choline:N-acetylaspartate ratios by approximately 15%. A study by Farchione and colleagues (Farchione, Moore, & Rosenberg, 2002) found a 32.5% increase in choline levels of the left, but not the right, dorsolateral prefrontal cortex of depressed children and adolescents, as compared with healthy controls. This increase tended to be more pronounced in patients with a family history of MDD. No significant differences were noted between the groups for N-acetylaspartate and creatine. A study by Kusumakar and colleagues (Kusumakar, MacMaster, Gates, Sparkes, & Khan, 2001) reported a significantly lower left amygdala choline:creatine ratio in depressed adolescents than in healthy controls. Bilateral amygdala N-aectylaspartate:creatine ratios and right amygdala choline:creatine ratios did not significantly differ between the two groups. Left amygdala choline:creatine ratios tended to be negatively associated with depression severity scores for the clinical group. In addition, an investigation by Rosenberg and others (Rosenberg et al., 2004) comparing pediatric patients with obsessive–compulsive disorder (OCD), MDD, and healthy controls found that both patients with OCD and those with MDD exhibited significant reduction of glutamatergic concentrations in the anterior cingulated cortex, as compared with controls Glutamatergic concentrations did not significantly differ between the two diagnostic groups. Rosenberg and colleagues (Rosenberg et al., 2005) reported reduced anterior cingulated glutamate, but not glutamine, in depressed pediatric patients as compared with controls. A study by Mirza and colleagues (Mirza et al., 2004) reported that depressed pediatric patients exhibited a 19% decrease in anterior cingulate glutamatergic levels, but not in occipital levels, as compared with healthy controls. This decrease in anterior cingulate glutamate was significantly associated with the degree of functional impairment.

The Stress Response System

The stress response system, consisting of the LHPA axis described earlier, has been an important focus of research on the neurobiological correlates of depression. LHPA hyperactivity is believed to contribute to depression mainly through hippocampal damage sustained because of chronic exposure to elevated glucocorticoid levels, which is consistent with often noted decreases in hippocampal volumes (Davidson et al., 2002). In addition, research has shown that central administration of CRF may trigger symptoms characteristic of depression such as anxiety and neurovegetative symptoms, suggesting that LHPA axis hyperactivity may influence brain regions other than the hippocampus, such as the hypothalamus (Nestler et al., 2002).

Although LHPA hyperactivity constitutes one of the most often replicated findings in the adult depression literature and may be observed in approximately 50% of depressed adult patients (Nestler et al., 2002; Gunnar & Vazquez, 2006), LHPA axis patterns are less clear in depressed pediatric populations (Andersen & Navalta, 2004). As described by Steingard (2000), studies investigating endocrine markers of LHPA functioning have yielded mixed findings. For example, Kutcher and colleagues (Kutcher et al., 1991) found evidence for higher nocturnal growth hormone secretion, higher levels of thyroid-stimulating hormone, but no significant difference in cortisol levels between depressed adolescents and healthy controls. These results, however, were not replicated in later investigations (DeBellis et al., 1996). Children of depressed mothers have been found to have increased stress hormone levels, both at baseline and in response to laboratory stressors (Bonari et al., 2004). In an investigation focusing on the hormonal response of depressed abused, depressed nonabused, and healthy nonabused children, Kaufman et al. (1997) found that depressed abused children experiencing chronic stressors exhibited greater ACTH secretion to a corticotropin-releasing hormone challenge than depressed abused children currently experiencing stable life circumstances, or depressed nonabused and healthy children. Birmaher et al. (2000) also found that children with a family history of mood disorders showed blunted growth hormone secretion response as compared with healthy controls not at risk for mood disorders. Luby et al. (2003) found evidence for alteration in LHPA functioning in depressed preschoolers, reflected in increased cortisol levels, as compared with children with psychiatric disorders other than depression and healthy controls.

Finally, hormonal influences have been proposed as key explanatory factors in the observed sex differences in depression prevalence rates. Sex differences in the prevalence of major depression have been well established, with female: male ratios approximately 2:1. Longitudinal and retrospective studies have shown that this disparity between the sexes appears to emerge around the time of puberty (Parker & Brotchie, 2004), sparking interest in the potential neurohormonal forces possibly contributing to such a striking gap. In their review of the literature, Parker and Brotchie (2004) reported that the disparity between the sexes in depressive symptomatology emerges at Tanner Pubertal Stage III. For example, Angold and colleagues (Angold, Costello, & Worthman, 1998) found that although boys tended to exhibit higher depression rates than girls before reaching Tanner Stage III, the reverse was true once Tanner Stage III was reached. The age at which Tanner Stage III was reached did not significantly predict depression rates. Furthermore, a related study indicated that the emergence of sex differences in depression rates with Tanner Stage III could not be attributed to changes in body morphology and their associated psychosocial consequences (Angold, Costello, Erkanli, & Worthman, 1999). Sex steroids, androgen and estrogen, were found to be more significantly associated with the increase in depression rates in adolescent girls (Angold et al., 1999).

In addition, Parker and Brotchie (2004) found that although adrenarche may lead to the decreased vulnerability of boys to depression during the transition from childhood to adolescence, hormonal changes occurring in girls may render them more vulnerable to depression, in part through increased vulnerability to stress (Parker & Brotchie, 2004). Female gonadal hormones have been found to have significant regulatory properties for major neurotransmitter systems, including serotonin, norepinephrine, and GABA (Parker & Brotchie, 2004), all three of which have been associated with depressive illness. More specifically, estrogen and progesterone appear to have opposing effects on brain chemistry. For example, estrogen decreases monoamine oxidase (MAO) activity, increases neurotransmission, and enhances mood, and progesterone increases MAO activity, decreases neurotransmission, and has a negative impact on mood (Parker & Brotchie, 2004). Through their impact on the neurotransmitter systems described above, as well as innervations within the limbic system, cyclical fluctuations of estrogen and progesterone throughout women's reproductive years are believed to confer vulnerability to anxiety, stress, and depression. The authors note that neurobiological explanations of sex differences in depression prevalence rates must be considered in the context of psychosocial forces at play in determining men's and women's social roles and mental health (Parker & Brotchie, 2004). However, as was demonstrated by Angold and colleagues (Angold, Worthman, & Costello, 2003), research with children and adolescents has demonstrated the primary role of sex steroids in the emergence of gender differences in early adolescence, suggesting that hormonal factors may be of crucial importance in the maintenance of such disparities during adulthood.

TRACING THE EMERGENCE AND ONSET OF BIOLOGICAL VULNERABILITIES

As described above, decades of research on the neurobiological bases of depression have allowed for the accumulation of knowledge concerning specific anatomical, functional, and neurochemical vulnerabilities that may play an etiologically significant role in the emergence, onset, and course of depression. Structural and functional anomalies of the frontal lobes, amygdala, hippocampus, and other brain regions have been implicated, together with possible dysregulation of the stress–response system and a contribution of gonadal hormones. Evidence for a strong continuity between pediatric depressive illness and adult forms of depression, along with the increasing attention of neurobiological studies to pediatric populations over approximately the last 10 years, have shifted the focus toward early identification of neurobiological anomalies associated with depression. The question that naturally follows this shift in emphasis is, At what point do the neurobiological anomalies observed in depressed adults, adolescents, and children become apparent? How early can neurobiological risk factors be identified? It is clear that depressed children and adolescents show neurobiological patterns similar to those of their adult counterparts. How early these patterns emerge may be crucial for prevention strategies and therefore merits careful consideration.

A fascinating group of studies have employed electroencephalographic (EEG) recordings in order to investigate the brain activity of children at risk of developing depression owing to a positive history of maternal depression. A significant portion of this work has focused on children in their first years of life. For example, Diego and colleagues (Diego, Field, Jones, & Hernandez-Reif, 2006; Diego et al., 2002) investigated the impact of depressed mothers' intrusive and withdrawn interaction styles on infants' frontal brain electrical activity. Results indicated that right frontal activation was greater in infants of depressed mothers than in infants whose mothers were not depressed. Right frontal activation was greatest for infants whose mothers were both depressed and withdrawn. Although depression and intrusiveness in mothers was associated with greater relative left frontal activity infants, greater relative right frontal activity in infants was associated with depression and withdrawn behaviors in mothers (Diego et al., 2006). Infants of depressed and intrusive mothers were also shown to give more attention to and exhibit greater relative right frontal asymmetric activity in response to facial expressions of surprise and sadness (Diego et al., 2002). Investigating the relationship between cortisol levels, withdrawn behaviors, and brain activity in 6-month-old infants, Buss and colleagues (Buss et al., 2003) found evidence for a significant positive association between cortisol levels and increased right frontal asymmetric activity. Infants' behavioral signs of sadness during a laboratory stranger-approach situation were also associated with increased right frontal asymmetric electrical activity. The authors noted that the observed asymmetry could be attributed to both left frontal hypoactivation and right frontal hyperactivation, with cortisol response being more strongly associated with left frontal hypoactivation, and sadness being associated with both left frontal hypoactivation and right frontal hyperactivation (Buss et al., 2003). Furthermore, Jones and colleagues (Jones, Field, Fox, Davalos, & Gomez, 2001), focusing on brain electrical correlates of emotions in infants of depressed mothers, similarly found evidence of greater right frontal activity in infants of depressed mothers. Infants of depressed mothers could also be described as exhibiting greater levels of negative facial expressions and fewer positively valenced facial expressions (Jones et al., 2001). In addition, Dawson and colleagues (Dawson et al., 1999) noted decreased left frontal electrical activity relative to right frontal activity in infants of depressed mothers in the context of various laboratory-based social interactions. A second study by Dawson and colleagues (Dawson et al., 2003), focusing on the preschool period, found evidence for a mediating role of children's frontal brain activity and environmental stressors in the relationship between maternal depression and preschoolers' behavioral problems. Similarly, focusing on children of mothers with childhood-onset depression, Forbes and colleagues (Forbes et al., 2006) recently reported that the internalizing and externalizing behaviors problems of 3- to 9-year-old children of mothers with childhood-onset depression were significantly associated with brain symmetry activity patterns. Finally, Tomarken and colleagues (Tomarken, Dichter, Garber, & Simien, 2004) reported that adolescents of depressed mothers showed a relative left frontal hypoactivation at resting state. Investigations of children and adolescents at risk of developing depression owing to a positive history of maternal depressive illness have therefore revealed relatively consistent specific brain electrical patterns, often in children as young as 6 months of age.

AN INTEGRATIVE FRAMEWORK: BRIDGING BIOLOGY AND THE ANALYTIC COUCH

As indicated in the introduction to this chapter, biological vulnerabilities underlying adult and pediatric manifestations of depression are most likely not sufficient to explain the full etiological picture at the root of depression onset and course. Rather, they are part of an intrinsically complex chain of etiological events including psychological and environmental risk factors in addition to constitutional factors. A clear relationship has been demonstrated between life stressors and the onset or exacerbation of depressive or internalizing symptoms. For example, in a longitudinal study focusing on the emergence and progression of internalizing symptoms in adolescence, Rueter and colleagues (Rueter, Scaramella, Wallace, & Conger, 1999) demonstrated that family stressors, more specifically parent–adolescent disagreements, indirectly predicted later anxiety or depressive disorder onset through effects on prodromal internalizing symptomatology. Although the idea that there are individual differences in vulnerability to life stressors may seem quite intuitive and almost obvious, recent research has provided evidence for some biological underpinnings of such differences. Caspi and colleagues (Caspi et al., 2003), using a prospective, longitudinal design spanning ages 3–26, found that the presence of one or two short alleles of the 5-HTT promoter polymorphism rendered individuals more vulnerable to the depressogenic effects of stressful life events, as compared with the homozygous long alleles. Similarly, investigating the relationship between stressful life events, major depression or generalized anxiety disorder episodes, and functional polymorphism of the serotonin transporter (5-HTT) in an adult twin population, Kendler and colleagues (Kendler, Kuhn, Vittum, Prescott, & Riley, 2005) found that individuals with the SS variant of the serotonin transporter were more sensitive to the depressogenic effects of mild to moderate stressful life events than individuals with the SL or LL variants. The impact of 5-HTT polymorphism appeared to be relatively specific to major depression, as no such interaction was found for generalized anxiety disorder. The likelihood of differential vulnerability to the depressogenic effects of environmental stressors due to serotonin polymorphism has also been observed in an adolescent population (Eley et al., 2004).

Furthermore, the interaction of neurobiological forces and stressors does not appear to be limited to contemporary events, but to early life experiences as well. In their review of the literature, Heim, Plotsky, and Nemeroff (2004) underscore the importance of early life stressors and their potential contribution to the development of depression. Events noted in their description of early life stressors include sexual/emotional/physical abuse, loss of a parent, and illnesses, among others. They report that not only are early life stressors associated with an increased risk and earlier onset of depression, but that animal models and some human studies have shown that early life stressors, such as maternal separation, are associated with hormonal, neurochemical, and brain structural changes, many of which are quite similar to the neurobiological findings associated with depression. For example, monoaminergic dysfunction and alterations of the prefrontal circuitry as well as limbic structures have been noted (Heim et al., 2004). These authors therefore suggest that some subtypes of depression may be characterized by the presence of early life stressors, the effect of which is mediated by neurobiological components. For example, they report that adult and child studies have shown that decreased hippocampal volumes may be characteristic only of depressed patients with a history of abuse in childhood (Heim et al., 2004). This fascinating body of work emphasizes the importance of placing both psychosocial and neurobiological factors potentially contributing to the risk, onset, and development of depression within a mutually informative, interactive, developmental framework. Perhaps then our newly developed imaging techniques and the "analytic couch" can and should happily coexist.

A tentative etiological model integrating neurobiological and psychosocial contributing factors to depression is presented in Figure 5.2. The first step of the model represents the family agglomeration of mental disorders, whereby depression and other affective disorders are known to run in families. A positive family history of depression of the mother may then influence children's prenatal environment by increasing the likelihood of maternal prenatal depression and its neurochemical and behavioral correlates. As evidenced by research described above, on the brain electrical patterns of infants of depressed mothers, and by reviews of the correlates of prenatal depression, the prenatal environment may in turn have a great impact on young infants' brain structure, function, and chemistry, as well as on young children's more general neurohomornal functioning. A positive family history of depression and prenatal depression are also likely to influence the early postnatal environment, increasing the odds of maternal postpartum depression and impacting parenting style and the parent–child relationship. The early environment is then in constant bidirectional interaction with the children's neurobiological functioning.

The interaction of children's neurobiological makeup and their environment can then give rise to personality patterns that may render them more or less vulnerable to depression. For example, Canli and colleagues (Canli et al., 2001), using fMRI technology, investigated the brain functional correlates of emotion processing associated with different personality characteristics or traits in healthy women—more specifically, neuroticism and extraversion. Results indicated that activation of frontal and temporal cortical regions, as well as subcortical structures, to emotionally positively valenced pictures was significantly correlated with extraversion, and that left temporal and frontal cortical activation to negatively valenced pictures significantly correlated with neuroticism. Both neuroticism and extraversion are known to predict onset of depression in youth and adults (e.g., Tackett & Krueger, 2005), so it seems reasonable to investigate the neural underpinnings tying together personality and depression.

Finally, individuals' neurobiological functioning, together with their developmental history and ensuing personality, may give rise to depressive symptomatology when contemporary triggers, such as stressful life events, occur. As illustrated by the dashed line linking depressive symptomatology and family history of mental health and psychopathology in Figure 5.2, the cycle of generational transmission of depression can repeat itself once children suffering from depression become parents themselves.

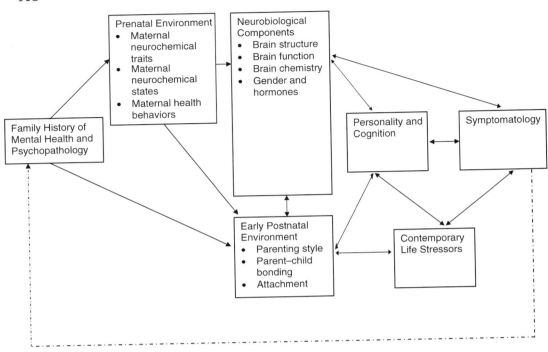

FIGURE 5.2. Integrative etiological model of depression.

CONCLUSIONS

Neurobiological studies have revealed anatomical, functional, and neurochemical anomalies associated with both early-onset and adult-onset depressive disorder. These results, however, show subtle fluctuations, with considerable overlap in volumetric, functional, or neurochemical distributions being observed between patients and controls. Perhaps contributing somewhat to the equivocal nature of available empirical evidence is the important fact that many of the neurobiological anomalies described in this chapter may not be specific to depression itself. As we described in the introduction to the chapter, depression most often occurs in the context of other comorbid conditions such as anxiety. It may be that many disorders, which we think of as distinct, in fact share similar biological etiological mechanisms and that the same phenotype may result from a number of etiological mechanisms, with multiple pathways. Attempting to isolate the neurobiological correlates of behavior-based disorders, which in fact co-occur more often than they present themselves separately, is relatively unlikely to yield reliable markers of any specific disorder. A lot more work therefore needs to be done before neurobiological findings can be used as diagnostic markers of depression and other disorders. Diagnostic subgroups of depression based on the presence or absence of specific neurobiological markers should, however, be used in research with the aim of identifying etiologically homogeneous clinical populations.

The involvement of certain brain regions, including the prefrontal cortex, the hippocampi, and the amygdala, has been repeatedly found in both pediatric and adult populations. The emerging literature on the neurobiological correlates of pediatric depressive illness therefore points toward some continuity between adolescent-onset depression and adult forms of the disorder, and potentially between childhood-onset and adult depression. Such findings are consistent with the observed continuity in symptoms and course between juvenile-onset and later-onset cases (e.g., see Avenevoli, Knight, Kessler, & Merikangas, Chapter 2, this volume). Furthermore, research focusing on very young children presenting with a significantly increased risk of developing depression and other difficulties owing to a positive history of maternal depression has shown that some of the neurobiological anomalies associated with depression in children, adolescents, and adults may actually be observable within the first few months of life, and that some of these anomalies may start to emerge during the prenatal period. Such findings point to the crucial importance of preventative strategies, including prenatal interventions focusing on the treatment and management of maternal depression during the perinatal period.

Also highlighted by the literature on the neurobiological bases of depression is the importance of environmental factors and their interaction with biological vulnerabilities. As described above, individuals' biological and genetic makeup can render them more vulnerable to depression. Stressful life events, however, may also alter neurobiology, creating different neurobiological subtypes of depression. Future investigations focusing on the interactive nature of biology and environmental forces may shed significant light on potential subtypes of depression, their respective onsets and courses, and the best preventative and treatment approaches to be used.

REFERENCES

Andersen, S. L., & Navalta, C. P. (2004). Altering the course of neurodevelopment: A framework for understanding the enduring effects of psychotropic drugs. *International Journal of Developmental Neuroscience, 22,* 423–440.

Andreasen, N. C. (1999). A unitary model of schizophrenia. *Archives of General Psychiatry, 56,* 781–787.

Angold, A., Costello, E. J., Erkanli, A., & Worthman, C. M. (1999). Pubertal changes in hormone levels and depression in girls. *Psychological Medicine, 29,* 1043–1053.

Angold, A., Costello, E. J., & Worthman, C. M. (1998). Puberty and depression: The role of age, pubertal status, and pubertal timing. *Psychological Medicine, 28,* 51–61.

Angold, A., Worthman, C. M., & Costello, E. J. (2003). Puberty and depression. In C. Hayward (Ed.), *Gender differences at puberty* (pp. 137–164). Cambridge, UK: Cambridge University Press.

Benkelfat, C., Ellenbogen, M. A., Dean, P., Palmour, R. M., & Young, S. N. (1994). Mood-lowering effect of tryptophan depletion: Enhanced susceptibility in young men at genetic risk for major affective disorders. *Archives of General Psychiatry, 51,* 687–697.

Beyer, J. L., & Krishnan, K. R. R. (2002). Volumetric brain imaging findings in mood disorders. *Bipolar Disorders, 4,* 89–104.

Birmaher, B., Dahl, R. E., Williamson, D. E., Perel, J. M., Brent, D. A., Axelson, D. A., et al. (2000). Growth hormone secretion in children and adolescents at high risk for major depressive disorder. *Archives of General Psychiatry, 57,* 867–872.

Bonari, L., Pinto, N., Ahn, E., Einarson, A., Steiner, M., & Koren, G. (2004). Perinatal risks of untreated depression during pregnancy. *Canadian Journal of Psychiatry, 49,* 726–735.

Bonte, F. J. (1999). Brain blood flow SPECT: Posterior flow deficits in young patients with depression. *Clinical Nuclear Medicine, 24,* 696–697.

Bonte, F. J., Trivedi, M. H., Devous, M. D., Harris, T. S., Payne, J. K., Weinberg, W. A., et al. (2001). Occipital brain perfusion deficits in children with major depressive disorder. *Journal of Nuclear Medicine, 42,* 1059–1061.

Booij, L., Van der Does, W., Benkelfat, C., Bremner, D., Cowen, P. J., Fava, M., et al. (2002). Predictors of mood response to acute tryptophan depletion: A reanalysis. *Neuropsychopharmacology, 27*, 852–861.

Botteron, K. N., Raichle, M. E., Drevrets, W., Heath, A., & Todd, R. D. (2002). Volumetric reduction in left subgenual prefrontal cortex in early onset depression. *Biological Psychiatry, 51*, 342–344.

Buss, K. A., Schumacher, J. R. M., Dolski, I., Kalin, N. H., Goldsmith, H. H., & Davidson, R. J. (2003). Right frontal brain activity, cortisol, and withdrawal behavior in 6-month-old infants. *Behavioral Neuroscience, 117*, 11–20.

Canli, T., Zhao, Z., Desmond, J. E., Kang, E. J., Gross, J., & Gabrieli, J. D. E. (2001). An fMRI study of personality influences on brain reactivity to emotional stimuli. *Behavioral Neuroscience, 115*, 33–42.

Carlson, N. R. (2001). *Physiology of behavior* (7th ed.). Boston: Allyn & Bacon.

Casey, B. J., Giedd, J. N., & Thomas, K. M. (2000). Structural and functional brain development and its relation to cognitive development. *Biological Psychiatry, 54*, 241–257.

Caspi, A., Sugden, K., Moffitt, T. E., Taylor, A., Craig, I. W., Harrington, H., et al. (2003). Influence of life stress on depression: Moderation by a polymorphism in the 5-HTT gene. *Science, 301*, 386–389.

Davidson, R. J., Pizzagalli, D., Nitschke, J. B., & Putnam, K. (2002). Depression: Perspectives from affective neuroscience. *Annual Review of Psychology, 53*, 545–574.

Dawson, G., Ashman, S. B., Panagiotides, H., Hessl, D., Self, J., Yamada, E., et al. (2003). Preschool outcomes of children of depressed mothers: Role of maternal behavior, contextual risk, and children's brain activity. *Child Development, 74*, 1158–1175.

Dawson, G., Frey, K., Panagiotides, H., Yamada, E., Hessl, D., & Osterling, J. (1999). Infants of depressed mothers exhibit atypical frontal electrical brain activity during interactions with mother and with a familiar, nondepressed adult. *Child Development, 70*, 1058–1066.

DeBellis, M. D., Dahl, R. E., Perel, J. M., Birmaher, B., Al Shabbout, M., Williamson, D. E., et al. (1996). Nocturnal ACTH, cortisol, growth hormone, and prolactin secretion in prepubertal depression. *Journal of the American Academy of Child and Adolescent Psychiatry, 35*, 1130–1138.

Diego, M. A., Field, T., Hart, S., Hernandez-Reif, M., Jones, N., Gullen, C., et al. (2002). Facial expressions and EEG in infants of intrusive and withdrawn mothers with depressive symptoms. *Depression and Anxiety, 15*, 10–17.

Diego, M. A., Field, T., Jones, N., & Hernandez-Reif, M. (2006). Withdrawn and intrusive maternal interaction style and infant frontal EEG asymmetry shifts in infants of depressed and nondepressed mothers. *Infant Behavior and Development, 29*, 220–229.

Drevets, W. C. (2000). Neuroimaging studies of mood disorders. *Biological Psychiatry, 48*, 813–829.

Drevets, W. C., Price, J. L., Simpson, J. R., Todd, R. D., Reich, T., Vannier, M., et al. (1997). Subgenual prefrontal cortex abnormalities in mood disorders. *Nature, 386*, 824–827.

Eley, T. C., Sugden, K., Corsico, A., Gregory, A. M., Sham, P., McGuffin, P., et al. (2004). Gene–environment interaction analysis of serotonin system markers with adolescent depression. *Molecular Psychiatry, 9*, 908–915.

Farchione, T. R., Moore, G. J., & Rosenberg, D. R. (2002). Proton magnetic resonance spectroscopic imaging in pediatric major depression. *Biological Psychiatry, 52*, 86–92.

Forbes, E. E., Shaw, D. S., Fox, N. A., Cohn, J. F., Silk, J. S., & Kovacs, M. (2006). Maternal depression, child frontal asymmetry, and child affective behavior as factors in child behavior problems. *Journal of Child Psychology and Psychiatry and Allied Disciplines, 47*, 79–87.

Ghaziuddin, N., King, C. A., Welch, K., Zaccagnini, J., Weidmer-Mikhail, E., Mellow, A. M., et al. (2000). Serotonin dysregulation in adolescents with major depression: Hormone response to meta-chlorophenylpiperazine (mCPP) infusion. *Psychiatry Research, 95*, 183–194.

Giedd, J. N. (2004). Structural magnetic resonance imaging of the adolescent brain. *Annals of the New York Academy of Sciences, 1021*, 77–85.

Gunnar, M. R., & Vazquez, D. (2006). Stress neurobiology and developmental psychopathology. In D. Cicchetti & D. J. Cohen (Eds.), *Developmental psychopathology: Vol. 2. Developmental neuroscience* (2nd ed., pp. 533–577). Hoboken, NJ: Wiley.

Hardan, A., Birmaher, B., Williamson, D. E., Dahl, R. E., Ambrosini, P., Rabinovich, H., et al. (1999). Prolactin secretion in depressed children. *Biological Psychiatry, 46,* 506–511.

Heim, C., Plotsky, P. M., & Nemeroff, C. B. (2004). Importance of studying the contributions of early adverse experience to neurobiological findings in depression. *Neuropsychopharmacology, 29,* 641–648.

Iosifescu, D. V., Renshaw, P. F., Lyoo, I. K., Lee, H. K., Perlis, R. H., Papakostas, G. I., et al. (2006). Brain white-matter hyperintensities and treatment outcome in major depressive disorder. *British Journal of Psychiatry, 188,* 180–185.

Jones, N., Field, T., Fox, N. A., Davalos, M., & Gomez, C. (2001). EEG during different emotions in 10-month-old infants of depressed mothers. *Journal of Reproductive and Infant Psychology, 19,* 295–312.

Kaufman, J., Birmaher, B., Perel, J., Dahl, R. E., Moreci, P., Nelson, B., et al. (1997). The corticotropin-releasing hormone challenge in depressed abused, depressed nonabused, and normal control children. *Biological Psychiatry, 42,* 669–679.

Kendler, K. S., Kuhn, J. W., Vittum, J., Prescott, C. A., & Riley, B. (2005). The interaction of stressful life events and a serotonin transporter polymorphism in the prediction of episodes of major depression: A replication. *Archives of General Psychiatry, 62,* 529–535.

Killgore, W. D., & Yurgelun-Todd, D. (2006). Ventromedial prefrontal activity correlates with depressed mood in adolescent children. *Neuroreport, 17,* 167–171.

Kotsoni, E., Byrd, D., & Casey, B. J. (2006). Special considerations for functional magnetic resonance imaging of pediatric populations. *Journal of Magnetic Resonance Imaging, 23,* 877–886.

Kowatch, R. A., Devous, M. D., Harvey, D. C., Mayes, T. L., Trivedi, M. H., Emslie, G. J., et al. (1999). A SPECT HMPAO study of regional cerebral blood flow in depressed adolescents and normal controls. *Progress in Neuro-psychopharmacology and Biological Psychiatry, 23,* 643–656.

Kusumakar, V., MacMaster, F. P., Gates, L. L., Sparkes, S., & Khan, S. C. (2001). Left medial temporal cytosolic choline in early onset depression. *Canadian Journal of Psychiatry, 46,* 959–964.

Kutcher, S., Malkin, D., Silverberg, J., Marton, P., Williamson, P., Malkin, A., et al. (1991). Nocturnal cortisol, thyroid stimulating hormone, and growth-hormone secretory profiles in depressed adolescents. *Journal of the American Academy of Child and Adolescent Psychiatry, 30,* 407–414.

Lai, T.-J., Payne, M. E., Byrum, C. E., Steffens, D. C., & Krishnan, K. R. (2000). Reduction of orbital frontal cortex volume in geriatric depression. *Biological Psychiatry, 48,* 971–975.

Leyton, M., Ghadirian, A. M., Young, S. N., Palmour, R. M., Blier, P., Helmers, K. F., et al. (2000). Depressive relapse following acute tryptophan depletion in patients with major depressive disorder. *Journal of Psychopharmacology, 14,* 284–287.

Liotti, M., & Mayberg, H. S. (2001). The role of functional neuroimaging in the neuropsychology of depression. *Journal of Clinical and Experimental Neuropsychology, 23,* 121–136.

Luby, J. L., Heffelfinger, A., Mrakotsky, C., Brown, K., Hessler, M., & Spitznagel, E. (2003). Alterations in stress cortisol reactivity in depressed preschoolers relative to psychiatric and no-disorder comparison groups. *Archives of General Psychiatry, 60,* 1248–1255.

Lyoo, I. K., Lee, H. K., Jung, J. H., Noam, G. G., & Renshaw, P. F. (2002). White matter hyperintensities on magnetic resonance imaging of the brain in children with psychiatric disorders. *Comprehensive Psychiatry, 43,* 361–368.

MacMaster, F. P., & Kusumakar, V. (2004a). MRI study of the pituitary gland in adolescent depression. *Journal of Psychiatric Research, 38,* 231–236.

MacMaster, F. P., & Kusumakar, V. (2004b). Hippocampal volume in early onset depression. *BMC Medicine, 2,* 2.

MacMillan, S., Szeszko, P. R., Moore, G. J., Madden, R., Lorch, E., Ivey, J., et al. (2003). Increased amygdala:hippocampal volume ratios associated with severity of anxiety in pediatric major depression. *Journal of Child and Adolescent Psychopharmacology, 13,* 65–73.

Miller, E. K., & Cohen, J. D. (2001). An integrative theory of prefrontal cortex function. *Annual Review of Neuroscience, 24,* 167–202.

Mirza, Y., Tang, J., Russell, A., Banerjee, S. P., Bhandari, R., Ivey, J., et al. (2004). Reduced anterior cingulate cortex glutamatergic concentrations in childhood major depression. *Journal of the American Academy of Child and Adolescent Psychiatry, 43,* 341–348.

Nestler, E. J., Barrot, M., Dileone, R. J., Eisch, A. J., Gold, S. J., & Monteggia, L. M. (2002). Neurobiology of depression. *Neuron, 34,* 13–25.

Nolan, C. L., Moore, G. J., Madden, R., Farchione, T., Bortoi, M., Lorch, E., et al. (2002). Prefrontal cortical volume in childhood-onset major depression: Preliminary findings. *Archives of General Psychiatry, 59,* 173–179.

Parker, G. B., & Brotchie, L. (2004). From diathesis to dimorphism: The biology of gender differences in depression. *Journal of Nervous and Mental Disorders, 192,* 210–216.

Pihl, R. O., Vant, J., & Assaad, J. M. (2003). Neuropsychological and neuroendocrine factors. In C. A. Essau (Ed.), *Conduct and oppositional defiant disorders: Epidemiology, risk factors, and treatment* (pp. 163–189). Mahwah, NJ: Erlbaum.

Rajkowska, G., Miguel-Hidalgo, J. J., Wei, J., Dilley, G., Pittman, S. D., Meltzer, H. Y., et al. (1999). Morphometric evidence for neuronal and glial prefrontal cell pathology in major depression. *Biological Psychiatry, 45,* 1085–1098.

Rosenberg, D. R., MacMaster, F. P., Mirza, Y., Smith, J. M., Easter, P. C., Banerjee, S. P., et al. (2005). Reduced anterior cingulate glutamate in pediatric major depression: A magnetic resonance spectroscopy study. *Biological Psychiatry, 58,* 700–704.

Rosenberg, D. R., Mirza, Y., Russell, A., Tang, J., Smith, J. M., Banerjee, S. P., et al. (2004). Reduced anterior cingulate glutarnatergic concentrations in childhood OCD and major depression versus healthy controls. *Journal of the American Academy of Child and Adolescent Psychiatry, 43,* 1146–1153.

Rosso, I. M., Cintron, C. M., Steingard, R. J., Renshaw, P. F., Young, A. D., & Yurgelun-Todd, D. A. (2005). Amygdala and hippocampus volumes in pediatric major depression. *Biological Psychiatry, 57,* 21–26.

Rueter, M. A., Scaramella, L., Wallace, L. E., & Conger, R. D. (1999). First onset of depressive or anxiety disorders predicted by the longitudinal course of internalizing symptoms and parent–adolescent disagreements. *Archives of General Psychiatry, 56,* 726–732.

Ryan, N. D., Birmaher, B., Perel, J. M., Dahl, R. E., Meyer, V., al-Shabbout, M., et al. (1992). Neuroendocrine response to L-5-hydroxytryptophan challenge in prepubertal major depression: Depressed vs. normal children. *Archives of General Psychiatry, 49,* 843–851.

Schall, J. D. (2004). On building a bridge between brain and behavior. *Annual Review of Psychology, 55,* 23–50.

Stein, M. B., Fuetsch, M., Müller, N., Höfler, M., Lieb, R., & Wittchen, H. U. (2001). Social anxiety disorder and the risk of depression: A prospective community study of adolescents and young adults. *Archives of General Psychiatry, 58,* 251–256.

Steingard, R. J. (2000). The neuroscience of depression in adolescence. *Journal of Affective Disorders, 61,* S15–S21.

Steingard, R. J., Renshaw, P. F., Hennen, J., Lenox, M., Cintron, C. B., Young, A. D., et al. (2002). Smaller frontal lobe white matter volumes in depressed adolescents. *Biological Psychiatry, 52,* 413–417.

Steingard, R. J., Renshaw, P. F., Yurgelun-Todd, D., Appelmans, K. E., Lyoo, I. K., Shorrock, K. L., et al. (1996). Structural abnormalities in brain magnetic resonance images of depressed children. *Journal of the American Academy of Child and Adolescent Psychiatry, 35,* 307–311.

Steingard, R. J., Yurgelun-Todd, D. A., Hennen, J., Moore, J. C., Moore, C. M., Vakili, K., et al. (2000). Increased orbitofrontal cortex levels of choline in depressed adolescents as detected by in vivo proton magnetic resonance spectroscopy. *Biological Psychiatry, 48,* 1053–1061.

Stockmeier, C. A. (2003). Involvement of serotonin in depression: Evidence from postmortem and imaging studies of serotonin receptors and the serotonin transporter. *Journal of Psychiatric Research, 37*, 357–373.

Strakowski, S. M., Adler, C. M., & DelBello, M. P. (2002). Volumetric MRI studies of mood disorders: Do they distinguish unipolar and bipolar disorder? *Bipolar Disorders, 4*, 80–88.

Tackett, J. L., & Krueger, R. F. (2005). Interpreting personality as a vulnerability for psychopathology: A developmental approach to the personality-psychopathology relationship. In B. L. Hankin & J. R. Z. Abela (Eds.), *Development of psychopathology: A vulnerability–stress perspective* (pp. 199–214). Thousand Oaks, CA: Sage.

Thomas, K. M., Drevets, W. C., Dahl, R. E., Ryan, N. D., Birmaher, B., Eccard, C. H., et al. (2001). Amygdala response to fearful faces in anxious and depressed children. *Archives of General Psychiatry, 58*, 1057–1063.

Thompson, R. A., & Nelson, C. A. (2001). Developmental science and the media: Early brain development. *American Psychologist, 56*, 5–15.

Tomarken, A. J., Dichter, G. S., Garber, J., & Simien, C. (2004). Resting frontal brain activity: Linkages to maternal depression and socio-economic status among adolescents. *Biological Psychology, 67*, 77–102.

Tutus, A., Kibar, M., Sofuoglu, S., Basturk, M., & Gönül, A. S. (1998). A technetium-99m hexamethylpropylene amine oxime brain single-photon emission tomography study in adolescent patients with major depressive disorder. *European Journal of Nuclear Medicine, 25*, 601–606.

Van der Does, A. J. W. (2001). The mood-lowering effect of tryptophan depletion: Possible explanation for discrepant findings. *Archives of General Psychiatry, 58*, 200–201.

Young, S., Smith, S., Pihl, R., & Ervin, F. (1985). Tryptophan depletion lowers mood in normal males. *Psychopharmacology, 87*, 173–177.

6 New Behavioral Genetic Approaches to Depression in Childhood and Adolescence

Jennifer Y. F. Lau and Thalia C. Eley

Several major scientific discoveries of the twentieth century have conspired to make genetics a strong contender in explaining individual differences in many aspects of behavior. Such discoveries include the extension of Mendel's laws of heredity to account for complex patterns of inheritance, the unraveling of the molecular structure of DNA (deoxyribonucleic acid), and most recently the completion of the first draft of the DNA sequence of the human genome. It is therefore not surprising that there has been a steady accumulation of behavioral genetic studies aimed at disentangling the role of nature and nurture in complex psychiatric disorders, including emotional ones such as depression. This interest has also begun to extend to conditions occurring earlier in development, such as in childhood and adolescence. Thus, rather than relying solely on extrapolation from adult findings, these studies began somewhat with a *tabula rasa*, or blank slate, to provide data from which conclusions about the heritability of early-onset conditions can be drawn.

This chapter offers an overview of behavioral genetic studies of depressive disorders and related symptoms in children and adolescents. The first two sections present an outline of the principles and assumptions of behavioral genetic methodology, discussing respectively the main quantitative and molecular designs utilized to explore the contributions of genes and the environment to behavioral phenotypes. Following this, we describe how these techniques have been applied to developmental research on depressive outcomes. Collectively, the findings from quantitative genetic studies support a heritable basis for pediatric depression in addition to substantial environmental contributions, but the data also implicate complex trends in the size and nature of these effects relative to age and development, sex, and the severity of the condition. Discussion of these trends constitutes a major part of this section. The next section focuses on the identity of specific genes and the associated neurobiological systems that have been implicated in depressive disorders by molecular studies. As there are comparatively fewer studies published with respect to child and adolescent depression, most of the work reviewed will be from studies of adults. In the final two sections, we focus on some novel questions dominating the agenda of recent quantitative and molecular research made possible by advances in analytic techniques. Rather than simply identifying the *level* of genetic and environmental influence, recent studies have begun to pose questions about *how* genetic and environmental risks are expressed through intermediate pathways to affect the phenotype. There are two main approaches, which are discussed in turn. The first addresses the interplay between genetic and environmental factors in these phenotypes, whereas the second aims to identify specific risk markers, also termed *endophenotypes*, which potentially mediate the risk effects associated with the distal genotype on the behavioral signs and symptoms of the phenotype. Consideration of these questions has encouraged collaborative links between behavioral genetic designs and those of other mainstream approaches, including neuroscience and psychology.

QUANTITATIVE GENETIC METHODOLOGY

Behavioral genetic designs belong to the category of methodological approaches examining variation between individual members of a population. Typically, such approaches explain variability in a dependent or outcome variable by variation in a second set of independent variables or predictors. What is unique to behavioral genetic designs is that variance in a phenotype is specifically attributed to genes and the environment (for an introduction to behavioral genetics, see Plomin, DeFries, McClearn, & McGuffin, 2001). More crucially, the direction of causation between genes and behavior is assumed to be one-way, so that naturally occurring variation in the sequencing of DNA molecules that characterize an individual's genotype, affects behavior. Behaviors in turn cannot alter genetic variation except in unusual circumstances, such as in exposure to high levels of ionizing radiation that may lead to genetic mutation. To the extent that genetic influences do not account for all variation in a phenotype, the rest is assigned to environmental factors (and measurement error), of which there are two types: shared and nonshared. The first refers to aspects of an environment that make family members resemble one another, and the second are factors that make family members dissimilar. Partitioning individual variation in behavioral phenotypes into these contributions constitutes one core component of behavioral genetic research. To this end, quantitative designs that capitalize on the different genetic relationships between family members to infer genetic and environmental effects are well established. These designs assume that the degree of behavioral resemblance between two related individuals varies as a function of their genetic relatedness and the level at which they share family (shared) environments. Differences in the expression of a phenotype are attributed to individual-specific (nonshared) environmental factors. The most common study designs applied to depressive phenotypes are family, twin, and adoption studies.

Family Studies

Family studies investigate the degree of clustering of depressive conditions among genetically related family members. A higher-than-chance incidence of depression among first-degree relatives is taken as tentative support for heredity. However, such conclusions are limited by the fact that first-degree relatives are also more likely to share the same family environment as well as genetics. Thus, these studies are unable to differentiate shared genetic from shared environmental explanations.

Twin Studies

Twin studies are undoubtedly the more widely used of the designs. In brief these exploit naturally occurring differences in the genetic relationship between monozygotic (MZ) and dizygotic (DZ) twins. MZ twins originate from the same fertilized ovum, and thus share all of their genetic material (A). DZ twins are created by the simultaneous fertilization of different ova and therefore, like full siblings, share on average only half of the segregating genes (½A). In addition to genetics, both types of twins also share their family (shared) environment (C). As both these sources can contribute to the phenotypic similarity observed between twins, MZ and DZ twin correlations can be re-expressed to reflect these terms. Thus, correlations between MZ twins (rMZ) are equal to A + C, whereas correlations between DZ twins (rDZ) are ½A + C. It follows that any difference in twin correlations between MZ and DZ pairs provides a rough estimate of genetic effects (A), and that any resemblance in MZ twins not due to genetic effects are accounted for by the shared family environment (C). As family members (including twins) also differ from one another in their expression of the phenotype, these differences attributed to nonshared environmental effects and calculated by differences between MZ twins on a phenotype: 1 −rMZ. Applying model-fitting techniques to these structural equations can yield parameter estimates that best fit the data.

Although these comparisons offer a simple method to signpost genetic and environmental contributions on different measures, conclusions drawn from twin analyses are not without limitations, which include consideration of the equal environments assumption and chorionicity, presence of assortative mating, and the generalizability of findings (see Plomin et al., 2001, for further details). A key assumption of the twin method is that MZ and DZ twins experience a shared environment to the same degree, but this can be violated in at least two ways. First, prenatally MZ twins are more likely to share gestational environments that are similar to one another, as compared with DZ twins. Approximately two-thirds of MZ twins develop in the same chorion, the sack within the placenta where the fetus develops, whereas all DZ twins develop in separate sacks. Second, in their postnatal environments, MZ twins may be perceived and treated more alike by others, in comparison to DZ twins, owing to the closer physical resemblance. As both scenarios can result in an amplified concordance for a trait among MZ twins relative to DZ twins, this can artificially inflate heritability estimates. To minimize the impact of these violations, it is critical to demonstrate that differences in environmental exposure between MZ and DZ twins are not systematically related to the increased similarity between MZ twins in behavioral outcomes. Detailed observations have attested to this. First, MZ twins who are monochorionic (develop in the same sack) are no more alike in terms of their risk for psychopathology than those who are dichorionic (develop in separate sacks; Riese, 1999). Second, aspects of increased postnatal environmental sharing between MZ twins, such as sharing a bedroom for a greater length of time during childhood, do not predict a subsequent similarity in the risk for depression (Cardno et al., 1999). Third, where parents have mistaken MZ twins as DZ twins (or vice versa), these variations in parental treatment have not influenced twin resemblance for depressive symptoms (Kendler, Neale, Kessler, Heath, & Eaves, 1994). Fourth, it has been argued that increased similarity in environmental exposure between MZ twins may be driven by genetic resemblance mediated through behavior rather than environmentally induced. This suggestion is derived from findings that many aspects of the social environment, such as perceptions of parenting, life events, and peer groups, are genetically influenced (Plomin & Bergeman, 1991). If this were true, exposure to more similar environments would fundamentally reflect genetic effects and thus the impact of this exposure on overall heritability estimates would be correctly taken as such.

Assortative mating refers to the well-documented finding that "birds of a feather flock together," or the tendency of individuals with similar phenotypes to mate more frequently than expected by chance. The presence of this phenomenon can alter genotypic frequencies, and thus genetic variance in families. In turn, this may result in corresponding increases in the proportion of predisposing genes shared between DZ twins, beyond the expected 50%. This may then inflate the resemblance between DZ twins, which serves to underestimate genetic effects. Although assortative mating has been documented among affective disorders, it is typically reported more in bipolar disorder than in major depression (Mathews & Reus, 2001).

The final issue concerning the validity of twin designs is whether twins are representative of the general (nontwin) population. Twins may have atypical obstetric and perinatal histories and suffer from birth complications and low birth weights more frequently than singletons (Phillips, 1993), and these differences can lead to variations in behavioral, emotional, and cognitive development in twins, as compared with singletons. However, existing studies addressing this issue indicate that twins are largely indistinguishable from nontwins in terms of behavioral and emotional problems, including depressive symptoms (Moilanen et al., 1999). A last caveat that applies to the findings of all quantitative designs is that the estimates derived relate to a particular population of genotypes at a specific time in its historical context. As such, extraneous variables such as evolution or culture, which may change gene frequencies, the expression of genetic effects, or the frequencies of environmental events, can potentially impact the findings (Neale & Maes, 2001). Together these limitations imply that any derived estimates of heritability should not be taken as absolutes, but rather as indications of the role of genes in different phenotypes. As shown in the following discussion, the twin design can be extended to more complex model-fitting approaches to test hypotheses of the nature of genetic and environmental contributions and possible risk mechanisms in depression.

Adoption Studies

The adoption design offers yet another method of disentangling genetic from environmental influences, drawing upon the differential relationships that occur between adoptive family members, biological (birth) family members, and nonadoptive (control) biological family members. In adoptive families, the adoptee shares his or her rearing environment but not his or her genes, with other family members. In contrast, the adoptee shares only genetic material, but not the rearing environment, with members of his or her biological family. Finally, individuals in nonadoptive biological families share both their environment and their segregating genes with other family members. Thus, the adoption design produces three different pairings: pairings between "environmental" relatives, between "genetic" relatives, and between "environmental + genetic" relatives. Similar to the twin design, correlations between dyads within these different pairings can be reexpressed to reflect the degree of shared genetic and/or environmental components. The comparison of correlations is then used to yield estimates of genetic and shared environmental influence. A particularly noteworthy feature of this design is that the estimate of shared environment is directly inferred from the relationship between members of the adoptive family, rather than seen as the nongenetic residual variance contributing to twin similarity in the twin design.

Although such designs offer a powerful means for separating environmental from genetic effects, they have also been criticized in at least three ways (see Plomin et al., 2001 for further details). First, there is the issue of the representativeness of adopted individuals, and their adoptive and biological parents, of the general population, which affects the generalizability of these findings. A counterargument to this is that any variation between adopted individuals and nonadopted controls is more likely to yield mean rather than variance differences, the latter of which is critical for estimating genetic and environmental effects. Moreover, evidence from the Colorado Adoption Project (DeFries, Plomin, & Fulker, 1994) indicates that biological and adoptive parents are reasonably representative of nonadoptive control parents, as are adopted children relative to their nonadopted counterparts. A second issue relates to the fact that biological (birth) mothers also provide the prenatal environment of their adopted-away children; thus, any mother–offspring resemblance could be attributed to this rather than shared genes. This possibility can be tested by examining the similarity between biological fathers and their offspring, thus eliminating the potential confounding effects of the prenatal environment. The final issue concerns selective placement, that is, when adopted parents are chosen on the basis of their similarity to the biological parents. For example, children of biological parents with high IQs could be matched with adoptive parents who also score highly on this dimension. Such matching could obscure the clean separation into genetic and environmental effects. More specifically, similarity between offspring and their adoptive parents would be inflated as a result of genetic mediation, whereas increased resemblance between offspring and biological parents may be attributable to environmentally mediated effects. Fortunately, there is little evidence to suggest selective placement for psychological traits and disorders, other than IQ.

MOLECULAR GENETIC METHODOLOGY

Although quantitative designs are critical in demonstrating the heritability of particular phenotypes, they make no assumptions about the identity of specific genes that are involved. Furthermore, as they are reliant on indirect means of assessing genetic liability, these effects are considered "latent" or unmeasured. In contrast, molecular genetic approaches examining the effects of DNA polymorphisms, that is, stretches of DNA containing variation in the sequencing of base pair molecules, on the observable behaviors of the phenotype, yield direct evidence for the causal role of genes (for more details on molecular genetic methods, see Eley & Craig, 2005, and Eley & Rijsdijk, 2005). It has been recognized that depression, like other complex phenotypes, shows a mode of transmission that is consistent with the contribution of multiple genes, each of small effect size. These are known as quantitative trait loci (QTLs) and refer specifically to genes involved in determining individual differences of continuously measured traits, of which the extreme ends are assumed to comprise disordered individuals. Such dimensional phenotypes differ from classic Mendelian traits, which are typically under the influence of a single gene whose presence (or absence) determines the manifestation of the phenotype. In contrast, QTLs are neither necessary nor sufficient for the phenotype to occur. The main implications these differences have for identifying actual genes are that classical designs used for single-gene disorders can no longer be appropriately applied to complex phenotypes. Rather, designs with greater statistical power to detect their effects are needed. This requirement has precipitated an exponential growth in new study designs and analytic strategies. Together with more efficient techniques to procure and analyze DNA, and an increased amount of information on variation within the human genome, these developments have stimulated a proliferation of molecular genetic studies aimed at locating susceptibility genes for behavioral disorders, including depression. Nevertheless, to date, these have largely been studies of adult populations.

The two most common strategies used to identify specific genes are linkage and association designs. Both methods utilize genetic markers that are stretches of DNA that vary between members of a population. Such variation gives rise to different versions, or alleles, across individuals. If there are multiple types of the allele, these are known as polymorphisms. As each individual possesses two alleles at a given locus, the particular combination of a person's alleles defines his or her genotype. Individuals can be homozygous (two copies of the same allele) or heterozygous (different alleles). Such markers of genetic variation may have functional significance; that is, they may impact upon mechanisms occurring at the molecular or cellular level, such as in the transcription of a particular enzyme. This in turn may influence the functioning of certain neurobiological systems, which can have implications for behavior. In this way, the upstream consequences of genetic variation may ultimately result in the development of behavioral signs and symptoms. Although some genetic markers may be directly implicated in pathways leading to the phenotype of interest, others may merely be located proximally to the disease gene, a principle that is exploited in linkage studies. Ultimately, the aim of molecular genetics is to identify gene–trait and gene–disorder relationships by examining relationships between different genetic markers and levels of a phenotypic trait or disorder within families (linkage) and within populations (association).

Linkage Studies

Linkage studies test for the coinheritance of a genetic marker with a disease (or high levels of a phenotypic trait) within families. In other words, a genetic marker is linked to a disease if it is more prevalent among affected than among unaffected family members. Linkage may occur because the marker is itself the susceptibility gene, or because it is located within close proximity to the gene of interest. As the probability of recombination decreases for alleles that are positioned closer, that is, where there is a lesser chance of crossover of alleles in neighboring loci during meiosis, such alleles are often inherited together. In other words, even if the marker is not directly implicated in the etiology of the disorder, demonstrating that it is in linkage with high levels of the phenotypic trait can potentially narrow the search for the susceptibility locus to a particular chromosomal region.

Traditional linkage analyses involve calculating a function of the probability of recombination between a known marker position and the unknown location of a predisposing gene, called the LOD (logarithmic odds) score. A high LOD score indicates a low rate of recombination, which in turn suggests that the marker is close to the disease allele. This translates to meaning a higher degree of linkage for that marker. Although these methods can be very powerful, they are reliant on the specification of a known model of inheritance of the phenotype of interest. For complex phenotypes such as depression, for which the inheritance mode is far from certain, the statistical power is considerably reduced. As a result, nonparametric (model-free) methods are needed and often applied. A common alternative is to simply examine whether there is an excess of marker–allele sharing between pairs of affected relatives. Exemplifying this approach is the sib-pair design, which compares the number of shared alleles between concordant siblings (both members are affected) and discordant siblings (only one member is affected). As siblings can either share no alleles, one allele, or both alleles at a given locus, one would expect that in concordant pairs, in which both members manifest the disorder, there is a significantly increased sharing of alleles, relative to discordant pairs.

Typically, large linkage studies have capitalized on genome-wide scans in which markers are uniformly distributed throughout the entire genome and each is tested for the degree of linkage to a measured trait. In this sense, these methods are systematic, yet in another they are also considered exploratory, with no prior theory guiding the search. Although their purpose lies in narrowing the number of chromosomal regions that potentially contain the genes of interest, a specific limitation of nonparametric linkage methods is that often very broad areas are identified. Thus, it is possible that a marker may appear to be tightly linked to a locus, but in reality may fall many kilobases away on the actual chromosome. This makes it difficult to delineate the precise location of the disease gene. Furthermore, confirming replication between studies is problematic. The use of linkage studies is optimal when complemented by other methods that can further restrict the search to more specific locations within the chromosomal region.

Association Studies

Association studies offer a far more accurate method for identifying the locations of specific genes. They are also more powerful in detecting genes of modest effect size. Whereas linkage methods rely on within-family inheritance patterns, association studies simply compare the frequencies of genetic markers at a particular chromosomal region in unrelated affected and unaffected individuals, often in the context of a case-control design. A significant association is reported if a genetic marker occurs at significantly higher frequencies in the affected group, as compared with the control group. These associations between allelic markers and susceptibility to a disease in a population may represent a special case of linkage between genetic variants that have been retained over many generations within the population. In linkage disequilibrium, apparently "unrelated" individuals may share common ancestors from whom the susceptibility gene was inherited together with allelic markers that were in close proximity. Over time, this relationship is preserved and evident among the affected individuals of the population, thus accounting for the significance of associations.

The simplicity of association designs has made them particularly attractive in relation to complex disorders and traits. Furthermore, the choice of alleles to examine can be guided by findings from linkage studies of markers within a specific region, or by polymorphisms that have a possible role in the biological etiology of the disorder (e.g., being one aspect of a neurotransmitter system). These designs are termed "candidate gene approaches" and differ from linkage studies that are more atheoretical in nature. Despite their popularity, there are two main caveats that may apply to the findings of association studies and that require careful consideration. The first of these is population stratification, whereby other sources of genetic variability between affected cases and controls could spuriously account for observed associations. The most common instance of this occurs when differences associated with ethnicity—most notably, physical characteristics such as eye color—are present. If the affected cases and controls are not carefully matched for their population of origin, one could potentially obtain a significant association between a gene for eye color and the disorder, if the former is more prevalent among the affected group relative to the unaffected group. One approach to avoid these methodological confounds is to consider within-family associations in which there is no variation due to ethnicity. Examples of this include comparing frequencies of alleles within discordant sibling pairs, or the proportions of transmitted versus nontransmitted alleles in offspring from their biological parents (Transmission-Disequilibrium Test). A second design-related caveat concerns high rates of Type 1 errors or false positives that may result from multiple testing of the different possible candidate genes. Bonferroni corrections can correct for these errors, by adjusting the alpha level of each individual test downward so that the overall risk for a number of tests remains the same. However, as individual QTLs are likely to have small effect sizes, such corrections can potentially result in there being no significant associations identified. A possible compromise is to use these tests in the context of well-powered and thus large samples or within internal replication samples.

QUANTITATIVE GENETIC STUDIES OF DEPRESSION

Findings from family and twin studies generally converge on the conclusion that early-onset depression symptoms are both familial and heritable, with large contributions from environmental factors (for a review, see Rice, Harold & Thapar, 2002a). Family studies have revealed significantly elevated rates of major depression in first-degree relatives of child probands (Birmaher, Ryan, Williamson, Brent, & Kaufman, 1996) and among the offspring of depressed parents (Weissman, Warner, Wickramaratne, Moreau, & Olfson, 1997), relative to family members of healthy and psychiatric controls. Similarly, twin studies have documented a profile of moderate genetic influences, weaker shared environmental effects, and large nonshared environmental contributions. Given these findings, it is surprising that the results of adoption studies stand in stark contrast. Of the two published studies, both have reported patterns of results suggesting negligible genetic and shared environmental effects (Eley, Deater-Deckard, Fombonne, Fulker, & Plomin, 1998; van den Oord, Boomsma, & Verhulst, 1994). As yet there are few convincing explanations for these conflicting findings. One suggestion has been that participants of both adoption designs were fairly young (10–15 and 9–12 years) and genetic effects may be rather minimal in this age range, as discussed next. Another possibility is that genetic influences demonstrated among twins may be expressed only in exposure to specific environments, a topic that is discussed in a subsequent section. These findings both suggest caution in the interpretation of findings from twin and family studies and highlight a need for further investigations using such alternative designs.

In spite of these caveats concerning the results of twin studies, perhaps one of their greatest strengths lies not in providing overall indices of heritability, but rather in serving as a springboard for the interpretation of the nature and role of genes and the environment in behavioral phenotypes. Indeed, this usage of the twin design as an exploratory tool has hinted that the genetic and environmental influences on vulnerability to depression may not be straightforward. Instead, complex patterns across age, development, and sex and among individuals with more severe forms of the phenotype have been revealed. Each of these "moderators" of genetic and environmental influence is considered.

Age and Developmental Trends

Cross-sectional comparisons of the magnitude of genetic and environmental indices across samples of different ages have suggested larger genetic and smaller shared environmental effects in adolescents than in children (Thapar & McGuffin, 1994; Hewitt, Silberg, Neale, Eaves, & Erickson, 1992; Eley & Stevenson, 1999; Silberg et al., 1999; Silberg, Rutter, & Eaves, 2001; Rice, Harold, & Tharpar, 2002b; Scourfield et al., 2003). Although these results may have important implications for the well-documented increases in rates of depression during adolescence, there are at least three reasons why these conclusions are premature. First, it is unclear whether age-related changes occur in both males and females. Whereas two studies have reported larger genetic effects in adolescent females (Hewitt et al., 1992; Silberg et al., 1999; Silberg, Rutter, & Eaves, 2001), another found increases in adolescent males only (Eley & Stevenson, 1999). A fourth study showed greater genetic effects among both males and females (Scourfield et al., 2003). These discrepant findings emphasize the importance of considering age-related changes in the context of sex effects. Second, there is some difficulty in reconciling these age trends with reports of substantial genetic influences in early childhood (54–76% at 3 years) as compared with middle childhood (34–48% between 7 and 12 years) (Boomsma, van Beijsterveldt, & Hudziak, 2005; van der Valk, van den Oord, Verhulst, & Boomsma, 2003). Furthermore, there are also decreasing genetic effects over time during adolescence ($a = 48\%$ at wave 1; $a = 22\%$ at wave 2; O'Connor, McGuire, Reiss, Hetherington, & Plomin, 1998, O'Connor, Neiderhiser, Reiss, Hetherington, & Plomin, 1998). Thus, changes in heritability and shared environment across development appear to be anything but linear and may even reflect a U-shaped curve. Finally, a different pattern of results has been found to characterize severe populations, such that genetic influences become smaller and shared environmental factors larger in adolescent high-scorers (e.g., Deater-Deckard, Reiss, Hetherington, & Plomin, 1997; Eley, 1997; Gjone, Stevenson, Sundet, & Eilertsen, 1996; Rice et al., 2002b). Far from providing any simple answers, these discrepant findings with respect to age point to a need for additional research.

Although cross-sectional comparisons of genetic and environmental influences across age groups provide useful insights into age-related changes, another method for studying developmental differences is to examine genetic and environmental continuity and change across time. That is, longitudinal twin data allow an estimation of the extent to which the same genetic and environmental factors contribute to depression symptoms at different time points (continuity) and/or whether there are new genetic and environmental factors in operation at a later time point (change). Such studies are informative in respect to developmental processes unfolding over time and form a parallel line of inquiry to age comparisons.

Two of the earlier studies utilizing this design demonstrated that whereas genetic factors contributed to the stability of symptoms over a period of 2–3 years, new environmental effects were responsible for change (O'Connor, Neiderhiser, et al., 1998; Silberg et al., 1999). Whereas both these studies focused on transitions during adolescence, a further three studies examining different age ranges found results deviating from this pattern. Using a sample that spanned childhood and adolescence (5–14 years), Scourfield and colleagues (2003) demonstrated an opposite pattern of effects, notably the emergence of "new" genetic influences over a 3-year period, with shared and some nonshared environmental influences remaining stable. Similarly, although some genetic influences persisted across time between ages 3 and 7, contributing to stability, new genetic factors specific to each age were also observed in a second study of childhood problems (van der

Valk et al., 2003). Finally, our own work has explored genetic and environmental continuity and change at three time points in adolescence and young adulthood, in which the average ages of the sample were 14 years, 5 months; 15 years; and 17 years, 8 months (Lau & Eley, 2006). Results showed a rather consistent profile of genetic effects across time (45%, 40%, and 45% at each time point, respectively), with decreasing shared environmental (19%, 9%, and 0%) but increasing nonshared environmental (36%, 51%, and 55%) effects. Decomposing these influences into the effects of "stable" and "new" factors, genes contributed primarily to the continuity of symptoms across time, although new genetic factors were evident at the second time point, which corresponds roughly to midadolescence. New nonshared environmental effects emerged at each time point, and overall these factors contributed to change rather than stability of symptoms.

It is not immediately obvious as to why there are differences between these studies. They may be due to design-related artifacts, such as the measure used to assess depression, to the informant or rater, the sex composition of the sample, or the length of follow-up. A more intriguing alternative is that there are genuine differences between the distinct developmental transition periods assessed in each study (early childhood to middle childhood, middle childhood to adolescence, within adolescence, and adolescence to young adulthood), which are driven by developmentally sensitive etiological influences. The possibility that new genes and new environmental influences come "online" at different stages to account for developmental changes requires further investigation.

Sex Effects

As with age differences, there is some indication of sex-related differences in the size of genetic and environmental influences on depressive symptoms between males and females, but the direction of these differences has been difficult to decipher. Four studies show greater genetic effects among adolescent females (Boomsma et al., 2000; Jacobson & Rowe, 1999; Silberg et al., 1999; Scourfield et al., 2003), whereas two others report larger estimates in adolescent males (Rice et al., 2002b; Eley & Stevenson, 1999). Among children, there is some consensus that females show larger genetic effects (Eley & Stevenson, 1999; Scourfield et al., 2003; Happonen et al., 2002; van der Valk et al., 2003), although this has not always been replicated (Hewitt et al., 1992; van der Valk et al., 2003). Still other studies have found no sex differences in either age group (Bartels et al., 2003; Bartels et al., 2004; Lau, Rijsdijk, & Eley, 2006; Gjone & Stevenson, 1997; Thapar & McGuffin, 1994). Together, these studies provide only modest evidence of sex differences in the heritability of depression. Although some studies reflect more complex interactions with age, the direction of these effects remains frustratingly unclear.

Extreme Scoring Individuals

There are now at least six articles reporting on genetic and environmental influences of extreme depression; five have assessed high scores on measures of depression (Deater-Deckard et al., 1997; Eley, 1997; Gjone et al., 1996; Rende, Plomin, Reiss, & Hetherington, 1993; Rice et al., 2002b), and one has analyzed clinically significant data (Glowinski, Madden, Bucholz, Lynskey, & Heath, 2003). Results of the former analyses are reasonably consistent in suggesting that, as compared with individuals scoring in the normal range, there are nonsignificant trends for genetic effects to be lower and shared environmental factors to be greater among high scorers (Deater-Deckard et al., 1997; Eley, 1997; Rende et al., 1993; Rice et al., 2002b). Unexpectedly, this pattern does not extend to the clinically significant sample, which demonstrated heritability and shared environmental effects comparable to those of normal-ranged individuals. Given that this latter study constitutes only one of its kind, further replications will be needed before these differences are interpreted.

The articles analyzing extreme groups also hint at age-related trends, such as that genetic influences are sizably larger and shared environmental effects smaller in high-scoring children, whereas nonsignificant decreases in genetic effects and increases in shared environmental effects characterize older high-scoring individuals (Gjone et al., 1996; Rice, Harold, & Thapar, 2003). Together, these results suggest that etiological influences in the development of severe depression are somewhat different between childhood and adolescence. These two studies also considered sex differences in group heritability and shared environmental effects, with neither study reporting significant differences. Thus, at present, until further study, etiological mechanisms operating at the extremes may be considered similar for girls and boys.

Summary

An increased effort to recruit large epidemiological samples of child and adolescent twins and siblings over the last two decades has permitted the exploration of more intricate trends in genetic and environmental effects on depressive symptoms in relation to age and development, sex, and severity of symptoms. Although the findings from behavioral genetic studies have not been definitive, they provide a potential platform for explaining certain epidemiological findings in the presentation of depression. Most notably, changes in the size of genetic and environmental factors or the emergence of "new" influences may provide possible explanations of observed age- and sex-related trends in prevalence rates during midpuberty. In addition, establishing the level of genetic and environmental effects in high-scoring individuals (those presumably at increased risk for disorder) in relation to those falling in the normal range, can offer insight into whether the former set of individuals represent an etiological disjunction. This can in turn contribute to resolving the conflicting categorical and dimensional conceptualizations of depression.

MOLECULAR GENETIC STUDIES OF DEPRESSION

The results of 2 genome-wide scans of unipolar depression in adults have only recently been published (for a more detailed review, see Huezo-Diaz, Tandon, & Aitchison, 2005, and Levinson, 2005). Although the studies tend to differ in the definition of the phenotype, they are reasonably consistent in utilizing the nonparametric sib-pair design. Results have implicated broad regions within chromosomes 1, 2, 3, 4, 5 6, 7, 8, 10, 11, 12, 15, and 18 as containing putative susceptibility genes. Despite there being some overlap between studies the areas identified (chromosomes 1, 4, 6, 7, 8, 11 and 12) are still too broad to pinpoint exact locations (Huezo-Diaz et al., 2005; Levinson, 2005).

Although conclusions from linkage studies have not been very fruitful, association studies, which often rely on a priori knowledge that a particular genetic system is involved in the pathogenesis of depression to narrow their searches, have been comparatively more rewarding. By far the most popular neurobiological system targeted in locating candidate genes is the serotonergic (5-HT) neurotransmitter system, a choice fueled largely by prevailing physiological theories holding that the activity of monoaminergic neurotransmitters is somewhat compromised in individuals with depression (for a review on the neurobiology of depression, see Hirschfeld, 2000). In short, these neuro-transmitters, including serotonin, represent the chemically induced transmission mechanisms by which neurons connecting different regions of the brain, particularly those involved in emotion regulation, communicate. There are now a number of consistent findings linking deficient serotonin levels and vulnerability to depression in adults. Among these are pharmacological studies of certain antidepressant drugs that may alleviate symptoms through the alteration of the functioning of this system and studies of indirect markers of serotonergic activity, such as the density of receptor-binding sites or quantities of metabolites and by-products in depressed individuals, which are suggestive of abnormalities of the system (Charney, Menkes, & Heninger, 1981; Coppen, Eccleston, & Peet, 1973; Drevets et al., 1999; Lopez, Chalmers, Little, & Watson, 1998). Yet in spite of this large body of evidence in support of the role of serotonin in depression, it is not yet known which of the multiple regulatory processes involved in chemical transmission is responsible for the deficiency in levels (Manji, Drevets, & Charney, 2001). Thus, from a molecular genetic perspective, studies have had to concentrate on a number of genes known to code for different steps involved in the transmission process. These have included identifying genetic variants located within the serotonin transporter gene, serotonin receptor genes, and genes that code the monoamine oxidase type A (MAOA) and tryptophan hydroxylase (TPH-1) enzymes. These attempts have been met with both positive and negative results, replications, and nonreplications (for more details on individual studies, see Huezo-Diaz et al., 2005, and Levinson et al., 2005). Thus far, there are good theoretically driven reasons for examining genetic variants involved in the release and regulation of serotonin, but the field is still in its infancy and studies of children and adolescents have been rare.

Expansions into other candidate gene systems have included other members of the monoamine family such as the noradrenergic and dopaminergic pathways, which may be involved in the brain reward systems (Huezo-Diaz et al., 2005); the hypothalamic pituitary adrenal axis, which is responsible for activating hormonal responses to acute and chronic stressors (Villafuerte et al., 2002); and different neurotrophic factors such as brain-derived neurotropic factor, which are implicated by more recent theories on the effects of neuroprotection and cellular resilience on the development of depression (Manji et al., 2001). Despite this relatively rich data base of information on the functional significance of particular genes, conclusions on their application in molecular genetic designs are far from definitive.

Identifying QTLs has proven challenging across almost all complex traits, and reports of high false positive rates and poor replicability across studies tend to characterize the field in general. The main reason for this is that complex phenotypes such as depression are multifactorial. This implies that not only are there multiple genes of small effect size accounting for the phenotype, but there are also important contributions by different aspects of the social environment across time. Such complexity can give rise to three issues that contribute towards the difficulty in the replication of linkage and association studies. First, because QTLs are probabilistic rather than deterministic, affected sibling pairs may not all share all chromosomal segments that contain them. Conversely, they may share many segments by chance. Second, there may be heterogeneity in the etiology of a phenotype. As phenotypes are defined essentially at the behavioral level (rather than by etiology), the same repertoire of symptoms may represent different genetic underpinnings or the sole effects of environmental adversity (phenocopies), which could lead to no differences observed in the comparison between groups. Finally, as there may be interplay between genetic and environmental influences (gene–environment interaction), there may be individuals who carry the susceptibility gene but who do not manifest the pheno-type inasmuch as they have not encountered the appropriate environmental event (reduced penetrance). Similarly, there may be interactions between different genetic loci (epistasis) that cannot be easily captured by studying genes independently. Although these potential issues somewhat dampen the excitement surrounding molecular genetics, the development of more sophisticated techniques to obtain and analyze DNA have made the collection of genotype information a very real possibility for many researchers. Indeed, it is the gradual inclusion of genotype data within large longitudinal samples that already have high-quality psychosocial and phenotypic data at their disposal, that promises to revolutionize the field of psychiatric genetics. Nowhere is the introduction of these appli-cations more exciting than within pediatric samples. This first wave of studies can further address questions on the role of development, providing a lens to view the dynamic expression of genetic and environmental factors across time.

GENE–ENVIRONMENT INTERPLAY AND DEPRESSIVE CONDITIONS

Until recently genetic and environmental factors were inaccurately depicted in behavioral genetic designs as having additive and independent effects on measured phenotypes. The result was that effects arising from gene–environment interplay were often incorporated within main genetic and environmental effects in quantitative designs, but essentially ignored in molecular genetic analyses. Advances in analytical techniques, however, have ensured a growing body of literature that supports the importance of genetic influences on environmental risk exposure (gene–environment correlation) and genetic influences on the susceptibility to environmental risks (gene–environment interaction) in relation to depressive phenotypes. Examining these processes of interplay thus reflects one approach to understanding risk mechanisms leading to emotional outcomes. The conceptual basis and empirical evidence of each is discussed.

Gene–Environment Correlations

Statistically, correlations between genes and the environment arise when the number of individuals carrying a particular genotype (genotypic frequencies) are not randomly dis-tributed across levels of environmental risk but, rather, occur more frequently within a certain environmental stratum. Conceptually, this implies the presence of genetic influ-ences on exposure to an environmental condition. Gene–environment correlation (rG-E) can be manifested in three contexts (Scarr & McCartney, 1983). Passive gene–environment correlation comes about because of the sharing in biological families of both genes and environment. Thus, it occurs when the effects of parental genotypes are related to the family environments their children are exposed to. For example, offspring of depressed mothers are likely to receive both a genetic predisposition to this condition and the environmental effects of a depressogenic parenting style, which may characterize the interpersonal styles of such mothers. *Evocative rG-E* refers to the genetic propensity of some individuals to elicit or evoke certain reactions from others. These effects may be mediated through intermediate factors, such as temperament or cognitive style. Thus, infants who cry easily or show irritability may be more likely to elicit negative reactions from caregivers, which may then affect on parenting style. Finally, *active rG-E* occurs when individuals select, create, and modify their environmental experiences, according to particular genetically mediated dispositions. Behaviorally inhibited or shy individuals may be less likely to seek out friends, instead choosing to engage in solitary play, thus ultimately influencing socioemotional development.

Longstanding support for genetic influences on many aspects of the environment has been documented, but such studies have mainly relied on quantitative designs (Plomin & Bergeman, 1991). These studies have shown first that many "social" risks such as stressful life events aggregate in families (e.g., Rijsdijk et al., 2001), but, more impressive, that genetic influences have been found on an astonishing array of family environment variables, including family connectedness (Jacobson & Rowe, 1999), parent–child interaction as assessed by questionnaire (Plomin, Reiss, Hetherington, & Howe, 1994), observation (O'Connor, Hetherington, Reiss, & Plomin, 1995), or both (Pike, McGuire, Hetherington, Reiss, & Plomin, 1996), sibling interactions assessed by questionnaire alone (Plomin et al., 1994) or combined with observation (Pike et al., 1996), parental divorce (O'Connor, Caspi, DeFries, & Plomin, 2000), and life events (Thapar & McGuffin, 1996; Thapar, Harold, & McGuffin, 1998; Silberg et al., 1999). Collectively, these findings suggest that there is far more complexity in the origins of the family environment than previously thought. Yet what is most pertinent to the study of risk mechanisms in depression is not that genes influence environments per se, but that genetic vulnerability involved in the phenotype is expressed through exposure to high-risk environments. In other words, the genes that are involved in the development of symptoms should overlap to some extent with those influencing aspects of the child's environment. This has also been widely reported in many adolescent studies. To illustrate, we examined genetic and environmental influences on two social risk variables, maternal punitive discipline and negative life events, in our adolescent sample described previously (Lau & Eley, in press). Results showed moderate genetic effects on both measures (both at 31%), implicating the presence of gene–environment correlation. Next we explored genetic influences that are shared between each social risk measure and depressive symptoms. Consistent with other examples in the literature (e.g., Eaves, Silberg, & Erkanli, 2003; Pike et al., 1996; Rice et al., 2003; Silberg et al., 1999; Thapar et al., 1998), there was significant overlap in genetic influences between symptoms and each social risk. Together, these results suggest that genetic liability for the phenotype may be expressed partly through creation of certain environmental risks.

Although there is widespread evidence for gene–environment correlations, it has proved challenging to analytically distinguish between the three different types. Nevertheless, this taxonomy has been useful in speculating on the various psychosocial paths through which genetic effects may be expressed across development. For example, it has been suggested that passive and evocative forms may be more salient in infancy and childhood, whereas active processes become increasingly important in adolescence, when individuals play a more dynamic role in shaping their own experiences. Indeed, one study that has explored developmental differences compared the relative contributions of genetic and environmental factors to the relationship between negative life events and depression in two age groups: 8–11 and 12–17 years (Rice et al., 2003). Genes played a larger role in this association among older adolescents as compared with the child group, lending support to the notion that "active" gene–environment correlation, which presumably underlies the genetic effects on negative life events, is of stronger importance to symptoms in the older age group. The emergence of active processes may also reflect some of the new genetic influences that emerge in this age range (Lau & Eley, 2006; Scourfield et al., 2003).

Gene–Environment Interactions

Interactions refers to the differential effect of one variable at varying levels of another variable. As such, gene–environment interactions arise when environmental risk effects change as a function of genetic risk, or when genetic risks are expressed only in the presence of an environmental stressor. In terms of risk mechanisms, *interactions* may refer to genetic influences on reactivity to the environment or to what happens when a stressor elicits (latent) genetic susceptibilities. Demonstrating gene–environment interactions in depressive conditions has, for the most part, proven difficult, given that more statistical power and thus larger samples are required to detect these than main effects. Yet this has not prevented an accumulation of studies dedicated to finding these effects within both quantitative and molecular designs.

Family designs afford one possibility for exploring interactions. An earlier study of our adolescent sample exemplifies this approach, by examining the main and interactive effects of a composite index of parental familial vulnerability to anxiety, depression, and neuroticism and other social aspects of the family environment, on self-reported depressive symptoms in the adolescent offspring (Eley, Liang, et al., 2004). The composite index of vulnerability maximizes familial liability to emotional conditions and is likely to reflect the effects of shared genes among family members (Sham et al., 2000). A significant interaction emerged between this composite and parental educational level in regard to adolescent symptoms (see Figure 6.1). Specifically, individuals who displayed high levels of familial risk and whose parents lacked educational qualifications had the highest symptom scores. This implies that adolescents in families with high rates of depression are particularly at risk for depression themselves if their parents lack qualifications. This effect may be mediated by coping strategies and an ability to seek help, as these skills may be improved in families that have achieved educational qualifications.

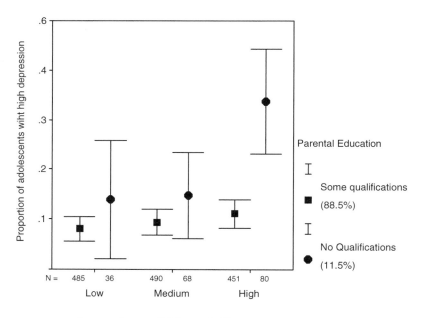

FIGURE 6.1. Parental educational influences on genetic risk to severe depression.

Although these results are certainly thought provoking in terms of specific pathways to adolescent depression, they are also limited by a failure to discount the alternative suggestion, that the familial composite reflects shared environmental influences rather than shared genes among family members. To disentangle these two sources, the twin design is again required, and variations of these analyses have permitted the two rather different tests of gene–environment interaction as demonstrated in one study of adolescent females (Silberg, Rutter, Neale, & Eaves, 2001). This study showed, first, that negative life events (an environmental risk) exacerbated genetic effects on self-reported depressive (and anxiety) symptoms. Second, individuals at genetic risk for depression (and anxiety), indexed by the presence of parental emotional disorders, were also more likely to exhibit depressive symptoms following recent negative life events. Thus, the first test indicated differences in genetic effects across levels of environmental risk, whereas the second showed genetic influences on reactivity to environmental risk.

An important point to consider in studies of interactions is whether there are confounding effects due to gene–environment correlation. Often, what are recognized as interactions may also be interpreted as genetic risks for depression that increase social adversity. In fact, the validity of interactions is premised on an assumption that there is no association between an individual's genetic makeup and his or her experience of particular environments. This assumption can therefore be violated when gene–environment correlations are present, as these occur by definition when individuals with a certain genotype are more likely to be exposed to particular environmental events. What this amounts to is that when testing for interactions, it must be very clear that the environmental variable examined is not influenced by genes that are also associated with behavioral outcomes. Should this be the case, this may signify a gene–environment correlation in the phenotype rather than an interaction. Yet, as gene–environment correlations and interactions are likely to coexist, a more sophisticated approach is to simultaneously assess and differentiate these effects (Purcell, 2002).

To this end, we explored whether genetic effects on depressive outcomes varied as a function of maternal punitive discipline and negative life events (G×E) after controlling for a finding of genetic effects on these variables. Results for both social risk measures indicated the joint presence of gene–environment correlation and interaction. Thus, genetic influences on adolescent depression were not only shared with those on punitive parenting or life events (gene–environment correlation), but they were also moderated by the presence of these risks (gene–environment interaction), such that genetic variance increased substantially with higher levels of each environmental risk. On the basis of these results, it can be seen that adolescents with higher genetic liability are more likely to be exposed to the double disadvantage of environmental risk (gene–environment correlation). Furthermore, under these high levels of adversity, genetic risks for depression have greater opportunity to be expressed (gene–environment interaction).

Perhaps the more precise method of assessing gene–environment interactions, which has recently created much excitement in the scientific community, is the use of specific measures of the environment and candidate genes in molecular studies. A groundbreaking study first showed an interaction between a functional polymorphism in the serotonin (5-HT) transporter promoter region and the effect of life events, in relation to depression symptoms in adults (Caspi et al., 2003). The 5-HT transporter gene is involved in regulatory processes during stress (Hariri et al., 2002), making it an excellent candidate for interaction with environmental stress. The polymorphism exists in two forms, a long and a short form. The short allele is less efficient than the longer allele, thus leading to differences in available serotonin in the brain (Lesch et al., 1996). Analyses revealed that the

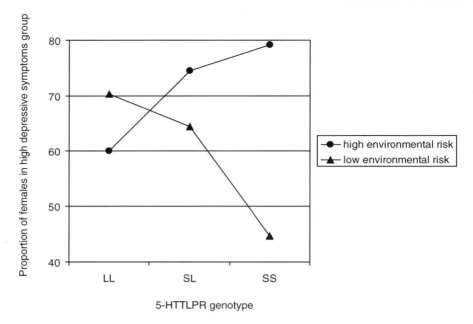

FIGURE 6.2. Impact of environmental risks on depressive symptom group by genotype in adolescent females.

effects of stressful life events were significantly stronger in individuals carrying one or two copies of the short form of the allele *s*, as shown by an increase in symptom frequencies and severity. This allele also moderated the longitudinal prediction from childhood maltreatment to adult depression. We subsequently replicated this finding in adolescent females, with an interaction between the same serotonin transporter regulatory region and a family-based measure of environmental risk (including social adversity, family life events, and parental employment level) (Eley, Sugden, et al., 2004). The effects of family-based environmental risk were significantly stronger in female adolescents who possessed at least one short allele (see Figure 6.2). Together these findings suggest that this allelic variant augments the effects of stress on emotional and behavioral symptoms.

The convergence of quantitative and molecular support has made the study of gene–environment interactions a topical area of research. However, these concepts are not entirely unfamiliar to psychologists, who have long used diathesis–stress theories to define the mechanisms by which latent predispositions are elicited by the occurrence of environmental stressors. Findings of gene–environment interaction may be viewed as an extension of these ideas by suggesting that genetic effects act on core processes associated with stress reactivity. This possibility is explored in greater detail in the next section.

INTERMEDIATE PHENOTYPES AS MEDIATORS OF GENETIC AND ENVIRONMENTAL RISK

Another approach to understanding genetic and environmental risk mechanisms in depression is to search for intermediate phenotypes that may reflect or even mediate the risks associated with these influences. "Endophenotypes" are risk markers or vulnerability traits that are more proximal to, and thus more directly influenced by, the genes relevant to a behavioral disorder than are its signs and symptoms (Gottesman & Gould, 2003). These genetic markers first caught the attention of molecular geneticists interested in elucidating specific disease genes. As endophenotypes were assumed to share one or more of the same genes that confer vulnerability to the disorder of interest and to reflect more simplistic genetic phenomena, it followed that their use would result in greater statistical power for the detection of susceptibility genes. A second but more subtle function of endophenotypes lies in illuminating the elusive pathways by which genes for behaviors are expressed. More specifically, they provide a means for identifying traits "upstream" of the products of gene expression but "downstream" from the clinical phenotype (Gottesman & Gould, 2003). As such, they can be identified at differing levels of analysis via neurophysiological, biochemical, endocrinological, neuroanatomical, cognitive, and neuropsychological measures. Several different sets of criteria have been proposed to help locate putative endophenotypes (e.g., Gottesman & Gould, 2003; Skuse, 2001; Waldman, 2005). Although there are variations between these suggestions, several key elements are apparent. First, the marker should co-occur with the disorder and its symptoms in the general population as well as in clinical groups. Although disease specificity and universality (applies to all) are ideal, these are not requirements, given that a common gene variant may affect multiple phenotypes (pleiotropic) and that there may be etiologically heterogeneous subgroups within the disorder. Second, the marker should be relatively state-independent rather than an epiphenomenon of the illness and measured with good reliability. Ideally, it should also possess temporal stability and be a developmental precursor to symptoms. The third and fourth criteria are that endophenotypes should show evidence of heritability and familial (genetic) overlap with the disorder of interest.

There are two possible approaches to identifying endophenotypes. Bottom-up accounts adopt a neuroscience explanation, beginning at the level of genes and progressing to gene expression, to protein function, to neurotransmitters, neural circuitry, and behavior. In comparison, top-down accounts work in the opposite direction, working backward from an individual's behaviors, to reported cognitions, psychological mechanisms, brain function, and genes. Any of these intermediate levels could reflect plausible candidate markers. Indeed, a recent review of putative endophenotypes for adult affective disorders identified a series of putative "psychopathological" and "biological" endophenotypes (Hasler, Drevets, Manji, & Charney, 2004). Each of these was subsequently assessed against the criteria discussed previously. In the former category, there was a mixture of cognitive and affective indices (mood bias toward negative emotions, impaired reward function, impaired learning and memory, impaired executive functions, stress reactivity) as well as behavioral dimensions (neurovegetative signs, diurnal variation, psychomotor change). The latter category consisted of abnormalities in the structure and function of brain regions that partake in the circuitry known to modulate emotional behaviors (amygdala and other limbic structures, prefrontal cortical regions, thalamus, and basal ganglia), alterations in certain neurobiological systems that allow reciprocal communications between these different regions (serotonin, dopamine and norepinephrine), altered hypothalamic–pituitary–adrenal (HPA) axis activity, and, finally, impairments in mechanisms that are involved in intracellular signaling pathways and that may be involved in neuroprotective effects and cellular resilience.

Although the mechanisms discussed here include risk factors that are well established in relation to the etiology of adult depression, very few studies have critically evaluated their potential as mediators of the distal genotype. By tabulating each candidate marker's fulfillment of the endophenotypic criteria, the authors demonstrated that impaired reward function, neuroticism (a measure of stress reactivity), tryptophan depletion (an index of serotonergic function), and dysfunctional cortisol responses (a marker of the abnormal HPA axis) met the majority of the requirements. Whereas each of these was hypothesized to reflect a different aspect of the genetic liability to depression, stress reactivity was proposed as a specific marker of gene–environment interaction. That is, neuroticism could constitute a genetically mediated diathesis influencing sensitivity to stressful events, thus underlying the observed interaction effects between genes and the environment.

Despite the finding of significant genetic effects on pediatric depression, the identification of endophenotypes has been somewhat lacking, falling behind that of other pediatric phenotypes such as ADHD, which have been the topics of various extensive reviews (Doyle, Faraone, et al., 2005; Doyle, Willcutt et al., 2005; Waldman, 2005). Given the relevance of gene–environment interactions in depression in younger samples, aspects of stress reactivity are particularly promising candidates. In our group, we have taken a top-down approach to the identification of these markers, with a particular interest in cognitive biases traditionally implicated in the development of these depressive behaviors. As some of these cognitive biases are considered to influence an individual's response to external, particularly negative events, we speculated that they may reflect genetic risk markers that were expressed through increased stress reactivity, thus accounting for gene–environment interactions. Given that these cognitive factors were identified through many existing and well-articulated cognitive models of depression, their association with depression was already established. Thus, the next steps we took in evaluating their potential as genetic markers were to explore their genetic and environmental structure and to examine the nature of their links with depressive conditions.

One of our first studies addressed these questions in relation to adolescent attributional style (Lau et al., 2006). According to the learned helplessness model (Abramson, Seligman, & Teasdale, 1978), later reformulated as the hopelessness theory (Alloy, Abramson, Metalsky, & Hartlage, 1988), attributional style is a risk factor for depression. Individuals who attribute negative events to internal (directed to the self), stable (likely to persist across time), and global (likely to affect many aspects of life) causes are thought to have increased risks for experiencing depression. These individuals may also possess an opposite pattern of attributions for positive events, such that these are interpreted using external, unstable, and specific reasons. This differential style of responding to environmental events is thought to be fully expressed in the presence of life events. Thus, attributional style is a stress–diathesis model and may be involved in moderating reactivity towards negative events. Given the robust evidence in favor of this model (e.g., Hankin, Abramson, & Siler, 2001), we set out to unravel its genetic and environmental etiology. Analyses of self-reported data on adolescent attributional style revealed that, like depressive symptoms, this cognitive factor was primarily influenced by genes (35%) and nonshared environmental effects (60%) (Lau et al., 2006). Moreover, common genetic and nonshared environmental influences between attributional style and concurrent depressive symptoms, which contributed to their phenotypic relationship, were found. Thus, making negative attributions is more than just a learned trait but is also heritable. More provocatively, these results are consistent with the interpretation that attributional style reflects some genetic liability to depression.

Also compatible with these findings, more recent analyses of our younger sample of 8-year-old twins show that another aspect of cognitive bias, threat perception, as indexed by a measure of the interpretation of ambiguous scenarios, was moderately heritable

(24%) but predominantly influenced by nonshared environmental influences (69%) (Eley et al., in press). Although genetic effects on depressive symptoms were marginally smaller (16%), with shared and nonshared environmental effects at 15 and 70%, respectively, genetic and environmental overlap between this bias and self-reported depressive symptoms was evident. Moreover, these shared components were influential in explaining the phenotypic correlation between them. As with attributional style, the interpretation of ambiguous situations is also thought to operate by influencing individual differences in the evaluation of threatening events.

Although identifying putative genetic markers from traditional psychological theories of pediatric depression has yielded positive results, not all cognitive biases are reflective of genetic effects or shared genetic links with symptoms. Instead, it is very plausible that some aspects of "response style" in reacting to environmental events are influenced primarily by the social environment. A recent example highlighting this possibility was a study of cognitive biases in regard to social relationships in our group of 8-year-olds (Gregory et al., in press). Specifically, the origins of negative perceptions and expectations of others and beliefs about others views of oneself, and their links with depressive (and anxiety) symptoms were explored. These "interpersonal cognitions" showed very little evidence of genetic influence, but rather were explained by nonshared and, to a lesser degree, shared environmental influences. Moreover, their relationship with depressive symptoms was mediated largely by environmental factors. This finding is somewhat unusual, given the previous findings of attributional style and threat perception; however, the authors reasoned that such social-cognitive biases may in fact reflect actual environmental experiences, such as social interactions operating within the family (parent–child attachment, family discord) or in the peer group (bullying, rejection). Thus, an initial interpretation of these results is that some cognitive biases mediate sources of environmental adversity in the development of depressive symptoms, rather than reflecting genetically mediated dispositions.

SUMMARY

With the exception of some discrepancies in the results of particular study designs, the application of behavioral genetic methodology to the study of pediatric depressive symptoms and disorders has highlighted the importance of studying both nature and nurture in these conditions, paralleling findings for many other childhood disorders. The pairing of more sophisticated conceptual questions with newer analytical tools has moved the field beyond examining the *extent* of genetic and environmental influences, however, to asking questions about the *nature* of these effects and *how* they may be expressed. Therefore, we have aimed to highlight not only the level of impact of genetic and environmental influences across various moderators, such as age and development and sex, and among extreme-scoring populations, but also their interplay in the development of symptoms. We have also explored the more exciting efforts aimed at identifying intermediate factors and processes by which genetic and environmental risks take effect on behavioral outcomes. A successful search for endophenotypes will necessarily involve integrating different levels of explanation that stem from other disciplinary approaches within genetic studies. Moreover, such integrative studies should be considered in the context of developmental change, that is, the differences in the interplay between factors across different stages of development. This is where collaboration between neuroscientists, psychologists, and behavioral geneticists will prove to be most fruitful, with the opportunity to piece together what at first seem to be rather discrepant parts of a puzzle in building an overall picture of the development of depression. At present, integrative studies have either selected top-down (behavior–cognitions–brains–genes) or bottom-up (genes–protein–function–behavior) approaches, but eventually studies need to attempt the more ambitious task of considering these approaches in parallel. Dialogue between these perspectives should meet at the level of the brain, highlighting potentially different avenues for intervention and prevention of the often lifelong and debilitating condition of depression.

REFERENCES

Abramson, L. Y., Seligman, M. E. P., & Teasdale, J. D. (1978). Learned helplessness in humans: Critique and reformulation. *Journal of Abnormal Psychology, 87,* 49–74.

Alloy, L. B., Abramson, L. Y., Metalsky, G. I., & Hartlage, S. (1988). The hopelessness theory of depression: Attributional aspects. *British Journal of Clinical Psychology, 27,* 5–21.

Bartels, M., Boomsma, D. I., Hudziak, J. J., Rietveld, M. J., Van Beijsterveldt, T. C., & van den Oord, E. J. (2004). Disentangling genetic, environmental, and rater effects on internalizing and externalizing problem behavior in 10-year-old twins. *Twin Research, 7*(2), 162–175.

Bartels, M., Hudziak, J. J., Boomsma, D. I., Rietveld, M. J., Van Beijsterveldt, T. C., & van den Oord, E. J. (2003). A study of parent ratings of internalizing and externalizing problem behavior in 12-year-old twins. *Journal of the American Academy of Child and Adolescent Psychiatry, 42*(11), 1351–1359.

Birmaher, B., Ryan, N. D., Williamson, D. E., Brent, D. A., & Kaufman, J. (1996). Childhood and adolescent depression: A review of the past 10 years: II. *Journal of the American Academy of Child and Adolescent Psychiatry, 35,* 1575–1583.

Boomsma, D. I., Beem, A. L., van den Berg, M., Dolan, C. V., Koopmans, J. R., Vink, J. M., et al. (2000). Netherlands twin family study of anxious depression (NETSAD). *Twin Research, 3*(4), 323–334.

Boomsma, D. I., van Beijsterveldt, C. E. M., & Hudziak, J. J. (2005). Genetic and environmental influences on anxious/depression during childhood: A study from the Netherlands Twin Register. *Genes, Brain and Behavior, 16,* 466–481.

Cardno, A. G., Marshall, E. J., Coid, B., MacDonald, A. M., Ribchester, T. R., Davies, N. J., et al. (1999). Heritability estimates for psychotic disorders: The Maudsley twin psychosis series. *Archives of General Psychiatry, 56*(2), 162–168.

Caspi, A., Sugden, K., Moffitt, T. E., Taylor, A., Craig, I. W., Harrington, H., et al. (2003). Influence of life stress on depression: Moderation by a polymorphism in the 5-HTT gene. *Science, 301,* 386–389.

Charney, D. S., Menkes, D. B., & Heninger, G. R. (1981). Receptor sensitivity and the mechanism of action of antidepressant treatment: Implications for the etiology and therapy of depression. *Archives of General Psychiatry, 38,* 1160–1180.

Coppen, A., Eccleston, E. G., & Peet, M. (1973). Total and free tryptophan concentration in the plasma of depressive patients. *Lancet, 2,* 60–63.

Deater-Deckard, K., Reiss, D., Hetherington, E. M., & Plomin, R. (1997). Dimensions and disorders of adolescent adjustment: A quantitative genetic analysis of unselected samples and selected extremes. *Journal of Child Psychology and Psychiatry, 38,* 515–525.

DeFries, J. C., Plomin, R., & Fulker, D. W. (1994). *Nature and nurture during middle childhood.* Cambridge, MA: Blackwell.

Doyle, A. E., Faraone, S. V., Seidman, L. J., Willcutt, E. G., Nigg, J. T., Waldman, I. D., et al. (2005). Are endophenotypes based on measures of executive functions useful for molecular genetic studies of ADHD? *Journal of Child Psychology and Psychiatry, 46*(7), 774–803.

Doyle, A. E., Willcutt, E. G., Seidman, L. J., Biederman, J., Chouinard, V. A., Silva, J., et al. (2005). Attention-deficit/hyperactivity disorder endophenotypes. *Biological Psychiatry, 57,* 1324–1335.

Drevets, W. C., Frank, E., Price, J. C., Kupfer, D. J., Holt, D., Greer, P. J., et al. (1999). PET imaging of serotonin 1A receptor binding in depression. *Biological Psychiatry, 46,* 1375–1387.

Eaves, L., Silberg, J., & Erkanli, A. (2003). Resolving multiple epigenetic pathways to adolescent depression. *Journal of Child Psychology and Psychiatry, 44,* 1006–1014.

Eley, T. C. (1997). Depressive symptoms in children and adolescents: Etiological links between normality and abnormality: A research note. *Journal of Child Psychology and Psychiatry, 38,* 861–866.

Eley, T. C., & Craig, I. W. (2005). Introductory guide to the language of molecular genetics. *Journal of Child Psychology and Psychiatry, 46,* 1039–1041.

Eley, T. C., Deater-Deckard, K., Fombonne, E., Fulker, D. W., & Plomin, R. (1998). An adoption study of depressive symptoms in middle childhood. *Journal of Child Psychology and Psychiatry, 39,* 337–345.

Eley, T. C., Gregory, A. M., Lau, J. Y. F., McGuffin, P., Napolitano, M., Rijsdijk, F. V., et al. (in press). In the face of uncertainty: A genetic analysis of ambiguous information, anxiety and depression in children. *Journal of Abnormal Child Psychology.*

Eley, T. C., Liang, H., Plomin, R., Sham, P., Sterne, A., Williamson, R., et al. (2004). Parental familial vulnerability, family environment, and their interactions as predictors of depressive symptoms in adolescents. *Journal of the American Academy of Child and Adolescent Psychiatry, 43,* 298–306.

Eley, T. C., & Rijsdijk, F. (2005). Introductory guide to the statistics of molecular genetics. *Journal of Child Psychology and Psychiatry, 46*(10), 1042–1044.

Eley, T. C., & Stevenson, J. (1999). Exploring the covariation between anxiety and depression symptoms: A genetic analysis of the effects of age and sex. *Journal of Child Psychology and Psychiatry, 40,* 1273–1284.

Eley, T. C., Sugden, K., Gregory, A. M., Sterne, A., Plomin, R., & Craig, I. W. (2004). Gene–environment interaction analysis of serotonin system markers with adolescent depression. *Molecular Psychiatry, 9,* 908–915.

Gjone, H., & Stevenson, J. (1997). The association between internalizing and externalizing behaviour in childhood and early adolescence: Genetic or environmental common influences. *Journal of Abnormal Child Psychology, 54,* 277–286.

Gjone, H., Stevenson, J., Sundet, J. M., & Eilertsen, D. E. (1996). Changes in heritability across increasing levels of behaviour problems in young twins. *Behavior Genetics, 26,* 419–426.

Gladstone, T. R., & Kaslow, N. J. (1995). Depression and attributions in children and adolescents: A meta-analytic review. *Journal of Abnormal Child Psychology, 23,* 597–606.

Glowinski, A. L., Madden, P. A., Bucholz, K. K., Lynskey, M. T., & Heath, A. C. (2003). Genetic epidemiology of self-reported lifetime DSM-IV major depressive disorder in a population-based twin sample of female adolescents. *Journal of Child Psychology and Psychiatry, 44*(7), 988–996.

Gottesman, I. I., & Gould, T. D. (2003). The endophenotype concept in psychiatry: Etymology and strategic intentions. *American Journal of Psychiatry, 160,* 636–645.

Gregory, A. G., Rijsdijk, F., Lau, J. Y. F., Napolitano, M., McGuffin, P., & Eley, T. C. (in press). Interpersonal cognitions and associations with depressive symptoms in school-aged twins. *Journal of Abnormal Psychology.*

Hankin, B. L., Abramson, L. Y., & Siler, M. (2001). A prospective test of the hopelessness theory of depression in adolescence. *Cognitive Therapy and Research, 25,* 607–632.

Happonen, M., Pulkkinen, L., Kaprio, J., Van der Meere, M. J., Viken, R. J., & Rose, R. J. (2002). The heritability of depressive symptoms: Multiple informants and multiple measures. *Journal of Child Psychology and Psychiatry, 43*(4), 471–479.

Hariri, A. R., Mattay, V. S., Tessitore, A., Kolachana, B., Fera, F., Goldman, D., et al. (2002). Serotonin transporter genetic variation and the response of the human amygdala. *Science*, 297, 400–403.

Hasler, G., Drevets, W. C., Manji, H. K., & Charney, D. S. (2004). Discovering endophenotypes for major depression. *Neuropsychopharmacology*, 29(10), 1765–1781.

Hewitt, J. K., Silberg, J. L., Neale, M. C., Eaves, L. J., & Erickson, M. (1992). The analysis of parental ratings of children's behavior using LISREL. *Behavior Genetics*, 22(3), 293–317.

Hirschfeld, R. M. (2000). History and evolution of the monoamine hypothesis of depression. *Journal of Clinical Psychiatry*, 61(Suppl. 6), 4–6.

Huezo-Diaz, P., Tandon, K., & Aitchison, K. J. (2005). The genetics of depression and related traits. *Current Psychiatry Reports*, 7(2), 117–124.

Jacobson, K. C., & Rowe, D. C. (1999). Genetic and environmental influences on the relationships between family connectedness, school connectedness, and adolescent depressed mood: Sex differences. *Developmental Psychology*, 35, 926–939.

Kendler, K. S., Neale, M. C., Kessler, R. C., Heath, A. C., & Eaves, L. J. (1994). Parental treatment and the equal environment assumption in twin studies of psychiatric illness. *Psychological Medicine*, 24(3), 579–590.

Lau, J. Y. F., & Eley, T. C. (2006). Changes in genetic and environmental influences on depressive symptoms across adolescence and young adulthood. *British Journal of Psychiatry*, 189, 422–427.

Lau, J. Y. F. & Eley, T. C. (in press). Disentangling gene environment correlations and interactions in adolescent depression. *Journal of Child Psychology and Psychiatry*.

Lau, J. Y. F., Rijsdijk, F., & Eley, T. C. (2006). I think, therefore I am: A twin study of attributional style in adolescents. *Journal of Child Psychology and Psychiatry*, 47, 696–703.

Lesch, K. P., Bengel, D., Heils, A., Zhang Sabol, S., Greenburg, B. D., Petri, S., et al. (1996). Association of anxiety-related traits with a polymorphism in the serotonin transporter gene regulatory region. *Science*, 274, 1527–1531.

Levinson, D. F. (2005). The genetics of depression: A review. *Biological Psychiatry*, 60(2), 84–92.

Lopez, J. F., Chalmers, D. T., Little, K. Y., & Watson, S. J. (1998). Regulation of serotonin 1A, glucocorticoid, and mineralocorticoid receptor in rat and human hippocampus: Implications for the neurobiology of depression. *Biological Psychiatry*, 43, 547–573.

Manji, H. K., Drevets, W. C., & Charney, D. S. (2001). The cellular neurobiology of depression. *Nature Medicine*, 7(5), 541–547.

Mathews, C. A., & Reus, V. I. (2001). Assortative mating in the affective disorders: A systematic review and meta-analysis. *Comprehensive Psychiatry*, 42(4), 257–262.

Moilanen, I., Linna, S. L., Ebeling, H., Kumpulainen, K., Tamminen, T., Piha, J., et al. (1999). Are twins' behavioural/emotional problems different from singletons'? *European Child and Adolescent Psychiatry*, 8(Suppl. 4), 62–67.

Neale, M. C., & Maes, H. M. (2001). *Methodology for genetic studies of twins and families*. Dordrecht, the Netherlands: Kluwer Academic.

O'Connor, T. G., Caspi, A., DeFries, J. C., & Plomin, R. (2000). Are associations between parental divorce in children's adjustment genetically mediated? An adoption study. *Developmental Psychology*, 36, 429–437.

O'Connor, T. G., Hetherington, E. M., Reiss, D., & Plomin, R. (1995). A twin-sibling study of observed parent–adolescent interactions. *Child Development*, 66, 812–829.

O'Connor, T. G., McGuire, S., Reiss, D., Hetherington, E. M., & Plomin, R. (1998). Co-occurrence of depressive symptoms and antisocial behavior in adolescence: A common genetic liability. *Journal of Abnormal Psychology*, 107, 27–37.

O'Connor, T. G., Neiderhiser, J. M., Reiss, D., Hetherington, E. M., & Plomin, R. (1998). Genetic contributions to continuity, change, and co-occurrence of antisocial and depressive symptoms in adolescence. *Journal of Child Psychology and Psychiatry*, 39, 323–336.

Phillips, D. I. (1993). Twin studies in medical research: Can they tell us whether diseases are genetically determined? *Lancet*, 341(8851), 1008–1009.

Pike, A., McGuire, S., Hetherington, E. M., Reiss, D., & Plomin, R. (1996). Family environment and adolescent depressive symptoms and antisocial behavior: A multivariate genetic analysis. *Developmental Psychology, 32,* 590–603.

Plomin, R., & Bergeman, C. S. (1991). The nature of nurture: Genetic influences on "environmental" measures. *Behavioral and Brain Sciences, 14,* 373–427.

Plomin, R., DeFries, J. C., McClearn, G. E., & McGuffin, P. (2001). *Behavioral genetics* (4th ed.). New York: Worth.

Plomin, R., Reiss, D., Hetherington, E. M., & Howe, G. W. (1994). Nature and nurture: Genetic contributions to measures of the family environment. *Developmental Psychology, 30,* 32–43.

Purcell, S. (2002). Variance components models for gene–environment interaction in twin analysis. *Twin Research, 5,* 554–571.

Rende, R. D., Plomin, R., Reiss, D., & Hetherington, E. M. (1993). Genetic and environmental influences on depressive symptomatology in adolescence: Individual differences and extreme scores. *Journal of Child Psychology and Psychiatry, 34,* 1387–1398.

Rice, F., Harold, G., & Thaper, A. (2002a). The genetic aetiology of childhood depression: A review. *Journal of Child Psychology and Psychiatry, 43,* 65–80.

Rice, F., Harold, G. T., & Thapar, A. (2002b). Assessing the effects of age, sex and shared environment on the genetic aetiology of depression in childhood and adolescence. *Journal of Child Psychology and Psychiatry, 43,* 1039–1051.

Rice, F., Harold, G. T., & Thapar, A. (2003). Negative life events as an account of age-related differences in the genetic aetiology of depression in childhood and adolescence. *Journal of Child Psychology and Psychiatry, 44,* 977–987.

Riese, M. L. (1999). Effects of chorion type on neonatal temperament differences in monozygotic pairs. *Behavior Genetics, 29,* 87–94.

Rijsdijk, F. V., Sham, P. C., Sterne, A., Purcell, S., McGuffin, P., Farmer, A., et al. (2001). Life events and depression in a community sample of siblings. *Psychological Medicine, 31,* 401–410.

Scarr, S., & McCartney, K. (1983). How people make their own environments: A theory of genotype → environmental effects. *Child Development, 54,* 424–435.

Scourfield, J., Rice, F., Thapar, A., Harold, G. T., Martin, N., & McGuffin, P. (2003). Depressive symptoms in children and adolescents: Changing aetiological influences with development. *Journal of Child Psychology and Psychiatry, 44,* 968–976.

Sham, P. C., Sterne, A., Purcell, S., Cherny, S. S., Webster, M., Rijsdijk, F. V., et al. (2000). GENE-SiS: Creating a composite index of the vulnerability to anxiety and depression in a community-based sample of siblings. *Twin Research, 3,* 316–322.

Silberg, J., Pickles, A., Rutter, M., Hewitt, J., Simonoff, E., Maes, H., et al. (1999). The influence of genetic factors and life stress on depression among adolescent girls. *Archives of General Psychiatry, 56,* 225–232.

Silberg, J. L., Rutter, M., & Eaves, L. (2001). Genetic and environmental influences on the temporal association between earlier anxiety and later depression in girls. *Biological Psychiatry, 49,* 1040–1049.

Silberg, J., Rutter, M., Neale, M., & Eaves, L. (2001). Genetic moderation of environmental risk for depression and anxiety in adolescent girls. *British Journal of Psychiatry, 179,* 116–121.

Skuse, D. S. (2001). Endophenotypes and child psychiatry. *British Journal of Psychiatry, 178,* 395–396.

Thapar, A., Harold, G., & McGuffin, P. (1998). Life events and depressive symptoms in childhood—shared genes or shared adversity: A research note. *Journal of Child Psychology and Psychiatry, 39*(8), 1153–1158.

Thapar, A., & McGuffin, P. (1994). A twin study of depressive symptoms in childhood. *British Journal of Psychiatry, 165,* 259–265.

Thapar, A., & McGuffin, P. (1996). Genetic influences on life events in childhood. *Psychological Medicine, 26,* 813–820.

van den Oord, E. J., Boomsma, D. I., & Verhulst, F. C. (1994). A study of problem behaviors in 10-

to 15-year-old biologically related and unrelated international adoptees. *Behavior Genetics*, *24*, 193–205.

van der Valk, J. C., van den Oord, E. J., Verhulst, F. C., & Boomsma, D. I. (2003). Genetic and environmental contributions to stability and change in children's internalizing and externalizing problems. *Journal of the American Academy of Child and Adolescent Psychiatry*, *42*(10), 1212–1220.

Villafuerte, S. M., Del-Favero, J., Adolfsson, R., Souery, D., Massat, I., Mendlewicz, J., et al. (2002). Gene-based SNP genetic association study of the corticotropin-releasing hormone receptor-2 (CRHR2) in major depression. *American Journal of Medical Genetics*, *114*(2), 222–226.

Waldman, I. D. (2005). Statistical approaches to complex phenotypes: Evaluating neuropsychological endophenotypes for attention-deficit/hyperactivity disorder. *Biological Psychiatry*, *57*, 1347–1356.

Weissman, M. M., Warner, V., Wickramaratne, P., Moreau, D., & Olfson, M. (1997). Offspring of depressed parents: 10 years later. *Archives of General Psychiatry*, *54*, 932–940.

7 Emotion Regulation and Risk for Depression

C. Emily Durbin and Daphna M. Shafir

Contemporary etiological models of mood disorders have proposed that the central abnormalities in internalizing disorders are localized in processes related to emotion, such that difficulties with emotion and/or its regulation are at the core of the pathophysiology of depression. Empirical evidence implicating abnormalities in emotional systems in depression has derived from a number of sources, including the fields of neuroscience (Davidson, 1998), developmental psychology (Zeman, Shipman, & Suveg, 2002), and personality psychology (Clark, 2005). Affective science, a domain of study focused on emotion phenomena, their development, and neural and psychological correlates, has begun to emerge as a distinct field of inquiry (Davidson, Jackson, & Kalin, 2000), yielding promise to further the methodological sophistication and theoretical clarity of research on emotion. In turn, it is likely that advancement in our understanding of emotion will contribute significantly to the literature on the etiology, developmental course, and maintenance of mood disorders across the lifespan. However, despite burgeoning interest in the concept of emotion regulation and its relevance to psychopathology, there remain a number of unresolved questions regarding the construct of emotion regulation, its measurement, and developmental trajectory. Successfully addressing these basic issues will be a vital part of the larger attempt to map the emotion and emotion regulation processes implicated in mood disorders.

It is evident in the language we use to describe our emotional experience that humans have intentions to regulate aspects of our emotional experience (including the subjective, physiological, and expressive components of emotion), and that intentions to regulate our emotions may arise from personal or interpersonal goals or a recognition of sociocultural norms regarding emotion (Tsai, Chentsova-Dutton, Freire-Bebeau, & Przymus, 2002; Markus, Kitayama, & VandenBos, 1996). These intentions motivate strategic engagement in behaviors aimed at changing some aspect of our emotional experience. The construct of emotion regulation is intuitively appealing to those interested in understanding and treating depression, because it seems to tap an important component of healthy adaptation that appears disrupted in depressed individuals and points toward specific targets for intervention. Furthermore, disruption in emotion regulation offers a face valid explanation for some of the functional difficulties associated with depression. Unfortunately, many of the early explorations of emotion regulation abnormalities in psychopathology simply inferred the presence of emotion dysregulation from behavioral or emotional problems. However, more recent work has begun to directly test the nature of emotion regulation deficits in disordered samples, as well as to build on the basic literature on emotion in nondisordered individuals. The aim of this work is to build more rigorous conceptualizations of emotion regulation that focus on defining precisely what is regulated in emotion regulation, to what end, and by what mechanisms.

We begin this chapter by reviewing prototypical definitions of emotion regulation, as well as criticisms that have been made of those definitions, and exploring the implications of these alternative conceptualizations for notions of the role of emotion regulation in the etiology and development of mood disorders. Next, we summarize plausible models of the association between emotion regulation and depression in children. Finally, we review the existing empirical literature on emotion regulation as it relates to the developmental psychopathology of mood disorders.

CLARIFYING THE CONSTRUCT OF EMOTION REGULATION

Varying definitions of emotion regulation have been proffered (Campos, Frankel, & Camras, 2004; Cole, Martin, & Dennis, 2004; Gross, 1998a; Thompson, 1994), but all have in common a recognition that the capacity to coordinate the action of emotional systems in tune with the changing demands of the environment is an important component of adaptive human functioning (Campos, Mumme, Kermoian, & Campos, 1994). Most definitions also assume that there are evolutionary origins for the psychological processes tasked with allowing for the flexible modulation of ongoing emotional experience. However, working definitions of emotion regulation have also varied along several dimensions, including (but not limited to) (1) the identified goal or function of emotion regulation processes with respect to psychological adjustment; (2) the extent to which emotion regulation is viewed as distinct from the processes of emotion itself; (3) whether they focus exclusively on negative emotions or consider both positively and negatively valenced emotions; (4) the explicitness with which the regulated components of emotion are identified; and (5) their developmental specificity.

The definitions offered by Gross (1998a) and Thompson (1990) are particularly illustrative of the different ways in which emotion regulation has been conceptualized. Gross's definition is similar to lay concepts; he described emotion regulation as "processes by which individuals influence which emotions they have, when they have them, and how they experience and express these emotions" (Gross, 1998a, p. 275). Several features of this definition are notable. It is applicable to both positive and negative emotions and implies the presence of self-regulatory mechanisms that are independent of those responsible for the generation of emotion. This framing of emotion regulation implies a significant strategic component and assumes that these regulatory processes are capable of acting directly and successfully on emotional experience. In terms of developmental specificity, Gross's definition appears to describe relatively mature capabilities that may not be available early in life.

In contrast, Thompson offered a view of emotion regulation that does not presuppose the success of strategies thought to serve a regulatory function. Thompson (1994) defined emotion regulation as extrinsic and intrinsic processes that serve to monitor, evaluate, and alter emotional reactions, including mechanisms that act on the causes of emotion as well as those that alter the parameters that define an emotional response (e.g., valence, intensity, time course, and expressive components). This conceptualization differs from Gross's in that it does not imply that all putative emotion regulation processes actually change emotional experience. In fact, Thompson highlighted the challenge of emotion regulation, noting that these processes are called upon to impact affective systems that are evolutionarily ancient. Furthermore, Thompson's definition broadens regulation processes to those external to the person, and makes explicit that regulation may serve goals other than the pursuit of particular emotional experiences (i.e., pleasant affect). According to Thompson (1990), one developmental function of the acquisition and elaboration of emotion regulation skills is that these processes allow emotion to become involved in the organization and shaping of higher-order behavior. In that respect, emotion regulation is seen as adaptive to the extent that it facilitates goal achievement; pleasant emotional experience may in fact be secondary to this function. Therefore, emotion regulation may conceivably involve the generation or maintenance of negative emotion, or the suppression or mitigation of positive emotion. As noted by Cole et al. (2004), emotions are subject to regulation, but are also themselves regulating. Emotions shape multiple domains of an individual's functioning, as well as influence the behavior of others in his or her environment.

Both Gross's and Thompson's definitions of emotion regulation appear to suggest that emotion regulation mechanisms are independent of the processes involved in the production of emotions. In contrast, Campos et al. (2004) argued that emotion regulation is composed of the same processes that give rise to emotion, such that one cannot distinguish cleanly between the unfolding of an "unregulated" emotion and the regulatory processes that come online after the onset of an emotional response. They described emotion regulation as coterminous with emotion, with both involving the selection of goal-oriented responses, monitoring the effectiveness of these responses, and modifying them in the service of attaining goals in the person's environment.

Campos et al.'s (2004) model of emotion regulation raises an important point for understanding the role of emotion regulation in mood disorders. If emotion and emotion regulation processes are the same, or even only partially overlapping, one cannot understand the role of emotion regulation in the etiology and maintenance of mood disorders without also exploring abnormalities in basic emotional processes not typically conceived of as regulatory. If this model is correct, then observational or self-report measures purporting to tap emotion regulation difficulties could in fact reflect the outcome of abnormalities in any part of the larger system responsible for the generation, unfolding, and modulation of emotion. Emotion regulation problems in depression may be secondary to more general abnormalities in emotional systems, rather than specific problems in the strategic selection and implementation of regulation strategies (e.g., rumination, reappraisal, etc.).

MEASUREMENT ISSUES IN EMOTION REGULATION

In addition to core definitional problems in the study of emotion regulation, the field also faces considerable measurement and design challenges. Observations that the presence of putative emotion regulation behaviors (e.g., distraction) co-occur with indicators of emotional arousal do not demonstrate that these behaviors are actually regulatory in the sense that they alter the underlying emotional processes. Rather, they could simply be an indicator of increased emotional intensity (they are part of the phenomena of emotion), or they could indicate an attempt at regulation that is in fact ineffective (separate from the emotion, but not actually altering its course or intensity). Buss and Goldsmith (1998) applied temporal contingency analyses to fine-grained coding of fear and anger and emotion regulation behaviors in infants to test whether the occurrence of putative regulatory behaviors did indeed result in subsequent changes in emotion intensity. They examined a number of possible regulators, including approach, withdrawal, distraction, and social referencing behaviors. They found limited support for the notion that the regulatory behaviors examined did in fact change the intensity of either fear or anger. Rather, findings were more consistent with the argument that these "regulatory" behaviors marked greater intensity of the emotional response and therefore are perhaps best viewed as part of the emotion itself. Findings such as these bolster Campos et al.'s (2004) position that emotion and emotion regulation are part and parcel of the same set of processes. Moreover, they demonstrate that our intuitions regarding which behaviors function to regulate emotion may not be borne out empirically. Unfortunately, Buss and Goldsmith's (1998) is the only study to use coding and statistical analyses that disentangle emotion and regulation behaviors in an observational study. It is not clear from this single study whether emotion regulation behaviors would emerge as distinct processes in an older sample of children or adolescents.

DISTINCTIONS BETWEEN EMOTION, EMOTION REGULATION, AND TEMPERAMENT

If one takes seriously the notion that emotion regulation problems are indicative of broader systemic difficulties in emotional systems, then it is important to fit emotion regulation within a broader nomological network of constructs relevant to the etiology and course of mood disorders. Modern models of child temperament and adult personality emphasize the centrality and lifespan continuity of emotion-related traits (Goldsmith & Campos, 1990; Shiner, 2000). Temperament is typically defined as individual differences in basic emotional reactivity and in the processes that moderate that reactivity (Rothbart & Bates, 1998). Therefore, temperament/personality may provide a framework for modeling the relationship between emotion regulation and depression. Two core traits present in most structural models of temperament/personality (John & Srivastava, 1999) are relevant to emotion and represent the "Big Two" of adult personality and child temperament: Negative Emotionality/Neuroticism (NE) and Positive Emotionality/Extraversion (PE). The facets of PE include the propensity to experience positive emotions (such as joy), as well as social dominance, vigor, reward seeking and consumption, and behavioral engagement. NE includes the tendency toward negative emotions (such as sadness, anger, and fear), as well as difficulty regulating those states, and high reactivity to stress (Watson & Clark, 1997; Clark & Watson, 1999). The frequent and intense negative mood states that define NE/Neuroticism might emerge from greater difficulty dampening or managing negative emotional reactions in those high in NE, and/or from a lower threshold for elicitation or greater intensity of elicitation of negative emotions. Similarly, low trait PE may be associated with difficulty upregulating positive emotions, or a higher threshold for elicitation or lower intensity of positive emotions.

Individual differences in PE and NE have been identified as possible diatheses for mood disorders. Clark, Watson, and Mineka's (1994) tripartite model proposed that high NE reflects a predisposition to multiple forms of psychopathology (including mood disorders), whereas low PE specifically predisposes a person to depression. Consistent with the tripartite model, self-reported low levels of PE and high levels of NE have been linked concurrently to depression in both adult and child clinical samples (Watson, Clark, & Carey, 1988; Brown, Chorpita, & Barlow, 1998; Lonigan, Carey, & Fitch, 1994; Chorpita & Daleiden, 2002). More important, PE and NE have been prospectively linked to the development of depression in adults (Hirschfeld et al., 1989; Kendler, Neale, Kessler, Heath, & Eaves, 1993; Clayton, Ernst, & Angst, 1994).

Longitudinal studies of child temperament have also documented links between early childhood measures of low PE and high NE and the later development of depression. Observational ratings of children's levels of positive and negative emotions and other subtraits of PE and NE obtained during the preschool/early childhood period have been shown to predict depressive symptoms and mood disorders in adulthood (Caspi, Moffitt, Newman, & Silva, 1996; van Os, Jones, Lewis, Wadsworth, & Murray, 1997; Block, Gjerde, & Block, 1991). Thus, individuals who later develop mood disorders exhibit abnormalities in emotionality in childhood, which suggests that these traits are early markers of depression and possibly are causally related to its development. An important avenue for future developmental psychopathology research will be to test whether these early diatheses interact with developmentally salient stressors, such as pubertal onset (Ge, Conger, & Elder, 2001), loss events (Monroe, Rohde, Seeley, & Lewinsohn, 1999), or school transitions, to predict mood disorders in children and adolescents. Consistent with the notion that emotionality traits are a diathesis for depression, PE and NE have a genetic basis and exhibit stability over developmental time (Roberts & DelVecchio, 2000; Pedlow, Sanson, Prior, & Oberklaid, 1993; Rothbart, Ahadi, & Evans, 2000). Moreover, the finding that emotion and emotion regulation abnormalities characteristic of depression may appear well prior to the emergence of frank mood disorders has implications for intervention and prevention efforts.

Studies using observational and laboratory measures of emotion in children identified as being at risk for depression also support the claim that emotion expression and regulation processes may be part of a diathesis for depression. For instance, the offspring of parents with mood disorders are characterized by low PE and high behavioral inhibition (a trait with elements of both PE and NE) in laboratory tasks designed to measure individual differences in emotionality and emotion regulation (Durbin, Klein, Hayden, Buckley, & Moerk, 2005; Kochanska, 1991; Rosenbaum et al., 2000). However, none of these studies have attempted to tease apart whether observed differences in children's emotional behavior are driven by differences in emotion regulation processes or by more basic elements of emotional reactivity. In one study (Durbin et al., 2005) preschoolers of mothers with a history of depression also exhibited higher levels of context-inappropriate negative emotions, which were defined as negative emotions occurring in contexts designed to elicit positive emotions, or negative emotions unusual for their situational context, such as anger (rather than fear) in response to the appearance of an unfamiliar male. High levels of these incongruous emotional reactions are consistent with difficulty in regulating emotional reactions to situational demands among children at risk for depression (Durbin et al., 2005), but are also consistent with other mechanisms.

If one views emotion and emotion regulation as part and parcel of the same set of processes, then this literature is consistent with the claim that children with or at risk for mood disorders are characterized by abnormalities in emotion regulation. However, it is also possible that these children simply differ from their low-risk peers in nonregulation aspects of emotion, such as (for example) the threshold for elicitation of particular emotions, the intensity of their emotional reactions, or the time course of their emotional reactions. Individuals who experience more frequent and/or intense emotional reactions may simply have more emotional material to regulate, so that regulatory difficulty represents not a deficit, but the greater challenge involved in modifying more intense and/or frequent emotions. If NE and PE emerge from individual differences in reactivity to emotion-eliciting stimuli, then it stands to reason that individuals high in these traits may be highly reactive to their environments, which may result in greater frequency of perturbations of their affective systems and therefore greater need for regulation. Thus, one can see high NE or low PE individuals as differing from individuals with average levels of these traits in their success at regulating negative or positive emotions, or in the amount of those emotions they are prone to experience, or some combination of both. Although the relevant literature is sparse, one study in adults suggested that self-reports of particular emotion regulation strategies (suppression and reappraisal) were modestly correlated with self-reports of PE and NE (Gross & John, 2003). This suggests that emotionality traits and specific emotion regulation behaviors are discriminable at the self-report level, but does not demonstrate that they in fact emerge from distinct processes.

Rather than impede emotion regulation, it is possible that high levels of PE and NE may actually promote the development of emotion regulation capacities. Fox and Calkins (2003) argued that temperamental emotionality may influence the development of emotion regulation skills by providing opportunities for external agents to support and shape a child's regulation of his or her emotions. If this is the case, then children who experience or express more frequent and/or intense emotions will have greater opportunities to learn emotion regulation skills (to the extent that their environment provides such education). One might predict that high PE and NE would interact with aspects of the social environment to predict depression, so that high levels of these traits would be associated with elevated risk for depression only if effective instruction in regulation was not provided by caregivers or other socializing agents. Empirical studies using prospective designs to test this hypothesis in child samples would provide an important test of the developmental association between NE, PE, and emotion regulation behaviors.

Campos et al.'s (2004) model of emotion regulation takes into account individual differences in the elicitation of emotion. They argued that emotion regulation processes may be centered on an individual set point or personal baseline state that could differ considerably across individuals, so that the end point of regulation is not uniform. One plausible determinant of this baseline set point is temperamental differences in emotionality. It is possible that individuals at risk for depression have baseline set points for the experience of positive emotions and of negative emotions that differ from those of individuals at low risk. To the extent that this set point is undesirable (less than euthymic), regulatory processes may not be successful at achieving a preferred state, or reaching such a state may require more exertion of or more flexibility of regulatory behaviors for at-risk individuals than for individuals with a euthymic set point.

Thus, it is plausible that individuals at risk for depression use similarly effective regulatory strategies as individuals at low risk, so that the overall effectiveness of these strategies for changing the magnitude or duration of an emotion is similar, but that for individuals at high risk, the regulation tactics leave them further from a euthymic state. For instance, the retrieval of positive autobiographical events following a mood induction improves the mood of nondysphoric adults, but it does not elevate the mood of dysphoric adults (Joormann & Siemer, 2004). The differential usefulness of this strategy could be due to the way in which these positive events are accessed and utilized, or perhaps this mood repair strategy is simply inadequate to counteract particularly negative mood states. If emotion regulation strategies such as these prove ineffective at attaining euthymic mood, dysphoric individuals may eventually succumb to learned helplessness (Seligman, 1975) concerning emotion regulation strategies, becoming less likely to engage in strategic attempts at mood regulation. Thus, high levels of NE or low levels of PE may result in a failure to acquire a broad repertoire of emotion regulation skills or in a reduction over time in the variety of skills in that repertoire.

High levels of PE or NE may also impact the selection of emotion regulation strategies from one's repertoire; more intense emotional reactions may bias one toward the selection of regulation strategies that are less effective. As noted by Compas, Connor-Smith, and Jaser (2004), the effect of temperament traits on depression risk may be partially mediated by coping/emotion regulation strategies, so that temperament traits influence the selection and implementation of coping strategies. One emotion regulation strategy that may be influenced by temperamental NE is rumination, which is defined as repetitive thinking about depressive symptoms and their causes and consequences (Nolen-Hoeksema, 1991). Perhaps rumination reflects a passivity regarding the ability to change one's negative emotions, coupled with a persistent focus on one's emotions. High NE would be expected to be associated with more intense and frequent negative emotions, thus leading to lower expectations that one can modulate negative feelings, and possibly greater rumination, which in turns feeds back to increase the likelihood of persistence of the emotion and its recurrence in the future. Thus, there are numerous mechanisms by which individual differences in temperamental emotionality traits may explain the link between emotion regulation variables and depression.

In addition to PE and NE, some developmentalists have argued for the relevance of a third temperament construct to risk for depression, namely effortful control. *Effortful control* refers to individual differences in the domain of executive functioning capacities, including the ability to inhibit dominant responses and to shift attention (Rothbart et al., 2000), which would thus be expected to influence broad classes of self-regulatory capacities, including emotion regulation. Effortful control processes first become evident near the end of the first year of life, grow rapidly during the toddler years, and become more organized and elaborated as a trait into early childhood and beyond (Kochanska, Murray, & Harlan, 2000). This suggests that individual differences in the developmental trajectory of effortful control may be related to differences in the emergence, flexibility, and success of emotion regulation strategies in children and adolescents. Kieras, Tobin, Graziano, and Rothbart (2005) found that young children who scored high on laboratory measures of effortful control (EC) exhibited more regulation of emotion following a disappointment paradigm than children who scored lower on EC indices. High EC children showed similar amounts of positive affect following receipt of a desired and an undesired gift, whereas low EC children showed more positive affect to the desired gift than to the undesired gift.

Block and Block (1980) described two personality constructs relevant to emotional/behavioral regulation and effortful control processes in general: ego control and ego resiliency. *Ego control* refers to the extent to which a person regulates his or her behavioral tendencies; low levels are associated with impulsivity, poor planning, and failure to inhibit previously rewarded behaviors. Extremely high levels of ego control, in contrast, are characterized by excessive restraint and a lack of spontaneity. Thus, one might expect high levels to be associated with excessive regulation of emotional responses; such overcontrol could reduce negative emotions, but could also dampen positive emotions. Low levels of ego control should be associated with diminished ability to enact emotion regulation behaviors, and therefore with greater frequency and/or intensity of both negative and positive emotions. Block and Block's second construct, *ego resiliency*, refers to the ability to adaptively modify one's temperamental level of ego control in a contextually appropriate manner that maximizes fitness with environmental demands. Presumably, high levels of ego resiliency would be associated with the capacity to regulate emotions smoothly and within the boundaries expected in different environments. Low levels, in contrast, may be predicted to result in similar levels of emotion regulation regardless of context and difficulty modulating one's regulation of emotion to serve other goals.

Very few other theorists have incorporated the notion of contextual flexibility of emotion regulation or other aspects of the construct of ego resiliency into models of adaptive emotion regulation. Moreover, constructs such as effortful control and ego control and resiliency point to the importance of examining whether mood disorders are specifically associated with problems in the regulation of emotion or emotion-guided behavior, or more generally characterized by difficulty in the regulation of a broader set of behaviors. From a developmental perspective, it will be important to understand how the development of emotion regulation abilities unfolds in the context of broader self-regulatory capacities, as well as to test when and by what mechanisms children develop the ability to flexibly modify their levels of emotion.

SPECIFIC EMOTION REGULATION CONSTRUCTS LINKED TO DEPRESSION

Although a number of crucial questions regarding the conceptualization of emotion regulation remain, the presence of competing frameworks for understanding this domain should stimulate theoretically motivated empirical work. This should involve developing a more refined taxonomy of the processes involved in the regulation of emotion, one that explicitly identifies the causal effect of putative regulation strategies on particular emotions, and that begins to lay out the underlying mechanisms (neural, physiological, behavioral, interpersonal) that constitute particular emotion regulation strategies. In order to advance our understanding of the relationship between emotion and depression, it is necessary to examine which particular components of emotion and/or its regulation are implicated in the etiology of depression. There are a number of parameters of emotion and emotion regulation that could potentially be involved in increasing risk for depression, such as (1) the extent to which a person strategically engages in emotion regulation and in which contexts he or she employs these strategies; (2) the typical intensity of the emotions the person has to regulate; (3) the distance between the person's desired hedonic state and his or her typical emotional state; (4) the variability (number and breadth) of emotion regulation strategies available to the person; (5) the effectiveness with which available regulation strategies are implemented; (6) the ability to monitor the effectiveness of each strategy employed; (7) the capacity to switch strategies if the first applied is ineffective; and (8) the extent to which emotion regulation strategies deplete other psychological resources that themselves are implicated in depression. Research focused on parsing emotion regulation constructs into these or other relatively narrow components may allow for more precise localization of the emotion regulation abnormalities associated with risk for depression. To date, the bulk of the literature has focused on the use of specific emotion regulation strategies. Below we review those strategies that have received most attention in the empirical literature.

Rumination

Response styles theory, originated by Nolen-Hoeksema (1987, 1991, 1998), posits that a person's reaction to depressive symptoms will ultimately increase or blunt further depressive symptoms. Specifically, a ruminative style that involves repetitive thinking about depressive mood and its causes and consequences has been linked to subsequent increases in depressive symptoms in adults, even after covarying initial depression levels (Just &

Alloy, 1997; Nolen-Hoeksema, 2000). Rumination is typically experienced as an "automatic response" that is intrusive and difficult to control (Silk, Steinberg, & Morris, 2003), so that it may represent an overlearned or less strategically employed emotion regulation behavior. Response theory contrasts rumination with other emotion regulation behaviors (such as distraction) that are thought to be less likely to perpetuate depressed mood. Nolen-Hoeksema (1998) has asserted that rumination plays a causal role in the maintenance and exacerbation of depressed mood, and it has been argued that sex differences in the prevalence of depressive disorders may be explained by the greater utilization of a ruminative response style among women (Butler & Nolen-Hoeksema, 1994; Nolen-Hoeksema, Larson, & Grayson, 1999). In addition, early adolescent girls engage in much more corumination—extensively discussing issues, revisiting problems, and focusing on negative feelings within relatively healthy and intimate relationships—than their male peers (Rose, 2002). This sex difference could partially explain why adolescent girls have more social support from intimate friendships yet more internalizing symptoms than do boys.

Of the few studies of response theory in adolescent and preadolescent samples, results have been similar to those seen in studies of adults. In one study, rumination predicted concurrent and future (6-week follow-up) depression scores even after covarying initial depression scores and other cognitive vulnerability factors, including negative attributional style (Schwartz & Koenig, 1996). Similar results were found in other samples (Abela, Brozina, & Haigh, 2002; Silk et al., 2003). As in adult samples, sex differences in response style are evident in adolescent samples (Ziegert & Kistner, 2002; Schwartz & Koenig, 1996). However, in a study of nonclinical adolescents, rumination did not account for a significant portion of variance in depression symptoms after covarying the effects of worry (Muris, Roelofs, Meesters, & Boomsma, 2004). This overlap points to the difficulty of conceptualizing rumination as an emotion regulation construct; the existing empirical literature is equally consistent with the claim that rumination is an epiphenomenon of negative affect, rather than a response to negative mood. Inconsistent with response theory, there has been little evidence for an association between distraction and depression in children and young adolescents (Garber, Braafladt, & Weiss, 1995; Glyshaw, Cohen, & Towbes, 1989; Kenealy, 1989; Plancherel, & Bolognini, 1995; Wierzbicki, 1989). Moreover, one study found that disengagement (denial, avoidance, escape, or wishful thinking) was related to higher, rather than lower, depressive symptoms and problem behavior in adolescents (Silk et al., 2003). In summary, there is considerable evidence linking the tendency to engage in ruminative strategies in response to depressed mood to indicators of severity of depression (symptoms, chronicity), but less evidence to support the notion that rumination represents an emotion regulation diathesis for mood disorders, rather than a correlate of high trait negative affect.

High Levels of Dispositional Emotion Regulation and Suppression of Emotion

Although many conceptions of the role of emotion regulation in depression suggest that it is a failure to regulate negative moods that leads to depression, it is also possible that excessive or rigidly applied emotion regulation can increase risk for mood disorders. Muraven and Baumeister (2000) argue that self-regulation is an effortful process that has a finite capacity, so that regulation in one psychological domain depletes resources available for subsequent regulation attempts. Thus, excessive regulation of emotion may make it more difficult for children (or adults) to engage in other executive or regulatory processes. As suggested by Block and Block's (1980) claim that both ego control and ego resiliency are important to healthy functioning, it is possible that excessive attempts to control or regulate emotional responses may be related to maladaptation, including depression or other forms of psychopathology. Gross and Levenson (1997) showed that adults who were asked to suppress their emotional reactions to evocative film clips exhibited increased sympathetic activation, as compared with those who did not attempt to suppress their emotions, suggesting that inhibition/suppression of emotion may result in physiological costs to the individual.

Gross and John (2003) noted that suppression may inhibit overt indicators of emotional reactivity (such as facial expressions) while failing to reduce other components of the emotional response (such as the subjective or physiological aspects). Reliance on suppression as a strategy may result in a more effortful process whereby the person has to engage in persistent management of his or her emotional displays without reaping the benefits of further processing or interpretation of these emotions. Gross and John (2003) argued that suppression may be problematic because, like other emotion regulation strategies implemented after the elicitation of an emotion, it acts primarily on the outputs of emotion systems, rather than their underlying components. In fact, suppression does not appear to be as effective as other strategies in terms of reducing subjective negative emotions (Gross, 1998b) and may even result in impairments in social interaction (Butler et al., 2003) or in memory for social information (Richards & Gross, 2000). It is important to note that in many studies of suppression, participants are asked to engage in deliberate attempts to dampen an emotion without more specific elaboration as to how this dampening is to be achieved. It is plausible that developmentally early attempts at strategic emotion regulation may take an analogous form, with children intending to reduce an unwanted state without specific skills or knowledge of how to achieve this reduction. Thus, suppression may be a developmental precursor for more process-oriented regulation strategies that reduce emotional intensity via a particular mechanism (such as distraction, reframing, etc.). Excessive attempts to regulate may be even more resource depleting for children than for adolescents or adults, who may have more practiced strategies for regulating their emotions than do children.

Overregulation of some components of emotion—whether via suppression or other regulation behaviors—may be more than effortful; it may be potentially detrimental in terms of important developmental achievements. To the extent that children engage in high levels of regulation of their emotions, they may forestall important learning experiences by which emotion promotes the acquisition of social cognition, interpersonal skills, or cognitive abilities. For instance, Abe and Izard (1999) point out that the experience of anger may promote perspective taking, the development of assertiveness, and negotiation of social rules, and shame and guilt may foster moral development and the learning of social standards. Therefore, dispositional overregulation of emotion may impede the development of a broader range of skills important to psychological and social adjustment in general and potentially set in motion depressogenic processes (such as low assertiveness or other interpersonal difficulties).

THEORETICAL PERSPECTIVES ON THE ROLE OF EMOTION REGULATION IN DEPRESSION

In addition to determining which emotion regulation strategies or components are correlated with depression, the literature must begin to turn to testing models of the causal relationship between the two constructs. Klein, Wonderlich, and Shea (1993) proposed a number of models of the association between personality traits and depression that provide a useful analogue for thinking about the relationship between emotion regulation and depression. These authors described several personality–depression models that could also characterize the causal relationship between emotion regulation and depression: common cause, predisposition, pathoplasty, complications, and concomitants. The common cause model proposes that emotion regulation difficulties and depression co-occur owing to partial or full overlap of their etiological factors. The common cause model is consistent with claims that the genetic and/or environmental processes causally related to emotion regulation problems are also implicated in the development of depression; thus, if this model is accurate, then (1) emotion regulation measures and depression should have shared correlates and (2) emotion regulation problems should exist in the absence of frank mood pathology. The common cause model would be supported by data indicating that particular environmental or genetic variables associated with depression in children are also related to emotion regulation problems. One obvious putative common cause could be temperamental emotionality traits (if these are indeed distinct from emotion regulation processes), although others (such as aspects of the early home environment) are also plausible common causes.

The predisposition model asserts that emotion regulation problems directly increase risk for depression, but that the etiological processes that give rise to emotion regulation problems are distinct from those involved in depression. This model implies that intervention efforts that directly target emotion regulation variables could decrease the likelihood of a person's developing depression. This contrasts with the common cause model, wherein manipulating one construct (emotion regulation) does not result in a change in the other (depression). The pathoplasty model states that emotion regulation problems alter the course or expression of depression after onset, so that particular emotion regulation strategies or deficits are associated with a more chronic or serious course of the disorder. For example, this would be consistent with findings that depressed individuals high in trait rumination have a more chronic course of the disorder than those low in rumination.

Two of Klein et al.'s (1993) models propose an alternative causal ordering, such that depression influences emotion regulation problems. First, the complication model (sometimes termed the scar model) asserts that depression changes emotion regulation skills, and that these changes persist even after the depressive disorder remits. Finally, the concomitants model argues that emotion regulation is altered during depressive episodes, but returns to a baseline state following remission of depression; this model implies that problems with emotion regulation are sequelae of depression, rather than causal factors that produce depression. There are no existing empirical data to test these two models against the alternatives. Clearly, these models are not exhaustive; one can imagine combining models to propose hybrids, or to incorporate reciprocal causation or feedback loops. However, they do provide a theoretical framework for understanding how emotion regulation may be implicated in mood disorders.

To further the empirical literature on the role of emotion regulation in the developmental psychopathology of depression, it will be necessary to conduct studies that can distinguish between alternative models of the association between the two constructs. To date, most of the literature has been limited to cross-sectional correlational studies. However, the predominant model of the role of emotion regulation in depression seems to be that emotion regulation problems precede and are causally related to the development of mood disorders; testing this claim appropriately requires prospective designs. In general, direct tests comparing two or more of these models require more sophisticated designs than cross-sectional comparisons of depressed versus nondepressed groups. Studies of child and/or adolescent samples, particularly those utilizing longitudinal designs, will be especially important and can be powerful in discriminating among these causal models.

MAPPING THE NATURE OF EMOTION REGULATION CONTRIBUTIONS TO DEPRESSION

Regulation of Positive Emotions

Although considerable attention has been paid to the regulation of negative emotions (particularly sadness, or more commonly, depressed mood) in mood disorders, less has been given to the regulation of positive emotions. Processes involved in the upregulation of positive mood may be particularly important for understanding mood disorders for five reasons. First, one emotion regulation strategy for a negative emotion or mood (such as depression) may be to replace it with a positive emotion or mood, as positive moods may buffer the effects of negative emotions (Tugade & Fredrickson, 2004; Meehl, 1975). Second, positive emotions may engender more creative thinking (Fredrickson, 1998), thereby allowing for more effective or flexible selection of strategies for regulating moods or responding to stressful situations. Third, anhedonia, or diminished interest and pleasure, is a central feature of depression, one that distinguishes it from anxiety disorders (Clark et al., 1994). Thus, understanding the regulation of positive moods may shed some light on processes specific to mood disorders relative to other forms of psychopathology with which they are comorbid. Fourth, difficulties with regulation of positive versus negative emotions may define distinct subtypes of depression. For instance, Davidson, Pizzagalli, Nitschke, and Putnam (2002) surmised, on the basis of the literature on adults, that there may be two distinct subtypes of depression based on difficulties with emotion regulation. The first would be characterized by a failure to anticipate positive outcomes and to generate behavior in the pursuit of reward. It is conceivable that this subtype may be associated with the inability to upregulate positive emotions. The second subtype described by Davidson, Pizzagalli, Nitschke, and Putnam (2002) is evidenced by individuals with difficulties in suppressing or overriding negative affect. Extension of such theorizing and tests of its applicability to children and adolescents are warranted. Finally, bipolar disorder may be characterized by poorly regulated positive affect (Liebenluft, Charney, & Pine, 2003), such as an inability to downregulate positive moods or to modulate the effect of positive mood on behavior and decision making. Understanding more about the regulation of positive emotions may therefore have the potential to illuminate the pathogenesis of both bipolar and unipolar mood disorders.

Given the findings regarding the link between temperamental PE and depression reviewed earlier, it seems likely that regulation of both positive and negative moods could play a role in the etiology of depression. However, there is a paucity of empirical data on the regulation of positive emotions, and the existing literature on regulation of negative emotions may not generalize to positive emotions. Whether strategies that are successful in the regulation of negative emotions are similarly effective for positive emotions is an empirical question. Watson (2000) noted that traditional models of negative emotions and their regulation provide a poor fit for understanding positive emotions and moods. He argued that positive moods are distinct from negative emotions/moods in that they usually lack clear onsets or offsets, are more influenced by biological factors than by environmental precipitants, and vary more widely than negative moods. Therefore, measuring positive mood regulation may require somewhat different strategies than measuring the regulation of negative moods/emotions. It is important to note that Watson was concerned primarily with mood regulation in adults; more work focusing on the regulation of positive emotion in children and adolescents is necessary. Concerning emotion regulation in children, Buss and Goldsmith (1998) proposed that there may be specificity regarding the discrete emotions for which a particular regulatory behavior is effective, or that the same regulatory behavior could impact different emotions in dissimilar ways. Contrasting positively and negatively valenced states may be a first step toward determining whether such specificity exists.

Truly Developmental Models of Emotion Regulation in Depression

Because most of the research linking emotion regulation difficulties to depression has been conducted with adult samples, we know little about when this association emerges, whether and how it changes over developmental time, or whether emotion regulation variables interact with developmental transitions to increase or decrease risk for depression. In childhood, when emotion regulation repertoires are still being fleshed out, individual differences in emotion regulation may be only weakly (if at all) predictive of depression. In late adolescence or adulthood, when most individuals would be expected to have acquired mature emotion regulation repertoires, individual differences in these strategies may be more strongly associated with depression. Alternatively, it is possible that emotion regulation may play an even stronger role in childhood depression than in adult depression, with children who lag behind in the acquisition of emotion regulation skills at particularly high risk for developing a mood disorder. One might also predict that emotion regulation deficits could interact with stressful developmental transitions to increase risk for depression to the extent that transitions produce changes in the intensity, frequency, or nature of emotions that need to be regulated.

Another important developmental issue regarding models of the association between emotion regulation and depression concerns the extent to which emotion regulation strategies exhibit continuity across the lifespan. If emotion regulation variables represent a diathesis for depression, then they would be expected to have some degree of temporal stability. Empirical data are lacking regarding the stability of emotion regulation variables, their developmental specificity, and mean level changes across development. In addition, although some simple regulatory behaviors (such as attention redirection) are available across the age span (Mangelsdorf, Shapiro, & Marzolf, 1995), other, more cognitively complex strategies, likely do not appear until later in development (e.g., reappraisal). It will be important to understand the developmental precursors of these more mature emotion regulation mechanisms, and whether early emotion regulation strategies exhibit heterotypic continuity with more mature emotion regulation skills (coherence across development between diverse, but phenotypically similar behaviors, owing to the action of an underlying latent trait that produces conceptually similar, but developmentally specific behaviors across development). In addition, it is likely that there are even more basic precursors to the development of emotion regulation skills, such as the ability to perceive and label one's own emotional state; understanding the role of these cognitive mechanisms in emotional development may shed light on the core components of emotion regulation. Basic research on developmental trajectories of emotion regulation skills will be necessary in order to interpret findings differentiating depressed from nondepressed children.

A truly developmental perspective on the role of emotion regulation in depression would also incorporate a fuller understanding of the function of particular emotions across development and would stimulate hypotheses regarding the benefits and costs of emotion regulation in particular circumstances. Many theories of emotion regulation reflect a hedonic stance, assuming that the primary motivation underlying emotion regulation is the desire to avoid negative emotions or moods and to experience positive emotions or moods (Larsen, 2000). However, from a developmental perspective, negative emotions may be desirable in that they facilitate certain emerging skills and may foster interpersonal resources, such as social support. Similarly, positive emotions may be undesirable in some contexts. In evolutionary terms, one would expect the development of emotion regulation skills to serve the goals of promoting the individual's adaptive abilities in his or her particular environment, rather than maximizing the person's hedonic state (Watson, 2000). It will be important to develop hypotheses regarding how particular emotion regulation strategies may fit well or poorly in particular environmental contexts and what underlying processes mediate between emotion regulation constructs and pathways to mood disorder onset and maintenance.

DEVELOPMENT OF EMOTION REGULATION

As compared with individual differences in temperamental emotionality, which appear very early in life (Caspi, 2000) and exhibit considerable stability (Roberts & DelVecchio, 2000; Durbin, Hayden, Klein, & Olino, 2007), emotion regulation skills are believed to come online later in development (Thompson, 1990). In particular, prototypical instances of emotion regulation, wherein a person experiencing an emotion reflects on that state and decides voluntarily how to respond to it, is a relatively late developmental achievement (Campos et al., 2004). However, if one takes a broader view of emotion regulation, it is clear that even young children have mechanisms for regulating their emotional reactions (Mangelsdorf et al., 1995), even though these behaviors may be less strategically employed. In addition to internal psychological resources, early emotion regulation may also be achieved through the action of external agents, such as caregivers (Campos et al., 1994; Thompson, 1990). With maturation, children's repertoires of emotion regulation abilities should become more varied and their application of emotion regulation strategies more flexible, resulting in the "coregulation" performed by child and caregiver gradually giving way to more independent regulation shouldered by the child.

Early in life, the immaturity of the frontal lobe capacities required for exerting inhibitory control limits the child's resources to regulate emotional arousal, even for the simplest strategies (Mangelsdorf et al., 1995). Shifting of visual attention is a core regulatory skill available to young infants, and the ability to disengage attention has been linked to maternal reports of lower negative emotions in their infants (Johnson, Posner, & Rothbart, 1991). With age, emerging maturation of underlying emotional systems, as well as development of attentional control, language, social referencing, memory, symbolic representation, perspective taking, and pretend play afford the child the opportunity to expand his or her regulation repertoire and exercise these behaviors in new domains. Through the first several years of life, children's executive attention capabilities undergo considerable change (Posner & Rothbart, 2000). With maturation, the most basic regulatory skills of self-soothing and shifting of attention, which are limited in their effectiveness, can become supplemented with more nuanced, complex, and goal-oriented regulatory skills. With cognitive development comes a better understanding of the causes of emotion, allowing the child to regulate his or her emotions by avoiding or terminating situations that may elicit undesirable emotions, or by explicitly altering the cognitions that may bring about or heighten particular emotions. Thus, the child becomes increasingly capable of modulating his or her emotional state by manipulating the circumstances that evoke emotion, rather than simply changing its intensity once evoked. These mechanisms fall under the rubric of what Campos et al. (1994) referred to as input regulation strategies. It is notable that the frontal lobe regions implicated in the development of executive functioning and behavioral control continue to develop well into adolescence (Sowell, Thompson, Holmes, Jernigan, & Toga, 1999).

CAREGIVER INFLUENCES ON EMOTION REGULATION

Given the role of caregivers in early emotion regulation, it is plausible that emotion regulation difficulties may originate in inappropriate modeling, deficient modeling, or problematic regulation by caregivers in early development, or perhaps by an inability of the caregiver to cede control of regulation to the child when developmentally appropriate. A variety of social-familial influences have been proposed to contribute to children's emerging emotion regulation skills (Saarni, 1999; Calkins, 1994; Fox & Calkins, 2003). Reviewing the literature on parent–infant affective interaction, Goodman (2002) suggested that maternal expressions of negative affect or lack of contingency between maternal and infant affect could impair emotional development by failing to support the child's regulation of emotional arousal. Thus, early dyadic interaction involving affective interchanges may serve a modeling function whereby the parent intervenes to regulate the child's affective state by matching and mismatching the child's affect (Tronick, Cohn, & Shea, 1986). Thompson (1990) suggested that well-regulated affective interchanges between caregiver and child serve to increase an infant's tolerance for emotionally arousing interactions that occur in other contexts.

In addition to microlevel, moment-by-moment influences on child affect, it is possible that more global aspects of parent–child interaction such as the attachment relationship or parenting styles may also contribute to the development of children's emotion regulation capacity and/or their use of specific emotion regulation strategies. Maughan and Cicchetti (2002) proposed that caregivers can impact children's emotion regulation skills by directly shaping their children's interpretations of their environments, in particular emotion-eliciting aspects of an environment. Thompson (1990) noted that caregivers directly impact children's emotion regulation by engaging in discourse about emotion and its causes, as well as using verbal coaching to support a child's emotion regulation. As the child becomes more independent, the parent continues to play a supportive role, but likely begins to reduce his or her level of overt control over the child's emotional expressions. Failure to cede this control may be problematic. For example, Calkins, Smith, Gill, and Johnson (1998) found that mothers who were high in controlling parenting behaviors had children who were less effective at regulating their own emotions.

The evidence reviewed above is consistent with the claim that parent–child interaction qualities can influence children's emotionality and emotion regulation. Unfortunately, the designs of these studies have not been sufficient to conclude that the observed effects are in fact mediated by environmental mechanisms, rather than by genetic influences operating to make parents and children similar in emotion regulation and related traits. Furthermore, it is important to explore whether parent-to-child effects act over and above stable characteristics of the child (such as temperament) or above evocative effects of child behavior/traits on the parent's behavior. Nonetheless, the studies do demonstrate intriguing associations between parent behavior and children's emotions. For instance,

Spinrad, Stifter, Donelan-McCall, and Turner (2004) found longitudinal associations between mothers' use of emotion regulation strategies in response to toddlers' behavior during cleanup and prohibition tasks in the laboratory and children's observed self-regulation during a laboratory disappointment task at age 5. Two maternal regulation strategies at the toddler assessment were predictive of children's negative affect at age 5—maternal questioning of a child's emotional reactions (invalidating the child's response) and relenting to the child's complaints about the prohibition. These findings could be interpreted as evidence that caregivers who are insensitive to their children's emotions or who respond to children's emotions by terminating prohibitions may interfere with their children's ability to develop their own internal emotion regulation skills. Although it is possible that the greater negative affect observed at age 5 was a result of poorer regulation of negative emotions in these children, it could also be evidence for the stability of negative affect across the toddler-to-early-school-age period (children who responded negatively to the prohibition at the toddler assessment may have also responded negatively to the disappointment task at age 5). Similarly, mothers' acquiescence to children's demands and/or questioning of their children's emotional reactions at the toddler laboratory visit may have been partially elicited by high levels of negative affect in the children. Further research will be necessary to tease apart these alternative hypotheses.

It is important to note that many of the social-familial factors that have been theorized to be involved in the development of children's emotion regulation skills have also been implicated in risk for depression in children, including attachment (Carlson & Sroufe, 1995), marital conflict (Katz & Gottman, 1994), and aspects of the parent–child relationship (Goodman & Gotlib, 1999; Cicchetti & Toth, 1998). Taken together, these lines of research provide support for the common cause model, which proposes that emotion regulation difficulties and depression may emerge from a similar set of etiological processes. Of particular note, the parenting of depressed mothers has been shown to be characterized by styles that may contribute to the development of poor emotion regulation in offspring, including understimulation, harsh parenting, and low levels of positivity (Lovejoy, Graczyk, O'Hare, & Neuman, 2000; Cohn, Campbell, Matias, & Hopkins, 1990).

GENDER DIFFERENCES IN EMOTION REGULATION AND ITS DEVELOPMENT

Gender differences in emotion regulation constructs have been observed in adult samples (e.g., Gross & John, 2003). This raises the obvious question as to when these differences first emerge and whether they can account for gender differences in the prevalence of mood disorders. Although there is a smaller body of literature on such difference in children, there is evidence that boys and girls differ in regard to some emotion regulation variables. First, as noted above, adolescent girls engage in more rumination than do boys (Ziegert & Kistner, 2002). Second, girls appear more likely than boys to exhibit positive affect or reduced levels of negative affect following standardized laboratory tasks meant to elicit disappointment or boredom, which has been interpreted as girls exhibiting greater regulation of their negative affect in response to the task (Cole, Zahn-Waxler, & Smith, 1994; Cole, Teti, & Zahn-Waxler, 2003). However, it is important to note that disappointment paradigms may be more successful at tapping children's strategic management of emotion displays than their regulation of underlying emotional arousal.

It is possible that gender differences in emotion regulation have their origins in differential treatment of emotions in boys versus girls. There is some evidence to suggest that parents respond differently to particular emotions depending on the gender of the child. For instance, Cole et al. (2003) examined sequential affective expressions in preschoolers and their mothers participating in a laboratory waiting task designed to elicit anger and boredom. They found that mothers were more likely to respond positively to boys' expressions of anger than to those of girls, but were more likely to respond contingently with positive affect to girls' positive affect, as compared with boys'. There is also evidence that parents preferentially reinforce sadness in girls and anger in boys (Block, 1983; Eisenberg et al., 2001). These findings suggest that social-familial influences may shape gender differences in emotion expression, and by extension, may also impact emotion regulation in boys and girls.

NEURAL AND PHYSIOLOGICAL CORRELATES OF EMOTION REGULATION AND THEIR DEVELOPMENT IN CHILDHOOD AND ADOLESCENCE

Evidence implicating emotion regulation difficulties in depression also derives from studies using measures of neural activity in brain regions thought to be involved in emotion. It should be noted that the predominance of this evidence has derived from studies of adult samples. The most well-replicated findings relevant to depression concern asymmetries in left versus right frontal lobe activation in positively versus negatively valenced states. It has been argued that the left and right prefrontal cortex are lateralized with respect to emotion, such that left-sided activation is involved in positive affect, appetitive motivation, and approach-related behavior, and right-sided activation is associated with negative affect, behavioral inhibition, and withdrawal-related behavior (Davidson, 1998). Thus, frontal lobe activation may reflect underlying processes related to the experience and regulation of emotion. A number of studies utilizing electroencepalography (EEG) have demonstrated asymmetric activation in frontal lobes in depressed individuals, characterized by reduced left (relative to right) activation (e.g., Bruder et al., 1997; Debener et al., 2000). These findings are generally interpreted as reflecting greater negative than positive affect and more reliance on withdrawal or avoidance regulation strategies (as compared with active, approach regulation strategies) in depressed individuals. Reduced left frontal activation has also been linked to behavioral inhibition in preschoolers (Davidson, 1998; Fox et al., 1995) and has been observed in the young offspring of depressed mothers (Dawson, Frey, Panagiotides, Osterling, & Hessl, 1997; Field, Fox, Pickens, & Nawrocki, 1995). Thus, there is some evidence that patterns of brain activity associated with depression in adults are also associated with risk factors for depression in children.

More recent work has focused on identifying particular neuroanatomical regions that may be involved in emotion and emotion regulation. Davidson, Pizzagalli, and Nitschke (2002) suggested that the right and left regions of the prefrontal cortex (PFC) play a role in emotion because they are involved in overriding automatic responses in the service of facilitating goal-oriented behavior. They argued that the chronic negative affect and amotivational behavior that often characterizes depression may be related to hypoactivation in PFC regions. Therefore, depressed individuals, who are prone to experiencing negative emotions that bias behavior toward rumination, avolition, or passivity, have difficulty regulating these emotions in order to mobilize and maintain representations of important goals and to initiate and sustain activity in the pursuit of such goals.

Davidson, Pizzagalli, and Nitschke (2002) described two other regions potentially implicated in emotion regulation. First, these authors suggested that hippocampal dysfunction may play a role in poor contextual modulation of emotion in depression. Second, subdivisions of the anterior cingulate cortex (ACC) have been proposed to be involved in monitoring conflict between the current state of the organism and incoming information that holds motivational and emotional cues. Connections between the ACC and PFC may inform the PFC's selection from various response options and its facilitation of goal-directed behavior (Davidson, Pizzagalli, & Nitschke, 2002). The ACC–PFC circuit comes into play when there is a conflict between environmental demands and a person's mood, and facilitates initiation of behavior appropriate to those demands, even in the face of negative mood. It is important to note that development of the ACC and dorsolateral PFC has been linked to the emergence of attentional control over emotional responses (Rothbart & Derryberry, 1997), suggesting that these regions are implicated in emotion regulation processes. It should also be noted that neuroscience approaches to understanding emotion and emotion regulation have been employed nearly without exception in adult samples. It will be crucial for future research to expand this work to child and adolescent samples, perhaps by utilizing convergent neural and psychological measures to map systems involved in the regulation of emotion or in punishment and reward processing (Forbes & Dahl, 2005).

Two other physiological variables that have been linked to emotion may play a role in its regulation. Vagal tone, which is thought to reflect parasympathetic influence on heart rate variability via the vagus nerve (Porges, 1996), has been conceptualized as an indicator of emotion regulation. Porges (1996) proposed that suppression of vagal tone is a physiological strategy for controlling arousal. Vagal tone has been linked to indicators thought to tap emotion and behavior regulation (e.g., Calkins & Dedmon, 2000). Cortisol levels, a measure of hypothalamic–pituitary–adrenal (HPA) axis functioning, have also been linked to both emotion and depression (e.g., Adam, 2006; Chrousos & Gold, 1992). Further research exploring the normal functioning of these systems, their developmental trajectory, and their association with risk for depression may provide a window into the processes underlying emotion regulation and its relationship to mood disorders.

EMPIRICAL FINDINGS REGARDING EMOTION REGULATION IN DEPRESSED CHILDREN AND ADOLESCENTS

An empirical literature on emotion regulation in children and adolescents is just beginning to emerge. The majority of studies have been conducted with nonclinical samples and have typically been limited to self- or parent-report measures of emotion regulation constructs. However, the existing data provide some support for the claim that emotion regulation processes may be altered in children with or at risk for the development of mood disorders. Specifically, three patterns have been most commonly found: inhibition of expression, poor control of expression, and nonnormative expression (Southam-Gerow & Kendall, 2001).

Evidence linking emotion regulation measures to child depression indices has emerged from studies employing parent reports, laboratory measures, and child self-reports. Given the lack of theoretical consensus regarding how emotion regulation should be conceptualized, it is not surprising that the operationalization of emotion regulation has varied widely across studies. As a result, it is difficult to draw firm conclusions regarding the link between depression and emotion regulation from the existing literature. In general, the most common design involves concurrent parent report measures of emotion regulation and child psychopathology constructs. For example, Rydell, Berlin, and Bohlin (2003) reported on associations between parental reports of child emotionality, emotion regulation, and adaptation in early elementary age children. They found that children with high levels of parent-reported internalizing problems were also reported to be high in poorly regulated fear, whereas those high in externalizing behavior problems were reported to have difficulty regulating positive emotions.

Eisenberg et al. (2001) reported on a study of concurrent associations between parent-reported symptoms and laboratory measures of emotion regulation. They compared four groups of children: one defined by high internalizing (mood and anxiety) symptoms, one scoring high on externalizing symptoms, one high on both internalizing and externalizing, and a control group low on both dimensions. The child participants completed a battery of laboratory tasks tapping behavioral and emotional regulation. Control children exhibited greater signs of regulation in several tasks than did the externalizing group (e.g., being asked to sit still, to complete a puzzle without peeking at the answer, receiving a disappointing prize). The internalizing group exhibited more regulation in laboratory tasks than the externalizing group, but generally did not differ from the control group on these measures. Of note, the laboratory tasks employed to tap regulation in this study may have done a better job of assessing regulation of impulsivity or noncompliance than of assessing emotional reactions, and thus may have been weaker tests of regulation processes involved in internalizing (as compared with externalizing) disorders. Externalizing children (and the comorbid group) were rated as exhibiting lower effortful regulation and higher impulsivity. In terms of parent-report measures of regulation, children high in internalizing symptoms were generally rated as low on effortful control indices, but were rated high in what the authors termed *involuntary control* (behavioral constraint and lower impulsivity). The authors interpreted these involuntary control indices as reflecting a lack of flexibility and spontaneity among the children high in internalizing problems, perhaps similar to the low levels of ego resiliency described by Block and Block (1980).

Cognitive paradigms allow for tests of basic processing of emotional stimuli and may be useful for isolating more specific components that play a role in the regulation of emotion. Ladouceur et al. (2005) used a modification of the *n*-back task designed to tap processing of emotional information in a sample of children and adolescents. In the original *n*-back task used to assess working memory, participants are asked to view a sequence of letters presented on a screen and to monitor such things as when the same letter appeared two letters prior in the presentation. In Ladouceur et al.'s (2005) study, children between the ages of 8 and 16 completed an "emotional *n*-back task" modification in which letter stimuli from the original task were superimposed on neutral, negative, or positive photographs. The authors presumed that the presence of emotionally evocative pictures would distract from the working memory task, such that the children must "regulate" by moving their attention from the photographs to the letter stimuli. Children from four groups participated (current anxiety disorder, current major depressive disorder [MDD], current comorbid anxiety disorder and mood disorder, and a normal control group free of lifetime psychopathology and negative for lifetime mood disorder in their first-degree relatives). There was a significant group by emotional *n*-back condition interaction; MDD and comorbid anxiety/mood disorder groups were significantly slower to respond to target stimuli in the negative, relative to the neutral, condition. In comparing reaction times to the positive relative to the neutral condition, the normal control group had longer reaction times to the positive condition, whereas the other (diagnostic) groups did not. The authors interpreted these findings as reflecting a difficulty among the depressed groups in inhibiting processing of the emotional content of the background negative pictures, leading to longer reaction times for this condition. In contrast, the normal group appeared to be biased toward processing positive content. Although this task seems to be tapping processing of task-irrelevant emotion-eliciting stimuli, it does not directly involve the regulation of emotional reactions.

Other studies have utilized child self-reports of emotion regulation, although these have generally been limited to adolescent samples. For example, Garnefski, Kraaij, and van Etten (2005) examined the association between adolescents' self-reported emotion regulation strategies and internalizing and externalizing problems (measured using the Child Behavior Checklist; CBCL). They found that internalizing problems were associated with higher levels of reported self-blame, rumination, and catastrophizing, and lower levels of positive reappraisal, suggesting the use of less adaptive emotion regulation strategies among children high in internalizing problems. Higher externalizing scores were weakly associated with higher catastrophizing, as well as greater blaming of others and positive refocusing. Thus, there were both overlap and specificity in the emotion regulation strategies reported by children high in internalizing and in externalizing symptoms. Silk et al. (2003) found that adolescents who reported more intense and labile emotions and less effective regulation of these emotions exhibited greater depressive symptoms. In particular, disengagement and rumination strategies were associated with higher levels of depressive symptoms. These studies suggest that internalizing psychopathology is associated with self-reported use of emotion regulation strategies believed to be less effective. However, they do not demonstrate that these strategies in fact regulate emotions rather than accompany them, or that these emotion regulation behaviors are causally related to depression.

EMPIRICAL FINDINGS IN CHILDREN OF DEPRESSED MOTHERS

Children of depressed parents exhibit numerous psychological problems and are at elevated risk for mood disorders themselves (Downey & Coyne, 1990; Goodman & Gotlib, 1999; Goodman & Tully, Chapter 17, this volume). Some theorists have proposed that this association may be partially mediated through impairments in the parent–child relationship (Goodman & Gotlib, 1999; Cicchetti & Toth, 1998), which may also play a role in the development of children's emotion regulation abilities (Goodman, 2002). Thus, one would expect children of depressed mothers to exhibit emotion regulation abnormalities. Garber, Braafladt, and Zeman (1991) presented mothers and their children with hypothetical emotion-eliciting scenarios and asked them to generate strategies for regulating emotion in those situations. Dyads with a depressed mother were compared with control dyads with a nondepressed mother. The depressed dyads named fewer overall strategies for regulating emotions, and coders rated their strategies as less effective than those of the control group. This suggests that one source of familial transmission of depression may be parental modeling of ineffective emotion regulation strategies.

Silk, Shaw, Skuban, Oland, and Kovacs (2006) examined a sample of young children (ages 4–7) of mothers with a history of childhood-onset depression and children of never depressed parents. The children were observed at ages 4, 5, and 7 in a delay of gratification task. Behaviors identified as possible emotion regulation strategies were coded in the delay task, including active distraction (shifting attention from the delay task to other activities), focusing on the object of delay, passive waiting (not engaging in any activity), information gathering (asking questions about the delay or the object), and physical comfort seeking from the mother. Children of mothers with a history of depression did not differ from those of never depressed mothers in active distraction, passive waiting, or information gathering. However, the children of depressed mothers did engage in greater focusing on the object of delay, as compared with the control group. It is unclear whether this behavior reflects a strategy for regulating emotion elicited by the delay, or is an index of the extent to which children were interested in the object of delay, or the degree of negative emotion they experienced in response to the task.

ASSOCIATION BETWEEN EMOTION REGULATION AND OTHER RISK FACTORS FOR DEPRESSION

Emotion regulation deficits appear not to be specific to depressive disorders. It has been suggested that externalizing disorders are also associated with difficulty appropriately regulating negative moods. For example, children with conduct disorder are described as having difficulty regulating anger (Cole, Zahn-Waxler, Fox, Usher, & Welsh, 1996). An important avenue for future research will be to examine whether internalizing and externalizing disorders are differentially associated with problems in the regulation of particular emotions (e.g., anger in externalizing disorders, sadness in mood disorders) and whether they differ in the kinds of problematic emotion regulation strategies employed (e.g., rumination in depression, blaming others in externalizing disorders). In addition to externalizing disorders, other forms of psychopathology have also been linked to problems with emotional regulation. Suveg and Zeman (2004) found that children who met the *Diagnostic and Statistical Manual of Mental Disorders*, fourth edition (DSM-IV) criteria for an anxiety disorder reported having difficulty in managing worry, sadness, and anger experiences, as well as having little confidence in their ability to regulate negative emotions. Borderline personality disorder has also been conceptualized as a disorder of emotion dysregulation (Putnam & Silk, 2005).

Moreover, emotion regulation problems may be one outcome of adverse early home environments associated with psychological disorders in children. In particular, maltreatment has been linked to psychological problems, including depression (Cicchetti & Manly, 2001), as well as to emotion regulation difficulties and related constructs (Shields & Cicchetti, 1998; Pollak, Vardi, Bechner, & Curtin, 2005). Children with a history of prolonged abuse or neglect demonstrate deficits in their ability to pose emotional expressions (Camras et al., 1988; During & McMahon, 1991), are more inhibited in their emotional expressions during conflict situations, as compared with nonmaltreated peers (Camras & Rappaport, 1993), and report themselves to be lower in emotion regulation abilities (Shipman, Zeman, Penza, & Champion, 2000).

These findings suggest that emotion regulation problems may not be specific to mood disorders, but serve as a general risk factor for psychological problems in childhood and adolescence (e.g., Chaplin & Cole, 2005). This implies that it will be important to examine whether emotion regulation deficits in children or adolescents with depression are accounted for by the presence of comorbid psychopathology, including externalizing disorders, or by shared early home environment risk factors, such as abuse or neglect. Future work should focus on examining whether there are specific emotion regulation domains that discriminate between different at-risk or pathological groups.

SUMMARY

The fields of affective science and developmental psychopathology hold promise for furthering our understanding of the etiology of mood disorders. Tentative links between risk for depression and abnormalities in emotion and the regulation of emotion in children are beginning to emerge. Basic research refining the construct of emotion regulation, its relationship to emotional processes, and its developmental trajectory can provide a benchmark for testing models of the role of emotion in the development of mood disorders. Although such research holds great potential for broadening and clarifying current theories about the development of mood disorders, it is still in its infancy.

A number of core questions regarding the role of emotion regulation in the development of depression remain to be answered. In particular, the question of whether emotion regulation is experimentally and phenomenologically discriminable from emotion itself is crucial, with implications that would alter our understanding of emotional dysfunction. When dysfunction does emerge, is it due to an excess of emotions to be regulated, reliance on poor emotion regulation strategies, or less effective utilization of adaptive strategies? Among depressed people and those at risk for developing depression, what is the relative importance of the expression and regulation of positive versus negative emotions, and do individual differences in these processes lead to different pathways to the disorder? In addition, it will be important to explore whether emotion regulation variables interact with aspects of the environment to promote or decrease risk for depression. Finally, integrating basic research on the development of emotion and its regulation with theories and methods from developmental psychology will likely yield significant gains in our understanding of the etiological significance of emotional abnormalities to the development of depression.

REFERENCES

Abe, J. A., & Izard, C. E. (1999). The developmental function of emotions: An analysis in terms of differential emotions theory. *Cognition and Emotion*, *13*, 523–549.

Abela, J. R. Z., Brozina, K., & Haigh, E. P. (2002). An examination of the response styles theory of depression in third- and seventh-grade children: A short-term longitudinal study. *Journal of Abnormal Child Psychology*, *30*, 515–527.

Adam, E. K. (2006). Transactions among adolescent trait and state emotion and diurnal and momentary cortisol activity in naturalistic settings. *Psychoneuroendocrinology*, *31*, 664–679.

Block, J. H. (1983). Differential premises arising from differential socialization of the sexes: Some conjectures. *Child Development*, *54*, 1335–1354.

Block, J. H., & Block, J. (1980). The role of ego-control and ego resiliency in the organization of behavior. In W. A. Collins (Ed.), *Minnesota Symposium on Child Psychology* (Vol. 13, pp. 39–101). Hillsdale, NJ: Erlbaum.

Block, J. H., Gjerde, P. F., & Block, J. H. (1991). Personality antecedents of depressive tendencies in 18-year-olds: A prospective study. *Journal of Personality and Social Psychology*, *60*, 726–738.

Brown, T. A., Chorpita, B. F., & Barlow, D. H. (1998). Structural relationships among dimensions of the DSM-IV anxiety and mood disorders and dimensions of negative affect, positive affect, and autonomic arousal. *Journal of Abnormal Psychology*, *107*, 179–192.

Bruder, G. E., Stewart, J. W., Mercier, M. A., Agosti, V., Leite, P., Donovan, S., et al. (1997). Outcome of cognitive-behavioral therapy for depression: Relation to hemispheric dominance for verbal processing. *Journal of Abnormal Psychology*, *106*, 138–144.

Buss, K. A., & Goldsmith, H. H. (1998). Fear and anger regulation in infancy: Effects on the temporal dynamics of affective expression. *Child Development, 69,* 359–374.

Butler, E. A., Egloff, B., Wilhelm, F. H., Smith, N. C., Erickson, E. A., & Gross, J. J. (2003). The social consequences of expressive suppression. *Emotion, 3,* 48–67.

Butler, L. D., & Nolen-Hoeksema, S. (1994). Gender differences in responses to depressed mood in a college sample. *Sex Roles, 30,* 331–346.

Calkins, S. D. (1994). Origins and outcomes of individual differences in emotional regulation. In N. A. Fox (Ed.), *Emotion regulation: Behavioral and biological considerations. Monographs of the Society for Research in Child Development, 59*(2–3), Series 240, 53–72. Chicago: University of Chicago Press.

Calkins, S. D., & Dedmon, S. A. (2000). Physiological and behavioral regulation in two-year-old children with aggressive/destructive behavior problems. *Journal of Abnormal Child Psychology, 28,* 103–118.

Calkins, S. D., Smith, C. L., Gill, K. L., & Johnson, M. C. (1998). Maternal interactive style across contexts: Relations to emotional, behavioral and physiological regulation during toddlerhood. *Social Development, 7,* 350–369.

Campos, J. J., Frankel, C. B., & Camras, L. (2004). On the nature of emotion regulation. *Child Development, 75,* 377–394.

Campos, J. J., Mumme, D. L., Kermoian, R., & Campos, R. G. (1994). A functionalist perspective on the nature of emotion. In N. A. Fox (Ed.), *The development of emotion regulation: Biological and behavioral considerations* (pp. 284–249). *Monographs of the Society for Research in Child Development, 59*(2–3).

Camras, L., & Rappaport, S. (1993). Conflict behaviors of maltreated and nonmaltreated children. *Child Abuse and Neglect, 17,* 455–464.

Camras, L., Ribordy, S., Hill, J., Martino, S., Spaccarelli, S., & Stefani, R. (1988). Recognition and posing of emotional expressions by abused children and their mothers. *Developmental Psychology, 24,* 776–781.

Carlson, E. A., & Sroufe, L. A. (1995). Contributions of attachment theory to developmental psychopathology. In D. Cicchetti & D. Cohens (Eds.), *Manual of developmental psychopathology: Vol. I. Theory and methods* (pp. 581–617). New York: Wiley.

Caspi, A. (2000). The child is the father of the man: Personality continuities from childhood to adulthood. *Journal of Personality and Social Psychology, 78,* 158–172.

Caspi, A., Moffitt, T. E., Newman, D. L., & Silva, P. A. (1996). Behavioral observations at age 3 years predict adult psychiatric disorders. *Archives of General Psychiatry, 53,* 1033–1039.

Chaplin, T. M., & Cole, P. M. (2005). The role of emotion regulation in the development of psychopathology. In B. L. Hankin & J. R. Z. Abela (Eds.), *Development of psychopathology: A vulnerability–stress perspective* (pp. 49–74). Thousand Oaks, CA: Sage.

Chorpita, B. F., & Daleidan, E. L. (2002). Tripartite dimensions of emotion in a child clinical sample: Measurement strategies and implications for clinical utility. *Journal of Consulting and Clinical Psychology, 70,* 1150–1160.

Chrousos, G. P., & Gold, P. W. (1992). The concepts of stress and stress system disorders. *Journal of the American Medical Association, 267,* 1244–1252.

Cicchetti, D., & Manly, J. T. (2001). Operationalizing child maltreatment: Developmental processes and outcomes. *Development and Psychopathology, 6,* 533–549.

Cicchetti, D., & Toth, S. (1998). The development of depression in children and adolescents. *American Psychologist, 55,* 221–241.

Clark, L. A. (2005). Temperament as a unifying basis for personality and psychopathology. *Journal of Abnormal Psychology, 114,* 505–521.

Clark, L. A., & Watson, D. (1999). Temperament: A new paradigm for trait psychology. In L. A. Pervin & O. P. John (Eds.), *Handbook of personality: Theory and research* (2nd ed., pp. 399–423). New York: Guilford Press.

Clark, L. A., Watson, D., & Mineka, S. (1994). Temperament, personality, and the mood and anxiety disorders. *Journal of Abnormal Psychology, 103,* 103–116.

Clayton, P. J., Ernst, C., & Angst, J. (1994). Premorbid personality traits of men who develop unipolar or bipolar disorders. *European Archives of Psychiatry and Clinical Neuroscience, 243,* 340–346.

Cohn, J. F., Campbell, S. B., Matias, R., & Hopkins, J. (1990). Face-to-face interactions of postpartum depressed and nondepressed mother–infant pairs at two months. *Developmental Psychology, 26,* 15–23.

Cole, P., Martin, S., & Dennis, T. (2004). Emotion regulation as a scientific construct: Methodological challenges and directions for child development research. *Child Development, 75,* 317–333.

Cole, P. M., Teti, L. O., & Zahn-Waxler, C. (2003). Mutual emotion regulation and the stability of conduct problems between preschool and early school age. *Development and Psychopathology, 15,* 1–18.

Cole, P. M., Zahn-Waxler, C., Fox, N. A., Usher, B. A., & Welsh, J. D. (1996). Individual differences in emotion regulation and behavior problems in preschool children. *Journal of Abnormal Psychology, 105,* 518–529.

Cole, P. M., Zahn-Waxler, C., & Smith, K. D. (1994). Expressive control during disappointment: Variations related to preschoolers' behavior problems. *Developmental Psychology, 30,* 835–846.

Compas, B. E., Connor-Smith, J., & Jaser, S. S. (2004). Temperament, stress reactivity, and coping: Implications for depression in childhood and adolescence. *Journal of Clinical Child and Adolescent Psychology, 33,* 21–31.

Davidson, R. J. (1998). Affective style and affective disorders: Perspectives from affective neuroscience. *Cognition and Emotion, 12,* 307–330.

Davidson, R. J., Jackson, D. C., & Kalin, N. H. (2000). Emotion, plasticity, context and regulation. *Psychological Bulletin, 126,* 890–906.

Davidson, R. J., Pizzagalli, D., & Nitschke, J. B. (2002). The representation and regulation of emotion in depression: Perspectives from affective neuroscience. In I. H. Gotlib & C. L. Hammen (Eds.), *Handbook of depression* (pp. 219–244). New York: Guilford Press.

Davidson, R. J., Pizzagalli, D., Nitschke, J. B., & Putnam, K. (2002). Depression: Perspective from affective neuroscience. *Annual Review of Psychology, 53,* 545–574.

Dawson, G., Frey, K., Panagiotides, H., Osterling, J., & Hessl, D. (1997). Infants of depressed mothers exhibit atypical frontal brain activity: A replication and extension of previous findings. *Journal of Child Psychology and Psychiatry and Allied Disciplines, 38,* 179–186.

Debener, S., Beauducel, A., Nessler, D., Brocke, B., Heilemann, H., & Kayser, J. (2000). Is resting anterior EEG alpha asymmetry a trait marker for depression? Findings for healthy adults and clinically depressed patients. *Neuropsychobiology, 41,* 31–37.

Downey, G., & Coyne, J. C. (1990). Children of depressed parents: An integrative review. *Psychological Bulletin, 108,* 50–76.

Durbin, C. E., Hayden, E. P., Klein, D. N., & Olino, T. M. (2007). Stability of laboratory assessed temperamental emotionality traits from ages 3 to 7. *Emotion, 7,* 388–399.

Durbin, C. E., Klein, D. N., Hayden, E. P., Buckley, M. E., & Moerk, K. C. (2005). Temperamental emotionality in preschoolers and parental mood disorders. *Journal of Abnormal Psychology, 114,* 28–37.

During, S., & McMahon, R. (1991). Recognition of emotional facial expression by abusive mothers and their children. *Journal of Clinical Child Psychology, 20,* 132–139.

Eisenberg, N., Cumberland, A., Spinrad, T., Fabes, R. A., Shepard, S. A., Reiser, M., et al. (2001). The relations of regulation and emotionality to children's externalizing and internalizing problem behavior. *Child Development, 72,* 1112–1134.

Field, T., Fox, N. A., Pickens, J., & Nawrocki, T. (1995). Relative right frontal EEG activation in 3- to 6-month-old infants of depressed mothers. *Developmental Psychology, 31,* 358–363.

Forbes, E. E., & Dahl, R. E. (2005). Neural systems of positive affect: Relevance to understanding child and adolescent depression? *Development and Psychopathology, 17,* 827–850.

Fox, N. A., & Calkins, S. D. (2003). The development of self-control of emotion: Intrinsic and extrinsic influences. *Motivation and Emotion, 27,* 7–26.

Fox, N. A., Coplan, R. J., Rubin, K. H., Porges, S. W., Calkins, K. H., Long, J. M., et al. (1995). Frontal activation asymmetry and social competence at four years of age. *Child Development, 66,* 1770–1784.

Fredrickson, B. L. (1998). What good are positive emotions? *Review of General Psychology, 2,* 300–319.

Garber, J., Braafladt, N., & Weiss, B. (1995). Affect regulation in depressed and nondepressed children and young adolescents. *Development and Psychopathology, 7,* 93–115.

Garber, J., Braafladt, N., & Zeman, J. (1991). The regulation of sad affect: An information-processing perspective. In J. Garber & K. A. Dodge (Eds.), *The development of emotion regulation and dysregulation* (pp. 208–240). New York: Cambridge University Press.

Garnefski, N., Kraaij, V., & van Etten, M. (2005). Specificity of relations between adolescents' cognitive regulation strategies and internalizing and externalizing psychopathology. *Journal of Adolescence, 28,* 619–631.

Ge, X., Conger, R. D., & Elder, G. H. (2001). Pubertal transition, stressful life events, and the emergence of gender differences in adolescent depressive symptoms. *Developmental Psychology, 37,* 404–417.

Glyshaw, K., Cohen, L. H., & Towbes, L. C. (1989). Coping strategies and psychological distress: Prospective analyses of early and middle adolescents. *American Journal of Community Psychology, 17,* 607–623.

Goldsmith, H. H., & Campos, J. J. (1990). The structure of temperamental fear and pleasure in infants: A psychometric perspective. *Child Development, 61,* 1944–1964.

Goodman, S. H. (2002). Depression and early adverse experiences. In I. H. Gotlib & C. L. Hammen (Eds.), *Handbook of depression* (pp. 245–267). New York: Guilford Press.

Goodman, S. H., & Gotlib, I. H. (1999). Risk for psychopathology in the children of depressed mothers: A developmental model for understanding mechanisms of transmission. *Psychological Review, 106,* 458–490.

Gross, J. J. (1998a). The emerging field of emotion regulation: An integrative review. *Review of General Psychology, 2,* 271–299.

Gross, J. J. (1998b). Antecedent- and response-focused emotion regulation: Divergent consequences for experience, expression, and physiology. *Journal of Personality and Social Psychology, 74,* 224–237.

Gross, J. J., & John, O. P. (2003). Individual differences in two emotion regulation processes: Implications for affect, relationships, and well-being. *Journal of Personality and Social Psychology, 85,* 348–362.

Gross, J. J., & Levenson, R. W. (1997). Hiding feelings: The acute effects of inhibiting negative and positive emotion. *Journal of Abnormal Psychology, 106,* 95–103.

Hirschfeld, R. M., Klerman, G. L., Lavori, P., Keller, M. B., Griffith, P., & Coryell, W. (1989). Premormid personality assessments of first onset of major depression. *Archives of General Psychiatry, 46,* 345–350.

John, O. P., & Srivastava, S. (1999). The big five trait taxonomy: History, measurement, and theoretical perspectives. In L. A. Pervin & O. P. John (Eds.), *Handbook of personality: Theory and research* (Vol. 2, pp. 102–139). New York: Guilford Press.

Johnson, M. H., Posner, M. I., & Rothbart, M. K. (1991). Components of visual orienting in early infancy: Contingency learning, anticipatory looking and disengaging. *Journal of Cognitive Neuroscience, 3,* 335–344.

Joormann, J., & Siemer, M. (2004). Memory accessibility, mood regulation, and dysphoria: Difficulties in repairing sad mood with happy memories? *Journal of Abnormal Psychology, 113,* 179–188.

Just, N., & Alloy, L. B. (1997). The response styles theory of depression: Tests and an extension of the theory. *Journal of Abnormal Psychology, 106,* 221–229.

Katz, L. F., & Gottman, J. M. (1994). Patterns of marital interaction and children's emotional development. In R. D. Parke & S. G. Kellam (Eds.), *Exploring family relationships with other social contexts* (pp. 49–74). Hillsdale, NJ: Erlbaum.

Kendler, K. S., Neale, M. C., Kessler, R. C., Heath, A. C., & Eaves, L. J. (1993). A longitudinal twin study of personality and major depression in women. *Archives of General Psychiatry, 50,* 853–862.

Kenealy, P. (1989). Children's strategies for coping with depression. *Behaviour Research and Therapy, 27,* 27–34.

Kieras, J. E., Tobin, R. M., Graziano, W. G., & Rothbart, M. K. (2005). You can't always get what you want: Effortful control and children's response to undesirable gifts. *Psychological Science, 16,* 391–396.

Klein, M. H., Wonderlich, S., & Shea, M. T. (1993). Models of the relationship between personality and depression: Toward a framework for theory and research. In M. H. Klein, D. J. Kupfer, & M. T. Shea (Eds.), *Personality and depression: A current view* (pp. 1–54). New York: Guilford Press.

Kochanska, G. (1991). Patterns of inhibition to the unfamiliar in children of normal and affectively ill mothers. *Child Development, 62,* 250–263.

Kochanska, G., Murray, K., & Harlan, E. T. (2000). Effortful control in early childhood: Continuity and change, antecedents, and implications for social development. *Developmental Psychology, 36,* 220–232.

Ladouceur, C. D., Dahl, R. E., Williamson, D. E., Birmaher, B., Ryan, N. D., & Casey, J. (2005). Altered emotional processing in pediatric anxiety, depression, and comorbid anxiety–depression. *Journal of Abnormal Child Psychology, 33,* 165–177.

Larsen, R. J. (2000). Toward a science of mood regulation. *Psychological Inquiry, 11,* 129–141.

Leibenluft, E., Charney, D. S., & Pine, D. S. (2003). Researching the pathophysiology of pediatric bipolar disorder. *Biological Psychiatry, 53,* 1009–1020.

Lonigan, C. J., Carey, M. P., & Finch, A. J. (1994). Anxiety and depression in children and adolescents: Negative affectivity and the utility of self-reports. *Journal of Consulting and Clinical Psychology, 62,* 1000–1008.

Lovejoy, M. C., Graczyk, P. A., O'Hare, E., & Neuman, G. (2000). Maternal depression and parenting behavior: A meta-analytic review. *Clinical Psychology Review, 20,* 561–592.

Mangelsdorf, S. C., Shapiro, J. R., & Marzolf, D. (1995). Developmental and temperamental differences in emotion regulation in infancy. *Child Development, 66,* 1817–1828.

Markus, H. R., Kitayama, S., & VandenBos, G. (1996). The mutual interaction of culture and emotion. *Psychiatric Services, 47,* 225–266.

Maughan, A., & Cicchetti, D. (2002). Impact of child maltreatment and interadult violence on children's emotion regulation abilities and socioemotional adjustment. *Child Development, 73,* 1525–1542.

Meehl, P. E. (1975). Hedonic capacity: Some conjectures. *Bulletin of the Menninger Clinic, 39,* 295–306.

Monroe, S. M., Rohde, P., Seeley, J. R., & Lewinsohn, P. M. (1999). Life events and depression in adolescence: Relationship loss as a prospective risk factor for first onset of major depressive disorder. *Journal of Abnormal Psychology, 108,* 606–614.

Muraven, M., & Baumeister, R. F. (2000). Self-regulation and depletion of limited resources: Does self-control resemble a muscle? *Psychological Bulletin, 126,* 247–259.

Muris, P., Roelofs, J., Meesters, C., & Boomsma, P. (2004). Rumination and worry in nonclinical adolescents. *Cognitive Therapy and Research, 28,* 539–554.

Nolen-Hoeksema, S. (1987). Sex differences in depression: Evidence and theory. *Psychological Bulletin, 101,* 259–282.

Nolen-Hoeksema, S. (1991). Responses to depression and their effects on the duration of depressive episodes. *Journal of Abnormal Psychology, 100,* 569–582.

Nolen-Hoeksema, S. (1998). Ruminative coping with depression. In J. Heckhausen & C. S. Dweck (Eds.), *Motivation and self-regulation across the life span* (pp. 237–256). New York: Cambridge University Press.

Nolen-Hoeksema, S. (2000). The role of rumination in depressive disorders and mixed anxiety/depressive symptoms. *Journal of Abnormal Psychology, 109,* 504–511.

Nolen-Hoeksema, S., Larson, J., & Grayson, C. (1999). Explaining the gender difference in rumination. *Journal of Personality and Social Psychology, 77,* 1061–1072.

Pedlow, R., Sanson, A., Prior, M., & Oberklaid, F. (1993). Stability of maternally reported temperament from infancy to 8 years. *Developmental Psychology, 29,* 998–1007.

Plancherel, B., & Bolognini, M. (1995). Coping and mental health in early adolescence. *Journal of Adolescence, 18,* 459–474.

Pollak, S. D., Vardi, S., Bechner, A. M. P., & Curtin, J. J. (2005). Physically abused children's regulation of attention in response to hostility. *Child Development, 76,* 968–977.

Porges, S. W. (1996). Physiological regulation in high-risk infants: A model for assessment and potential intervention. *Development and Psychopathology, 8,* 43–58.

Posner, M. I., & Rothbart, M. K. (2000). Developing mechanisms of self regulation. *Development and Psychopathology, 12,* 427–441.

Putnam, K. M., & Silk, K. R. (2005). Emotion dysregulation and the development of borderline personality disorder. *Development and Psychopathology, 17,* 899–925.

Richards, J. M., & Gross, J. J. (2000). Emotion regulation and memory: The cognitive costs of keeping one's cool. *Journal of Personality and Social Psychology, 79,* 410–424.

Roberts, B. W., & DelVecchio, W. F. (2000). The rank-order consistency of personality traits from childhood to old age: A quantitative review of longitudinal studies. *Psychological Bulletin, 126,* 3–25.

Rose, A. (2002). Co-rumination in the friendships of girls and boys. *Child Development, 73,* 1830–1843.

Rosenbaum, J. F., Biederman, J., Gersten, M., Hirschfeld-Becker, D. R., Kagan, J., Snidman, N., et al. (2000). A controlled study of behavioral inhibition in children of parents with panic disorder and depression. *American Journal of Psychiatry, 157,* 2002–2010.

Rothbart, M. K., Ahadi, S. A., & Evans, D. E. (2000). Temperament and personality: Origins and outcomes. *Journal of Personality and Social Psychology, 78,* 122–135.

Rothbart, M., & Bates, J. (1998). Temperament. In W. Damon (Series Ed.) & N. Eisenberg (Vol. Ed.), *Handbook of child psychology: Vol. 3. Social, emotional, and personality development* (5th ed., pp. 105–176). New York: Wiley.

Rothbart, M. K., & Derryberry, D. (1997). Reactive and effortful processes in the organization of temperament. *Development and Psychopathology, 9,* 633–652.

Rydell, A.-M., Berlin, L., & Bohlin, G. (2003). Emotionality, emotion regulation, and adaptation among 5- to 8-year-old children. *Emotion, 3,* 30–47.

Saarni, C. (1999). *The development of emotional competence.* New York: Guilford Press.

Schwartz, J. A., & Koenig, L. J. (1996). Response styles and negative affect among adolescents. *Cognitive Therapy and Research, 20,* 13–36.

Seligman, M. P. (1975). *Helplessness: On depression, development, and death.* San Francisco: Freeman.

Shields, A., & Cicchetti, D. (1998). Reactive aggression among maltreated children: The contributions of attention and emotion regulation. *Journal of Clinical Child Psychology, 24,* 381–395.

Shiner, R. L. (2000). Linking childhood personality with adaptation: Evidence for continuity and change across time into late adolescence. *Journal of Personality and Social Psychology, 78,* 310–325.

Shipman, K. L., Zeman, J., Penza, S., & Champion, K. (2000). Emotion management skills in sexually maltreated and nonmaltreated girls: A developmental psychopathology perspective. *Development and Psychopathology, 12,* 47–62.

Silk, J. S., Shaw, D. S., Skuban, E. M., Oland, A. A., & Kovacs, M. (2006). Emotion regulation strategies in offspring of childhood-onset depressed mothers. *Journal of Child Psychology and Psychiatry, 47,* 69–78.

Silk, J. S., Steinberg, L., & Morris, A. S. (2003). Adolescents' emotion regulation in daily life: Links to depressive symptoms and problem behavior. *Child Development, 74,* 1869–1880.

Southam-Gerow, M., & Kendall, P. (2001). Emotion regulation and understanding: Implications for child psychopathology and therapy. *Clinical Psychology Review, 22*, 189–222.

Sowell, E. R., Thompson, P. M., Holmes, C. J., Jernigan, T. L., & Toga, A. W. (1999). In vivo evidence for post-adolescent brain maturation in frontal and striatal regions. *Nature Neuroscience, 2*, 859–861.

Spinrad, T. L., Stifter, C. A., Donelan-McCall, N., & Turner, L. (2004). Mothers' regulation strategies in response to toddlers' affect: Links to later emotion self-regulation. *Social Development, 13*, 40–55.

Suveg, C., & Zeman, J. (2004). Emotion regulation in children with anxiety disorders. *Journal of Clinical Child and Adolescent Psychology, 33*, 750–759.

Thompson, R. A. (1990). Emotion and self-regulation. In R. A. Thompson (Ed.), *Nebraska Symposium on Motivation, 1988: Vol. 36. Socioemotional development* (pp. 25–52). Lincoln: University of Nebraska Press.

Thompson, R. A. (1994). Emotion regulation: A theme in search of a definition. *Monographs of the Society for Research in Child Development, 59*(2–3, Serial No. 240).

Tronick, E. Z., Cohn, J., & Shea, E. (1986). The transfer of affect between mothers and infants. In T. B. Brazelton & M. W. Yogman (Eds.), *Affective development in infancy* (pp. 11–25). Westport: Ablex.

Tsai, J. L., Chentsova-Dutton, Y., Freire-Bebeau, L., & Przymus, D. E. (2002). Emotional expression and physiology in European Americans and Hmong Americans. *Emotion, 2*, 380–397.

Tugade, M. M., & Fredrickson, B. L. (2004). Resilient individuals use positive emotions to bounce back from negative emotional experiences. *Journal of Personality and Social Psychology, 86*, 320–333.

van Os, J., Jones, P., Lewis, G., Wadsworth, M., & Murray, R. (1997). Developmental precursors of affective illness in a general population birth cohort. *Archives of General Psychiatry, 54*, 625–631.

Watson, D. (2000). Basic problems in positive mood regulation. *Psychological Inquiry, 11*, 205–209.

Watson, D., & Clark, L. A. (1997). Extraversion and its positive emotional core. In R. Hogan & J. A. Johnson (Eds.), *Handbook of personality psychology* (pp. 767–793). San Diego: Academic Press.

Watson, D., Clark, L. A., & Carey, G. (1988). Positive and negative affectivity and their relation to anxiety and depressive disorders. *Journal of Abnormal Psychology, 97*, 346–353.

Wierzbicki, M. (1989). Children's perceptions of counter-depressive activities. *Psychological Reports, 65*, 1251–1258.

Zeman, J., Shipman, K., & Suveg, C. (2002). Anger and sadness regulation: Predictions to internalizing and externalizing symptoms in children. *Journal of Clinical Child and Adolescent Psychology, 31*, 393–398.

Ziegert, D. I., & Kistner, J. A. (2002). Response styles theory: Downward extension to children. *Journal of Clinical Child and Adolescent Psychology, 31*, 325–334.

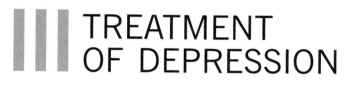

III TREATMENT OF DEPRESSION

8 Cognitive-Behavioral Treatment of Depression during Childhood and Adolescence

Mark A. Reinecke and Golda S. Ginsburg

Major depression during childhood and adolescence is an important clinical problem and a significant social concern. At any given time, 1–3% of children, and 5–7% of adolescents meet the diagnostic criteria for major depression (Essau & Dobson, 1999; Lewinsohn, Hops, Roberts, Seeley, & Andrews, 1993). Depression during childhood is associated with significant psychosocial impairment and puts youth at risk for both substance abuse and suicide (Brent, 1995; Shaffer et al., 1996). Moreover, it tends to co-occur with other psychiatric illnesses—comorbidity is the rule rather than the exception—which can complicate the treatment process and is associated with poorer treatment outcomes (Curry et al., 2006). Of particular concern is the fact that depression among children and adolescents is both chronic and recurrent. The median length of a depressive episode during adolescence is 9 months, and it puts youth at risk for repeated episodes of depression during adulthood (Kovacs, Obrosky, Gatsonis, & Richards, 1997; Reinecke & Curry, 2008; Weissman et al., 1999).

In addressing these concerns, a range of pharmacological and psychosocial interventions have been developed for treating depressed youth (Brent, Gaynor, & Weersing, 2002; Curry, 2001). Outcome studies suggest that cognitive-behavioral approaches may be efficacious for treating depression among adolescents (Fonagy, Target, Cottrell, Phillips, & Kurtz, 2002; Moore & Carr, 2000; Reinecke, Ryan, & DuBois, 1998; Weisz, McCarty, & Valeri, 2006). Outcome research with depressed prepubertal youth, although more limited, also is encouraging. Cognitive-behavioral therapy (CBT) for depression among youth is active, problem-focused, and collaborative. It involves the strategic use of empirically supported techniques to address cognitive, behavioral, and social factors that underlie and maintain a child's distress. Based on a cognitive-behavioral formulation (Nezu, Nezu, & Lombardo, 2004; Persons, 1989; Rogers, Reinecke, & Curry, 2005), interventions are selected that address the full range of cognitive, behavioral, somatic, and social symptoms of depression. In the cognitive domain, children and adolescents learn to solve problems more effectively and to apply cognitive techniques to change maladaptive, negatively valenced beliefs, attitudes, and thoughts that contribute to their depression. Within the behavioral domain, they are encouraged to participate in activities that provide them with a sense of accomplishment and enjoyment and to reestablish trusting, supportive relationships with others. Social skills and assertiveness training are used to address behavioral problems that exacerbate and maintain their depression, and direct attempts are made to facilitate the development of close, secure relationships with parents and other family members. Within the physiological domain, anxious and agitated youth are taught to use relaxation imagery, meditation, and other techniques to regulate their moods.

Our goal in CBT with depressed youth is not limited, however, to providing them with tools and techniques for managing negative moods. Rather, it is to provide them, and their caregivers, with feelings of efficacy and hope. Cognitive therapists endeavor to provide them with a rationale for understanding depression, strategies for coping with life's problems, and a sense of optimism. An explicit goal, as such, is to empower both the child and the parent. It is to give them a vision of a more positive future and tools for bringing this about.

In this chapter we review cognitive-behavioral models of depression during childhood, and treatment strategies derived from them. We discuss empirical support for the efficacy and effectiveness of these approaches and briefly review limitations and shortcomings in this literature. We conclude with a discussion of future directions for clinical innovation.

COGNITIVE THERAPY IN PRACTICE: GENERAL PRINCIPLES

Cognitive therapy was initially developed as a treatment for major depression among adults (Beck, 1963, 1983; Beck, Rush, Shaw, & Emery, 1979). Incorporating both cognitive and behavioral strategies, the approach has received a great deal of empirical and clinical interest over the past 30 years. It is a well-supported intervention for treating unipolar depression among adults (Gloaguen, Cottraux, Cucherat, & Blackburn, 1998; Hollon & Najavits, 1988; Hollon, Thase, & Markowitz, 2002), and substantial evidence exists in support of many of the key components of cognitive models of psychopathology (Clark & Beck, 1999; Haaga, Dyck, & Ernst, 1991; Ingram, Miranda, & Segal, 2006). More recently, attempts have been made to apply these models to understanding depression among children and adolescents (Spence & Reinecke, 2004). As Leahy (1988) and Lewinsohn and Clarke (1999) have noted, however, developmental factors need to be taken into account in treating depressed youth.

What are the essential features of CBT in practice? Cognitive therapy with children and adolescents, as with adults, is time limited, problem focused, and strategic. Treatment typically is not open-ended or long-term. Rather, it is brief and attempts to quickly bring about symptomatic improvement. Although no specific number of sessions is set, one endeavors to bring about meaningful change within 12–16 sessions. Treatment is active and highly focused. The cognitive-behavioral therapist directly attempts to rectify cognitive deficits, distortions, and deficiencies that may be contributing to the child's depression, and develops the child's social skills and affect regulation abilities. As in cog-

TABLE 8.1. Characteristics of CBT with Youth

1. Time limited, brief
2. Problem oriented, focused, strategic
3. Collaborative therapeutic rapport
4. Empirically based, "personal scientist"
5. Structured and active (agenda, homework)
6. Clear and consistent focus on cognitive contents and
   processes, and on developing social and affect regulation skills

nitive therapy with adults, the therapeutic relationship in CBT with youth (and their parents) is both supportive and collaborative. Working with the child and his or her parents, the therapist attempts to understand the child's phenomenal experience, the meanings the child and parents ascribe to events, and how he or she attempts to cope with daily challenges.

Depressed youth tend to demonstrate negative views of themselves, others, and their futures. They see themselves as flawed, unlovable, undesirable, and ineffective and see others as critical, rejecting, and uncaring. At the same time, they view their future as bleak and feel incapable of bringing about desired outcomes. These negativistic beliefs and attitudes are seen by the therapist as objects to be understood and explored, rather than as facts to be accepted. Working with the child or adolescent, the therapist endeavors to understand the experiences that have led to the development of these beliefs and to test their utility and validity. Beliefs are acquired and function in a social context. With this in mind, child cognitive therapists also work to understand *caregivers'* beliefs, attitudes, expectations, attributions, and values and how these influence their caregiving practices and the child's developing sense of him- or herself and others. As in CBT with adults, sessions with youth are structured and active. Specific concerns or problems are identified, as are cognitive, behavioral, social, and environmental factors that may maintain them. Based on an understanding of the outcome literature, the therapist then selects empirically supported strategies or "modules" (Curry & Reinecke, 2003) to address these factors and introduces them to the child and his or her parents. As in CBT with depressed adults, sessions are organized in accord with an agenda that is developed by the child and the therapist, and every session concludes with a "homework assignment" for the child or parent to practice during the subsequent week. The defining characteristics of CBT with youth are summarized in Table 8.1.

VULNERABILITY FOR DEPRESSION

Studies indicate that a range of cognitive, biological, social, and environmental factors interact in placing youth at risk for depression (Ingram et al., 2006; Spence & Reinecke, 2004). The practice of CBT with depressed youth is based on the assumption that by rectifying factors implicated in vulnerability for depression, one can alleviate dysphoria and reduce the risk of relapse or recurrence. Treatment, then, is formulation-based and prescriptive (Rogers et al., 2005). Interventions are selected based on an understanding of cognitive, social, and environmental variables that are contributing to a child's distress (Reinecke & Simons, 2005). The techniques and strategies used, as a result, are individually tailored and strategic.

Cognitive models of vulnerability for depression tend to take the form of diathesis–stress formulations. That is, they assume that the onset of a depressive episode is precipitated by the interaction of a stressful life event (typically an interpersonal loss or a failure) and a preexisting cognitive vulnerability. Such cognitive vulnerabilities, however, are not active at all times. Like software on a computer that has not been "booted up," they are seen as latent or dormant much of the time. Vulnerable and nonvulnerable youth, as such, may not be distinguishable unless confronted with a stressful life event. Experimentally, it often is necessary to activate cognitive diatheses by exposing an individual to a "priming" experience (such as listening to sad music) for the specific vulnerability to become apparent (Gotlib & Krasnoperova, 1998). Cognitive vulnerabilities are typically seen as taking the form of depressogenic schemas or tacit beliefs (Beck, 1963, 1983). Schemas are stable, organized cognitive structures that include representations of the self and others and serve to guide the processing of information (including perception, encoding, retrieval, and problem solving). They are based on prior experiences and have an affective valence.

Depressed youth tend, as a group, to demonstrate many of the same cognitive and perceptual biases and distortions that characterize the thought of depressed adults. Specifically, they demonstrate negative thoughts about themselves, the world, and their future, a tendency to selectively attend to negative events and to recall experiences associated with loss or rejection. Like depressed adults, they demonstrate maladaptive schema (Hammen & Goodman-Brown, 1990; Hammen & Zupan, 1984; Prieto, Cole, & Tageson, 1992; Reinecke & DuBois, 2001; Taylor & Ingram, 1999), which may lead them to attribute negative meanings to their experiences. They tend, for example, to view themselves as unlovable, undesirable, or flawed and to view others as unreliable, unsupportive, and uncaring. Depressed youth often anticipate rejection and tend to ruminate about their predicaments. Like depressed adults, depressed youth demonstrate deficits in rational problem solving, as well as deficits in problem-solving motivation. Specifically, they tend to anticipate that their attempts to solve life's problems will not be successful, and consequently avoid addressing problems directly or approach them in an impulsive, careless manner. Many depressed youth maintain perfectionistic standards, which can impede treatment and place them at risk for relapse. Finally, depressed youth tend, as a group, to demonstrate a negative attributional style. That is, they tend to view losses or failures as stemming from personal characteristics that are broad, stable, and unchanging. They may, for example, attribute a failure on a math exam to the fact that they "are just plain stupid," rather than to the fact that did not study sufficiently, that there were other external factors that may have contributed to their poor performance, and that they have specific difficulties with this course (but have done well in other areas). In summarizing the literature on cognitive vulnerability for depression, Ingram et al. (2006) state, "Data from studies examining the cognitive characteristics of children who are at risk for depression support the idea that these children have negative cognitive structures available . . . [which take the form of] negative self-schemas that, when accessed, are linked to the appearance of self-devaluing and pessimistic thoughts, as well as to dysfunctional information processing" (p. 79). Each of these cognitive and perceptual factors may be implicated in a child's depression and may serve as a target for clinical intervention; see Table 8.2.

Interpersonal factors also are implicated in the development and maintenance of depression (Hammen, 1992; Ingram et al., 2006). Relationships between depressed youth and their parents often are characterized by conflict, problems with attachment, communications difficulties, and rejection (Barber, 1996; Beardslee, Versage, & Gladstone,

TABLE 8.2. Cognitive Targets of Cognitive-Behavioral Intervention

1. Automatic thoughts (self, world, future) and images
2. Perceptions
3. Cognitive distortions
4. Memories
5. Schemas, assumptions
6. Goals, wishes, plans, standards (perfectionism)
7. Problem solving (rational skills, problem-solving motivation)
8. Attributions

1998; Billings & Moos, 1983; Kenny, Moilanen, Lomax, & Brabeck, 1993; Parker, 1993; Rapee, 1997). At the same time, depressed youth tend to withdraw from others and behave in ways that alienate others and contribute to a loss of social reinforcement. Depressed youth tend, as a group, to demonstrate social skills deficits and experience difficulties with peers (Altmann & Gotlib, 1988; Panak & Garber, 1992; Peterson, Mullins, & Ridley-Johnson, 1985; Rudolph, Hammen, & Burge, 1994). The family and peer environments of depressed youth are often stressful and unsupportive and so serve as a context for the development of negative schemas about themselves and others. In addition, depressed youth often behave in ways that magnify and perpetuate negative social interactions, creating a pernicious feed-forward cycle resulting in additional rejection, loss, and depression. Social learning models of depression (Lewinsohn, 1975) posit that depression stems from a loss of perceived reinforcement. This can result from a loss of positive reinforcement (e.g., being complimented by a coach on a strong performance or receiving a good grade) or an increase in negative outcomes (e.g., being criticized by a parent or failing a quiz). An explicit goal of CBT is to increase the availability and salience of positive reinforcement and decrease negative reinforcement or punishment. Social and behavioral difficulties are an important focus of treatment in CBT with depressed youth (see Table 8.3). Inasmuch as families of depressed youth tend to be characterized by more conflict and less support, cognitive therapists work with both children and parents to break these negativistic cycles and create more positive, supportive relationships.

Finally, studies suggest that depressive episodes are often precipitated by stressful life events (Monroe & Hadjiyannakis, 2002). Children and adolescents are particularly sensitive to social loss, and depressive episodes are often triggered by arguments, conflicts, or loss in relationships with parents or peers. Recent research suggests that there may be associations between major and minor stressful life events and depression among youth

TABLE 8.3. Behavioral Targets of Cognitive-Behavioral Intervention

1. Social skills
2. Communication skills
3. Conflict resolution, negotiation
4. Maladaptive coping (alcohol or drug use, cutting and parasuicidal behavior)
5. Attachment difficulties

TABLE 8.4. Social and Environmental Targets of Cognitive-Behavioral Intervention

1. Stressors (major and minor)
2. Supports (family, peer, community)
3. Cues, reinforcers

(Compas, Grant, & Ey, 1994; Goodyer, Wright, & Altham, 1988; Goodyer, Herbert, & Altham, 1998). Not all youth who experience a stressful life event, however, become clinically depressed. Responses to negative life events appear to be moderated by the availability of social supports, problem-solving skills, and cognitive factors associated with resilience (e.g., cognitive flexibility, stable self-concept). As noted, contemporary cognitive-behavioral theories of vulnerability to depression (Abramson, Metalsky, & Alloy, 1989; Beck, Rush, Shaw, & Emery, 1979; Gotlib & Hammen, 1992; Spence & Reinecke, 2004) are typically presented in the form of diathesis–stress models in which risk for depression is seen as stemming from the interaction of stressful life events and preexisting cognitive vulnerabilities. Given the prominence of stress in most theories of depression, cognitive-behavioral therapists work with parents of depressed youth to reduce levels of stress at home, to develop social supports, and to support the use of adaptive coping skills (see Table 8.4).

Depression is a complex disorder. As noted earlier, a wide range of factors—intrapsychic, social, environmental, and biological—are implicated in its etiology and maintenance. Moreover, these factors appear to influence one another in complex ways (Gotlib & Hammen, 1992; Harrington, Wood, & Verduyn, 1998). Simple, linear models for understanding mood and adaptation during childhood and adolescence, as a consequence, will likely prove inadequate. With this in mind, we propose that any comprehensive clinical model of depression must account for the full range of vulnerability, risk, and resilience factors that are associated with the disorder, and that clinical interventions may usefully target the full range of factors associated with risk. The goal of CBT, as such, is to help depressed adolescents to become aware of negative beliefs, attitudes, expectations, and attributions and to substitute them with more adaptive beliefs and constructions. Behaviorally, CBT therapists work to assist adolescents to behave in ways that will elicit positive reinforcement, to limit behavior that elicits negative reinforcement, and to reduce the use of maladaptive coping strategies (such as alcohol or substance abuse and avoidant or impulsive problem solving). By flexibly combining cognitive and behavioral strategies, CBT attempts to rapidly facilitate behavioral and emotional change.

CBT WITH CHILDREN AND ADOLESCENTS

Several cognitive-behavioral treatment protocols for treating depressed youth have been developed during recent years (Brent & Poling, 1997; Clarke, Lewinsohn, & Hops, 1990; Stark et al., 2006; Curry & Reinecke, 2003; Treatment for Adolescents with Depression Study (TADS) Team, 2004; Weisz, Southam-Gerow, Gordis, & Connor-Smith, 2003). Each emphasizes the acquisition of cognitive and behavioral skills that can used to manage depressed affect. Based on cognitive-mediation models (Dobson & Dozois, 2001; Reinecke & Freeman, 2003), these protocols are founded on the assumption that cognitive processes, mood, behavior, and environmental factors transactionally influence one another over the course of development, and that by changing beliefs, attitudes, and thoughts, one can affect a change in one's mood and behavior. To accomplish this, children and adolescents are encouraged to develop specific goals for treatment and learn to monitor their moods. They are encouraged to engage in pleasant activities, to reestablish supportive relationships with peers and family members, and to engage in activities that provide a sense of accomplishment or mastery. Specific skills, including relaxation, conflict resolution and negotiation, identification of cognitive distortions or biases, identification of maladaptive thoughts, rational disputation of maladaptive thoughts, and developing realistic counter-thoughts often are taught. Early treatment manuals tended to be highly structured and encouraged therapists to teach specific skills to all patients in a specific order. Protocols developed during recent years, however, allow for therapists to tailor their interventions to the needs of individuals by including mandatory or standard skills, which all youth are taught, and elective skills, which are introduced when needed. Recently developed "modular" approaches to cognitive-behavioral therapy (Curry & Reinecke, 2003; Rohde, Feeny, & Robins, 2005) are prescriptive in the sense that they permit clinicians to select therapeutic techniques based on the specific cognitive and behavioral vulnerabilities of individual patients. They offer therapists strategies and techniques that can be modified and shaped to meet the needs of youth with different levels of cognitive and emotional development, different presenting concerns, and different family and community contexts.

COGNITIVE THERAPY IN PRACTICE: SPECIFIC STRATEGIES

As discussed earlier, depressed children, like depressed adults, manifest negative views of themselves, their world, and their future. These negative thought patterns increase the probability that they will become depressed when they encounter a stressful life event, such as a loss or a failure. These maladaptive cognitive patterns are acquired and consolidated in a social context. Early experiences of abuse, neglect, or emotional unresponsiveness can lead children to believe that they are undesirable or unlovable, that they cannot count on others to reliably protect or support them, and that others are potentially rejecting and uncaring. These early beliefs or "working models" (Bowlby, 1969, 1970) are subsequently internalized as maladaptive schemas about the self and others (Gotlib & Hammen, 1992; Ingram et al., 2006; Reinecke & Rogers, 2001). A range of strategies are brought to bear to change these beliefs and to develop more adaptive information-processing skills. By working with parents to improve relationships at home, and with youth to improve relationships with peers, cognitive-behavior therapy endeavors to change the social environments that support the development of maladaptive beliefs. A list of specific therapeutic interventions is presented in Table 8.5.

Two cognitive-behavioral paradigms developed for treating depressed adults have been successfully modified for use with children and adolescents and have greatly influenced contemporary clinical practice. Aaron Beck's cognitive therapy tradition focuses on changing maladaptive beliefs, attitudes, and schemas, whereas Peter Lewinsohn's behavioral tradition emphasizes the development of social skills, activity scheduling, and relaxation training as a means of increasing the rate and salience of reinforcements in the child's life.

Beck's cognitive therapy of depression directly endeavors to change maladaptive information-processing strategies and beliefs. Beck (1983) hypothesized that depression-prone individuals possess "dysfunctional attitudes" or schemas about themselves (seeing

TABLE 8.5. Cognitive-Behavioral Interventions

1. Rationale
2. Goal setting
3. Mood monitoring
4. Activity scheduling
   a. Pleasant activities
   b. Social activities
   c. Mastery activities
5. Problem solving
   a. Rational problem solving
   b. Problem-solving motivation
6. Automatic thoughts
   a. Rational disputation
   b. Adaptive self-statements
7. Cognitive distortions
8. Affect regulation
9. Social skills
10. Assertiveness
11. Negotiation/communication and compromise
12. Parent–child interaction
    a. Attachment security
    b. Parent training
13. Taking stock and relapse prevention

themselves as flawed, unlovable, defective), their world (seeing it as dangerous, rejecting, and unsupportive), and their future (seeing it as hopeless, they are unable to bring about desired outcomes). This negativistic belief system, when activated, influences perceptual, memory, and interpretive processes, resulting in a negatively biased understanding of the individual's experiences. Depression-prone children may, for example, be more likely to notice and recall situations in which they had failed at school or not been invited to a sleepover, and to overlook or minimize situations in which they had been successful or enjoyed playing with friends. Interventions based in this tradition attempt to overcome these depressogenic cognitive and perceptual biases.

The Coping with Depression course (Clarke et al., 1990) is a behaviorally based psychoeducational group intervention based on the assumption that depressed youth experience low rates of positive reinforcement and that they behave in ways that may contribute to a loss of social support. In this course, adolescents are taught that thoughts, emotions, and behaviors reciprocally influence one another and that by changing one's thoughts, perceptions, and behaviors, it is possible to influence one's mood. Positive thoughts lead to positive behaviors and positive moods in an "upward spiral," whereas depressive thoughts lead to negativistic behavior and dysphoric mood in a "downward spiral." Thus, adolescents are taught cognitive, behavioral, and social skills as a means of facilitating clinical improvement.

In practice, there are important points of contact between these treatment approaches. They are technically similar, differing primarily in emphasis. Beck's approach, though decidedly cognitive in nature, encourages participation in enjoyable, reinforcing activities and encourages individuals to participate in social activities as a means of changing maladaptive beliefs. At the same time, Lewinsohn's approach includes many cognitive components and actively endeavors to develop individuals' ability to recognize and appreciate reinforcers in their environment and how negativistic beliefs can influence their behavior. Here, however, change in cognition is in the service of increasing rates of reinforcement. The cognitive-behavioral protocols we have discussed have many features in common, and an argument can be made that effective treatments flexibly use many of their shared components (Evans et al., 2005). Several of these treatment modules are discussed in turn.

Psychoeducation

Effective treatments tend to be psychoeducational in nature. Children and adolescents typically are referred for treatment by their parents, who are confused by their children's difficulties and are unsure what can be done to solve them. Parents are often frustrated and frightened by the recurring nature of their child's problems, and by their inability to rectify them. With this in mind, CBT therapists typically begin treatment by educating youth and their parents about depression and CBT. Using the child's and the parent's descriptions of their concerns, the therapist presents an integrative model of depression and the cognitive-behavioral model of treatment. The therapist notes how depression is multiply determined, and how cognitive, behavioral, emotional, biological, and environmental factors interact in contributing to the child's distress. Whenever a new technique is introduced, the therapist begins by presenting a rationale. It is important that patients and their parents understand the strategy and how it may be helpful for them. When needed, research findings may be discussed (e.g., benefits of CBT versus medication, suicidal ideations and medications, risk of relapse), and popular books (e.g., *More Than Moody*, *Mind over Mood*), websites (e.g., *www.cognitivetherapy.com*, *www.academyofct.org*), and workbooks can be recommended.

Therapeutic Collaboration

The therapeutic relationship in CBT is collaborative in nature (Beck et al., 1979). The CBT therapist is neither nondirective (as in Rogerian, supportive, or psychodynamic psychotherapy), nor highly directive (as in behavior therapy). Rather, the therapist is active and works *with* the patient to understand his or her difficulties and how the youth understands his or her world. The youths' (and their parents') thoughts, attitudes, beliefs, attributions, expectations and assumptions are treated as hypotheses to be examined to determine their validity and utility. It is vitally important for children and their parents to feel that their therapist appreciates their concerns and perspectives. The parental belief that the therapist does not understand them or appreciate their views is a strong predictor of premature termination of treatment. With this in mind, we typically conclude each session by asking parents and children if they feel they have been understood that day and if there is anything important that has been overlooked.

Depressed children and their parents often feel hopeless and helpless. With this in mind, the CBT therapist endeavors to communicate a sense of optimism and confidence. In contrast to dynamic psychotherapy, in which negative transference reactions toward the therapist within the therapy session are accepted and interpreted, in CBT therapists actively attempt to identify and address patients' negative thoughts and expectations about therapy. Patients and parents are encouraged to express any concerns they may have, so that negative feelings about the therapy can be addressed before they undermine the therapeutic rapport. Adolescents (and their parents) are unlikely to participate in activities that they believe will not be helpful. Inasmuch as feelings of pessimism are a defining characteristic of depression, CBT therapists attempt to model a realistic sense of optimism within the therapy session.

Goal Setting

Cognitive-behavioral therapy is strategic and problem focused. *Every* statement, question, and intervention during the therapy session is directed toward gathering information, clarifying or changing a thought or a belief, or developing an adaptive behavioral skill. An important function of the therapist is to maintain the therapeutic focus and provide structure. The therapist, the child, and his or her caregivers begin treatment by discussing their goals for therapy. Establishing treatment goals is no small task, as the objectives of children and those of parents often have little in common. Parents, for example, often want their child to be more polite and compliant, to get along better with siblings, and to improve his or her school performance. Adolescents, in contrast, often feel that they have no problems (other than their parents' nagging them) and want to be left alone. Neither the parent nor the teen, however, may acknowledge that the adolescent is clinically depressed and has been experiencing suicidal ideations. Our initial goal as therapists, then, is to guide the parent and the child in developing a list of goals that all can agree upon. The goals should be meaningful, specific, and concrete (i.e., decrease depressive symptoms, decrease frequency of arguments). The therapist then works with the child and the parents to monitor progress in achieving these goals over the course of treatment.

Homework

Patient activity is a strong predictor of therapeutic outcome. It may be argued, then, that homework assignments are a crucial component of CBT. As in CBT with adults, children and adolescents are strongly encouraged to engage in at least one task each week that will allow them to test the validity or utility of a belief, gather information, or develop a new skill. *Every* CBT session concludes with developing a homework assignment. Inasmuch as the term *homework* often has negative connotations for children and adolescents, one can simply give it another name (e.g., "something to try this week"). Children and adolescents often are not compliant in completing their therapeutic homework assignments. It can be helpful, then, to recruit parents to serve as a "coaches" for completing assignments at home and to identify cognitive or environmental "chocks" or "blocks" that impede completion. If, for example, a teen believes that "it won't work . . . nothing helps," he or she will be unlikely to attempt the assignment. The validity of these beliefs can be tested (as one would test any automatic thought), and more adaptive beliefs (e.g., "I haven't tried this before . . . it's worth a shot . . . can't hurt to try") can be suggested. Providing a rationale for the assignment, collaboratively developing the task, recognizing and rewarding attempts to complete homework assignments, and reflecting on positive outcomes of completing homework assignments can all improve compliance (Friedberg & McClure, 2005; Hudson & Kendall, 2005).

Mood Monitoring

CBT is founded on the assumption that, by changing cognitions, it is possible to change one's mood. Before children and adolescents can understand relations between thoughts and mood, however, they must be able to monitor their moods. They need to be able to distinguish and label different emotional states, discriminate levels of intensity of mood, and appreciate how moods can change over time. Children and adolescents are taught to track how they are feeling (we recommend monitoring *both* positive and negative moods), so that they will be able relate these moods to situations that make them feel better or worse and to identify accompanying thoughts. By monitoring positive and negative moods, they come to appreciate that they don't "always feel bad" and that their moods are "movable" or changeable. Children and adolescents practice rating moods on a 0–10 "feelings thermometer," with the patient providing anchors for various points on the scale. After a child becomes proficient at rating his or her moods, the child is asked to record situations in which he or she felt this way and the events that led to changes in his or her mood. Finally, children practice recording the thoughts that accompanied each situation. As they come to recognize that there are some activities that lead them to feel worse, and others that are associated with feeling better, they are encouraged to increase the activities that make them feel better. Mood monitoring, then, serves as a foundation for a new clinical skill, activity scheduling.

Activity Scheduling

Depressed children, like depressed adults, tend to engage in relatively few activities that give them a sense of pleasure or accomplishment. They tend to withdraw from other people, and often stay in their bedrooms and engage in solitary activities (such as listening to music, watching TV, surfing the Web, or playing videogames). With this in mind, the CBT therapist talks with the parent and child about the importance of participating in activities that are fun and that provide a sense of competence or achievement. Again, this is no small task. Depressed youth often experience difficulty in identifying activities they would enjoy (i.e., "Nothing is fun"), and parents frequently feel it is inappropriate to "reward" their child with pleasant activities before the child's demeanor and behavior improve. It is thus quite important to share the rationale for the intervention with the family and to keep its primary function (alleviating depression, rather than improving compliance) in mind. The therapist begins by working with the child to develop a list of activities that he or she may enjoy. Activities on the list should be genuinely enjoyable to the child or adolescent, safe, active, inexpensive, readily available, legal, and (preferably) social. If the patient experiences difficulty in identifying potentially enjoyable activities, the therapist can "prime the pump" by giving the child a copy of Peter Lewinsohn's "Pleasant Activities Checklist." A copy of this list is available as a pdf file at *www.ori.org*. Although the list was developed for use with adults and is somewhat dated, teenagers often find it interesting, even amusing, to complete. We simply ask them to read the list and circle any item to which they may respond, "If I did this, I might like it." From the responses, we collaboratively develop a list of 10 activities they would like to pursue. Once this list has been compiled, we count the number of times they have engaged in these activities over the past week in order to generate a baseline. We also ask them to rank their moods during the days of these activities. The patients, with the support of their parents, are then asked to increase the number of pleasant activities they participate in each day and to note the corresponding change in their moods. A similar approach can be used to increase participation in activities that are associated with feelings of mastery or competence. We typically encourage patients to participate in one or two pleasant and mastery activities per day. Whether it is a cause or consequence of depression, depressed youth tend, as a group, to engage in few activities that are enjoyable or that provide a sense of competence. Systematically scheduling and participating in pleasurable activities, and completing tasks that provide a sense of accomplishment, provide a powerful tool for alleviating depression.

Social Interaction

Interpersonal factors—including social withdrawal, excessive dependency, social inhibition, and impaired social skills—can put individuals at risk for depression and increase the likelihood of relapse and recurrence (Joiner, 2002). Depressed youth tend to withdraw from others and to behave in ways, both subtle and obvious, that alienate peers and family members. They tend, as a group, to avoid eye contact, seldom smile or laugh, ask few questions, slouch, seek reassurance from others, direct conversations to themselves and their problems, solicit negative feedback from others, and complain. Dysphoric individuals tend, as well, to behave in an obsequious, dependent manner that may cause or maintain their depression. Studies indicate that interpersonal skill deficits such as these can interfere with individuals' ability to gain positive social reinforcement and can, under some circumstances, put them at risk for depression (Joiner, 2002). Social skills training can be used to help children and adolescents who experience difficulty in making and keeping friends (Clarke et al., 1990). Through modeling, role play, discussion, and guided practice, depressed youth develop skills for meeting, greeting, and talking with others, for maintaining appropriate eye contact, and for entering and leaving conversations. They are encouraged not to excessively seek reassurance from others and to assiduously avoid soliciting negative feedback. Specific negative thoughts that may interfere with social relationships (e.g., "Nobody will like me," "I have *no* personality," "Nobody cares . . . they're all snobs and idiots") are identified and addressed through rational disputation.

Problem Solving

Depressed children and adolescents often demonstrate poor problem-solving skills and low problem-solving motivation. They view their problems as unsolvable and so either avoid addressing them or approach them in an impulsive, careless manner. Depressed youth often experience difficulty in identifying problems, generating possible solutions, evaluating them, and implementing them. Problem-solving training can be quite helpful in addressing these difficulties. Youth are taught strategies for confronting and resolving problems that would otherwise lead them to feel depressed and powerless. The CBT therapist begins by acknowledging that everyone has problems and suggesting that the only thing that discriminates the easily solvable from the overwhelming is the availability of strategies for managing them. The therapist then presents problems that other children and adolescents might encounter (e.g., lost or broken toy, poor grades, curfew, problems with friends, chores, a lost dog), and the patient is encouraged to identify a specific problem and to generate a range of possible solutions that might be tried. The therapist and the patient then discuss the pros and cons of the various solutions (including short- and long-term consequences) and select the best course of action. Once the child becomes comfortable with generating and evaluating solutions for others' problems, a formal model of problem solving is introduced. Using the acronym RIBEYE, youth are taught to approach problems in a thoughtful, systematic manner. RIBEYE stands for Relax, Identify the problem, Brainstorm possible solutions, Evaluate their strengths and weaknesses, say Yes to one (or two), and Encourage yourself for success. Beginning with simple problems, the therapist guides the child through the process of solving problems in his or her life. As this is accomplished, the patient is encouraged to address more significant problems and to practice using RIBEYE at home and at school. It is important to keep in mind that problem solving training is designed to teach youth *how to think about* problems and stressful life events, rather than what to think. The focus is not on rectifying maladaptive beliefs, but on providing skills for managing life's challenges. As Frauenknecht and Black (2004) note, our goal is to teach problem-solving skills that can be used in a range of settings. This is done by providing the child with graduated experiences in therapy (using modeling and role play) and integrating this with *in vivo* practice. The generalization of skills is most likely to occur when explicit attempts are made to bring it about.

Affect Regulation

Clinically depressed youth frequently manifest deficits in the ability to modulate negative moods. When confronted by events that would, for many, lead to mild feelings of sadness, vulnerable youth can rapidly become severely despondent. They lack the requisite cognitive, behavioral, and social skills needed to effectively regulate their moods. As a consequence, they are often described by parents and others as "moody" or "volcanic." Such depressed youth are taught specific strategies for coping with emotionally arousing situations. Using a blank emotions thermometer, the therapist asks the adolescent to describe his or her feelings when he or she is "about to lose it . . . When your feelings are going out of control." The patient is then asked to identify thoughts, physiological sensations, and behavioral cues that occur just before his or her mood escalates to this level. These cues are typically feelings of agitation, tension, and thoughts such as "I can't take this!" As anchors are placed on the thermometer, the patient comes to identify cues indicating that his or her mood is beginning to escalate and that he or she will need to take action to prevent an outburst. The therapist and the teen then work collaboratively to develop a list of cognitive, behavioral, and social strategies that can be introduced before the mood escalates. Such strategies include performing relaxation exercises, leaving the situation, using adaptive self-statements (e.g., "It's no big deal, there's nothing here I can't handle"), seeking social support, and using distraction. Many depressed youth, when they experience mild feelings of sadness, tend to reflect on their emotions and their predicaments. This perseverative process of self-focused attention and tendency to ruminate can magnify their feelings of dysphoria and can place individuals at risk for longer and more severe depressive episodes (Nolen-Hoeksema, 1991; Nolen-Hoeksema & Morrow, 1991). Therefore, ruminative youth are taught to direct their attention away from their inner emotional states and to engage in solution-focused thinking. Using rational problem-solving skills, they learn to cope more effectively with stressful life events and challenges that are contributing to their distress. By anticipating situations that may lead to an emotional outburst, an adolescent can prepare for them.

Automatic Thoughts and Cognitive Distortions

In CBT for depression, a great deal of emphasis is put on teaching adolescents to identify and change maladaptive thoughts and to challenge errors in thinking. Certain cognitive distortions (i.e., perfectionism) are particularly troubling in that they can exacerbate feelings of depression and put individuals at increased risk for relapse. It is important, then, to teach youth to recognize and change these thought patterns.

Before individuals can change what they think, however, they must become aware of what they are thinking. Beck et al. (1979) recommended using a process of guided discovery to assist depressed adults to identify negative thoughts and cognitive errors. Similar procedures can be used with children and adolescents. Based on Socratic questioning, guided discovery is a process by which a therapist, by patiently asking a series of gentle questions, guides the patient to recognize errors in his or her logic and to see how maintaining a particular belief may be maladaptive. By avoiding direct confrontation, the therapist maintains a collaborative rapport and demonstrates how, through careful questioning, the patient can come to a new, more adaptive way of thinking about his or her predicament. The therapist is doing more, however, than working to change a specific maladaptive belief or cognitive distortion. Rather, the therapist is modeling a rational way of thinking and a systematic way of approaching life's problems. Maintaining a Socratic, collaborative stance is particularly important with children and adolescents, as direct attempts to challenge a belief may be taken as a reprimand and may lead children to defensively attempt to "prove they are right." Simply pointing out a child's maladaptive thoughts and cognitive distortions (e.g., "*Nobody* likes me," "I'm too stupid to do *anything*") and suggesting alternative, more positive, thoughts is not likely to be effective. Rather, the child or teen must recognize that his or her negative beliefs are, in fact, untrue, and develop skills for evaluating the validity of his or her thoughts that can be used in a range of situations. To promote the generalization of these skills to new settings, the CBT therapist encourages children and adolescents to apply cognitive techniques, learned in the therapy session, to problems they encounter at home and at school as part of their homework.

Building on the patient's understanding of mood monitoring, we ask the patient to recall thoughts that he or she has experienced in depressing situations in the past. Most youth have little difficulty with this and readily share why they are upset by events in their lives. One need only ask, "What was going through your mind then?" or "What was the most upsetting thing about this?" Should difficulties arise in identifying negative thoughts, they can be asked to complete objective rating scales of common negative thoughts. The Children's Automatic Thoughts Questionnaire can be quite helpful with school-age children, and the Young–Brown Schema Questionnaire is useful with older adolescents in identifying possible maladaptive beliefs. In a similar manner, teens can be provided with a list of common cognitive distortions and, after reviewing it, be given a set of brief hypothetical vignettes illustrating them. This provides the adolescents with an opportunity to identify cognitive distortions and maladaptive thoughts in others' lives and to reflect on how they may experience them in their own lives. As they become adept at identifying maladaptive thoughts during sessions, teens are asked to complete a three-column mood log at home as a homework task.

Developing Adaptive Counter-Thoughts

Once adolescents have an understanding of negative thoughts and cognitive distortions, and of how these can maintain negative moods, they are taught how to change them by "talking back" to their thoughts. As in CBT with adults, depressed children and adolescents are encouraged to view their thoughts and beliefs as hypotheses to be tested, rather than as facts. They learn to pay particular attention to information that may be inconsistent with these beliefs and to revise their thoughts based on new information.

Once teenagers have become aware of their negative thoughts and recognize how they may influence their moods, they are taught to evaluate them though rational disputation. This is an advanced cognitive skill, and the argument has been made that it is necessary for youth to possess hypothetico-deductive reasoning (formal operational thought) before they can use it effectively. Briefly, the therapist and the adolescent subject automatic thoughts to logical analysis by (1) examining evidence for and against the belief, (2) determining if there is another, more adaptive, way of understanding the experience that is more consistent with the evidence, and (3) identifying alternative courses of action or possible solutions for remaining problems.

We introduce the concept of rational disputation to youth with an analogy—"Contrasting Coaches." Most children and adolescents have participated in a sport, and we inquire which they would prefer after they have made a mistake: Coach A, who yells and berates them for their failure, and who admonishes them not to make such a bonehead mistake again, or Coach B, a supportive coach who notes what led to the mistake, demonstrates how to overcome it, encourages them not to get down about it, and reinforces their efforts to improve? Children invariably select Coach B, allowing us to discuss how we "coach ourselves" through losses, failures, and problematic situations. Are we self-punitive, negative, perfectionistic, and self-critical; or positive, balanced, and solution focused? If you were to adopt a more positive, solution-focused stance, how would you feel? How would you act?

Using automatic thoughts that the adolescent has identified, the CBT therapist then teaches the adolescent specific strategies for rectifying maladaptive thoughts. The child learns that evaluating evidence is the key to resolving life's problems. Upsetting thoughts are seen as questions or hypotheses to be tested, and evidence is sought to ascertain their validity and utility. Specifically, the child is taught to ask:

1. What is the evidence that supports the thought?
2. Is there any contradictory evidence? Is there any evidence I have overlooked, or anything that might lead me to think the thought may not be true?
3. Is there another way of looking at the situation?
4. If the negative thought is true, is it really such a big deal?
5. What is the solution? What can be done to handle this?

Through role playing and role reversal, the therapist can model getting "stuck" in a negative automatic thought and seek the patient's help in thinking about the problem in new ways. Difficulties most often occur at two points in this sequence—at Question 3, when adolescents are asked to develop an alternative, more adaptive, understanding of events, and at Question 5, when they are asked to consider new courses of action and how adopting a new perspective would influence their behavior and to reflect on how new ways of behaving would affect their mood. In light of these considerations, homework assignments center on developing helpful counter-thoughts and on listing ways in which they can be applied in daily life. It can be helpful, as well, to examine whether maintaining a negative belief may be functional in the child's life. Several years ago we worked with a depressed young woman who, whenever she was complimented, would negate the compliment and criticize herself. If complimented on her clothes, for example, she would respond "No, it's really ugly, my clothes are terrible," leading her to feel worse. Interestingly, her self-criticisms were often followed by additional compliments from her friends (e.g., "No, it really is a cool sweatshirt, I like it!"), reinforcing the patient's statement and initiating yet another round of self-criticism. When asked why she did this, she commented, "Mom always told me not to get too proud . . . If I'm hard on myself, it keeps other people from doing it." Her depressogenic self-criticism was, from her perspective, reasonable and adaptive. Moreover, it was being reinforced by her peers and her mother. These ancillary beliefs—that one should "never act proud" and "others will criticize me"—became the focus of additional rational disputation.

It is worth noting that cognitive therapists are not simply encouraging youth to think positively or to adopt a "positive mental attitude." Rather, our goal is to develop their ability to think flexibly and adaptively and to use newly developed capacities for hypothetico-deductive reasoning in ways that allow for greater freedom of action as well as a sense of efficacy and hope. Adaptive counter-thoughts, as such, must not only be positive; they must be reasonable.

Relaxation Training

Depressed children and adolescents often become tense and anxious when confronted with stressful life events or social situations. These feelings of anxiety and tension can reduce their awareness of reinforcers and can interfere with their ability to use the cognitive and behavioral skills they have learned. Relaxation training can be particularly helpful, then, for children or adolescents who report feeling tense or "stressed out" or who have a history of a comorbid anxiety disorder. Treatment begins by asking children to monitor situations in which they feel anxious and the thoughts they are experiencing in those settings. As they become aware of anxiety-provoking situations, they are asked to note how their anxiety is manifested physically. Do they, for example, experience feelings of tension, headaches, sweating, or stomachaches? They are then taught simple relaxation techniques, including controlled breathing, guided imagery (e.g., relaxing on a warm beach), muscle relaxation, and adaptive self-statements (e.g., "No problem here . . . nothing I can't handle"). The techniques can be audiotaped so that a teen can practice them at home. As in CBT for anxiety disorders, youth are encouraged not to avoid anxiety-provoking situations, but to confront them. Through guided practice, they come to see that exposure and mastery are the keys to overcoming one's fears. As one anxious teenager succinctly noted, "If you're afraid of dogs, sooner or later you've got to pet the puppy!"

Taking Stock and Relapse Prevention

The final phase of CBT with depressed youth focuses on consolidating the skills they have learned over the course of treatment and preventing relapse. The therapist, the patient, and his or her parents review the gains that have been made and determine which cognitive and behavioral skills have been most helpful. There is an emphasis on identifying associations between the use of these skills and the positive changes that have been observed. The specific problems and concerns that precipitated the referral for therapy are reviewed, and ways of coping with similar events, should they occur, are discussed. Because depression is a recurrent disorder and feelings of sadness are a normal part of every life, the possibility that the patient will experience feelings of dysphoria at some point in the future is discussed. Strategies for managing these feelings are reviewed, as are ways of managing "high-risk" situations he or she may encounter. Maintenance therapy sessions to prevent relapse and follow-up booster sessions are scheduled.

IS CBT EFFECTIVE WITH DEPRESSED YOUTH?

Controlled outcome studies completed over the past 25 years indicate that individual and group CBT can be useful in treating depression among children and adolescents, and that these gains may be maintained over time (for thoughtful reviews, see Curry, 2001;

Fonagy et al., 2002; Harrington, Whittaker, Shoebridge, & Campbell, 1998; Lewinsohn & Clarke, 1999; Moore & Carr, 2000; Reinecke et al., 1998; Weisz et al., 2006).

The first controlled trial of CBT with depressed youth was completed by Butler, Meizitis, Friedman, and Cole (1980), who assigned 54 depressed youth to group CBT, a social skills group, a support group (which served as an attention-placebo control), or a waiting-list control. Youth in the two active treatment groups showed clinically significant gains relative to those in the two control groups. Interestingly, participants in the social skills group fared better that those receiving CBT.

Several years later, Reynolds and Coats (1986) completed a study in which 30 moderately dysphoric adolescents were randomly assigned to group CBT, relaxation training, or a waiting-list control condition. Youth receiving one of the active treatments demonstrated a significant reduction in depressive symptoms relative to those in the control condition. These gains were maintained over a brief (5-week) follow-up period. Differences were not observed, however, between adolescents who had received CBT and those who had received relaxation training.

Shortly thereafter, Stark, Reynolds, and Kaslow (1987) published the results of a study of 28 depressed adolescents. Youth were assigned to self-instructional training (SIT), a problem-solving skills training (PSST) group, or a waiting-list control condition. Adolescents who received active treatment demonstrated significantly greater reductions in severity of depression than did controls. These gains were maintained over an 8-week follow-up period.

Several years later, Lewinsohn, Clarke, Hops, and Andrews (1990) evaluated the efficacy of the Coping with Depression (CWD) course, a group CBT protocol that emphasizes the development of social skills, relaxation, and maintaining social relationships as a means of alleviating depression among adolescents. Fifty-nine high school students meeting the criteria for a depressive disorder were randomly assigned to either group CBT, group CBT supplemented by parent training, or a waiting-list control condition. Adolescents who received CBT demonstrated significant reductions in depression relative to those in the control condition. These gains were maintained over a 2-year follow-up period. Clinical improvement was similar in the two CBT conditions. The addition of a parent training component, then, did not appear to facilitate clinical improvement. The Coping with Depression Course has been refined over the past 15 years and can be quite effective for treating mild to moderate depression. A copy of the CWD protocol can be obtained from the authors at *www.kpchr.org/public/acwd/acwd.html*.

That same year, Lerner and Clum (1990) published the results of a comparative outcome study examining the relative efficacy of group social problem-solving therapy and supportive psychotherapy for treating adolescents who were suicidal. They found that problem-solving therapy was more effective than supportive psychotherapy for reducing severity of depression, alleviating feelings of pessimism, and reducing feelings of loneliness at posttreatment and at 3-month follow-up.

Kahn, Kehle, Jenson, and Clark (1990) published the results of a study of the effectiveness of group CBT, relaxation training, and self-modeling interventions for treating depressive symptoms among 10- to 14-year-old students. Participants were randomly assigned to one of the three active treatment groups, or to a waiting-list control. Youth who received an active treatment demonstrated a significant reduction in severity of depression relative to those in the control condition. These gains were maintained at 1-month follow-up. Few differences were observed, however, between outcomes for the three active treatments.

Several years later, Wood, Harrington, and Moore (1996) examined the relative effectiveness of brief (6-session) individual CBT and relaxation training for treating clinically depressed adolescent outpatients. At the conclusion of the acute treatment phase, youth receiving CBT were more likely to have remitted than those in the control condition. These differences were not apparent at 3-month follow-up, though, owing to the continued improvement of youth who had received relaxation training.

In a second study, Kroll, Harrington, Jayson, Fraser, and Gowers (1996) found that depressed adolescents who continued to receive CBT after remission demonstrated lower rates of relapse and recurrence than did those in a control group who discontinued CBT after their depression had lifted.

Based on earlier work by Beck and colleagues (1979), Brent and Poling (1997) developed a CBT protocol emphasizing rational disputation of maladaptive beliefs. The effectiveness of this treatment was examined in a randomized controlled trial comparing CBT, systemic behavioral family therapy (SBFT), and nondirective supportive therapy (NST) for treating clinically depressed adolescents (Brent et al., 1997). One hundred and seven adolescents were randomly assigned to one of the three active treatments. Adolescents who received CBT demonstrated higher rates of remission from depression than did youth who received either SBFT or NST (60% versus 38% or 39%, respectively). Moreover, youth who received CBT evidenced a more rapid response than those in the other two groups.

Clarke, Rohde, Lewinsohn, Hops, and Seeley (1999) replicated earlier findings reported by Lewinsohn et al. (1990) in an investigation of the efficacy of two versions of the CWD cognitive-behavioral group intervention. One hundred and twenty-three adolescents (ages 14–18) meeting the criteria of the *Diagnostic and Statistical Manual of Mental Disorders*, third edition, revised (DSM-III-R) for major depressive disorder and/or dysthymia were randomly assigned to one of three conditions—adolescent-only group therapy, adolescent group therapy supplemented by a parent treatment component, or a waiting-list control group. At the conclusion of the acute treatment phase, adolescents in both treatment groups improved significantly more than controls in depressive symptomatology reported on the self-report Beck Depression Inventory (BDI; Beck, Ward, Mendelson, Mock, & Erbaugh, 1961), though not on the clinician-rated Hamilton Rating Scale for Depression (HAM-D; Hamilton, 1960). Although the magnitude of the difference between active treatments and the waiting-list control was smaller than had been observed in the original (Lewinsohn et al., 1990) study, adolescents in both active treatment groups recovered from episodes of depression at a significantly higher rate than did controls. At 2-year follow-up, the authors also found that booster sessions did not reduce the rate of recurrence for depression, but appeared to accelerate recovery among adolescents who were still depressed at the end of the acute phase. The possibility exists, then, that youth who remain mildly depressed at the conclusion of acute treatment may benefit from additional outpatient CBT.

Finally, Rosselló and Bernal (1999) evaluated the efficacy of cognitive-behavioral therapy and interpersonal psychotherapy (IPT) for treating depressive symptoms in a sample of Puerto Rican adolescents (13–18 years of age) meeting DSM-III-R criteria for major depressive disorder and/or dysthymia. Seventy-one participants were randomly assigned to one of the active, individual treatments or a waiting-list control group. In comparison with controls, adolescents in both treatment conditions reported significant reductions in depressive symptoms. These gains were maintained at 3 months posttreatment. No differences in rates of improvement were apparent for adolescents in the two active treatment groups. IPT and CBT appear, as such, to have been equally effective in this trial.

Taken together, results from 11 early randomized controlled trials suggested that CBT may be efficacious for treating depression among adolescents. CBT was uniformly found to be more effective than a waiting-list or attention control, and therapeutic gains tended to be maintained over time. These findings were congruent with the results of research completed with dysphoric prepubertal children (e.g., Weisz, Thurber, Sweeney, Proffitt, & LeGagnoux, 1997).

Subsequent trials of CBT with depressed youth have tended to differ from earlier studies in several important ways. Recent studies have tended to use larger samples and have included adolescents who are more difficult to treat. Participants in recent studies generally report higher levels of depression and have a larger number of comorbid diagnoses than did participants in earlier trials. Recent studies have also tended to use more rigorous controls (e.g., pill placebo or medication management, rather than a waiting-list control). It is also noteworthy that the percentage of female participants in these studies has been somewhat higher than in earlier investigations, and that participants in recent studies have tended to be clinically referred outpatients rather than high school students or community participants. Furthermore, in each of these studies, analyses were conducted in accordance with intent-to-treat strategies, in contrast to several earlier studies in which analyses were limited to treatment completers.

A study by Clarke and colleagues (2002) is representative of more recent investigations of outcome. Briefly, they evaluated the effectiveness of a cognitive-behavioral intervention for treating depressed adolescents receiving services in a health maintenance organization (HMO). Eighty-eight participants (13–18 years old) who met DSM-III-R criteria for major depression and/or dysthymia were randomly assigned to receive typical HMO care or usual care plus a group cognitive-behavioral intervention. Participants in the usual care condition were permitted to receive mental health services provided by either the HMO or by outside health care providers. Participation in the CBT intervention did not yield a significant advantage in reducing symptoms of depression relative to usual care at posttreatment, or at 12- and 24-month follow-up assessments. Similarly, there was no difference between conditions in depression recovery rates.

Rohde, Clarke, Mace, Jorgensen, and Seeley (2004) compared a cognitive-behavioral group treatment with a life skills tutoring intervention for the treatment of depressed adolescents (ages 13–17 years). Ninety-one participants meeting DSM-IV criteria for major depressive disorder and conduct disorder were randomly assigned to either the cognitive behavioral intervention or the life skills tutoring group. Major depression recovery rates were significantly higher for adolescents in the cognitive-behavioral group, as compared with those receiving the life skills tutoring intervention, and youths in the cognitive-behavioral condition reported significantly greater reductions in depressive symptomatology. At both 6- and 12-month follow-up, recovery rates did not differ significantly between groups, however.

The Treatment for Adolescents with Depression Study Team (TADS; 2003, 2004, 2005) investigated the efficacy of cognitive-behavioral therapy, fluoxetine, and their combination for treating symptoms of depression among adolescents (12–17 years) with a primary DSM-IV diagnosis of major depressive disorder. Four hundred and thirty nine participants at 13 sites were randomly assigned to one of four conditions: CBT, medication management with fluoxetine (FLX), a combination of CBT with FLX (Combo), or matched pill placebo (PBO). Intent-to-treat (ITT) analyses of patients at 12 weeks postrandomization indicated that the combination of cognitive-behavioral therapy with FLX produced the greatest improvement in depressive symptoms, followed by treatment with FLX alone (TADS, 2004). The rate of response after 12 weeks of treatment for the combination of CBT and FLX was 71%, whereas for FLX alone it was 60.6%, for CBT alone it was 43.2%, and for PBO it was 34.8%. At 12 weeks, treatment with CBT alone was less effective than FLX alone and was not significantly more effective than PBO. Moreover, the remission rate was significantly higher for youth receiving a combination of FLX and CBT relative to either treatment alone or to PBO (Kennard et al., 2006), and youth receiving a combination of CBT and FLX demonstrated higher levels of functional improvement, global health, and quality of life than did youth receiving either mono-therapy (Vitiello et al., 2006). Analyses of time-to-response indicate that the probability of an early, sustained treatment response was approximately three times greater for youth receiving Combo treatment than PBO, and two times greater for FLX than PBO (Kratochvil et al., 2006). Taken together, these findings indicate that a combination of CBT and FLX may offer a greater opportunity for rapid alleviation of depressive symp-toms and improvement of functioning for moderately to severely depressed youth than FLX or CBT alone (March, Silva, Vitiello, & the TADS Team, 2006).

Given these results, the question naturally arises—is CBT alone effective for treating more severely depressed youth? After receiving 12 weeks of acute TADS treatment, the blind was broken on the two pill conditions (FLX and PBO), and treatment non-responders were offered a choice of treatments. Full- and partial- treatment responders in the three active treatment arms then received 6 weeks of consolidation treatment, fol-lowed by 18 weeks of maintenance treatment. At this point all treatments were discontin-ued and participants entered a 1-year follow-up phase. Data collected at the conclusion of Stage III (maintenance phase) indicated that treatment gains were maintained over time for all three active treatments. Moreover, CBT alone, FLX, and their combination yielded equivalent levels of clinical improvement in depressive symptomatology at 36-week follow-up. CBT alone appears, then, to be as effective as FLX or Combo treatment for alleviating depression among adolescents, but takes longer to bring this about.

Interestingly, youth receiving CBT demonstrated a somewhat greater and more rapid reduction in suicidal ideations than did youth receiving FLX. Although suicidal thinking improved in all TADS treatment arms, these improvements were greatest in the two CBT conditions (CBT alone and Combo; TADS Team, 2004; Emslie et al., 2006). Suicidal events were twice as common among adolescents receiving FLX alone than among those receiving CBT alone or Combo treatment, indicating that CBT may protect against suicidality in youth. These findings are potentially quite important and are worthy of rep-lication. They suggest that when suicidal ideations or a history of suicidal gestures are present, careful monitoring of suicidality and a referral for CBT would be appropriate.

Taken together, these findings suggest that CBT can be effective for treating mild to moderate depression in adolescents and that treatment gains tend to be maintained over time (at least over the short term). The mean acute posttreatment effect size in the Reinecke et al. (1998) meta-analysis of CBT with depressed adolescents was 1.02 (a large effect),whereas the mean acute treatment effect size of non-TADS studies in the Weisz et al. (2006) meta-analysis was .48 (a moderate effect). It is not yet clear why the TADS CBT protocol appeared to yield lower short-term effectiveness than had been observed in other studies. This may have stemmed from design characteristics of the study (such as the use of a more stringent control group or the relatively short time frame for the acute treatment phase), sample characteristics (e.g., more severe, higher levels of functional impairment, significant comorbidity), treatment characteristics (i.e., the TADS CBT protocol introduced a broad range of techniques over a short period of time, potentially reducing the potency of any one intervention), or a combination of factors. That said, controlled outcome studies indicate that CBT appears to be more effective than doing nothing, is more effective than an attention control, and is more effective than empathic and supportive encouragement. It has not been found, however, to be consistently more effective than other active, empirically supported treatments, such as IPT or treatment with antidepressant medications.

SHORTCOMINGS AND LIMITATIONS

Although the results of research completed to date are promising, there are important limitations and shortcomings that should give one pause. First, although a number of well-designed studies have been completed with depressed adolescents, few have compared CBT with other empirically supported treatments and only one has compared CBT with medication management. Moreover, controlled outcome research with clinically depressed prepubertal youth is almost entirely lacking, as are data on the effectiveness of CBT in community settings. Studies to date have, for the most part, been conducted in university or medical center settings and have used highly skilled clinicians. What we have, then, is an understanding of the efficacy of CBT under optimal conditions. What is needed are large, well-controlled studies of the effectiveness of CBT in community settings with heterogeneous clinical samples.

Although the acute treatment effect sizes reported in all but one of the published outcome studies are statistically significant, it appears that a substantial percentage of youth who receive CBT continue to experience significant depressive symptomatology and functional impairment after 12–18 weeks of treatment. Relatively few youth in any of the three TADS treatment conditions, for example, achieved full remission during the acute treatment phase. Although many youth benefit from CBT, many others demonstrate a less than optimal response. However good our treatments may be, they clearly are not good enough. There is a possibility that children and adolescents who have partially remitted may benefit from additional time in CBT. There is also a possibility that they may benefit from additional treatments (i.e., therapeutic augmentation) or more intensive treatment (i.e., a dose effect).

As noted, early-onset depression may be a particularly malignant subtype of major depression and may be conceptually similar to chronic depression in adults (Reinecke & Curry, 2008). Thus, combining CBT with medications may make some sense. Research with chronically depressed adults indicated that a combination of an interpersonally focused form of CBT and medications (in this case, nefazodone) was more effective than either treatment alone (Keller et al., 2000). Inasmuch as only one controlled trial has been completed examining the efficacy of combined CBT and medications with clinically depressed youth, further research on combined treatment is needed.

Although research suggests that CBT can be effective in reducing the risk of relapse in depressed adults, the effect of CBT on relapse and recurrence rates among depressed youth has not been established. Given the chronic, recurring course of early-onset depression, any intervention that can reduce the risk of relapse and improve the developmental trajectory of depressed youth would be of enormous clinical and social benefit. Additional research on the utility of maintenance CBT, and on strategies for targeting social and cognitive factors that appear to be associated with relapse (including perfectionism, negative attributional style, family conflict, and excessive reassurance seeking), is warranted.

The most important question for clinicians typically is not "Does this treatment work?" but "Which treatment for which patient under which conditions?" Although we can say with some confidence that CBT can, under some circumstances, be effective for treating depressed youth, our understanding of predictors and moderators of treatment response is rudimentary (Brent et al., 1998; Curry et al., 2006). As Curry and colleagues (2006) noted, "For the practicing clinician, moderators are more helpful . . . because they suggest directions for differential treatment selection and planning" (p. 1428). At present there is a paucity of data on patient characteristics that predict response to CBT treatment protocols or, at a finer-grained level, which patients will respond most strongly to which specific interventions. Modular CBT (Curry & Reinecke, 2003) is founded on the assumption that specific clinical interventions can be selected based on the individual needs of specific patients. The utility of matching interventions to patients based on an assessment of vulnerability factors, however, has not been demonstrated. A great deal of additional research will be needed before we can confidently match individual patients with specific empirically supported treatments. Most contemporary CBT protocols take the form of omnibus packages and include an array of techniques and interventions. Relatively little is known about which specific components of these programs are most strongly associated with a positive outcome and which strategies are necessary, sufficient, or supportive of clinical improvement. Although some dismantling studies have been conducted with depressed adults (Jacobson, Dobson, & Truax, 1996), relatively little work has been done using this strategy with depressed children and adolescents (Kazdin, 2001).

CONCLUSIONS

Early-onset depression is a serious condition that can severely damage the lives of children and their families. Fortunately, effective treatments, including CBT, are available. Taken together, the results of randomized controlled trials completed over the past 25 years allow us to propose tentative guidelines for treating depressed adolescents. Although we are not advocating the dissemination of any one CBT protocol, the body of existing evidence suggests that, for mildly to moderately depressed youth, 12–18 sessions of CBT (either individual or group) can be effective for reducing levels of depression and improving psychosocial adjustment. Medications can also be effective, but may be associated with a slight increase in suicidal ideations relative to placebo. Individual CBT has not consistently been found to be effective for the acute treatment of moderate to severe depression. Thus, a combination of CBT and fluoxetine appears to offer the best opportunity for rapid symptomatic and functional improvement for more severely depressed youth. Relapse rates after the discontinuation of antidepressant medications are unacceptably high, whereas relapse rates after CBT are substantially lower. Research completed with depressed adults suggests that CBT may be helpful for reducing the risk of relapse and that continuation of CBT with partially remitted patients may also be of benefit. Methodological problems with long-term follow-up studies make it difficult, however, to draw firm conclusions. With this in mind, we suggest that adolescents may wish to consider continuing with maintenance medications or to receive a trial of adjunctive CBT so that they can then be weaned from their medications. Finally, CBT is recommended whenever suicidal ideations or a history of suicidal gestures is apparent. It is worth noting, as well, that there are significant risks associated with not treating early-onset depression. Although depressive episodes wax and wane in intensity and tend to spontaneously remit, major depression among youth is a chronic and recurrent disorder and is associated with significant impairment and mortality.

REFERENCES

Abramson, L., Metalsky, G., & Alloy, L. (1989). Hopelessness depression: A theory based subtype of depression. *Psychological Review, 96,* 358–372.

Altmann, E., & Gotlib, I. (1988). The social behavior of depressed children: An observational study. *Journal of Abnormal Child Psychology, 16,* 29–44.

Barber, B. (1996). Parental psychological control: Revisiting a neglected construct. *Child Development, 67,* 3296–3319.

Beardslee, W., Versage, E., & Gladstone, T. (1998). Children of affectively ill parents: A review of the past 10 years. *Journal of the American Academy of Child and Adolescent Psychiatry, 37,* 1134–1141.

Beck, A. (1963). Thinking and depression: 1. Idiosyncratic content and cognitive distortions. *Archives of General Psychiatry, 9,* 324–333.

Beck, A. (1983). Cognitive therapy of depression: New perspectives. In P. Clayton & J. Barrett (Eds.), *Treatment of depression: Old controversies and new approaches* (pp. 265–284). New York: Raven Press.

Beck, A., Rush, A., Shaw, B., & Emery, G. (1979). *Cognitive therapy of depression.* New York: Guilford Press.

Beck, A., Ward, C., Mendelson, M., Mock, J., & Erbaugh, J. (1961). An inventory for measuring depression. *Archives of General Psychiatry, 4,* 561–571.

Billings, A., & Moos, R. (1983). Comparisons of children of depressed and nondepressed parents: A social-environmental perspective. *Journal of Abnormal Child Psychology, 11,* 463–485.

Bowlby, J. (1969). *Attachment and loss: Attachment.* New York: Basic Books.

Bowlby, J. (1970). *Attachment and loss: Separation, anxiety, and anger.* New York: Basic Books.

Brent, D. (1995). Risk factors for adolescent suicide and suicidal behavior: Mental and substance abuse disorders, family environmental factors, and life stress. *Suicide and Life Threatening Behavior, 25,* 52–63.

Brent, D., Gaynor, S., & Weersing, V. (2002). Cognitive-behavioral approaches to the treatment of depression and anxiety. In M. Rutter & E. Taylor (Eds.), *Child and adolescent psychiatry: Modern approaches* (pp. 921–937). London: Blackwell Scientific.

Brent, D., Holder, D., Kolko, D., Birmaher, B., Baugher, M., Roth, C., et al. (1997). A clinical trial for adolescent depression comparing cognitive, family, and supportive therapy. *Archives of General Psychiatry, 54,* 877–885.

Brent, D., Kolko, D., Birmaher, B., Baugher, M., Bridge, J., Roth, C., et al. (1998). Predictors of treatment efficacy in a clinical trial of three psychosocial treatments for adolescent depression. *Journal of the American Academy of Child and Adolescent Psychiatry, 37,* 906–914.

Brent, D., & Poling, K. (1997). *Cognitive therapy treatment manual for depressed and suicidal youth.* Pittsburgh: Star Center. (available from *brentda@msx.upmc.edeu*)

Butler, L., Meizitis, S., Friedman, R., & Cole, E. (1980). The effect of two school based intervention programs on depressive symptoms in preadolescents. *American Educational Research Journal, 17,* 111–119.

Clark, D., & Beck, A. (1999). *Scientific foundations of cognitive theory and therapy of depression.* New York: Wiley.

Clarke, G., Hornbrook, M., Lynch, F., Polen, M., Gale, J., O'Connor, E., et al. (2002). Group cognitive-behavioral treatment for depressed adolescent offspring of depressed parents in a health maintenance organization. *Journal of the American Academy of Child and Adolescent Psychiatry, 41,* 305–313.

Clarke, G., Lewinsohn, P., & Hops, H. (1990). *Instructors manual for the Adolescent Coping with Depression course.* Kaiser Permanente Center for Health Research website: *www.kpchr.org/public/acwd.html.*

Clarke, G., Rohde, P., Lewinsohn, P., Hops, H., & Seeley, J. (1999). Efficacy of acute group treatment and booster sessions. *Journal of the American Academy of Child and Adolescent Psychiatry, 38,* 272–279.

Compas, B., Grant, K., & Ey, S. (1994). Psychosocial stress and child and adolescent depression: Can we be more specific? In W. Reynolds & H. Johnston (Eds.) *Handbook of depression in children and adolescents* (pp. 509–523). New York: Plenum Press.

Curry, J. (2001). Specific psychotherapies for childhood and adolescent depression. *Biological Psychiatry, 49,* 1091–1100.

Curry, J., & Reinecke, M. (2003). Modular therapy for adolescents with major depression. In M. Reinecke, F. Dattilio, & A. Freeman (Eds.), *Cognitive therapy with children and adolescents* (2nd ed., pp. 95–127). New York: Guilford Press.

Curry, J., Rohde, P., Simons, A., Silva, S., Vitiello, B., Kratochvil, C., et al. (2006). Predictors and moderators of acute outcome in the Treatment for Adolescents with Depression Study (TADS). *Journal of the American Academy of Child and Adolescent Psychiatry, 45*(12), 1427–1439.

Dobson, K., & Dozois, D. (2001). Historical and philosophical bases of the cognitive-behavioral therapies. In K. Dobson (Ed.), *Handbook of cognitive-behavioral therapies* (2nd ed., pp. 3–39). New York: Guilford Press.

Emslie, G., Kratochvil, C., Vitiello, B., Silva, S., Mayes, T., McNulty, S., et al. (2006). Treatment for Adolescents with Depression Study (TADS): Safety results. *Journal of the American Academy of Child and Adolescent Psychiatry, 45,* 1440–1455.

Essau, C., & Dobson, K. (1999). Epidemiology of depressive disorders. In C. Essau & F. Petermann (Eds.), *Depressive disorders in children and adolescents: Epidemiology, course and treatment* (pp. 69–103). Northvale, NJ: Aronson.

Evans, D., Foa, E., Gur, R., Hendin, H., O'Brien, C., Seligman, M., et al. (Eds.). (2005). *Treating and preventing adolescent mental health disorders: What we know and what we don't know.* Oxford, UK: Oxford University Press.

Fonagy, P., Target, M., Cottrell, D., Phillips, J., & Kurtz, Z. (2002). *What works for whom?: A critical review of treatments for children and adolescents.* New York: Guilford Press.

Frauenknecht, M., & Black, D. (2004). Problem-solving training for children and adolescents. In E. Chang, T. D'Zurilla, & L. Sanna (Eds.), *Social problem solving: Theory, research, and training* (pp. 153–170). Washington, DC: American Psychological Association.

Friedberg, R., & McClure, J. (2005). Adolescents. In N. Kazantzis, F. Deane, K. Ronan, & L. Abate (Eds.), *Using homework assignments in cognitive behavior therapy* (pp. 95–116). New York: Routledge.

Gloaguen, V., Cottraux, J., Cucherat, M., & Blackburn, I. (1998). A meta-analysis of the effects of cognitive therapy in depressed patients. *Journal of Affective Disorders, 49,* 59–72.

Goodyer, I., Herbert, J., & Altham, P. (1998). Adrenal steroid secretion and major depression in 8- to 16-year-olds: III. Influence of cortisol/DHEA ratio at presentation on subsequent rates of disappointing life events and persistent major depression. *Psychological Medicine, 28,* 265–273.

Goodyer, I., Wright, C., & Altham, P. (1988). Maternal adversity and recent stressful life events in anxious and depressed children. *Journal of Child Psychology and Psychiatry, 29,* 651–667.

Gotlib, I., & Hammen, C. (1992). *Psychological aspects of depression: Toward a cognitive-interpersonal integration.* Chichester, UK: Wiley.

Gotlib, I., & Krasnoperova, E. (1998). Biased information processing as a vulnerability factor for depression. *Behavior Therapy, 29,* 603–617.

Haaga, D., Dyck, M., & Ernst, D. (1991). Empirical status of cognitive theory of depression. *Psycholological Bulletin, 110,* 215–236.

Hamilton, M. (1960). A rating scale for depression. *Journal of Neurology, Neurosurgery, and Psychiatry, 23,* 56–62.

Hamilton, M. (1967). Development of a rating scale for primary depressive illness. *British Journal of Social and Clinical Psychology, 6,* 278–296.

Hammen, C. (1992). The family-environment context of depression: A perspective on children's risk. In D. Cicchetti & S. Toth (Eds.), *Rochester Symposium on Developmental Psychopathology* (Vol. 4, pp. 145–153). Rochester, NY: University of Rochester Press.

Hammen, C., & Goodman-Brown, T. (1990). Self-schemas and vulnerability to specific life stress in children at risk for depression. *Cognitive Therapy and Research, 14,* 215–227.

Hammen, C., & Zupan, B. (1984). Self-schemas and the processing of personal information in children. *Journal of Experimental Child Psychology, 37,* 598–608.

Harrington, M., Wood, A., & Verduyn, C. (1998). Clinically depressed adolescents. In P. Graham (Ed.), *Cognitive-behaviour therapy for children and families* (pp. 156–193). Cambridge, UK: Cambridge University Press.

Harrington, R., Whittaker, J., Shoebridge, P., & Campbell, F. (1998). Systematic review of efficacy of cognitive behaviour therapies in childhood and adolescent depressive disorder. *British Medical Journal, 316,* 1559–1563.

Hollon, S., & Najavits, L. (1988). Review of empirical studies on cognitive therapy. In A. Frances & R. Hales (Eds.), *American Psychiatric Press review of psychiatry* (Vol. 7, pp. 643–666). Washington, DC: American Psychiatric Press.

Hollon, S., Thase, M., & Markowitz, J. (2002). Treatment and prevention of depression. *Psychological Science in the Public Interest, 3,* 39–77.

Hudson, J., & Kendall, P. (2005). Children. In N. Kazantzis, F. Deane, K. Ronan, & L. Abate (Eds.), *Using homework assignments in cognitive behavior therapy* (pp. 75–94). New York: Routledge.

Ingram, R., Miranda, J., & Segal, Z. (2006). Cognitive vulnerability to depression. In L. Alloy & J. Riskind, (Eds.), *Cognitive vulnerability to emotional disorders* (pp. 63–91). Mahwah, NJ: LEA.

Jacobson, N., Dobson, K., & Truax, P. (1996). A component analysis of cognitive behavioral treatment for depression. *Journal of Consulting and Clinical Psychology, 64,* 295–304.

Joiner, T. (2002). Depression in its interpersonal context. In I. Gotlib & C. Hammen (Eds.), *Handbook of depression* (pp. 295–313). New York: Guilford Press.

Kahn, J., Kehle, T., Jenson, W., & Clark, E. (1990). Comparison of cognitive-behavioral, relaxation, and self-modeling interventions for depression among middle-school students. *School Psychology Review, 19,* 196–211.

Kazdin, A. (2001). *Psychotherapy for children and adolescents: Directions for research and practice.* Oxford, UK: Oxford University Press.

Keller, M., McCullough, J., Klein, D., Arnow, B., Dunner, D., Gelenberg, A., et al. (2000). A comparison of nefazodone, the cognitive behavioral-analysis system of psychotherapy, and their combination for the treatment of chronic depression. *New England Journal of Medicine, 342,* 1462–1470.

Kennard, B., Silva, S., Vitiello, B., Curry, J., Kratochvil, C., Simons, A., et al. (2006). Remission and residual symptoms after short-term treatment in the Treatment of Adolescents with Depression Study (TADS). *Journal of the American Academy of Child and Adolescent Psychiatry, 45,* 1404–1411.

Kenny, M., Moilanen, D., Lomax, R., & Brabeck, M. (1993). Contributions of parental attachment to view of self and depressive symptoms among early adolescents. *Journal of Youth and Adolescence, 13,* 408–430.

Kovacs, M., Obrosky, D., Gatsonis, C., & Richards, C. (1997). First-episode major depressive and dysthymic disorder in childhood: Clinical and sociodemographic factors in recovery. *Journal of the American Academy of Child and Adolescent Psychiatry, 36,* 777–784.

Kratochvil, C., Emslie, G., Silva, S., McNulty, S., Walkup, J., Curry, J., et al. (2006). Acute time to response in the Treatment for Adolescents with Depression Study (TADS). *Journal of the American Academy of Child and Adolescent Psychiatry, 45,* 1412–1418.

Kroll, L., Harrington, R., Jayson, D., Fraser, J., & Gowers, S. (1996). Pilot study of continuation cognitive-behavioral therapy for major depression in adolescent psychiatric patients. *Journal of the American Academy of Child and Adolescent Psychiatry, 35,* 1156–1161.

Leahy, R. (1988). Cognitive therapy of childhood depression: Developmental considerations. In S. Shirk (Ed.), *Cognitive development and child psychotherapy* (pp. 187–204). New York: Plenum Press.

Lerner, M., & Clum, G. (1990). Treatment of suicide ideators: A problem-solving approach. *Behavior Therapy, 21,* 403–411.

Lewinsohn, P. (1975). The behavioral study and treatment of depression. In M. Hersen & R. M. Eisler (Eds.), *Progress in behavior modification* (pp. 19–64). New York: Academic Press.

Lewinsohn, P., & Clarke, G. (1999). Psychosocial treatments for adolescent depression. *Clinical Psychology Review, 19,* 329–342.

Lewinsohn, P., Clarke, G., Hops, H., & Andrews, J. (1990). Cognitive-behavioral treatment for depressed adolescents. *Behavior Therapy, 21,* 385–401.

Lewinsohn, P., Hops, H., Roberts, R., Seeley, J., & Andrews, J. (1993). Adolescent psychopathology, I: Prevalence and incidence of depression and other DSM-III-R disorders in high school students. *Journal of Abnormal Psychology, 102,* 133–144.

March, J., Silva, S., Vitiello, B., & the TADS Team. (2006). The Treatment for Adolescents with Depression Study (TADS): Methods and message at 12 weeks. *Journal of the American Academy of Child and Adolescent Psychiatry, 45,* 1393–1403.

Monroe, S., & Hadjiyannakis, K. (2002). The social environment and depression: Focusing on severe life stress. In I. Gotlib & C. Hammen (Eds.), *Handbook of depression* (3rd ed., pp. 314–340). New York: Guilford Press.

Moore, M., & Carr, A. (2000). Depression and grief. In A. Carr (Ed.), *What works with children and adolescents? A critical review of psychological interventions with children, adolescents, and their families* (pp. 203–232). London: Routledge.

Nezu, A., Nezu, C., & Lombardo, E. (2004). *Cognitive-behavioral case formulation and treatment design: A problem-solving approach.* New York: Springer.

Nolen-Hoeksema, S. (1991). Responses to depression and their effects on the duration of depressive episodes. *Journal of Abnormal Psychology, 100,* 569–582.

Nolen-Hoeksema, S., & Morrow, J. (1991). A prospective study of depression and posttraumatic stress symptoms after a natural disaster: The Loma Prieta earthquake. *Journal of Personality and Social Psychology, 61,* 115–121.

Panak, W., & Garber, J. (1992). Role of aggression, rejection, and attributions in the prediction of depression in children. *Development and Psychopathology, 4,* 145–165.

Parker, G. (1993). Parental rearing style: Examining the links with personality vulnerability factors for depression. *Social Psychiatry and Psychiatric Epidemiology, 28,* 97–100.

Persons, J. (1989). *Cognitive therapy in practice: A case formulation approach.* New York: Norton.

Peterson, L., Mullins, L., & Ridley-Johnson, R. (1985). Childhood depression: Peer reactions to depression and life stress. *Journal of Abnormal Child Psychology, 13,* 597–609.

Prieto, S., Cole, D., & Tageson, C. (1992). Depressive self-schemas in clinic and nonclinic children. *Cognitive Therapy and Research, 16,* 521–534.

Rapee, R. (1997). Potential role of childrearing practices in the development of anxiety and depression. *Clinical Psychology Review, 17,* 47–67.

Reinecke, M., & Curry, J. (2008). Chronic depression in youth. In M. Whisman (Ed.), *Cognitive therapy for complex and comorbid depression.* New York: Guilford Press.

Reinecke, M., & DuBois, D. (2001). Socioenvironmental and cognitive risks and resources: Relations to mood and suicidality among inpatient adolescents. *Journal of Cognitive Psychotherapy, 15,* 195–222.

Reinecke, M., & Freeman, A. (2003). Cognitive therapy. In A. Gurman & S. Messer (Eds.), *Essential psychotherapies: Theory and practice* (2nd ed., pp. 224–271). New York: Guilford Press.

Reinecke, M., & Rogers, G. (2001). Dysfunctional attitudes and attachment style among clinically depressed adults. *Behavioural and Cognitive Psychotherapy*, 29, 129–141.

Reinecke, M., Ryan, N., & DuBois, D. (1998). Cognitive-behavioral therapy of depression and depressive symptoms during adolescence: A review and meta-analysis. *Journal of the American Academy of Child and Adolescent Psychiatry*, 37, 26–34.

Reinecke, M., & Simons, A. (2005). Vulnerability to depression among adolescents: Implications for cognitive-behavioral treatment. *Cognitive and Behavioral Practice*, 12(2), 166–176.

Reynolds, W., & Coats, K. (1986). A comparison of cognitive-behavior therapy and relaxation training for the treatment of depression in adolescents. *Journal of Consulting and Clinical Psychology*, 54, 653–660.

Rogers, G., Reinecke, M., & Curry, J. (2005). Case formulation in TADS CBT. *Cognitive and Behavioral Practice*, 12(2), 198–208.

Rohde, P., Clarke, G., Mace, D., Jorgensen, J., & Seeley, J. (2004). An efficacy/effectiveness study of cognitive-behavioral treatment for adolescents with combined major depression and conduct disorder. *Journal of the American Academy of Child and Adolescent Psychiatry*, 43, 660–668.

Rohde, P., Feeny, N., & Robins, M. (2005). Characteristics and components of the TADS CBT approach. *Cognitive and Behavioral Practice*, 12(2), 186–197.

Rosselló, J., & Bernal, G. (1999). The efficacy of cognitive-behavioral and interpersonal treatments for depression in Puerto Rican adolescents. *Journal of Consulting and Clinical Psychology*, 67, 734–745.

Rudolph, K., Hammen, C., & Burge, D. (1994). Interpersonal functioning and depressive symptoms in childhood: Addressing the issues of specificity and comorbidity. *Journal of Abnormal Child Psychology*, 22, 355–371.

Shaffer, D., Gould, M., Fisher, P., Trautman, P., Moreau, D., Kleinman, M., et al. (1996). Psychiatric diagnosis in child and adolescent suicide. *Archives of General Psychiatry*, 53, 339–348.

Spence, S., & Reinecke, M. (2004). Cognitive approaches to understanding, preventing, and treating child and adolescent depression. In M. Reinecke & D. Clark (Eds.), *Cognitive therapy across the lifespan: Evidence and practice* (pp. 358–395). Cambridge, UK: Cambridge University Press.

Stark, K., Hargrave, J., Sander, J., Custer, G., Schnoebelen, S., Simpson, J., et al. (2006). Treatment of childhood depression: The ACTION treatment program. In P. C. Kendall (Eds.), *Child and adolescent therapy: Cognitive-behavioral procedures* (3rd ed., pp. 169–216). New York: Guilford Press.

Stark, K., Reynolds, W., & Kaslow, N. (1987). A comparison of the relative efficacy of self-control therapy and a behavioral problem-solving therapy for depression in children. *Journal of Abnormal Child Psychology*, 15, 91–113.

Taylor, L., & Ingram, R. (1999). Cognitive reactivity and depressotypic information processing in the children of depressed mothers. *Journal of Abnormal Psychology*, 108, 202–210.

Treatment for Adolescents with Depression Study (TADS) Team. (2003). Treatment for Adolescents with Depression Study (TADS): Rationale, design, and methods. *Journal of the American Academy of Child and Adolescent Psychiatry*, 42, 531–542.

Treatment for Adolescents with Depression Study (TADS) Team. (2004). Fluoxetine, cognitive-behavioral therapy, and their combination for adolescents with depression: Treatment for Adolescents with Depression Study (TADS) randomized controlled trial. *Journal of the American Medical Association*, 292, 807–820.

Treatment for Adolescents with Depression Study (TADS) Team. (2005). Treatment for Adolescents with Depression Study (TADS): Demographic and clinical characteristics. *Journal of the American Academy of Child and Adolescent Psychiatry*, 44, 28–40.

Vitiello, B., Rohde, P., Silva, S., Wells, K., Casat, C., Waslick, B., et al. (2006). Functioning and quality of life in the Treatment for Adolescents with Depression Study (TADS). *Journal of the American Academy of Child and Adolescent Psychiatry*, 45, 1419–1426.

Weissman, M., Wolk, S., Goldstein, R., Moreau, D., Adams, P., Greenwald, S., et al. (1999).

Depressed adolescents grown up. *Journal of the American Medical Association, 281,* 1707–1713.

Weisz, J., McCarty, C., & Valeri, S. (2006). Effects of psychotherapy for depression in children and adolescents. *Psychological Bulletin, 132,* 132–149.

Weisz, J., Southam-Gerow, M., Gordis, E., & Connor-Smith, J. (2003). Primary and secondary control enhancement training for youth depression: Applying the deployment-focused model of treatment development and testing. In A. Kazdin & J. Weisz (Eds.), *Evidence-based psychotherapies for children and adolescents* (pp. 165–183). New York: Guilford Press.

Weisz, J., Thurber, C., Sweeney, L., Proffitt, V., & LeGagnoux, G. (1997). Brief treatment of mild-to-moderate child depression using primary and secondary control enhancement training. *Journal of Consulting and Clinical Psychology, 65,* 703–707.

Wood, A., Harrington, R., & Moore, A. (1996). Controlled trial of brief cognitive-behavioural intervention in adolescent patients with depressive disorders. *Journal of Child Psychology and Psychiatry, 37,* 737–746.

9 Psychopharmacological Treatment of Depression in Children and Adolescents

Eric Fombonne and Suzanne Zinck

This chapter discusses the use of antidepressant medications to treat affective disorders in children and adolescents. Children and adolescents presented to a clinician with mood disturbances should benefit from a thorough evaluation. Evaluations should include a review of symptoms associated with depressive conditions and potential comorbid disorders; a medical examination identifying co-occurring medical diseases that may influence the onset, course, and treatment of the depressive condition; a detailed review of the patient's psychosocial context, searching for social or relational stressors that may be implicated in the onset and maintenance of depression; an evaluation of academic/school performance; and a detailed family history of affective and other psychiatric disorders. Following this initial assessment, a proper diagnostic formulation and a specific diagnosis should be provided within the class of depressive conditions (i.e., major depressive episode, dysthymic disorder, depression not otherwise specified, etc.). Furthermore, an evaluation of suicidality and suicidal risk should be performed for each adolescent, as the results of such an evaluation may influence subsequent treatment decisions. Careful evaluations of impairments associated with depressive symptomatology affecting the patient's well-being, his or her family relationships, peer relationships, leisure activities, and school functioning should also be performed. As depressive conditions vary in severity, the level of impairment may act as a guide for both initial treatment decisions and monitoring treatment efficacy.

Depressive disorders are very common, with prevalence increasing sharply during the adolescent years and strong continuity into adulthood (Fombonne, Wostear, Cooper, Harrington, & Rutter, 2001). Many depressive syndromes fall short of diagnostic criteria for major depression, but nevertheless impinge significantly on adolescents' well-being and development. However, most of the research on the treatment of depressive disorders in youths has concentrated on those meeting the criteria for major depressive disorder.

Consequently, most of the research reviewed in this chapter applies to youth with a diagnosis of major depression. The implications of most research findings on the treatment of major depression, encompassing both psychopharmacological and psychotherapeutical techniques, are commonly extended to less severe forms of depression in clinical practice.

The clinical management of any affective disorder in a youth usually involves a combination of approaches. Psychotherapeutical techniques are usually employed, either simple counseling or psychotherapies such as cognitive-behavioral therapy (see Reinecke & Ginsburg, Chapter 8, this volume) and interpersonal psychotherapy (Fombonne, 2002; see Young & Mufson, Chapter 12, this volume). The family is also usually involved in the treatment, which enables clinicians to educate parents about the youth's depressive condition, to work collaboratively with them, and sometimes to directly tackle family relationship difficulties that may be contributing to the onset or maintenance of depression. Working with the school and with other community partners who have meaningful roles in the life of the adolescent is also required. The use of medication is only one aspect of the management of child or adolescent depression. For the rest of this chapter, we assume that nonmedicinal aspects of management have been carefully considered and implemented. First, we review the various classes of antidepressant agents and remind the reader of key pharmacological principles. In the second section, we review the efficacy studies of the major classes of antidepressant medications that have thus far been subjected to rigorous research. Third, we illustrate the practical issues in treating young persons with antidepressants, following current guidelines from different professional organizations. Finally, in the last section, we address special issues such as the pharmacological management of treatment-resistant depression, what is known about the efficacy of combining psychotherapy and psychopharmacology, and the recent concerns raised about the increased risk of suicidal behaviors associated with the treatment of adolescents with antidepressants.

CLASSES OF ANTIDEPRESSANT DRUGS

In this section, before we describe the principal classes of antidepressant medications, we review basic pharmacological principles (pharmacokinetics and pharmacodynamics) that must be known by the prescriber. This knowledge guides the choice of medication and the use of these drugs in clinical practice.

Pharmacokinetics and Pharmacodynamics

Pharmacokinetics relates to the absorption and distribution of medications in various tissues, the associated metabolic pathways, and excretion mechanisms. Each medication varies with respect to these mechanisms, and knowledge of these mechanisms is important in selecting a drug and understanding the onset of action of the medication. Many drugs, especially antidepressants, need several days of administration before they attain a steady state, which is necessary to evaluate drug response. The absorption of a medication is influenced by several factors, including the packaging of the drug (slow-release drugs have a longer action and a lower concentration peak) and the ability of the drug to dissolve (which, when reduced, can lead to poor bioavailability). Furthermore, drugs are metabolized when they are absorbed by the gut wall. The more intensive this initial metabolism is, the less bioavailability there is. Medications distribute in various body tissues unevenly. Drugs that are lipid soluble have higher volume of distribution. Many drugs are metabolized in the liver, using the complex system of enzymes known as cytochromes. Different cytochromes metabolize different drugs, and knowledge of the cytochrome system is required to monitor drug response, especially to evaluate drug–drug interactions when patients are taking various medications. Some drugs can block the metabolic pathway of other drugs, leading to increased plasma levels of the other drugs. This occurs frequently with antidepressant medications, which can increase plasma levels of other psychotropic drugs (i.e., neuroleptics). In addition, there are genetic polymorphisms of the cytochrome enzymes, leading to individual variability in the efficiency of certain metabolic pathways. Some proportion of the population, generally small (less than 10% among European Americans), metabolize poorly. This may result in adverse or toxic effects occurring rapidly with relatively small doses. In contrast, intensive metabolizers require a higher dosage of the same medication to achieve a response. There is considerable individual variability in response to medication, and practitioners must monitor individual patients carefully with these parameters in mind. Excretion of drugs is usually by liver metabolism, although some medications (e.g., lithium) are excreted through the kidneys. Because many drugs interact with others (and not all of these interactions are well known and described), it is advised to use monotherapy when possible in the treatment of any psychiatric disorder. When using some medications, plasma monitoring and sampling may be available and useful (such as in treatments involving lithium, valproic acid, clozapine), but it is not routinely performed or useful in treating uncomplicated depressive disorders.

Pharmacodynamics relates to the mechanisms of actions of the drug on the central nervous system. Different drugs act on different transmitter systems, which rely on neurotransmitters such as noradrenalin, serotonin, norepinephrine, dopamine, histamine, or acetylcholine. For some psychiatric disorders, the involvement of particular receptors is well established (e.g., that of D_2-dopamine receptors in schizophrenia). For depression and other conditions, the involvement of some receptors is known (e.g., the involvement of the $5\text{-}HT_2\text{-}5\text{-}HT_1$ receptors in depression), but multiple receptors are probably involved in many psychiatric conditions. The action of a drug can vary, but a drug usually acts to increase the transmission of a given neurotransmitter over a synaptic cleft. This is achieved by increasing synthesis of the neurotransmitter or by blocking its reuptake from the synaptic cleft into the presynaptic neuron. Drugs may also act at the postsynaptic level by blocking receptors that have an affinity for particular transmitters, thereby modulating transmitter action on the postsynaptic neurons. Most antidepressant medications act on several receptors, and these actions are thought to be responsible for both their efficacy and the side effects associated with each drug.

Tricyclic Antidepressants

Tricyclic antidepressants (TCAs) have been used since the late 1950s in adult psychiatry, and numerous studies have shown their efficacy in treating adult depression. The most well-used TCAs are tertiary amines, including clomipramine, amitriptyline, and imipramine, and two of their active metabolites, desipramine and nortriptyline. TCAs act on two major neurotransmitter systems, the noradrenergic and the serotonergic systems. Clomipramine is the most potent serotonergic of all TCAs. TCAs act on serotonin receptors by blocking serotonin reuptake in the presynaptic neuron through the $5\text{-}HT_1$ receptor and by increasing serotoninergic activity through binding to postsynaptic $5\text{-}HT_2$ receptors. TCAs also bind to presynaptic $alpha_2$ receptors and postsynaptic $alpha_1$ receptors, increasing the amount of norepinephrine in the synaptic cleft. These represent the main action mechanisms of TCAs. TCAs are well absorbed and distribute widely into the body owing to their lipophilic properties. The metabolism of TCAs involves different cytochromes, and excretion occurs largely through renal clearance. TCAs interact with many other medications, psychotropic or not. TCAs also act at other sites, including muscarinic and histaminic receptors. These are responsible for anticholinergic side effects, which include dry mouth, tachycardia, blurred vision, constipation, and urinary retention. Antihistaminic effects are responsible for sedation. The cardiac toxicity of TCAs is well documented in adults and children. Increased heart rate, increased blood pressure, and changes in cardiac conduction illustrated in changes in electrocardiographic (EKG) parameters are known consequences. Strict guidelines for monitoring TCAs have been put in place for pediatric populations, especially after the sudden deaths of children undergoing treatment with TCAs , particularly desipramine, were reported in the early 1990s (Abramovicz, 1990; Biederman, 1991; Riddle, Geller, & Ryan, 1993). Because of their high toxicity index, TCAs are dangerous in overdoses, leading to tachycardia, hypotension, fatal arrhythmia, and seizures.

Selective Serotonin Reuptake Inhibitors

Selective serotonin reuptake inhibitors (SSRIs) were developed in the 1980s, with the first drug, fluoxetine, being marketed in 1987. Since then, other SSRIs have been discovered. SSRIs act mostly on serotonergic neurons by blocking the transporter system that reuptakes serotonin from the synaptic cleft into the presynaptic neuron. Blockade of this reuptake pump leads to an increased amount of serotonin in the synapse, increased stimulation of the postsynaptic neuron, and antidepressant action. Serotonin binds to several types of postsynaptic receptors ($5\text{-}HT_{1A}$, $5\text{-}HT_{2A}$, $5\text{-}HT_{2C}$, $5\text{-}HT_3$, $5\text{-}HT_4$, . . .) and regulates the release of serotonin in the synapse through a presynaptic autoreceptor ($5\text{-}HT_{1D}$). There are complex interactions between noradrenergic and serotoninergic neurons that have both receptors regulated by both neurotransmitters. Serotonergic neurons are abundant in the raphé nucleus, part of the brainstem, from where serotonergic neurons project to various parts of the brain. Projections target the frontal lobes (important for mood regulation), the basal ganglia (movement control, obsessions, and compulsions), the hypothalamus (regulating eating behavior and appetite), the limbic system (anxiety), sleep centers in the brainstem, and lower spinal neurons (involved in sexual function). Peripheral serotonin receptors are also abundant in the gut and regulate intestine motility and function. SSRIs vary in their activity on various types of postsynaptic or peripheral serotonin receptors, which explains their differential side effect profiles. In addition, although the action of SSRIs most affects serotonin transmission, SSRIs also have a variety of secondary pharmacological actions on other transmitters and their receptors (e.g., dopamine, acetylcholine, histamine, etc.). This may account for differences in response and tolerance of each SSRI by individual patients (Stahl, 2000).

The five most commonly used SSRIs are fluoxetine, paroxetine, fluvoxamine, sertraline, and citalopram. Citalopram is the most selective SSRI, whereas paroxetine and sertraline are the most potent inhibitors of the serotonin transporter system. These drugs vary in their metabolism; some (e.g., fluoxetine) have active metabolites and others (e.g., paroxetine) do not. In addition, their half-lives vary enormously, with fluoxetine having the longest and paroxetine and fluvoxamine among the shortest. These characteristics can influence the dosing schedule as well as patterns of drug discontinuation. When discontinued, drugs with short half-lives can generate unpleasant discontinuation syndromes. SSRIs vary in their use of cytochromes, leading to different patterns of drug–

drug interactions. SSRIs are safe drugs and lethal overdoses are rare, although some have been reported.

Other Classes of Antidepressants

There are other antidepressants, which either have different mechanisms of action or combine multiple mechanisms of action, as compared with the more selective actions of TCAs and SSRIs.

Monoamine oxydase inhibitors (MAOIs) were among the first drugs to be found to have antidepressant activity, and their discovery led to the development of the mono-amine hypothesis in understanding depressive disorders. Monoamine oxydase (MAO) is an enzyme distributed in the central nervous system and other organs. This enzyme catabolyzes norepinephrine, serotonin, and MAO inhibitors. By reducing this catabolic pathway, MAOIs increase the presence of norepinepherine and serotonin. The MAOIs of the first generation were difficult to use because of the irreversibility of their action and the fact that numerous drug–drug interactions and drug–food interactions were observed. In particular, food containing cheese, wine, and some vegetables could lead to large increases in blood pressure, and dietary noncompliance in some patients, especially ado-lescents, made these drugs difficult to employ. A more recent generation of MAOIs, referred to as reversible inhibitors of the monoamine oxydase (RIMAs), do not appear to have the same irreversible binding properties and therefore allow more flexibility in their use. *Venlafaxine* has been available for 10 years and is the first selective serotonin and norepinephrine reuptake inhibitor. As compared with TCAs, it has no affinity for muscarinic, cholinergic, or histaminic receptors and does not therefore lead to side effects associated with these mediators. At lower doses, venlafaxine is mostly a serotoninergic reuptake inhibitor. At higher doses, the activity on the noradrenergic system is improved.

Other drugs such as *nefazodone* and *trazodone* also act as serotonin reuptake inhibitors. These bind selectively to postsynaptic 5-HT receptors and to other transmit-ters, giving them a particular side effect profile, which is considered in their prescrip-tion. For example, nefazodone has been shown to improve sleep architecture and to have minimal sexual dysfunction associated with its use. Trazodone is often used for its sedative properties to induce and facilitate sleep in depressed patients. Both drugs have side effects that need to be monitored carefully. *Bupropion* is a novel antidepressant that exerts its action through inhibition of norepinephrine and dopamine reuptake. Because of its dopaminergic properties, it has been used in children with attention defi-cit disorders and has been recommended for depression comorbid with attention-deficit/hyperactivity disorder (ADHD). However, bupropion has significant side effects, including an increased risk of seizure. *Mirtazapine* is a novel antidepressant that has five different modes of action and a strong affinity for histaminic receptors. As a result, somnolence, increased appetite, and weight gain are common side effects. Other drugs, such as *reboxetine*, the first selective inhibitor of norepinephrine reuptake, exist but are not licensed in every country.

EFFICACY STUDIES

Up until the late 1970s, depressive disorders were hardly recognized in children and ado-lescents. It was only in the beginning of the 1980s that research into child and adolescent depression started to develop. The first attempts to treat juvenile affective disorders with medications before the 1980s relied mostly on a few case studies or open-labeled studies. These studies were difficult to interpret owing to the lack of precise diagnostic criteria for including subjects and other methodological weaknesses. The first randomized clinical trials (RCTs) were conducted with TCAs. Thirteen such RCTs were conducted between 1980 and 2001. When the SSRIs were made available, RCTs started to be conducted in the 1990s with children and adolescents. Several RCTs with SSRIs have now been published, allowing evaluation of their efficacy. In addition, some unpublished studies have recently been reviewed when concerns were raised about the safety of this medication (see below). With the exception of venlafaxine, for which one small randomized clinical study ($n = 40$) combining drug therapy and psychotherapy has been published (Mandoki, Tapia, Tapia, & Sumner, 1997), published controlled studies of other antidepressant drugs that are not part of the TCA or SSRI classes are unavailable. These other drugs are therefore not discussed in this section, as their use is mostly for second- or third-line choices for depressions that are difficult to treat and is reserved for specialized practitioners. First, methodological issues concerning RCTs of antidepressants in children and adolescents are addressed. Then the rest of this section summarizes studies that have evaluated the efficacy of TCAs and SSRIs.

Methodological Issues

Although the studies selected for this review are all RCTs, there are major methodological differences across the studies that are important to appreciate in order to understand the variance in their results. This issue is not unique to child psychopharmacology studies. Adult randomized clinical trials evaluating the efficacy of drugs have also yielded variable results. About half of the adult clinical trials for antidepressants do not support the efficacy of the active drugs.

Randomized clinical trials must be adequately powered to detect clinically significant differences between a drug and a placebo. Few single-site studies could recruit large enough samples over a reasonable period of time, so investigators have sometimes relied on multisite designs. First, multisite designs are usually associated with more variability in the results, pose complex logistic problems, incorporate sites where expertise in the evaluation of depressed patients and conduct of trials is more variable, with fidelity to the research design being more difficult to respect. As shown by Cheung, Emslie, and Mayes (2005), the tendency in multisite studies is for differences between drug and placebo effects to be lower as a direct function of the number of subjects included at each site. Second, the design of the studies has been variable in terms of treatment duration, titration of the medication, and other features. For example, some studies use placebo run-ins as a way to eliminate placebo responders when subjects improve at the end of the initial testing period. However, not all trials have used this approach, and placebo–response rates, like drug–response rates, have varied enormously (between 30 and 60%). A third source of variability in these studies is subject recruitment. Studies have included children, adolescents, or both. Considering a trend in many studies for adolescents to be more responsive to psychopharmacological interventions than children, it is important to keep in mind this age heterogeneity. Selection criteria for inclusion in studies have also varied in terms of instrumentation and exclusion of subjects based on comorbid conditions or degrees of suicidality. Fourth, many studies have included subjects whose major depression duration has been long (sometimes averaging 40–50 weeks). As a result, and in accordance with the natural history of this remitting psychiatric disorder, it could well be that subjects are included in studies at a point in the time course of the disorder where remission is on its way. If so, this would attenuate the power of each study to detect true differences between the active drug and the placebo. Fifth, some studies included inpatient and outpatient subjects, whereas others selected subjects referred to psychiatric centers or community-based clinics. The severity of the depressive disorders in subjects included in trials has also varied across studies. As severity is likely to be associated with the natural course of the disorder, lesser severity at initial presentation may be associated with higher placebo–response rates in some studies. Finally, another source of variability in the studies arises from the use of different outcome measures to evaluate efficacy. Several measures of depressive symptomatology have been used, both clinician-administered and self-report. In more recent trials, consensus has determined that the revised Childhood Depression Rating Scale (CDRS) (Poznanski et al., 1984) is the most sensitive measure to capture change in trials. Investigators have also used the pool of depressive items generated by semistructured diagnostic interviews such as the Schedule for Affective Disorders and Schizophrenia for School-Age Children (K-SADS; Ambrosini, 2000), other depressive checklists like the Children's Depression Inventory (CDI; Kovacs, 1985), the Beck Depression Inventory (BDI; Beck, Ward, Mendelson, Mock, & Erbaugh, 1961), the Mood and Feeling Questionnaire (Angold et al., 1995), the Hamilton Depression Rating Scale (HRDS; Hamilton, 1960). Not all of these measures have an established record of being sensitive to short-term changes in levels of depressive symptomatology. Even when the CDRS has been used, the criteria for defining improvement or remission have varied across studies, some investigators using a 20% decreased score as a standard of improvement, others having much more stringent criteria; this has been shown to affect the response rates quite dramatically (Cheung et al., 2005). Most studies have also used a clinician global categorical outcome measure based on the Clinical Global Improvement (CGI) scale, a crude classification of improvement by the clinician in broad categories (e.g., very much improved, much improved, etc.).

Efficacy Studies of TCAs

Six randomized clinical trials have been performed with children having a diagnosis of depressive disorder (Petti & Law, 1982; Kashani, Shekim, & Reid, 1984; Preskorn, Weller, Hughes, Weller, & Bolte, 1987; Puig-Antich et al., 1987; Geller, Cooper, McCombs, Graham, & Wells, 1989; Hughes, Preskorn, Weller, & Weller, 1990). Four of these studies investigated imipramine with dosages up to 5mg/kg/day and durations between 4 and 8 weeks. The other studies investigated the efficacy of amitriptyline and of nortriptyline. Most studies were lacking power, with sample sizes ranging from 6 to 50 (median sample size = 30). In five of these studies the comparisons did not show any superiority of the active drug over a placebo. In one study there was a small advantage for the imipramine over placebo (Preskorn et al., 1987). Among adolescent samples, five studies were published during the same period (Kramer & Feiguine, 1981; Geller, Cooper, Graham, & Marsteller 1990; Klein & Koplewicz, 1990; Kutcher, Boulos, Ward, & Marton, 1994; Kye, Waterman, Ryan, & Birmaher, 1996). As in the child studies, the sample sizes were small (range 20–60, median = 31) and the duration of the trials rarely exceeded 6 weeks. Desipramine was examined in two studies, amitriptyline in two, and nortriptyline in one. All five adolescent studies showed no superiority of the active compound over the placebo. Even though the power to detect differences was reduced in most studies, the pattern of results and changes in depressive checklist mean scores were very similar in both groups, suggesting there was indeed no advantage to treating depressed youths with tricyclics.

In a recent meta-analysis that incorporated a few more recent studies, Hazell, O'Connell, Heathcote, and Henry (2006) reviewed all RCTs of tricyclic medications in depressed subjects between the ages of 6 and 18. For each study, they selected the best outcome measure, either change in depression scores on a rating scale of depressive symptomatology or a categorical outcome defining improvement in each study. This allowed the pooling of results across studies, using effect size and odds ratios for averaging the results. The 13 trials selected in this meta-analysis involved 506 participants. When improvement was assessed as a categorical outcome, there was no advantage of TCAs over placebo (the pooled odds ratio was not significantly different from 1, estimated as 0.84 with 95% CI: 0.56–1.25). When the results were evaluated using reductions in symptom scores, a very small benefit was found for the active drugs over placebo (net effect size = −0.31, p = 0.05) suggestive of a very modest reduction of depressive symptomatology due to the active compound. This effect size appeared to be slightly higher (i.e., 0.47) in the subgroup of adolescents, which suggests a trend of better response to TCAs in older subjects in the pooled analysis.

In line with all the individual studies reporting adverse effects of the treatments, the meta-analysis of Hazell et al. (2006) indicated that, as compared with placebo-treated individuals, youths treated with TCAs reported four times more vertigo, seven times more orthostatic hypotension, six times more tremor, and five times more dry mouth. These adverse side effects were associated with early dropouts in many of the studies.

This lack of efficacy of TCAs in studies of depressed children and adolescents is not well understood. In some studies the sample selection included very heterogeneous groups of children presenting with not only depression, but also significant comorbid disorders, which may explain the lack of response to medication. In most studies it was also found that the response rate in the placebo-treated groups were very high, blurring any true differences between the two groups. As TCAs act by blocking the reuptake of norepinephrine, it is also possible that TCAs do not have the same efficacy in young subjects as in adults owing to the fact that the noradrenergic system is not fully mature before the end of the adolescent period. In addition, the influence of high levels of circulating sex hormones has been raised as a possible factor mitigating the response to TCAs. Finally, independent studies of childhood depression have demonstrated that childhood depression with prepubertal onset may have different correlates and outcomes (Harrington, Fudge, Rutter, Pickles, & Hill, 1990; Jaffee et al., 2002), suggesting that depression with a prepubertal onset may be heterotopic to adolescent and adult depression. Although this interpretation is consistent with a trend found in Hazell et al.'s (2006) meta-analysis, it does not explain why adolescent studies of TCAs have failed to document the same response rates that have consistently been found in adult studies.

As mentioned above, sudden deaths of children treated with tricyclics were reported in the early 1990s. These children were not necessarily treated for depressive conditions, but rather for ADHD syndromes, indicating that in the context of strenuous physical activities, TCAs could lead to fatal arrhythmias and death. This, combined with the lack of evidence of efficacy, has led to the disregard of TCAs as first-line drugs for the management of youth depression.

Efficacy Studies of SSRIs

Six studies investigating SSRI efficacy have been published, excluding one fluoxetine study that had a very small sample size and an unusual patient selection (Simeon, Dinicola, Ferguson, & Copping, 1990). Three studies evaluated fluoxetine, one paroxetine, one sertraline, and one citalopram. The major design characteristics and results of these studies are summarized in Table 9.1. Contrary to the TCA studies, most of these studies provided sufficient statistical power to detect reasonable differences. Table 9.1 provides the results of these studies using both a categorical outcome measure, the Clinical Global Improvement scale, and a dimensional outcome measure, the Childhood Depression Rating Scale or, in one study (Keller et al., 2001), the Hamilton Depression Rating Scale. The results generally indicate an advantage of the active drug over placebo, although the size of the difference in responses is usually not impressive. This is true both when categorical and dimensional outcome measures are considered.

From Table 9.1, it appears that fluoxetine, the most studied drug, is most consistently associated with efficacy. However, it is noteworthy that improvements with fluoxetine treatment were not always detected using self-report measures such as the Children's Depression Inventory (Kovacs, 1985) or impairment measures such as the Global Assessment Functioning Scale (Shaffer et al., 1983). Within studies, discrepancies have often been found between different outcome measures and have no clear interpretation. In the study by Keller et al. (2001), there was a third group treated with imipramine (unrepresented in Table 9.1) that showed no differences between imipramine and placebo, a higher dropout rate in the imipramine group due to side effects, and better efficacy of paroxetine over imipramine. In that study, the response rate to paroxetine over placebo was relatively unimpressive on main outcome measures, but secondary measures such as the K-SADS depressive item scale and rates of remission (66 vs. 46%, $p = .02$) indicated more clearly the advantage of the active drug. The study evaluating sertraline (Wagner et al., 2003) had a larger sample size, but concerns were raised because the authors had pooled results from two independent studies. Although the results in each independent study were largely negative, pooling the data indicated a statistically significant advantage for the active compound. However, the magnitude of the advantage was very small. Even though the pooling of data of these two studies may have been decided a priori, as in Cheung et al. (2005), it is noteworthy that this highly powered study is associated with effect sizes and likelihood of improvement that are of minimal clinical significance.

Unpublished clinical trials (two on paroxetine, one on citalopram, one on venlafaxine, one on nefazodone, and one on mirtazapine) have also been conducted and reviewed by the U.S. Food and Drug Administration (2004). These studies have shown both positive efficacy and absence of efficacy. At the same time, significant methodological weaknesses have sometimes made the results from such studies difficult to evaluate.

At the moment, data on the efficacy of SSRIs to treat child and adolescent depression are only emerging. It is important to highlight the fact that this is a new field of investigation, that the methodological issues reviewed above indicate the difficulty of conducting these studies, and that there are important sources of variability within and across investigations. Of note is the fact that active drug–response rates have often been comparable to those from adult studies, whereas placebo–response rates have tended to be higher, reducing the ability to detect meaningful differences.

At this time, a provisional conclusion as to the moderate efficacy of antidepressant drugs can be reached, especially for fluoxetine. However, there is no reason to predict that the efficacy of other SSRIs would be lower than that of fluoxetine. No study has compared head-to-head two different SSRIs. There is still an insufficiency of well-designed RCTs of antidepressants in young people, and it can be hoped that the methodological problems identified in the first generation of RCTs will be addressed in future research.

TABLE 9.1. Published Randomized Clinical Trials of SSRIs

Authors	Medication	Dose	Trial duration	Sample size		Ages (years)	Depression Checklist—outcome measures[a]	Clinical Global Improvement (active drug vs. placebo)
				Active drug	Placebo			
Emslie et al. (1997)	Fluoxetine	20 mg	8 weeks	48	48	7–17	−20.1 vs. −10.5 (p = .001)	56% vs. 33% (p = .02)
Keller et al. (2001)	Paroxetine	20–40 mg	8 weeks	93	87	12–18	−10.7 vs. −9.1 (p = .13)	66% vs. 48% (p = .02 par vs. pb)
Emslie et al. (2002)	Fluoxetine	10–20 mg	9 weeks	109	110	8–17	−22.0 vs. −14.9 (p = .001)	52.3% vs. 36.8% (p = .028)
Wagner et al. (2003)	Sertraline	50–200 mg	10 weeks	189	187	6–17	−22.8 vs. −20.2 (p = .01)	63% vs. 53% (p = .05)
March et al. (2004)	Fluoxetine	10–40 mg	12 weeks	109	112	12–17	−22.6 vs. −19.4 (p = .01)	61% vs. 35% (p = .001)
Wagner et al. (2004)	Citalopram	20–40 mg	8 weeks	89	85	7–17	−21.7 vs. −16.5 (p = .04)	47% vs. 45% (NS)

[a]Childhood Depression Rating Scale or Hamilton Depression Rating Scale (mean differences between end-point and baseline scores).

PRINCIPLES OF MANAGEMENT

When the decision has been made to include a psychopharmacological component in the management of a depressed youth, there are certain measures that must be taken. First, a comprehensive psychiatric assessment should be performed, including an evaluation of the family history of affective disorders and identifying possible risk for bipolar disorder in the child. Indicators of such a possibility are a positive family history of bipolar disorder, a very acute onset, psychomotor retardation, mood-congruent psychosis, and a previous hypomanic response to antidepressants. A thorough medical investigation should be performed, with adequate biological tests if a contributing medical disorder is suspected (e.g., hypothyroidy). Blood count, liver function and EKG results should be obtained in some circumstances, as well as results of pregnancy tests in females. It is good practice to use a depression symptom checklist to assess baseline symptomatology and to identify the symptoms that are generating the most impairment. Similarly, side effects checklists can be used at baseline in order to facilitate the subsequent interpretation of side effects, should they appear in the course of the treatment. In addition to self-report depression rating scales, the clinician can use simple measures such as the Clinical Global Improvement scale or impairment scales such as the Children's Global Assessment Scale (CGAS; Shaffer et al., 1983) or clinician-rated depression scales like the CDI (Kovacs, 1985) or the HRDS (Hamilton, 1960).

A drug must then be chosen from the five available SSRIs. Attention must be paid to the pharmacokinetic properties of the medications and to the patient's particular symptom profile, which may best be managed by a drug with a particular mechanism of action. Knowledge of coexisting drug treatments and of potential drug–drug interactions can also guide the selection of the most appropriate SSRI.

An initial target dose must then be chosen. A rule is to increase dosage slowly, in order to avoid emergent side effects at the beginning of the treatment. It is currently advised that, during the first month, weekly monitoring of patients taking SSRIs should be performed with particular attention to side effects and the emergence of behavioral activation or suicidality. The goals of therapeutic drug monitoring are to avoid toxicity, to evaluate compliance, to improve therapeutic response, to monitor drug–drug or food–drug interactions, and to adjust the drug dosage according to growth, development, and co-occurring medical conditions. Optimization of the treatment is an important task. Improvement can be achieved with the initial target dose, but greater improvement can be obtained by increasing the dosage slightly if the drug is well tolerated. As there is great individual variability in response to these medications, fine titration of the dosage must be performed for each individual in order to maximize efficacy and limit side effects.

Some side effects are common with SSRIs. Increased nervousness and anxiety at the beginning of the treatment, sexual side effects such as anorgasmia or decreased libido, gastrointestinal symptoms, nausea, weight gain, sedation, fatigue, headaches, and sweating are all common. Many of these side effects are transient, well tolerated, and disappear after some time. A progressive titration of the dose initially limits the impact of these side effects.

SSRIs exert their full effect after several weeks of treatment. Six to eight weeks are often necessary to obtain a full response. The response should be documented with the rating scale used at baseline in order to ascertain that sufficient decrease in depressive symptomatology has been achieved and that impairment due to depressive symptoms has decreased. While monitoring a patient using SSRIs, it is important to take a collaborative approach with the patient and his or her family and to evaluate compliance, which is a problem for some young people. Lack of compliance can lead to unpleasant symptoms due to discontinuation syndromes with some SSRIs.

When depression has lifted, it is recommended to maintain the patient on the same dose until remission has been achieved for at least several months. Discontinuation of medication too early can lead to unnecessary relapses. Although empirical studies on the optimal duration of SSRI treatment in youth depression are lacking, it is advisable to maintain treatment for at least 6 months, and sometimes for 9–12 months. This interval corresponds roughly to the average duration of episodes of depression in youths and adults. When there has been a sustained remission, discontinuation of the medication can be envisaged. As a rule, diminution of dosage should always be progressive over a period of time.

SPECIAL ISSUES

In this section, we discuss briefly some of the issues that can arise in the psychopharmacological management of juvenile depression.

Treatment-Resistant Depression

Response to an SSRI can vary from 50 to70%, meaning that a relatively high number of patients will not respond to a well-administered course of an SSRI. If so, it is advisable to change to another SSRI, as some patients in clinical practice respond to one SSRI but not another. When no improvement has been achieved with three properly conducted antidepressant drug trials, other strategies can be employed. Augmentation strategies consist of adding other medications (i.e., lithium, l-tryptophan, triodothironine, buspirone, etc.) to boost the efficacy of the antidepressant. These approaches must be implemented by practitioners with special expertise in psychopharmacology. Combination strategies consist of combining two different antidepressants. For example, some patients treated with SSRIs develop apathetic syndromes, which can be corrected by the addition of antidepressant drugs acting more selectively on the noradrenergic system. In some severe cases, the depression can present with psychotic symptoms, which may require the addition of neuroleptics, and when bipolar disorder is diagnosed, the addition of a mood stabilizer.

Safety

Concerns about the safety of SSRIs were initially raised in 2003 by a report from the Medicine and Healthcare Products Regulatory Agency (MHRA) in the United Kingdom. That agency issued a statement that paroxetine should not be used to treat patients under age 18. Following this initial report and further statements by the MHRA that, with the exception of fluoxetine, SSRIs were not suitable for treating children under age 18, a major investigation was conducted by the U.S. Food and Drug Administration (FDA; 2004). This entailed a systematic review of published and unpublished studies, reexamining the raw data of all RCTs, identifying events that might be categorized as suicide-related and reevaluating their severity. At the end of this review in October 2004, the FDA issued a black-box warning describing an increased risk of suicide-related events associated with the use of SSRIs in youth. The FDA reviewed 26 RCTs involving SSRIs used for treating depression and other disorders. Table 9.2 summarizes some of the

TABLE 9.2. Overall Relative Risks for Suicide-Related Events in Pediatric Trials, by Drug

Drug		Relative risk (95% CI)	
Trade name	Generic name	MDD trials	All trials
Celexa	Citalopram	1.37 (0.53–3.50)	1.37 (0.53–3.50)
Luvox	Fluvoxamine	—[a]	5.52 (0.27–112.55)
Paxil	Paroxetine	2.15 (0.71–6.52)	2.65 (1.00–7.02)
Prozac	Fluoxetine	1.53 (0.74–3.16)	1.52 (0.75–3.09)
Zoloft	Sertraline	2.16 (0.48–9.62)	1.48 (0.42–5.24)
Effexor XR	Venlafaxine	8.84 (1.12–69.51)	4.97 (1.09–22.72)
Remeron	Mirtazapine	1.58 (0.06–38.37)	1.58 (0.06–38.37)
Serzone	Nefazodone	No events	No events
Wellbutrin	Bupropion	—[a]	No events
Total		1.66 (1.02–2.68)	1.95 (1.28–2.98)

Note. CI, confidence interval; MDD, major depressive disorder. Data from Hammad, Loughren, and Racoosin (2006).
[a] No MDD trials of this drug.

results of the FDA assessment. Across studies, patients treated with SSRIs had a small, albeit significant, increase in suicidality or suicide-related events. It is important to note that the magnitude of the increase was small, as indicated by an average odds ratio of 2 against a baseline risk for these events in the placebo group of about 2%. Moreover, there was never a suicidal death reported in any of the trials reviewed by the FDA.

Several scientific bodies of different academies followed up on these findings. Most professional organizations have concluded that although the small increase in the risk of suicide-related events is important to note, the data do not favor the discontinuation of the use of these drugs in clinical practice. Rather, they pointed to the need to be more careful and systematic in the initiation of treatment with SSRIs in young people, recommending the monitoring of patients weekly over the first month and every 2 weeks over the following 2 months. Clinicians have continued to use these medications and have found them to be beneficial to several groups of patients with depression, anxiety, or other psychiatric disorders. Yet, as with any other medication, clinicians must consider the serious adverse events that can occur with these medications and carefully weigh the cost–benefit ratio of using a drug with each patient. Clinical practice sometimes takes place in contexts where other resources are unavailable (e.g., trained mental health professionals to deliver efficacious psychotherapies may not be available), and medications therefore remain a useful part of the armamentarium to address juvenile depression. A detailed account of the FDA review can be found on its website and in subsequent articles that have commented on the issue of SSRI safety in juvenile depression (*www.fda.gov/cder/drug/antidepressants/*).

Combining Psychotherapy and Psychopharmacology

At this time there is only one study that has evaluated the efficacy of combining psychotherapy (cognitive-behavioral therapy) and psychopharmacology (SSRIs, such as fluoxetine) in youth with depression (March et al., 2004). The study had a large sample, 439 patients, ages 12–17. The combination of fluoxetine and cognitive-behavioral therapy (CBT) achieved the highest rate of improvement (71%), as compared with fluoxetine alone (61%), CBT alone (43%), or placebo (35%). These preliminary results parallel those of adult studies, showing that the combination of the two modalities seems to be more efficacious. Interestingly, subjects who benefited from CBT, with or without fluoxetine, reported fewer suicide-related events. This suggests that psychotherapy may decrease suicidal risk. However, an unusual finding was that the CBT group was not superior to the placebo group, a result that conflicts with several studies of CBT that have established the robust efficacy of this psychotherapeutic technique. This indicates that the type of CBT or the fidelity to CBT in the study was suboptimal. The future will undoubtedly see more research in this area.

Managing Adolescent Depression in Primary Care Settings

A recent task force of mental health professionals from the United States and Canada reviewed the evidence and established guidelines for evaluating and treating adolescent depression in primary care settings (Cheung et al., in press). These guidelines include several recommendations for detecting depression in adolescents seen by general practitioners, pediatricians, or family doctors' offices, suggest tools that can be easily used to diagnose and evaluate depressive symptoms, and outline the basic principles of management, by a primary care clinician, of a noncomplicated depressive disorder in an adolescent. Among the potential treatments, prescriptions of SSRIs are discussed, with practical recommendations for the initiation and monitoring of treatment. In the context of epidemiological data indicating that depressive disorders in adolescents have an annual prevalence rate of about 4–5%, it is important that primary care physicians are well trained to detect and to treat mild- to moderate-intensity depression. The numbers of potential patients involved are too high for them to be treated exclusively in psychiatric settings. These guidelines, established for primary care practitioners for the first time, should enhance the management of depression at different levels of care and provide a role for psychopharmacological management within a framework that gives detailed attention to monitoring the response and safety of these drugs when administered to young people.

In conclusion, randomized clinical studies evaluating the efficacy of antidepressants in treating juvenile depression have given preliminary results. Evidence suggests that tricyclic antidepressants lack efficacy, and because of their high index of toxicity, these medications should not be used as a first-line treatment. Studies of SSRIs have provided mixed results, likely reflecting methodological variability within and across studies, that may in turn have reduced the ability to detect true differences. However, some studies have shown consistent trends and significant results in regard to the efficacy of some medications, especially fluoxetine. These findings have emerged from a small number of published and unpublished studies, and it should be kept in mind that adult studies have also often been negative. It has been common practice for regulatory agencies to license drugs when at least two different RCTs show efficacy. This is a stringent criterion, which, if used with child and adolescent studies, may be too limiting, given the relative dearth of research in this area. It is likely that the future will see better-designed RCTs that will address some of the methodological difficulties identified in this initial series of clinical trials and will, it is hoped, consolidate the preliminary encouraging results.

REFERENCES

Abramowicz, M. (1990). Sudden death in children treated with a tricyclic antidepressant. *Medical Letter on Drugs and Therapeutics, 32,* 53.

Ambrosini, P. (2000). The historical development and present status of the Schedule for Affective Disorders and Schizophrenia for School-Age Children (K-SADS). *Journal of the American Academy of Child and Adolescent Psychiatry, 39*(1), 49–58.

Angold, A., Costello, E. J., Messer, S. C., Pickles, A., Winder, F., & Silver, D. (1995). The development of a short questionnaire for use in epidemiological studies of depression in children and adolescents. *International Journal of Methods in Psychiatric Research, 5,* 237–249.

Beck, A., Ward, C., Mendelson, M., Mock, J., & Erbaugh, J. (1961). An inventory for measuring depression. *Archives of General Psychiatry, 4,* 561–571.

Biederman, J. (1991). Sudden death in children treated with a tricyclic antidepressant. *Journal of the American Academy of Child and Adolescent Psychiatry, 30*(3), 495–498.

Cheung, A. H., Emslie, G. J., & Mayes, T. L. (2005). Review of the efficacy and safety of antidepressants in youth depression. *Journal of Child Psychology and Psychiatry, 46*(7), 735–754.

Cheung, A., Zuckerbrot, R., Jensen, P., Laraque, D., Stein, R. E. K., and the GLAD-PC Steering Group. (in press). Guidelines for Adolescent Depression in Primary Care (GLAD-PC). *Pediatrics.*

Emslie, G. J., Heiligenstein, J. H., Wagner, K. D., Hoog, S. L., Ernest, D. E., Brown, E., et al. (2002). Fluoxetine for acute treatment of depression in children and adolescents: A placebo-controlled, randomized clinical trial. *Journal of the American Academy of Child and Adolescent Psychiatry, 41*(10), 1205–1215.

Emslie, G. J., Rush, A. J., Weinberg, W. A., Kowatch, R. A., Carmody, T., & Rintelmann, J. (1997). A double-blind, randomized, placebo-controlled trial of fluoxetine in children and adolescents with depression. *Archives of General Psychiatry, 54*(11), 1031–1037.

Fombonne, E. (2002). Interpersonal psychotherapy for adolescents. In H. Remschmidt (Ed.), *Psychotherapy in children and adolescents* (pp. 124–137). Cambridge, UK: Cambridge University Press.

Fombonne, E., Wostear, G., Cooper, V., Harrington, R., & Rutter, M. (2001). The Maudsley long-term follow-up study of adolescent depression: I. Psychiatric outcomes in adulthood. *British Journal of Psychiatry, 179,* 210–217.

Geller, B., Cooper, T. B., Graham, D. L., & Marsteller, F. A. (1990). Double-blind placebo-controlled study of nortriptyline in depressed adolescents using a "fixed plasma level" design. *Psychopharmacology Bulletin, 26*(1), 85–90.

Geller, B., Cooper, T. B., McCombs, H. G., Graham, D., & Wells, J. (1989). Double-blind, placebo-controlled study of nortriptyline in depressed children using a "fixed plasma level" design. *Psychopharmacology Bulletin, 25*(1), 101–108.

Hamilton, M. (1960). A rating scale for depression. *Journal of Neurology and Neurosurgery in Psychiatry, 23,* 56–62.

Hammad, T. A., Loughren, T., & Racoosin, J. (2006). Suicidality in pediatric patients treated with antidepressant drugs. *Archives of General Psychiatry, 63,* 332–339.

Harrington, R., Fudge, H., Rutter, M., Pickles, A., & Hill, J. (1990). Adult outcomes of childhood and adolescent depression. I. Psychiatric status. *Archives of General Psychiatry, 47*(5), 465–473.

Hazell, P., O'Connell, D., Heathcote, D., & Henry, D. (2006). Tricyclic drugs for depression in children and adolescents. *Cochrane Database of Systematic Reviews,* (3).

Hughes, C. W., Preskorn, S. H., Weller, E., & Weller, R. (1990). The effect of concomitant disorder in childhood depression on predicting treatment response. *Psychopharmacological Bulletin, 26,* 235–238.

Jaffee, S. R., Moffitt, T. E., Caspi, A., Fombonne, E., Poulton, R., & Martin, J. (2002). Differences in early childhood risk factors for juvenile-onset and adult-onset depression. *Archives of General Psychiatry, 58,* 215–222.

Kashani, J. H., Shekim, W. O., & Reid, J. C. (1984). Amitriptyline in children with major depressive disorder: A double-blind crossover pilot study. *Journal of the American Academy of Child Psychiatry, 23*(3), 348–351.

Keller, M. B., Ryan, N. D., Strober, M., Klein, R. G., Kutcher, S. P., Birmaher, B., et al. (2001). Efficacy of paroxetine in the treatment of adolescent major depression: A randomized, controlled trial. *Journal of the American Academy of Child and Adolescent Psychiatry, 40*(7), 762–772.

Klein, R., & Koplewicz, H. (1990). *Desipramine treatment in adolescent depression.* Paper presented at the Child Depression Consortium Meeting, Pittsburgh, PA.

Kovacs, M. (1985). The Children's Depression Inventory (CDI). *Psychopharmacological Bulletin, 21*(4), 995–998.

Kramer, A. D., & Feiguine, R. J. (1981). Clinical effects of amitriptyline in adolescent depression: A pilot study. *Journal of the American Academy of Child Psychiatry, 20*(3), 636–644.

Kutcher, S., Boulos, C., Ward, B., & Marton, P. (1994). Response to desipramine treatment in adolescent depression: A fixed-dose, placebo-controlled trial. *Journal of the American Academy of Child and Adolescent Psychiatry, 33*(5), 686–694.

Kye, C. H., Waterman, G. S., Ryan, N. D., & Birmaher, B. (1996). A randomized, controlled trial of amitriptyline in the acute treatment of adolescent major depression. *Journal of the American Academy of Child and Adolescent Psychiatry, 35*(9), 1139–1144.

Mandoki, M., Tapia, M. R., Tapia, M. A., & Sumner, G. S. (1997). Venlafazine in the treatment of children and adolescents with major depression. *Psychopharmacological Bulletin, 33*(1), 149–154.

March, J., Silva, S., Petrycki, S., Curry, J., Wells, K., Fairbank, J., et al. (2004). Fluoxetine, cognitive-behavioral therapy, and their combination for adolescents with depression: Treatment for Adolescents with Depression Study (TADS) randomized controlled trial. *Journal of the American Medical Association, 292*(7), 807–820.

Medicine and Healthcare Products Regulatory Agency. (2003). *Selective serotonin reuptake inhibitors (SSRIs): Overview of regulatory status and CSM advice relating to major depressive disorder (MDD) in children and adolescents including a summary of available safety and efficacy data.* London: Department of Health.

Petti, T. A., & Law, W. (1982). Imipramine treatment of depressed children: A double-blind pilot study. *Journal of Clinical Psychopharmacology, 2*(2), 107–110.

Poznanski, E. O., Grossman, J. A., Buchsbaum, Y., Banegas, M., Freeman, L., & Gibbons, R. (1984). Preliminary studies of the reliability and validity of the Childhood Depression Rating Scale. *Journal of the American Academy of Child Psychiatry, 23*(2), 191–197.

Preskorn, S. H., Weller, E. B., Hughes, C. W., Weller, R. A., & Bolte, K. (1987). Depression in prepubertal children: Dexamethasone nonsuppression predicts differential response to imipramine vs. placebo. *Psychopharmacology Bulletin, 23*(1), 128–133.

Puig-Antich, J., Perel, J. M., Lupatkin, W., Chambers, W. J., Tabrizi, M. A., King, J., et al. (1987). Imipramine in prepubertal major depressive disorders. *Archives of General Psychiatry, 44*(1), 81–89.

Riddle, M. A., Geller, B., & Ryan, N. (1993). Another sudden death in a child treated with desipramine. *Journal of the American Academy of Child and Adolescent Psychiatry, 32*(4), 792–797.

Shaffer, D., Gould, M. S., Brasic, J., Ambrosini, P., Fisher, P., Bird, H., et al. (1983). A children's global assessment scale (CGAS). *Archives of General Psychiatry, 40*(11), 1228–1231.

Simeon, J. G., Dinicola, V. F., Ferguson, H. B., & Copping, W. (1990). Adolescent depression: A placebo-controlled fluoxetine treatment study and follow-up. *Progress in Neuropsychopharmacology and Biological Psychiatry, 14*(5), 791–795.

Stahl, S. M. (2000). *Essential psychopharmacology: Neuroscientific basis and practical applications* (2nd ed.). New York: Cambridge University Press.

U.S. Food and Drug Administration. (2004). *Suicidality in children and adolescents being treated with antidepressant medications.* Washington, DC: FDA Public Health Advisory.

Wagner, K. D., Ambrosini, P., Rynn, M., Wohlberg, C., Yang, R., Greenbaum, M. S., et al. (2003). Efficacy of sertraline in the treatment of children and adolescents with major depressive disorder: Two randomized controlled trials. *Journal of the American Medical Association, 290*(8), 1033–1041.

Wagner, K. D., Robb, A. S., Findling, R. L., Jin, J., Gutierrez, M. M., & Heydorn, W. E. (2004). A randomized, placebo-controlled trial of citalopram for the treatment of major depression in children and adolescents. *American Journal of Psychiatry, 161*(6), 1079–1083.

10 Treatment of Childhood Depression

The ACTION Treatment Program

Kevin D. Stark, Jennifer Hargrave, Brooke Hersh,
Michelle Greenberg, Jenny Herren, and Melissa Fisher

Cognitive-behavioral therapy (CBT) is one of the most highly investigated psychosocial interventions for depressive disorders among youth. At the time of this writing, we were in the fifth year of a 5-year efficacy study of a gender- and age-specific CBT group intervention for depressed 9- to 13-year-old girls. Preliminary results of this investigation suggest that the ACTION treatment program is effective for girls who are experiencing major depressive disorder and/or dysthymic disorder. The girls' significant others work with the therapist to encourage the girls to apply the skills. In the ideal situation the girls learn coping, problem solving, and cognitive restructuring skills at the same time that their family environments are being changed through individual family sessions and a parent training group.

The main objectives of this chapter are to describe the underlying theory of the ACTION program and the treatment itself. In the ACTION treatment program, research and theory underlie the therapists' conceptualization of each case. The conceptualization enables the therapist to individualize a group treatment to meet the needs of each child. It helps bring the treatment to life as it determines the content of the treatment procedures and the choice of treatment procedures to be used.

GUIDING THEORY

From the perspective of CBT, it is recognized that there are multiple pathways to the development of a depressive disorder. Each child has his or her own unique pathway.

Depression is caused by disturbances in cognitive, interpersonal, neurochemical, and environmental functioning, as well as deficits in critical emotion regulation skills. Furthermore, there are reciprocal relationships between these disturbances. Thus, a disturbance in one area would affect, and be affected by, each of the other domains, and a depressive disorder can develop.

In the following sections, we first discuss the theoretical tenets that are the foundation of the ACTION treatment program, starting with the cognitive disturbances that underlie depressive disorders. Subsequently, disturbances in the other domains of functioning are described.

Cognitive Disturbances

Children are active constructors of their environments both in terms of their perceptions of the environment and with respect to their actions that impact the environment. They try to make sense of, or derive meaning from, their interactions with the environment, and especially from interactions with significant others. As children develop, they interpret events in terms of their meanings of the self. If a message about the self is communicated often enough and is accompanied by other learning experiences that communicate the same message, this self-view becomes internalized and structuralized as a core belief. Core beliefs about the self develop first and influence the development of additional beliefs. Beliefs serve as filters that eliminate belief-inconsistent information and efficiently process belief-consistent information that further strengthens the developing sense of self. Other critical core beliefs include those about the self within interpersonal relationships, the world in general, and the future.

It has been hypothesized (e.g., Beck, Rush, Shaw, & Emery, 1979; Cole & Turner, 1993)—and research (Stark, Schmidt, & Joiner, 1996) supports the notion—that a child's core beliefs are formed through early learning experiences and communications within the family (the cognitive interpersonal pathway; Stark, Laurent, Livingston, Boswell, & Swearer, 1999). The core beliefs about the self that underlie depression include (1) I am unlovable, (2) I am worthless, and (3) I am helpless (Beck et al., 1979). These beliefs can develop as a result of interactions that are characteristic of an insecure attachment, negative evaluative statements directed at the child by caregivers, a history of abuse and rejection (Puig-Antich et al., 1985), and parental overreliance on punitive procedures (Poznanski & Zrull, 1970). It is important to note that the child, through genetic predispositions and temperament factors, plays a role in constructing this environment.

Once developed, beliefs are in an active or latent state. A traumatic or stressful event that is related to the content of the belief may trigger its activation. Once activated, beliefs guide the information-processing system. Dysfunctional core beliefs produce a distortion in the child's perceptions of daily events and in the meanings that the child draws about him- or herself from these events. Experiences are viewed through the lense of one or more of the three aforementioned core beliefs, and information that is inconsistent is distorted to make it support the core belief. However, it is important to note that because the belief system of a child is developing, the child may be immersed in the events that are shaping the development of the core beliefs. Thus, the child's perceptions may not be distorted; rather, they may be a realistic reflection of the child's life. Therapists have to evaluate the child's beliefs to determine whether they are distorted or realistic. When they are realistic, the environment becomes the focus of treatment.

Intermediate beliefs are higher-order beliefs that guide a child's behavior and information processing, but they are not as central as the core beliefs. They are formed after core beliefs and support them. For example, a child with the core belief "I am helpless" may have an intermediate belief that she cannot do new things without someone's help. Thus, she is unwilling to try new things. When forced to try new things, she seeks help but gives up quickly when she cannot get the help. When the child thinks about new schoolwork, she believes that she cannot do it without help from her teacher. Another form of intermediate belief is a conditional assumption. Conditional assumptions take the form of "If, then" statements. For example, the conditional assumption "If I get close to someone, then that person will leave me" would impact the child's social life. Although intermediate beliefs do not play a superordinate role in the child's information processing, they are important targets for intervention inasmuch as they support depressive core beliefs, give rise to their own maladaptive cognitions, and guide maladaptive behaviors.

The most superficial level of cognition is automatic thought, the thoughts and images that permeate an individual's consciousness and reflect the underlying beliefs. Automatic thoughts are evident in a child's verbalizations during group meetings. When they stem from a distorted belief, the distortion is evident. For example, a child who is loved by his parents and liked by his peers may think and verbalize, "No one likes me."

Negative automatic thoughts and intermediate beliefs are useful targets for restructuring when they reflect a core belief that has been targeted for change. It may be most expedient to target core beliefs first, as that may lead to a change in the intermediate beliefs and automatic thoughts. However, because core beliefs develop early in life and are so firmly entrenched, they are also likely to be most resistant to change. Given this resistance, it is important to identify each child's core beliefs early in treatment so that extensive efforts can be made to change them to "I am lovable and loved," "I am worthy," and/or "I am efficacious." Given the amount of effort it takes to produce change in core beliefs and the fact that it is difficult for children to learn to identify their negative thoughts/beliefs and to change them, half of the sessions (10) in the ACTION program are devoted to teaching the girls how to evaluate the validity of their thoughts/beliefs and how to change them to be more positive and realistic. This process is described in a later section on cognitive restructuring.

Neurochemical Disturbances

Disturbances in cognition reciprocally interact with and affect brain chemistry through a stress reaction. Stress has both a direct impact on neurochemical/brain functioning and an indirect effect through the individual's perceptions of stress and the potential harm that he or she may experience. The depression-prone individual may believe that he or she does not possess the skills or abilities to cope. In addition, such individuals are more likely to perceive a wider variety of events as potentially harmful, which leads to greater stress. Stress appears to impact the hypothalamic-adrenal system, causing the adrenal glands to oversecrete hydrocortisone or cortisol. When stressed, hypothalamic neurons, regulated by norepinephrine neurons in the locus coeruleus, secrete corticotropin-releasing hormone, which stimulates the production of adrenocorticotropin (ACTH) by the pituitary. ACTH then stimulates the adrenal glands to produce cortisol. Stress-related hormones and neurotransmitters influence cerebral functioning (Kolb & Whishaw, 1996). This may lead to a disruption in the neurotransmitter system as well as produce symptoms of depression.

A biochemical disturbance would affect mood, vegetative functioning, and information processing and leave a youngster more vulnerable to the effects of stress. The disturbance in mood and information processing would feed back to and impact the biochemical disturbance, which would affect the child's behavior, and thus his or her relationships with others. The behaviors and reactions of significant others may be misperceived because of distortions in information processing, leading to a confirmation of, or the activation of, dysfunctional beliefs.

The biochemical disturbance may be genetically based or caused by prolonged stress. Regardless of its origin, it may be possible to intervene through the use of medication, psychotherapy, or a combination of the two. There is strong evidence that use of one of the selective serotonin reuptake inhibitors (SSRIs) is an effective treatment for some depressed youth (Emslie et al. 2002; Emslie et al., 1997) and that a combination of medication and CBT may be even more effective (March, 2004). Furthermore, although CBT and fluoxetine are equivalent in terms of the rate of effectiveness at 20 weeks following the start of treatment, fluoxetine produces change more quickly (Curry, personal communication, August 2006). Although there is some controversy about the use and safety of antidepressant medications with children and adolescents (for a review, see Stark, Hargrave, Schnoebelen, Simpson, & Molnar, 2005), a trial under the careful supervision of a psychiatrist is indicated for youth who do not respond to an initial trial of psychosocial interventions. For many depressed youth, a combination of an SSRI and CBT is the most effective intervention and the one that produces the most rapid response. It may also be clinically prudent to initiate a medication trial simultaneously with CBT when the child is experiencing a severe episode of depression and when the child has a family member who was successfully treated with an antidepressant.

Behavioral Disturbances

Within the behavioral realm, youth experience a number of disturbances that contribute to the development and maintenance of a depressive disorder. These include disturbances in interpersonal behaviors, deficits in the use of social skills, and a failure to engage in recreational activities. These types of behaviors lead to a reduction in reinforcement and are hypothesized to produce depression (Lewinsohn, 1974; Coyne, 1976).

Depressed youth experience interpersonal difficulties. They are less popular (see, e.g., Jacobsen, Lahey, & Strauss, 1983), less liked (see, e.g., Peterson, Mullins, & Ridley-Johnson, 1985), and more often rejected by peers (Kennedy, Spence, & Hensley, 1989). Depressed youth engage in less social interaction (Kazdin, Esveldt-Dawson, Sherick, & Colbus, 1985) and are less likely to have or maintain a "best friendship" (Puig-Antich et al., 1985). Consistent with Coyne's (1976) hypothesis, depressed children elicit negative reactions from adults (Mullins, Peterson, Wonderlich, & Reaven, 1986) and peers (Kennedy et al., 1989). Thus, depressed youth may not have the parental (Stark, Humphrey, Crook, & Lewis, 1990) or peer social support (see, e.g., Blechman, McEnroe, Carella, & Audette, 1986) necessary to help buffer the impact of stressful events. The extent to which children feel supported, safe, and secure predicts their use of adaptive mood regulation strategies (Kliewer & Lewis, 1995). Thus, the depressed youngster would fail to learn essential mood regulation skills.

Depression is associated with a lack of social skills (Kennedy et al., 1989; Wierzbicki & McCabe, 1988). Depressed youth may lack social skills or possesses them but fail to use them, owing to a cognitive disturbance (Felner, Lease, & Phillips, 1990; Sacco & Graves, 1984). Either of these conditions can lead to social neglect or rejection. It also is possible that the social skills disturbances are caused by depressive symptoms (Bell-Dolan, Reaven, & Peterson, 1993). For example, dysphoria and irritability permeate the depressed individual's interactions with peers and adults (Puig-Antich et al., 1985), who find this affect aversive and thus they progressively withdraw from and avoid interactions with the depressed individual (Mullins et al., 1986; Kennedy et al., 1989). Over time, this leads the depressed individual to become isolated, less active in general, and supports the belief "I am unlovable." Similarly, social withdrawal leads to isolation, inactivity, and a loss of a major source of reinforcement. Fatigue leaves the youngster feeling too tired to do anything. Over time, peers stop asking the young person to participate in activities because he or she "never wants to do anything." Sleep disturbance produces a similar outcome. Negative self-evaluations, hopelessness, and low self-esteem in general lead to a lack of self-confidence, which may result in the depressed child's being ignored or victimized by peers. To address these disturbances, it is important to help the depressed child to become socially and behaviorally activated to effect an improvement in mood and energy level and to increase the child's opportunities to obtain reinforcement.

Another behavioral disturbance is a failure to engage in recreational activities. This may be due to a lack of exposure to enjoyable activities within the family, the child's not having learned how to have fun, or the child's not valuing fun. Another possibility is that anhedonia and other symptoms of depression prevent the child from experiencing pleasure, and he or she does not seek out activities that other children enjoy. Regardless of the reason, a lack of enjoyable activities means that the child also lacks the relief from stress they provide, as well as a way to elevate mood, energy, and motivation.

Effective intervention has to be flexible enough to address possible deficits in social skills and performance. It may also be necessary to intervene in the family environment to provide education about the importance of interpersonal relationships and to solicit parental support for the child's being more socially active. In addition, the parents may have to assist the child with his or her attempts to identify recreational activities that bring the child pleasure and then to engage in them. It may be necessary for the family as a whole to engage in more recreational activities.

Disturbance in Affect Regulation

Depressive symptoms and disorders have been conceptualized as a failure to regulate affect (Cole & Kaslow, 1988). Depressed youth often lack developmentally appropriate skills for regulating negative affect. Understanding the normative progression of emotional regulation across development informs the creation of developmentally sensitive treatment models. Four trends characterize the typical development of affect regulation: (1) progression from other-regulation to self-regulation (Cole & Kaslow, 1988; Dunn & Brown, 1991; Rossman, 1992; Thompson, 1991), (2) expansion of children's emotion regulation repertoire with age (Kopp, 1989; Cole & Kaslow, 1988; Altshuler & Ruble, 1989; see Masters, 1991, for contradictory results), (3) a shift from more behavioral strategies to cognitive strategies (Altshuler & Ruble, 1989), and (4) an increased emphasis on situational characteristics (see Stark et al., 1999, for a description of the development of affect regulation).

Research supports the conceptualization of depression as a failure to regulate negative affect (Cole & Kaslow, 1988; Garber, Braafladt, & Weiss, 1995; Garber, Braafladt, & Zeman, 1991). Depressed children have difficulty altering negative affect once they are experiencing it. They also tend to generate more passive, less effective methods to regulate mood relative to nondepressed children and to hold lower expectations for the efficacy of strategies generated by others (Garber et al., 1991, 1995). Depressed children are also more likely to report using strategies that may exacerbate distress (Garber et al.,

1991, 1995). Specifically, depressed girls tend to avoid direct problem solving in interpersonal situations and depressed boys tend to act in aggressive ways that exacerbate interpersonal conflict. Depressed children also report significantly less engagement in pleasant activities, relative to nondepressed children (Garber et al., 1991). In addition to these ineffective behavioral coping strategies, depressed youth appear to possess less effective cognitive coping strategies. Saarni and Crowley (1990) suggest that school-age children's understanding of the link between thinking and feeling breaks down when they become overwhelmed. This breakdown parallels an aspect of cognitive theories that characterize depressed individuals as unable to disrupt dysfunctional, depressogenic thoughts. Other researchers have also observed a marked disruption in the generation and enactment of effective strategies during times of intense distress (Altshuler & Ruble, 1989; Dodge, 1991).

Children of depressed mothers tend to exhibit maladaptive affect regulation (Cicchetti, Ganiban, & Barnett, 1991) and so parent–child interaction is one possible pathway to these affect disturbances. Depressed mothers show deficits in the skills needed to foster adaptive affect regulation in their children. For example, they tend to exhibit more negative affect and less sensitive responding (Campbell, Cohn, & Meyers, 1995), and they avoid conflict with their children by withdrawing from confrontation or using unilateral enforcement strategies (Kochanska, Kuczynski, Radke-Yarrow, & Welsh, 1987). Depressed mothers react to negative affect in their children with more criticism and less encouragement of problem solving, which may hinder children's attempts to develop effective affect regulation strategies (Garber et al., 1991). The noncontingent child-directed speech of depressed mothers (Bettes, 1988; Breznitz & Sherman, 1987) may also be less effective in facilitating self-regulation. This leads us to the next depression-related domain: the family environment.

Disturbances in the Family Environment

Evidence from clinical observations and research suggests that many depressed youngsters come from families that are experiencing disturbances (Costello, Mustillo, Erkani, Keeler, & Angold, 2003; Sander & McCarty, 2005). Families of depressed youth are often characterized by greater chaos, abuse and neglect (Kashani, Ray, & Carlson, 1984), conflict (Forehand et al., 1988; Kane & Garber, 2004; Marmorstein & Iacono, 2004; Sagrestano, Paikoff, Holmbeck, & Fendrich, 2003), a more critical, punitive, and belittling or shaming parenting style (see, e.g., Arieti & Bemporad, 1980), greater communication difficulties (Puig-Antich et al., 1985), and a lower activity level (Stark et al., 1990) than families of nondepressed youth. The tone of the mother–child, and to a somewhat lesser extent the father–child, relationship is characterized as cold, hostile, tense, and at times rejecting (Puig-Antich et al., 1985). When affection is expressed, it is contingent upon behavior that is consistent with parental expectations (Cole & Rehm, 1986). One of the most consistent findings reported across studies using a variety of methods is a lack of support and approval from within the family (Sheeber & Sorensen, 1998; Stice, Ragan, & Randall, 2004). In addition to being related to depression, parent–child conflict appears to be a precipitant to suicidal behavior among adolescents (Brent et al., 1993). Strict affectionless control is related to depression and pathology in general (Nomura, Wickramaratne, Warner, Mufson, & Weissman, 2002). In addition to a correlational relationship between family disturbances and depression, a prospective relationship has been found between family disturbances and the development of depressive symptoms (Asarnow, Goldstein, Tompson, & Guthrie, 1993; Sheeber, Hops, Alpert, Davis, & Andrews, 1997) and to the recurrence of depressive episodes during adolescence (Sanford et al., 1995).

It is important to intervene with the families of depressed youth either through parent training or family therapy. The objectives are to eliminate any abuse or neglect, improve cohesion and supportiveness, decrease conflict, improve communication, and increase the family's involvement in recreational activities. The parents may benefit from learning positive behavior management skills, reducing their use of affection and emotional consequences as their behavior management strategies.

THE ACTION TREATMENT PROGRAM: AN EXAMPLE OF CBT FOR DEPRESSED YOUTH

Overview of Child Treatment

The ACTION program is a CBT small-group intervention designed for girls between 9 and 13 years old. It follows a structured therapist's manual (Stark, Simpson, et al., 2006) and workbook (Stark, Schnoebelen, et al., 2006). Groups consist of two to five girls, who meet twice a week for a total of 20 group meetings over 11 weeks. We prefer 1-hour meetings with groups of 9- and 10-year-olds, and 75-minute meetings with children 11 years old and older. Experience suggests that children and younger adolescents benefit from meeting twice a week rather than once a week.

In addition, there are two individual family meetings that take place between the 3rd and 4th, then the 9th and 10th group meetings, respectively (see Table 10.1 for a session-by-session outline). We also ask parents to participate in a parent training group that meets once a week for eight sessions of 90 minutes each (see Table 10.2 for a session-by-session outline).

The treatment materials can be adapted for use with individual clients, but it is important to note that preliminary results of our research indicate that some of the effectiveness of the program is attributable to the group format. The treatment is designed to be fun and engaging while teaching the youngsters a variety of skills that are applied to their depressive symptoms, interpersonal difficulties, and other stressors. The skills are taught to the girls through didactic presentations and activities; they are rehearsed during in-session activities and applied through therapeutic homework.

To make the intervention developmentally appropriate, activities are experiential in nature. Activities are used to build the rationale for treatment and for teaching the children how to use the therapeutic skills and strategies. Similarly, when a therapeutic skill is introduced, the girls complete an activity so that they can change their thinking. Experiencing the benefits of the treatment strategies combats their pessimism, increases treatment credibility, and provides them with a sense of personal efficacy. The application of skills outside the meetings is critical for successful treatment. Thus, skill application is monitored and recorded through completion of therapeutic homework, and homework completion is encouraged through an in-session reward system.

The treatment program is based on a self-regulation model in which youngsters use skills to achieve and to maintain a pleasant mood. They use negative thoughts or a change in mood as a sign to engage in coping, problem solving, and/or cognitive restructuring. There are four primary treatment components: (1) affective education, (2) coping skills training, (3) problem-solving training, and cognitive restructuring. A more complete description of each treatment component appears in the following sections. In general,

TABLE 10.1. Objectives by Meeting

Meeting No.	Objectives
1	Discuss parameters of meetings; introduce counselors and participants; establish rationale for treatment; discuss confidentiality; establish group rules; build group cohesion; establish within-group incentive system.
2	Introduce participants to chat time and agenda setting; establish pragmatics of completing homework; introduce mood meter and Take ACTION List; complete within-session coping activity.
3	Discuss importance of thinking about meetings and doing practice; introduce clients to various therapeutic components, including: focusing on the positive, Catch the Positive Diaries, affective education, and coping strategies.
Individual family meeting 1	Review therapeutic concepts; development of treatment goals.
4	Extend group cohesion; review participant goals and strategies; discuss application of coping strategies; complete coping skills activity within session.
5	Experience impact of coping skills activity within session; introduction, extension, and application of problem solving; introduction to brainstorming step of problem solving.
6	Demonstrate the role of cognition in emotion and behavior; introduce connection of thoughts to feelings; enactment of coping skills activity within session.
7	Apply problem solving to real-life situations; practice brainstorming activity; experience coping skills activity within session.
8	Apply problem solving to teasing; experience coping skills activity within session.
9	Apply problem solving to interpersonal problems; experience coping skills activity within session.
Individual family meeting 2	Review therapeutic concepts; identify common negative thoughts; individualize Catch the Positive Diaries; introduce cognitive restructuring.
10	Prepare for cognitive restructuring; experience coping skills activity within session; practice cognitive restructuring.
11	Introduce how perceptions are constructed; illustrate how depression distorts thinking; provide rationale for changing negative thoughts.
12	Practice identifying negative thoughts of group members; introduce client strengths through a self-map; practice cognitive restructuring.
13	Practice identifying negative thoughts; continue identifying strengths for the self-maps; practice cognitive restructuring with questions using alternative interpretations.
14	Continue identifying negative thoughts, adding strengths to the self-maps, and practicing cognitive restructuring.
15	Continue identifying negative thoughts and adding strengths to the self-maps; introduce examining evidence as a tool for cognitive restructuring.
16	Continue identifying negative thoughts and adding strengths to the self-maps; practice cognitive restructuring; prepare for termination.
17	Continue adding strengths to the self-maps; integrate and apply cognitive restructuring; continue preparing for termination.
18	Continue adding strengths to the self-maps; integrate and apply all of the learned skills; continue preparing for termination.
19	Draw conclusions from self-maps; empowerment activity for clients to continue using skills on their own; prepare for group termination.
20	Say good-bye to the group; say good-bye to negative thoughts and feelings; terminate.

TABLE 10.2. Objectives by Parent Meeting

Meeting No.	Objectives
1: parents only	Discuss parameters of meetings; introduce counselors and participants; establish rationale for treatment and model of depression; discuss confidentiality; discuss parents' role in treatment; introduce parents to coping skills; help parents to learn the principles of positive reinforcement.
2: joint meeting	Help parents to understand the child treatment; extend parents' understanding of positive reinforcement; demonstrate how to use compliments as reinforcers; help parents to understand the power of fun activities and to experience the mood-enhancing nature of fun activities.
3: parents only	Discuss parents' treatment goals for their daughters; teach the parents empathic listening skills; briefly introduce the parents to problem solving.
4: joint meeting	Practice management of child behavior through use of positive reinforcement; improve communication skills; extend parents' understanding and use of problem solving.
5: parents only	Encourage parents to use problem solving; teach parents conflict resolution skills.
6: joint meeting	Practice management of child behavior through use of positive reinforcement; provide parents with practice in using family meetings to manage conflict; improve parents' ability to help their daughters to change their negative thoughts.
7: parents only	Discuss and eliminate barriers to conflict resolution; help parents to understand the importance of negative thoughts; demonstrate the link between thinking and emotions; help parents to see the role they play in their daughters' negative thinking; help parents to become thought detectives.
8: joint meeting	Review major skills through playing a game; discuss how to handle depressive symptoms should they recur; express appreciation for family involvement in treatment; say good-bye.

the first 9 sessions focus primarily on affective education and teaching coping and problem-solving skills. Sessions 10 through 19 focus on learning and applying cognitive restructuring, improving the girls' core beliefs about the self, and continued use of coping and problem-solving strategies.

Case Conceptualization

The ACTION treatment program, like any other manualized intervention, cannot be effectively applied in a cookbook fashion. To be effective, the therapist must be able to develop a conceptualization of the specific child's depressive disorder and then use this as a road map to direct the therapy. Case conceptualization is an ongoing hypothesis-generating and testing process that begins prior to treatment, during the initial assessment, and continues throughout treatment. The therapist uses assessment data, historical information, thoughts verbalized during treatment, and the child's behavior patterns to develop and test hypotheses about the child's core beliefs. To determine which core belief(s) are operating for each child, the therapist listens to the child's self-references and the meanings the child draws from daily experiences. The beliefs are reflected in the themes and consistencies found in each child's thoughts. The meanings of events can be deduced by asking, "What does it mean about you if . . . ?" The therapist follows the child's answer with similar questions until the most basic meaning is uncovered. Beck

(1995) refers to this procedure as the "downward arrow" technique. When the therapist believes that she has identified a core belief, she asks the child whether it fits. The therapist then very actively looks for ways to change it.

The therapist individualizes treatment by developing a plan for how she is going to use the skills being taught within the session to address each child's dysfunctional beliefs, For example, a child may believe that she is helpless, and the skill to be taught in the upcoming meeting is coping through use of fun activities. After the therapist has the group experience the benefits of this coping strategy, she asks the girl how her effective use of the coping strategy fits with the belief that she is helpless and cannot help herself to manage her mood.

The case conceptualization can also guide the therapist's decision making during meetings. For example, a therapist may see a child's statement as (1) an opportunity to help her see how evidence contradicts a depressive belief or supports a more adaptive belief, (2) an opportunity to teach her how to use coping skills, or (3) an opportunity to use problem solving to change the situation. While the therapist is teaching the youngsters coping and problem-solving skills, she is also assessing their mastery of these skills and the presence of beliefs that prevent the successful use of these skills. This information becomes part of the case conceptualization.

Once a child's beliefs have been identified, the next step in the case conceptualization is identification of the environmental events that are maintaining the beliefs. To accomplish this, the therapist assesses the child's interactions with her caregivers, with significant others in her life, and with peers. During all interactions with parents, and especially during conjoint parent–child meetings, the therapist assesses the parents' behavior management, communication, conflict resolution, and emotion regulation skills. The degree of warmth and supportiveness in the parent–child relationship is also assessed. The presence of parental psychopathology is formally assessed during completion of pretreatment measures, and because many parents do not accurately report this information, ongoing assessment is maintained during interactions with the parents.

All of the aforementioned information is used to develop a case conceptualization and in developing treatment plans.

Goal Setting

CBT is a collaborative approach to therapy in which the participant is fully informed of the treatment objectives and the methods that will be employed to achieve these objectives. Central to this collaborative process is helping the participant to identify his or her goals for therapy. In the case of treating children, this may also involve helping parents to identify their goals for their child's treatment and for changing their family or parenting practices.

In the ACTION program, the therapist begins the goal-setting process by reviewing the pretreatment assessment information. This information is used to complete an initial case conceptualization that is translated into treatment goals: positively worded statements about desired outcomes. Between the third and fourth group meetings, the therapist meets individually with each child and her parents to discuss treatment goals. The therapist merges the goals that she has generated during case conceptualization, with the child's goals and concerns to develop a set of three or four collaboratively generated goals for treatment. In addition, the therapist describes the treatment procedures that will be used to help the child achieve these goals. Before the end of this goals meeting, the therapist asks the child if she would be willing to share her goals with the group. During the fourth group meeting, with each child's permission, the children share goals with each other and brainstorm how they can help each other to reach their goals. The strategies for helping each other are recorded on goals sheets so that the children can refer to them as needed. At the beginning of every other subsequent meeting, there is a "goals check-in" time to report progress toward goal attainment and to celebrate progress. As goals are achieved, the therapist helps the participants identify new goals.

Core Therapeutic Components

Affective Education

Affective education is the component of treatment in which the girls learn about depression and their own experiences of it. They are taught the CBT model of depression, including its causes, and how this model applies to them. They are provided with the rationale for treatment, and they learn how they are going to manage their own experiences of depression. The girls are provided with experiences that help them to become more self-aware, particularly in regard to therapeutically relevant experiences such as their depressive thoughts, unpleasant emotions, and other depressive symptoms. Participants are then taught to use these experiences as cues to engage cognitive strategies, problem solving, and/or coping skills as a means of managing the unpleasant emotions. Affective education is threaded throughout the program and is especially evident during the first few meetings.

Because of developmental limitations, children are taught a simplified model of depression in which sadness is caused by negative thoughts and undesirable outcomes. In order to manage depression, the girls learn three core strategies:

1. If the undesirable situation cannot be changed, use a coping strategy.
2. If the undesirable situation can be changed, use problem solving to improve it.
3. Catch negative thoughts and change them to more realistic and positive thoughts.

In order to use these three broad strategies, the youngsters have to recognize their unpleasant emotions, their negative thoughts, and that they are experiencing a problem. Youngsters identify their emotions by acting like "emotion detectives" who investigate their own experience of the "three B's": Body, Brain, and Behavior. Participants are taught greater awareness of their emotional experiences by tuning in to how their bodies are reacting, what they are thinking, and how they are behaving. During the meetings, when a child states that she is experiencing a particular emotion, the therapist asks her to describe what is happening in her body, what she is thinking, and how she is behaving. Simultaneously, the therapist may use a simple cookie-cutter drawing of a girl to illustrate what is happening in her body, brain, and behavior. As treatment progresses and the girls become more proficient at this process, they complete the drawings themselves. The girls also complete therapeutic homework assignments in which they identify their emotional experiences and independently assess their experiences of the three B's.

To help the girls recognize that a problem exists, they are taught to look for signs that they are experiencing a problem. Possible signs include a shift to unpleasant affect, the occurrence or potential occurrence of an undesirable outcome, and feeling anxious or worried about something.

A number of strategies and activities are used to help the girls learn about the distorted nature of depressive cognition. In addition, they learn how to become aware of negative thoughts. The methods for accomplishing this are described in the section on cognitive restructuring.

Coping Skills Training

A central objective of CBT for depression is to behaviorally activate the depressed youngster. In the ACTION program coping skills are used to achieve this therapeutic objective. Emotion-focused coping is taught both as a general strategy for enhancing mood and more specifically for when a child is experiencing an undesirable or stressful situation that she cannot change. Coping skills are taught and practiced during meetings 2–9. Coping skills training is emphasized at the beginning of treatment because these skills help the girls produce an immediate improvement in mood. This improvement in mood makes it easier for them to learn and benefit from the problem solving and cognitive restructuring that are taught later.

As part of the development of the ACTION treatment, a pilot study was completed in which teachers identified especially resilient 9- to 13-year-old students. These youngsters were placed in same-gender-and-age focus groups. The goal of the focus groups was to identify the naturally occurring coping strategies they use to manage sadness and anger/irritability. Five broad categories of coping skills emerged:

1. Do something fun and distracting.
2. Do something soothing and relaxing.
3. Seek social support.
4. Do something that expends lots of energy.
5. Change your thinking.

The girls experience the benefits of examples of coping skills from each of the five broad categories within the treatment sessions. The therapist chooses the coping skills to be taught and applied during each meeting, based on what she believes to be most needed by the group. For example, if the group appears to be very flat in affect, the therapist does something fun and energizing as a means of enlivening the group. It is important to note that the therapist may include coping skills training during any meeting when it would be helpful.

Children have to experience the benefits of coping skills before they will try to use them. When a coping strategy is taught, the therapist first asks the girls to rate their mood and then to participate in an activity in which they use one of the coping skills. For example, the girls may play with hula hoops for 5 minutes along with the therapist (fun and distracting), or they may play freeze tag (exerting energy), or wiggle their toes in sand while imaging a relaxing beach scene (soothing and relaxing); they may talk with one another about a stressor (talk to someone), or they may be asked to talk back to their negative thoughts (change your thinking). After completing the activity, they rerate their moods. Inevitably, their moods dramatically improve. The therapist processes the experience with them. Then the group generates a list of further specific activities from the particular general category (e.g., exerting energy) of coping strategies.

In addition to teaching coping strategies, the therapist helps the girls to identify situations in which it is most advantageous to use specific coping skills. For example, doing something fun and distracting can help lift mood, reduce anger, or reduce anxiety. Soothing and relaxing coping skills are emphasized as a means of reducing anger, irritability, and stress in general. In addition, they can be used to create a calm, pleasant emotional state. Expending energy is useful for generating more energy in general, reducing stress, elevating mood, and fostering better sleep hygiene. Talking to someone can be used as a way to calm down, to distract oneself from something that is upsetting, as a means of gaining perspective, and a way to feel more connected. Early in treatment, participants are taught to use simple coping statements as a means of managing mood. Coping statements are used by participants prior to and during the time they are acquiring more complex cognitive restructuring strategies. These statements are designed to help a child, at least temporarily, to combat depressive thinking. They are not to be confused with the more elegant cognitive restructuring procedures described in a later section of the chapter.

Although it is apparent that the youngsters can learn and benefit from using coping skills, therapeutic improvement is dependent on applying the skills outside the meetings. To facilitate this, therapeutic homework is assigned. This homework progresses from identifying changes in emotion and the accompanying thoughts, to noting a change in emotions, the context of the emotional change, and the coping skill used to improve mood. In general, participants have a relatively easy time learning coping skills and applying them to their depressive symptoms. By the midpoint in treatment, they give examples of how they use coping skills to improve their moods. In fact, they like some skills so much that it is difficult to get them to use other skills.

Catch the Positive Diary: A Tool to Promote Activation and Coping

As the name suggests, the Catch the Positive Diary (CPD) is designed to help the girls catch (attend to) positive events by helping them to self-monitor and record the occurrence of a variety of therapeutically important positive events. In treating depressed youth, the CPD is used to (1) activate a child through engagement in fun activities, (2) redirect the child's attention from negative to positive events, (3) increase the child's completion of therapeutically relevant activities, and (4) help the child find evidence that supports new, more adaptive beliefs and that counters negative beliefs. The CPD activates a change in the child's attention from negative to positive information, helping to restructure the child's maladaptive thoughts and beliefs.

The CPD is a chart listing positive events to be self-monitored, with a column for each day of the week. There is also a place for the child to rate her mood each day. The list of positive events increases and changes over the course of treatment, as the lists are tailored for the individual girls' case conceptualizations. Commonly occurring positive events may be included on the list as a means of directing a girl's attention to evidence that contradicts the belief that "nothing good ever happens to me." Thus, the girls may be instructed to add to their lists events such as receiving a compliment, getting a good grade, playing an instrument, doing a nice job on an art project, hearing something funny, laughing with friends, acting silly, hearing a song you like, dancing, and so forth. Depressed youth generally fail to notice these common positive and, as such, mood-enhancing events. Thus, self-monitoring of these events restructures core beliefs and the negative thoughts that arise from them. For example, a child may hold the distorted belief that she is unlovable. If the therapist has proof that she is loved, she helps the girl to construct a list of critical events that prove that she is loved. As these events occur, the child checks them off in her diary and the outcome of the assignment is processed during the next meeting. When such tasks are given to a child, it is useful to complete the list early in the meeting so that she can practice monitoring the occurrence of an event during the meeting. In this way the therapist can help her recognize examples of the target events.

Self-monitoring of enjoyable activities leads to an increase in the frequency of these activities.

To further motivate the girls, the therapist can graph each girl's mood and the number of recreational activities completed each day. The graph visually illustrates the relationship between the two as mood improves with increased engagement in fun activities. An overarching goal of the treatment program, and of the CPD, is to improve mood by increasing the frequency and types of coping skills used by the girls. As the other categories of coping skills are taught to the girls and the benefits are experienced in session, the girls' favorite examples of these coping skills are added to the list. Thus, the list expands from fun activities to include soothing and relaxing activities, activities that vigorously expend energy, social activities, and coping thoughts. The CPD is a very flexible tool that can be used for many therapeutic purposes.

Problem-Solving Training

As the girls acquire a better understanding of their emotions, they are taught that some of the undesirable situations that lead to unpleasant emotions can be changed. Problem solving is the strategy they use to plan for changing undesirable situations. The five-step problem-solving sequence is formally introduced during the fifth meeting. During this meeting, the group also creates a list of the problems that girls of their age typically face. Then the group goes through the list and determines which problems can be changed and which cannot. For problems that cannot be changed, the therapist asks which coping skill they would use to moderate the impact of such situations.

The problem-solving procedure used here is a modification of that described by Kendall (see, e.g., Kendall & Braswell, 1993). Through education, modeling, coaching, rehearsal, and feedback, children are taught to break down problem solving into five component steps. To help the girls remember, the therapist refers to the steps as the "5 P's"—(1) problem definition (**Problem**), (2) goal definition (**Purpose**), (3) solution generation (**Plans**), (4) consequential thinking (**Predict and Pick**), and (5) self-evaluation (**Pat on the back**). Steps are defined in a developmentally sensitive manner, and activities are used to illustrate the meaning and purpose of each step.

The negativity of depressed youth can interfere with their implementation of problem solving; however, there are some steps that can be taken to minimize the impact of this negativity. For example, the first step in the process—problem identification and definition—may be the most difficult step for depressed children to learn, as they often view a problem as a personal threat. To a depressed child, the existence of a problem means that there is something wrong with her or that the problem represents an impending loss. In addition, depressed children with a helpless core belief feel overwhelmed by problems and think that they cannot solve them. Thus, their sense of hopelessness has to be combated through concrete experience demonstrating that they can, in fact, overcome problems. The second step in the problem solving sequence is identifying the desired outcome for the problem. The key to helping depressed youth with the second step—identifying their goals—is to help them to choose constructive goals and to avoid destructive goals. Generating alternative solutions—the third step—is especially difficult for those with a core belief of helplessness, because they typically believe that nothing will work to help them. As depressed youth try to use consequential thinking—the fourth step—when faced with real-life problems, the therapist often has to help them recognize potential positive outcomes. It is necessary at this step to combat the youngsters' pessimism, as it is easier for them to generate reasons why a plan will not work rather than why it will. They often base their predictions on how they are feeling (emotional reasoning). The final step involves monitoring and evaluating the outcome of the plan. When the girls first start using problem solving, it is important for the therapist to process the outcome of a plan, as depressed youngsters are likely to minimize their successes, magnify their failed attempts, and attribute failures to themselves. The girls are taught to use coping statements for unsuccessful plans, as well as other coping skills, to help themselves deal with the unpleasant affect associated with a failed plan.

Once the girls have learned the problem-solving steps and the therapist and other group members have helped them generate a plan that has a high probability of being successful, the girls have to actually implement the plan in their real-life situations. A girl is more likely to try if she believes that the plan will work and if she believes that she has the ability to successfully implement it. Thus, it is important to address both of these issues with the girls as the plans are developed and the girls are assigned homework to implement them. It may be useful to ask a girl if she can foresee anything that would get in the way of her trying the plan. A problem-solving homework form can be completed during the meeting as the therapist and other group members help her work through the steps and develop the plan. She can then refer to this form as she tries to implement the plan. It is helpful to begin applying the problem solving to simpler problems with solutions that are more likely to be successful. Thus, the girl develops a history of success with problem solving, which increases the probability that she will use it in the future. Cognitive restructuring strategies can also be used to get the girls over the cognitive roadblocks that prevent them from using problem solving outside the meetings. These strategies are discussed next.

Cognitive Restructuring

ESTABLISHING THE RELATIONSHIP BETWEEN THOUGHTS AND MOODS

To effectively restructure a child's distorted thoughts and beliefs, it is necessary to first establish a relationship between negative thoughts and unpleasant mood and other depressive symptoms. It is possible to do this through a number of methods. Although cognitive restructuring is specifically taught to the children during the later sessions, it is possible to establish this relationship in the earlier meetings. During the earlier meetings the therapist watches for opportunities to educate the children about the relationship between their negative thoughts and unpleasant mood and other depressive symptoms. Whenever a child states how she feels, the therapist links the feeling to the thoughts she had. For example:

> CHILD: I felt horrible last night.
>
> THERAPIST: What were you thinking when you felt horrible?
>
> CHILD: That my only friend had dumped me.
>
> THERAPIST: Oh, I see. If you think that your only friend no longer likes you, you feel horrible. How would you have felt if you had thought that she was upset but that she would be over it tomorrow?

This procedure of using the child's own experiences to illustrate the link between thoughts and feelings is the most desirable way to build the child's understanding of this relationship. It is necessary to do this repeatedly throughout treatment.

A number of in-session activities are used to supplement the linking of the girls' thoughts and their emotions. Early in treatment, when the relationship between thoughts and feelings is still being established, the therapist writes thoughts on cutouts of "thought bubbles" and the names of various emotions on heart-shaped cutouts. These cutouts are placed inside a paper bag. The girls take turns pulling a cutout from the bag. If a thought bubble is chosen, then the girl is instructed to state the emotion that would go with it. If an emotion cutout is chosen, then the child is instructed to state the thought that is likely to cause that emotion. The other group members can help as needed or offer additional examples. The therapist can choose to complete some additional processing such as: "When was the last time you felt that way? What was happening? What were you thinking?" The therapist should try to make the thought and emotion cutouts real for the girls by using thoughts that the girls have verbalized during previous meetings and by using examples of the girls' emotional experiences as reported in previous meetings. These and other activities are designed to teach the girls through their own in-session experiences. They can then be used to extend the girls' understanding of the nature of cognition and its relationship to emotional adjustment.

ESTABLISHING THE RATIONALE FOR COGNITIVE RESTRUCTURING

It is important for the girls to understand that they construct their thoughts, that their thoughts may not be true, and that they can change them. To accomplish this, the therapist shows the girls a cartoon of a common situation that is open to multiple interpretations that is experienced by girls of their age. The girls are instructed to each write a very short story about what is happening in the cartoon. Typically, they come up with very different stories. They share their stories, and then the therapist processes the outcome with them.

> "How could all of you be looking at the same picture but see it in different ways? What does this tell us about the way we think?"
> "Which story is correct? What does that tell us about the way we think?"
> "Debbie, can you see the same thing Lisa saw? Shaniqua, can you see it the way Melissa did? So, you can change the way that you think about things?"
> "Who can tell us about a time when you thought something and it turned out that you saw it the wrong way—you misunderstood it?"
> "When you are depressed, what do you think happens to your thinking? Are your thoughts more positive or more negative?"
> "Did you know that often when you are depressed, your thoughts aren't true? They lie to you and make you see things in a negative way when this isn't true."

To illustrate the negative bias in depressive thinking, the girls are asked to complete a task in which each is given a large bead to put into her shoe between the sole and the bottom of her foot. Then each is given a Jolly Rancher to suck on. The girls are instructed to walk around and notice the discomfort of the bead. Then they are asked to concentrate on the fruity, sweet flavor of the candy.

THERAPIST: What happens when you concentrate on the candy?

CHILD: The bad feeling goes away.

THERAPIST: What happens when you concentrate on the bead?

CHILD: You forget about the candy and get annoyed at the bead.

THERAPIST: So two things are happening at the same time and you can notice one or the other, depending on which one you attend to? When someone is feeling depressed, which one do you think that person attends to?

CHILD: The bead.

THERAPIST: What happens to the good things, like the candy, that are happening at the same time?

CHILD: They are ignored.

THERAPIST: Right. When someone is feeling depressed, she is likely to notice only the unpleasant, negative, or unwanted things that are going on and then she misses the good things that are happening. So, if you noticed only the negative things that are going on, how would you feel?

CHILD: Really down.

THERAPIST: Right. What would happen if you also noticed the good things that were happening?

CHILD: You would feel good.

THERAPIST: Right, and how would you feel if you noticed both things?

CHILD: Okay.

THERAPIST: Yes. So, if you want to feel better, should you pay more attention to the beads in your life or the sweet things? Were you able to do this just a minute ago when you were walking around?

CHILD: Yes.

THERAPIST: Ah ha, so that is what we are going to work on. Noticing the sweet and good things.

To successfully use cognitive restructuring, it is necessary to teach the children two important points. First, that their thoughts often are not true. Second, that we are continually confronted with multiple ways of thinking about things and that we are making choices about what we want to think and believe. Children and adolescents believe that their thoughts are objective and reflect the truth. They do not understand that their thoughts are constructed, biased by their past learning history, and may be far from the truth. "Just because you think it, it doesn't mean that it is true." (Beck, 1995). This is a surprising revelation for children. The activities used within the group and examples from the children's lives are used to make this point ring true for the girls. Helping the girls to recognize that their depression lies to them through negative thoughts has therapeutic value in and of itself. In many situations, we can choose what we want to believe because there is no clear-cut, definitive way of thinking that is right. So, sometimes we have to look at the practical outcome of believing a negative thought and then weigh the advantages to choosing to believe an alternative viable and possibly true thought. Once again, real-life situations are used to make this point.

When the children understand that their thoughts affect their emotions, that their thoughts are constructed, and that thinking more realistically will help them feel better, they can begin to focus on their own negative thoughts.

IDENTIFYING NEGATIVE THOUGHTS

To independently restructure negative thoughts and the beliefs that underlie them, children must become aware of their own thoughts. Negative thoughts are easier to recognize when someone else expresses them; therefore, we begin by asking the girls to notice others' negative thoughts as a bridge to recognizing and identifying their own negative thoughts. To accomplish this, the therapist and the girls discuss how to recognize negative thoughts and then make a game of catching each other's. The girls are instructed to call out, "Negative thought," whenever someone expresses one through their in-group statements. The therapist purposely makes many negative statements to give the girls practice at doing this and to normalize being the recipient of the "negative thought" comment. Subsequently, the girls are asked to catch and record their own negative thoughts on homework forms, which they bring to the group.

COGNITIVE RESTRUCTURING STRATEGIES

The cognitive restructuring process involves identifying distorted thoughts and then providing the child with corrective learning experiences. Depressed youth are taught to recognize and then evaluate negative thoughts, using a number of cognitive restructuring strategies. A variety of in-session activities and therapeutic homework exercises are used to teach youngsters to be "Thought Judges," who evaluate the validity of their negative thoughts using two questions: (1) What is another way to think about it? and (2) What is the evidence? If a child's negative thought is realistic and reflects a situation that can be changed, then the youngster is encouraged to use problem solving to develop and follow a plan that produces improvement. If the situation is real but cannot be changed, then a coping strategy is used to manage her reaction to the situation.

Negative thoughts are restructured by the therapist throughout treatment as they are identified. During the first nine meetings, the therapist identifies negative thoughts and asks questions that lead to cognitive restructuring. Consequently, the girls are not required to do a lot of self-reflection outside the meetings. The girls are introduced to the cognitive restructuring procedure during meeting 6 so that they can better understand what the therapist has been helping them to do during the early meetings. Cognitive restructuring becomes the focus of treatment in meetings 10 to 20. This requires the youngsters to become more self-focused and to focus on negative thoughts that can exacerbate depressive symptoms. However, they can manage the upset that comes with increased self-focus by using coping and problem-solving skills taught earlier in treatment. The therapist helps to start the shift in thinking and serves as a model for how to do it.

Once a negative thought has been identified, the child is taught to ask one of the two "Thought Detective Questions" as a means of evaluating the thought's validity and developing adaptive thoughts to replace the negative ones. The girls learn the question that is best suited for different negative thoughts. "What's another way to think about it?" is the easiest cognitive restructuring question for children to learn. They use this question to generate alternative, plausible, and positive thoughts about a distressing situation. So this is a good question to use when the girls draw a negative conclusion from a situation from which many other viable conclusions could be drawn. "What's the evidence?" is used when the objective facts do not support the child's negative thought.

The standard cognitive restructuring procedure is difficult to teach children to use—once again reflecting a developmental difference between children and adults. A powerful tool in this case is an activity that the girls refer to as "Talking back to the Muck Monster." When the participants are having difficulty changing, or letting go of, negative thinking, we refer to this as being "stuck in the negative muck." The girls like and understand this metaphor. When they are stuck in the negative muck, it is the "Muck Monster" that is filling them with negative thoughts and holding them back from extricating themselves from the muck. Somewhat surprisingly, the girls consistently report having an image of the Muck Monster. They are eager to describe it, and they are asked to draw it in preparation for the activity. Therapists encourage this, as it depersonalizes negative thinking, creates emotional distance between the child and her depressive thinking, and creates a concrete opponent to defeat. Talking back to the Muck Monster is completed as many times as needed to help the girls learn how to restructure their negative thoughts between the 10th meeting and termination.

The therapist maintains a list of each girl's negative thoughts, which includes thoughts endorsed on the pretreatment assessment measures, verbalized during treatment meetings, and recorded on homework forms. This list represents the content of each girl's Muck Monster. During an individual meeting that occurs between meetings 10 and 11, the therapist discusses each girl's list with her in order to confirm that it "rings true" and to make her aware of these thoughts and beliefs, as well as their impact on emotions, behavior, and interpersonal relationships. The beliefs are written inside the girls' drawings of their Muck Monsters, and the thoughts that stem from the beliefs are written in thought bubbles around the Muck Monster.

To help the girls learn how to independently apply cognitive restructuring, they are asked to talk back to the Muck Monster using the two Thought Detective Questions. To accomplish this, an extra chair is brought to the group meetings for the Muck Monster. The therapist moves to the empty chair and holds a child's picture of the Muck Monster while she states one of the child's negative thoughts. The girl forcefully uses the two Thought Detective Questions to guide her talking back to the Muck Monster. Group members help her to do this by providing additional evidence or alternative interpretations. The girls may be encouraged to very forcefully talk back to the Muck Monster by yelling at it. Other group members assist and cheer her on as she forcefully evaluates negative thoughts and then replaces them with more realistic positive ones. Sometimes it is helpful to have one of the girls play the role of the Muck Monster and have her hold the drawing of the Muck Monster as she verbalizes her own negative thoughts, while the therapist forcefully talks back to the Muck Monster by using the two Thought Detective Questions. The girls enjoy this activity, and it helps them learn how to use cognitive restructuring. To provide the girls with additional help in applying cognitive restructuring outside the meetings, the workbook has forms that guide the process of catching, evaluating, and replacing negative thoughts.

Restructuring of negative thoughts is also completed indirectly through guided learning experiences incorporated into treatment. These learning experiences are chosen on the basis of the case conceptualization initially developed before treatment meetings begin and further refined over the ensuing meetings. Thus, at the same time that the therapist is refining the case conceptualizations, she is watching for opportunities to use the child's own experiences to help her process evidence that contradicts her negative beliefs and supports new, more adaptive beliefs. For example, a girl whose underlying core belief is "I'm unlovable," with an intermediate belief "No one likes me," states that the following events happened between meetings. She talked with a friend on the Internet. She had a friend sleep over during the weekend. She was invited to a birthday party. She and her mom baked Christmas cookies together. Her mom tucks her into bed and says prayers with her every night. Through Socratic questioning, each of these events can be used to help her see that she is liked by peers and loved by significant others. The therapist also gives the child specific homework assignments that provide her with learning experiences that contradict existing negative beliefs and build new, more adaptive beliefs.

BUILDING A POSITIVE SENSE OF SELF

The primary objective of cognitive restructuring is to help the children build positive core beliefs about themselves. Depressed children evaluate their performances, possessions, and personal qualities more negatively than nondepressed youth, and their self-evaluations tend to be negatively distorted (Kendall, Stark, & Adam, 1990). During the last eight meetings, additional activities are used to support a positive sense of self. This treatment component appears last because all of the other skills are used during the process.

One of the tools used to help youngsters develop a more positive sense of themselves is the "self-map." The self-map consists of a relatively large circle in the middle of a page with a series of smaller circles surrounding it. Each small circle has a line connecting it to the larger middle circle, and most of the smaller circles have labels such as "Friend," "Daughter," "Student," and the like. The large circle represents the child, and the smaller circles represent the multitude of characteristics that the child possesses. Each circle represents an area of the child's life and an aspect of self-definition. Overall, the self-map helps the girls to broaden their self-definitions and to recognize more strengths than they previously acknowledged. Participants are asked to fill in each bubble with relevant strengths. In addition, parents and teachers are interviewed by the therapist to identify their perceptions of the child's strengths in each of the domains. This information is provided to the girls by the therapist. We have found that this information can be very powerful, as the children enjoy receiving the compliments. In addition, group members provide each other with positive feedback for each circle. Once again, receiving this information from peers appears to be very powerful and believable.

The CPD is used as the children are asked to self-monitor evidence that supports the positive self-descriptions outlined on the self-maps. For example, a child may base much of her self-worth on her musical talent. She would be instructed to self-monitor her successes during class, individual instruction, practice, and concerts. In addition, emphasis would be put on her effort toward becoming a better musician, rather than on comparing herself with others. Furthermore, the personal pleasure she derives from playing her instrument would be emphasized.

In some instances, the children's negative self-evaluations are accurate and they can benefit from change. In such instances, the goal of treatment is to help the youngsters to translate personal standards into realistic goals and then to develop and carry out plans for attaining their goals. Following the translation process, the children prioritize the areas in which they are working toward self-improvement. Initially, a plan is formulated for producing improvement in an area where success is probable. The long-term goal is broken down into subgoals, and problem solving is used to develop plans that will lead to the attainment of subgoals and, eventually, the main goal. Prior to enacting their plans, the children try to identify possible impediments to carrying out the plans. Once again, problem solving is used to develop contingency plans for overcoming the impediments. Once the plans, including contingency plans, have been developed, the children self-monitor their progress toward change. Alterations to plans are made along the way.

Parent Training

Parent training (Stark, Simpson, Yancy, & Molnar, 2007a, 2007b) is designed to support the child treatment component by teaching parents how to reinforce their child's efforts to apply therapeutic skills and to apply the same skills themselves. Parents are taught a number of skills that are designed to remediate possible disturbances in family functioning. The parent-training meetings are completed in groups at their daughter's school after school hours. Meetings are conducted by the child's therapist and last approximately 90 minutes. There are eight group parent meetings and two individual family meetings completed over the 11 weeks that their daughters are participating in treatment (see Table 10.2). The individual family meetings occur between the third and fourth group meetings and again between the seventh and eighth group meetings. The daughters also participate in half of the parent meetings and both individual family meetings. The meetings are structured similarly to the child meetings. However, in addition, prior to reviewing the main points from the previous parent meeting, the girls provide the parents with a description of the skills they have learned and then try to teach the parents how to use them.

Skills Taught to the Parents

Parents are provided with information about depression in children and young teens, our model of depressive disorders, and how to successfully treat them. To create a more positive environment, parents are taught to manage their daughters' behavior through the use of reinforcement for desirable behavior. At the same time, they are instructed to decrease their use of punitive and coercive strategies. Teaching parents this more positive approach to managing their daughters' behavior creates a home environment that has a positive affective valence, and it sends the girls a positive message about themselves ("I am a good person") and about their parents ("They pay attention to me"). During the first two parent group meetings, parents learn the impact of positive reinforcement on their daughters and how to effectively use it. They apply it during meetings when their daughters are present. They are also instructed to monitor their use of positive reinforcement at home. During the second meeting, the girls help their parents develop a reward menu and identify areas in which they think they could benefit from some more parental encouragement. In addition, during this meeting, parents experience the power of doing fun things with their daughters as they play a game together. Parents are encouraged to help their daughters do more fun things as a coping strategy, and they are encouraged to do more recreational things as a family. During the third meeting, the parents are taught the deleterious effects of excessive use of punishment. They are helped to identify all of the forms of punishment they use and are encouraged to decrease the use of punishment and to replace it with positive reinforcement.

During the same week that the girls set their goals for treatment and collaboratively work with the therapist to identify the plans for obtaining their goals, the therapist conducts individual family meetings and collaborates with the parents to identify their goals for their daughter and their family. In addition, with the girl's permission, the therapist and the parents go over the child's goals for treatment and the plan for obtaining the goals. Parents are encouraged to support these goals, and actions they can take to help their daughter achieve her goals are discussed.

Parents are taught a variety of communication skills, including empathic listening as well as the following skills:

1. Keep it brief.
2. Don't blame.
3. Be specific.
4. Make feeling statements.
5. Give options if possible.

These skills are modeled by the therapists, role-played by the therapists and parents, and practiced during sessions by the parents and their daughters. The training begins with discussions on easy topics and then progresses to more emotionally laden topics.

Empathic listening is important because it communicates to the child that she is being listened to and understood, which leads to a sense of being loved and worthy. In addition, it is a cornerstone of good communication between the girls and their parents. The girls are taught to ask their parents if it is a good time to talk, when they are feeling upset or experiencing a problem. Likewise, the parents are taught to initiate a conversation with their daughter when they sense she is upset. Once the conversation is initiated, the parent clears his or her mind of distractions and then listens to the daughter without providing her with any quick comforts or solutions. The parent listens for the emotion or message that underlies the girl's statements. This can be very difficult for parents, as they may have a hard time just listening and an even harder time identifying the underlying emotions or broader meaning. It takes a good deal of role playing and coaching for the parents to be able to listen empathically. In some cases, it seems that the best that can be done is to teach a parent to become an active listener.

Parents are also taught the same five-step problem-solving procedure that the girls learn. Parents are taught to view misbehavior and any problems the family faces as merely problems to be solved. The girls teach their parents the steps and then play a game with their parents as a procedure for demonstrating the meaning of each step and how to apply each step to a simple situation—in this case, the game. Once the parents have been exposed to the steps and understand the process, the therapist divides the parents and daughters into family units and provides the families with a hypothetical family problem to be solved.

Elevated levels of conflict are commonly reported in families with depressed children (Stark et al., 1990) and it is related to the length of the depressive episode. Thus, parents are taught conflict resolution skills. More specifically, they are taught how to structure and use family meetings as a means of reducing conflict. The first step in a family meeting is to say something positive about each family member. Then the person who has called the meeting sets the agenda, states the issue, and gives examples of the personal impact of the point of conflict. Next, this person initiates a discussion about alternative behaviors that would solve the problem, and the family discusses potential outcomes for each alternative. Finally, a plan is chosen and initiated. The families role-play the meeting process with coaching from the therapists. Emphasis is placed on catching the conflict early before the upset gets so bad that it cannot be constructively managed. Over the course of the next few meetings, the therapist works with the parents to eliminate barriers to resolving conflict, such as parent beliefs.

Parents can play a significant role in helping their daughters to catch, to evaluate, and to restructure their negative thoughts and beliefs. During the second individual family meeting and during the seventh and eighth group parent meetings, the parents learn about the impact of negative thinking on their daughters' emotional well-being. They are taught to look at the messages they inadvertently send to their daughters through their own actions and through the things they say. During the individual family meeting, and while the individual families are grouped in their own constellations within the larger group meeting, the girls describe the impact of their specific negative thoughts on their emotions and the parents then help their daughters to "talk back" to the thoughts. Parents are encouraged to identify their own negative thoughts and to restructure them using the same procedures as their daughters use.

SUMMARY

The ACTION program is designed to teach girls to use unpleasant affect and other depressive symptoms as cues to employ coping, problem-solving, and cognitive restructuring skills. Affective education is used to teach the girls to recognize and identify their emotional experiences. Initially, treatment efforts are focused on pleasant emotions and positive experiences as a means of creating an improvement in mood. Subsequently, the girls are taught to use coping strategies in situations that they cannot change, problem solving when they can change a situation, and cognitive restructuring when their symptoms are caused by negatively distorted thinking. Consistent with principles of cognitive therapy, the treatment sessions are highly structured, with each segment of the meeting intended to have therapeutic value.

The ACTION program is designed to change the family environment through parent training. Parent training teaches parents to use positive reinforcement as the primary means of managing behavior and to decrease the use of punitive and coercive behavior management procedures. Parents are taught empathic listening as well as other communication skills. Family problem solving and conflict resolution skills are taught as a means of reducing stress due to conflict within the family. Another important aspect of the parent-training component is to help parents understand how they can support their daughters in the application of the ACTION skills in the home environment. Finally, parents are encouraged to apply the skills their daughters are learning to their own lives.

REFERENCES

Altshuler, J. L., & Ruble, D. N. (1989). Developmental changes in children's awareness of strategies for coping with uncontrollable stress. *Child Development, 60,* 1337–1349.

Arieti, S., & Bemporad, J. R. (1980). The psychological organization of depression. *American Journal of Psychiatry, 137,* 1360–1365.

Asarnow, J. R., Goldstein, M. J., Tompson, M., & Guthrie, D. (1993). One-year outcomes of depressive disorders in child psychiatric inpatients: Evaluation of the prognostic power of a brief measure of expressed emotion. *Journal of Child Psychology and Psychiatry, 34,* 129–137.

Beck, A. T., Rush, J., Shaw, B. F., & Emery, G. (1979). *Cognitive therapy of depression.* New York: Guilford Press.

Beck, J. (1995). *Cognitive therapy: Basics and beyond.* New York: Guilford Press.

Bell-Dolan, D. J., Reaven, N. M., & Peterson, L. (1993). Depression and social functioning: A multidimensional study of the linkages. *Journal of Clinical Child Psychology, 22,* 306–315.

Bettes, B. A. (1988). Maternal depression and motherese: Temporal and intonational features. *Child Development, 59*(4), 1089–1096.

Blechman, E. A., McEnroe, M. J., Carella, E. T., & Audette, D. P. (1986). Childhood competence and depression. *Journal of Abnormal Psychology, 95,* 223–227.

Brent, D. A., Perper, J. A., Mortiz, G., Allman, C., Friend, A., Roth, C., et al. (1993). Psychiatric risk factors for adolescent suicide: A case-control study. *Journal of the American Academy of Child and Adolescent Psychiatry, 32,* 521–529.

Breznitz, Z., & Sherman, T. (1987). Speech patterning of natural discourse of well and depressed mothers and their young children. *Child Development, 58,* 395–400.

Campbell, S. B., Cohn, J. F., & Meyers, T. (1995). Depression in first-time mothers: Mother–infant interaction and depression chronicity. *Developmental Psychology, 31,* 349–357.

Cicchetti, D., Ganiban, J., & Barnett, D. (1991). Contributions from the study of high-risk populations to understanding the development of emotion regulation. In J. Garber & K. Dodge (Eds.), *The development of emotion regulation and dysregulation* (pp. 15–48). New York: Cambridge University Press.

Cole, D. A., & Rehm, L. P. (1986). Family interaction patterns and childhood depression. *Journal of Abnormal Child Psychology, 14,* 297–314.

Cole, D. A., & Turner, J., Jr. (1993). Models of cognitive mediation and moderation in child depression. *Journal of Abnormal Psychology, 102,* 271–281.

Cole, P., & Kaslow, N. J. (1988). Interactional and cognitive strategies for affect regulation: Developmental perspective on childhood depression. In L. Alloy (Ed.), *Cognitive processes in depression* (pp. 310–343). New York: Guilford Press.

Costello, E. J., Mustillo, S., Erkani, A., Keeler, G., & Angold, A. (2003). Prevalence and development of psychiatric disorders in childhood and adolescence. *Archives of General Psychiatry, 60*(8), 837–844.

Coyne, J. C. (1976). Toward an interactional description of depression. *Psychiatry, 39,* 28–40.

Dodge, K. A. (1991). Emotion and social information processing. In J. Garber & K. Dodge (Eds.), *The development of emotion regulation and dysregulation* (pp. 159–181). New York: Cambridge University Press.

Dunn, J., & Brown, J. (1991). Relationships, talk about feelings, and the development of affect regulation in early childhood. In J. Garber & K. Dodge (Eds.), *The development of emotion regulation and dysregulation* (pp. 89–108). New York: Cambridge University Press.

Emslie, G. J., Heiligenstein, J. H., Wagner, K. D., Hoog, S. L., Ernest, D. E., Brown, E., et al. (2002). Fluoxetine for acute treatment of depression in children and adolescents: A placebo-controlled, randomized clinical trial. *Journal of the American Academy of Child and Adolescent Psychiatry, 41,* 1205–1215.

Emslie, G. J., Rush, A. J., Weinberrg, W. A., Gullion, C. M., Rintelmann, J., & Hughes, C. W. (1997). Recurrence of major depressive disorder in hospitalized children and adolescents. *Journal of the American Academy of Child and Adolescent Psychiatry, 36,* 785–792.

Felner, R. D., Lease, A. M., & Phillips, R. S. C. (1990). Social competence and the language of adequacy as a subject matter for psychology: A quadripartite trilevel framework. In T. P. Gullotta, G. R. Adams, & R. Montemayor (Eds.), *The development of social competence in adolescence* (pp. 245–264). Beverly Hills, CA: Sage.

Forehand, R., Body, G., Slotkin, J., Fauber, R., McCombs, A., & Long, N. (1988). Young adolescents and maternal depression: Assessment, interrelations and family predictors. *Journal of Consulting and Clinical Psychology, 56,* 422–426.

Garber, J., Braafladt, N., & Weiss, B. (1995). Affect regulation in depressed and nondepressed children and young adolescents. *Development and Psychopathology, 7,* 93–115.

Garber, J., Braafladt, N., & Zeman, J. (1991). The regulation of sad affect: An information-processing perspective. In J. Garber & K. A. Dodge (Eds.), *The development of emotion regulation and dysregulation* (pp. 208–240). New York: Cambridge University Press.

Jacobsen, R. H., Lahey, B. B., & Strauss, C. C. (1983). Correlates of depressed mood in normal children. *Journal of Abnormal Child Psychology, 11,* 29–40.

Kane, P., & Garber, J. (2004). The relations among depression in fathers, children's psychopathology, and father–child conflict: A meta-analysis. *Clinical Psychology Review, 24,* 339–360.

Kashani, J. H., Ray, J. S., & Carlson, G. A. (1984). Depression and depressive-like states in preschool-age children in a child development unit. *American Journal of Psychiatry, 141,* 1397–1402.

Kazdin, A. E., Esveldt-Dawson, K., Sherick, R. B., & Colbus, D. (1985). Assessment of overt behavior and childhood depression among psychiatrically disturbed children. *Journal of Consulting and Clinical Psychology, 53,* 201–210.

Kendall, P. C., & Braswell, L. (1993). *Cognitive-behavioral therapy for impulsive children* (2nd ed.). New York: Guilford Press.

Kendall, P. C., Stark, K. D., & Adam, T. (1990). Cognitive deficit or cognitive distortion in childhood depression. *Journal of Abnormal Child Psychology, 18,* 255–270.

Kennedy, E., Spence, S., & Hensley, R. (1989). An examination of the relationship between childhood depression and social competence amongst primary school children. *Journal of Child Psychology and Psychiatry, 30,* 561–573.

Kliewer, W., & Lewis, H. (1995). Family influences on coping processes in children and adolescents with sickle cell disease. *Journal of Pediatric Psychology, 20,* 511–525.

Kochanska, G., Kuczynski, L., Radke-Yarrow, M., & Welsh, J. D. (1987). Resolutions of control episodes between well and affectively ill mothers and their young children. *Journal of Abnormal Child Psychology, 15,* 441–456.

Kolb, B., & Whishaw, I. Q. (1996). *Fundamentals of human neuropsychology* (4th ed.). New York: Freeman.

Kopp, C. B. (1989). Regulation of distress and negative emotions: A developmental view. *Developmental Psychology, 25,* 343–354.

Lewinsohn, P. M. (1974). A behavioral approach to depression. In R. J. Friedman & M. M. Katz (Eds.), *The psychology of depression: Contemporary theory and research* (pp. 50–87). New York: Guilford Press.

March, J. (2004). The treatment for adolescents with depression study (TADS): Short-term effectiveness and safety outcomes. *Journal of the American Medical Association, 292,* 807–820.

Marmorstein, N. R., & Iacono, W. G. (2004). Major depression and conduct disorder in youth: Associations with parental psychopathology and parent–child conflict. *Journal of Child Psychology and Psychiatry, 45,* 377–386.

Masters, J. C. (1991). Strategies and mechanisms for the personal and social control of emotion. In J. Garber & K. Dodge (Eds.), *The development of emotion regulation and dysregulation* (pp. 182–207). New York: Cambridge University Press.

Mullins, L. L., Peterson, L., Wonderlich, S. A., & Reaven, N. M. (1986). The influence of depressive symptomatology in children on the social responses and perceptions of adults. *Journal of Clinical Child Psychology, 15,* 233–240.

Nomura, Y., Wickramaratne, P. J., Warner, V., Mufson, L., & Weissman, M. M. (2002). Family discord, parental depression and psychopathology in offspring: Ten-year follow-up. *Journal of the American Academy of Child and Adolescent Psychiatry, 41,* 402–409.

Peterson, A. C., Sarigiani, P. A., & Kennedy, R. E. (1991). Adolescent depression: Why more girls? *Journal of Youth and Adolescence, 20,* 247–271.

Peterson, L., Mullins, L. L., & Ridley-Johnson, R. (1985). Childhood depression: Peer reactions to depression and life stress. *Journal of Abnormal Child Psychology, 13,* 597–609.

Poznanski, E. O., & Zrull, J. (1970). Childhood depression: Clinical characteristics of overtly depressed children. *Archives of General Psychiatry, 23,* 8–15.

Puig-Antich, J., Lukens, E., Davies, M., Goetz, D., Brennan-Quattrock, J., & Todak, G. (1985). Psychosocial functioning in prepubertal major depressive disorders: I. Interpersonal relationships during the depressive episode. *Archives of General Psychiatry, 42,* 500–507.

Rossman, B. R. (1992). School-age children's perceptions of coping with distress: Strategies for emotion regulation and the moderation of adjustment. *Journal of Child Psychology and Psychiatry, 33,* 1373–1397.

Saarni, C., & Crowley, M. (1990). The development of emotional regulation: Effects on emotional state and expression. In E. A. Blechman (Ed.), *Emotions and the family: For better or for worse* (pp. 53–73). Hillsdale, NJ: Erlbaum.

Sacco, W. P., & Graves, D. J. (1984). Childhood depression, interpersonal problem-solving, and self-ratings of performance. *Journal of Clinical Psychology, 13,* 10–15.

Sander, J. B., & McCarty, C. A. (2005). Youth depression in the family context: Familial risk factors and models of treatment. *Clinical Child and Family Psychology Review, 8*, 203–219.

Sanford, M., Szatmari, P., Spinner, M., Munroe-Blum, H., Jamieson, E., Walsh, C., et al. (1995). Predicting the one-year course of adolescent major depression. *Journal of the American Academy of Child and Adolescent Psychiatry, 34*, 1618–1628.

Sargrestano, L. M., Paikoff, R. L., Holmbeck, G. N., & Fendrich, M. (2003). A longitudinal examination of familial risk factors for depression among inner-city African American adolescents. *Journal of Family Psychology, 17*, 108–120.

Sheeber, L., Hops, H., Alpert, A., Davis, B., & Andrews, J. (1997). Family support and conflict: Prospective relations to adolescent depression. *Journal of Abnormal Child Psychology, 25*, 333–344.

Sheeber, L., & Sorensen, E. (1998). Family relationships of depressed adolescents: A multimethod assessment. *Journal of Clinical Child Psychology, 27*, 268–277.

Stark, K. D., Hargrave, J. L., Schnoebelen, S., Simpson, J. P., & Molnar, J. (2005). Treatment of childhood depression. In P. C. Kendall (Ed.), *Child and adolescent therapy: Cognitive behavioral procedures* (3rd ed.). New York: Guilford Press.

Stark, K. D., Humphrey, L. L., Crook, K., & Lewis, K. (1990). Perceived family environments of depressed and anxious children: Child's and maternal figure's perspectives. *Journal of Abnormal Child Psychology, 18*, 527–547.

Stark, K. D., Laurent, J., Livingston, R., Boswell, J., & Swearer, S. (1999). Implications of research for the treatment of depressive disorders during childhood. *Applied and Preventive Psychology: Current Scientific Perspectives, 8*, 79–102.

Stark, K. D., Schmidt, K., & Joiner, T. E. (1996). Depressive cognitive triad: Relationship to severity of depressive symptoms in children, parents' cognitive triad, and perceived parental messages about the child him or herself, the world, and the future. *Journal of Abnormal Child Psychology, 24*, 615–625.

Stark, K. D., Schnoebelen, S., Simpson, J., Hargrave, J., Glenn, R., & Molnar, J. (2006). *Children's Workbook for ACTION.* Broadmore, PA: Workbook Publishing.

Stark, K. D., Simpson, J., Schnoebelen, S., Hargrave, J., Glenn, R., & Molnar, J. (2006). *Therapist's Manual for ACTION.* Broadmore, PA: Workbook Publishing.

Stark, K. D., Simpson, J., Yancy, M., & Molnar, J. (2007a). *Parent training manual for ACTION.* Broadmore, PA: Workbook Publishing.

Stark, K. D., Simpson, J., Yancy, M., & Molnar, J. (2007b). *Workbook for ACTION parent training manual.* Broadmore, PA: Workbook Publishing.

Stice, E., Ragan, J., & Randall, P. (2004). Prospective relations between social support and depression: Differential direction of effects for parent and peer support? *Journal of Abnormal Psychology, 113*, 155–159.

Thompson, R. A. (1991). Emotion regulation and emotion development. *Educational Psychology Review, 3*, 269–307.

Wierzbicki, M., & McCabe, M. (1988). Social skills and subsequent depressive symptomatology in children. *Journal of Clinical Child Psychology, 17*, 203–208.

11 Positive Psychotherapy for Young Adults and Children

Tayyab Rashid and Afroze Anjum

Think of Emma—a typical depressed adolescent; she is sad, empty, slow, has little appetite and low libido, sleeps a lot, and is anxious occasionally. On the basis of these symptoms, a *Diagnostic and Statistical Manual of Mental Disorders* (DSM-IV-TR; American Psychiatric Association, 2000) Axis I diagnosis will be given to her. A number of treatment options are available for Emma. She can spend months or even years in trying to access and then interpret the finer aspects of her internalized anger; she can learn to untwist her faulty thinking; she can learn to better understand her relational difficulties, and, of course, Emma can benefit from antidepressant medication. These options will help her to learn what is wrong with her, but what is right about her will be left high and dry. They can overlook certain facts, such as that Emma cares for her friends, occasionally savors natural and artistic beauty, often resolves interpersonal conflicts amicably, has risen to the occasion in the face of a trauma in the past, and loves creative writing, becoming totally absorbed in the process whenever she writes, albeit intermittently. Extensive and planned therapeutic effort will be spent in undoing Emma's guilt, shame, and thinking errors, but no systematic doses of optimism, hope, zest, or courage will be dispensed.

Psychotherapies that attend explicitly to the strengths as well as the weaknesses of clients like Emma are few and far between. We have created and piloted one such psychotherapy, which explicitly builds positive emotions, strengths, and meaning in clients' lives to promote happiness. We call this approach positive psychotherapy (PPT). This chapter describes the story of PPT. To make the case, we first discuss the pervasive power of negatives and the importance of attending to them in therapy. In doing so, we acknowledge and highlight the benefits of traditional therapies, which have primarily attended to negative emotions and characteristics of clients. However, we argue that therapy needs to go beyond negatives and should also explicitly focus on the positive emotions and strengths of a client. We survey theoretical notions of well-being, growth, positive emotions, and strengths, as well as interventions that have explicitly targeted happiness. Next, we introduce PPT and describe its theoretical assumptions, content, potential mechanism of action, and process. Although we believe that PPT may be an effective treatment for many disorders, depression is our primary empirical target here. We present results from preliminary studies, including two randomized controlled trials (RCTs) with depressed young adults and children. Finally, we conclude by highlighting potential clinical applications, ongoing studies, and limitations of PPT.

ENAMORED WITH NEGATIVES

We are enamored with the negative, bad, and evil. Machiavelli, Schopenhauer, Hegel, Darwin, Marx, and Freud—all have described the evil and negative undercurrent of human existence. Freud (1996) even asserted, "I have found little that is 'good' about human beings on the whole. In my experience most of them are trash." Not surprisingly, he thought (Freud, 1995) that human civilization is merely a sublimation of sexual and aggressive drives. Negatives almost seem to have seductive power because of their potency, intricacies, and valence. Pursuit of negatives is pervasive in academia, literature, and art. From *Desperate Housewives* to *Fear Factor*, the contemporary media thrive on negatives, as fear, violence, abuse, graft, greed, jealously, insecurity, and sexual infidelity are carefully and creatively juxtaposed in news, dramas, music, and films. In his opening line to *Anna Karenina*, Leo Tolstoy (1877/1999) wrote that although all happy families are alike, each unhappy family is unhappy in its own way. Accounts of evil, bad, and negatives arouse our curiosity more than stories of virtue, good, integrity, cooperation, altruism, and modesty. We ruminate about negative emotions for months, and sometimes for years, rather than savor positive moments. The pain of losing $100 stings us more than the pleasure we feel at gaining $100 (Kahneman & Tversky, 1984). Bad emotions, bad parents, and bad feedback have more impact than good ones. Bad impressions and stereotypes are quicker to form and more resistant to disconfirmation than good ones (Baumeister, Bratslavsky, Finkenauer, & Vohs, 2001). Much like mainstream culture, psychology has been fascinated with the darker side of human behavior. Social psychology focuses on racism, aggression, prejudice, and discrimination; cognitive psychology on processing errors, negative schemas, biases, and illusions; school psychology on dyslexia, dysgraphia, phonological problems, attentional deficits, and a host of developmental disorders; and clinical psychology on symptoms, disorders, trauma, and stress.

But why are we attracted more to negatives than to goods? Perhaps it is courtesy of our Pleistocene (ice age) brains that evolved from our firefighting needs. Seligman (2002) observes, "Negative emotions—fear, sadness and anger—are our line of defense against external threats, calling us to battle stations" (p. 30). Danger, loss, and trespass are threats to self-preservation. Throughout evolution, life has been a Darwinian fitness test of putting out fires, tackling trespassers and ensuring food, shelter, and a mate. However, the pain of preservation has yielded specific gains. David Buss (2000) maintains that psychological pain, depression, varieties of anxiety, fear, and phobias, and specific forms of anger and grievances solve specific adaptive problems such as sexual coercion (pain), inhabiting a subordinate position in the social hierarchy (depression), spousal infidelity (jealousy), and the blocking of one's goal-directed behavior (anger). Those who are attuned more to negatives survive. Thus, attending to negatives is adaptive. There is strong and accumulating evidence that negatives carry more weight and impact (e.g., Cottrell & Neuberg 2005; Hoorens, 1996; Rozin & Royzman, 2001; Wright, 1988) and that the human brain is wired to react more strongly to bad than to good (Ito, Larsen, Smith, & Cacioppo, 1998; Luu, Collins, & Tucker, 2000). There are more negative emotions than positive ones—twice as many, by one count (Nesse, 1991). Therefore, perception and analysis of negative states and traits comes naturally to us. In therapy, clients' negatives stand out more saliently than their positives. Moreover, clients often seek therapy because it is hard for them to let go of negatives easily. Negative emotions cause psychological pain, and coming to therapy is an attempt to mitigate this pain. Acknowledging the omnipresence of negatives and also being sensitive to the psychological pain of clients, PPT's basic premise is not to negate negatives but to approach them differently—undoing them by targeting strengths as well as symptoms. As Duckworth, Steen, and Seligman (2005) put it, this is a *"build-what's-strong"* approach to supplement the traditional *"fix-what's-wrong"* approach. PPT with Emma will entail using more frequently her social intelligence, kindness, appreciation of beauty, resiliency, and creativity, in addition to working on her depressive symptoms.

Dividends of Focusing on Negatives in Psychotherapy

Psychotherapy has made huge strides by focusing on negatives. Rigorous random assignment studies have demonstrated that psychotherapy helps significantly more than placebo and perhaps more long-lastingly than medications (Lambert et al., 2003; Shadish, Navarro, Matt, & Phillips, 2000; Seligman, 1995). Moreover, today there are empirically validated therapies for more than a dozen mental ailments, such as depression, schizophrenia, obsessive–compulsive disorder, panic disorder and so forth (Barrett & Ollendick, 2004; Kazdin & Weisz, 2003). A focus on negatives has also refined specific forms of psychotherapies, and we now have empirically validated treatments for specific disorders, such as exposure for phobias and posttraumatic stress disorder, cognitive-behavior therapy for depression, bulimia, headache, panic, and irritable bowel syndrome, and insight-oriented therapy for marital discord (Plante, 2005). Moreover, we have vastly increased our understanding of finer, yet important, aspects of psychotherapy such as therapeutic alliance, nuances of therapeutic communication, nonverbal language, therapist effects, treatment process, and the process of feedback to and from the client (Weinberger, 1995; Wampold, 2001). Nevertheless, the focus on pathology has mitigated symptoms effectively but has not necessarily enhanced happiness, which is left high and dry. Despite understanding the evolutionary, philosophical, social, and psychological underpinnings of the pervasive impact of negatives, we feel that there is little empirical justification for psychology's predominantly negative view of human nature, which influences psychotherapy significantly. Perhaps it is time we reexamine our assumptions regarding psychotherapy. Psychotherapy, in its present state, is far from being a comprehensive treatment. It effectively reduces symptoms but does not necessarily enhance happiness. Reduction or even remittance of symptoms does not automatically enhance happiness. In fact, there is a growing awareness that some psychotherapies confound response to treatment with full recovery. Moreover, therapy outcome researchers have expressed concern that quality of life needs to be included in the evaluation of treatment outcome (Gladis, Gosch, Dishuk, & Crits-Christoph, 1999). Therefore, psychological well-being needs to be incorporated into the definition of recovery (Fava, 1996). Ryff and Singer (1996) have suggested that an absence of well-being creates conditions of vulnerability to possible future adversities and that the path to lasting recovery lies not exclusively in alleviating symptoms but in engendering the positive. Psychotherapy needs to be a hybrid enterprise that includes alleviation of psychopathology as well as promotion of happiness.

Complete Mental Health

Human beings want to be happy, not just less afraid, sad, or anxious. More than two millennia ago, Aristotle thought that happiness was the whole aim and end of human existence. People rank the pursuit of happiness as one of their most cherished goals in life in almost every culture researchers have examined (Diener & Oishi, 2000). Duckworth et al. (2005) argue that persons who carry the weightiest psychological burden care about much more in their lives than just the relief of their suffering. Troubled persons want more satisfaction, contentment, and joy, not just less sadness and worry. They want to build their strengths, not just to lessen sadness—and they want lives imbued with meaning and purpose. The current *modus operandi* of psychotherapy, working largely on symptoms, does indeed make clients like Emma less sad and anxious but does not increase their satisfaction, contentment, joy, and happiness. Empirically, happiness and psychopathology are not opposite ends of a single continuum. Measures of psychopathology (e.g., depression) correlate modestly and negatively with various measures of happiness and well-being (Ryff & Keyes, 1995). Specifically, measures of happiness and well-being correlate on average −.51 with the Zung Depression Inventory (Zung, 1965) and −.55 with the Center for Epidemiologic Studies Depression Scale (CES-D; Radloff, 1977). Life satisfaction and happiness associate about −.40 to −.50 with scales of depression symptoms (Frisch, Cornell, Villanueva, & Retzlaff, 1992). In short, there is about 25% shared variance between common scales of depression and happiness and subjective well-being. The Midlife in the United States (MIDUS) study of 3,032 adults between the ages of 25 and 74 found that only 21.6% of the population are *flourishing*, that is, feeling positive emotions toward life and functioning well psychologically and socially (Keyes, 2003). Nearly 20% of the adults fit the criteria for *languishing*, a state in which an individual is devoid of positive emotion toward life, is not functioning well psychologically or socially, and has been depressed during the past year. The rest are somewhere between languishing and flourishing. Individuals who are flourishing have excellent health, miss fewer days at work, cut back on work on fewer days, and have fewer physical limitations in their daily lives, whereas languishing individuals tend to have emotional distress and psychological impairment at levels that are comparable to the impairment associated with a major depressive episode. Thus, complete mental health as suggested by Keyes and Lopez (2002) is not merely the absence of psychopathology, nor is it just the presence of high levels of well-being and happiness. It is a complete state consisting of (1) the absence of psychopathology and (2) the presence of happiness, well-being, and life satisfaction. Therefore, the current state of psychotherapy is half-baked as it targets only absence or reduction of symptoms. Psychotherapy should not only target the undoing of symptoms but also explicitly enhance happiness. It should not seek to move a client only from −8 to −2, but also to +8. Doing so, we hope, will not only treat psychological disorders effectively but will also prevent their future recurrence.

Potential for Prevention

Positive emotions and strengths are some of the best candidates to prevent psychopathology. Human strengths such as courage, future-mindedness, optimism, emotional and social intelligence, spirituality, honesty, and perseverance can act as buffers against psychological disorders. Traditional psychotherapies merely treat symptoms, but not necessarily prevent them from recurring. To appreciate the difference between treatment and prevention, consider an example. The substantial drop in cardiovascular disease in the United States, the United Kingdom, and other developed countries has not arisen primarily from the availability of better individual treatments. Rather, it has arisen largely from efforts to educate the public about health promotion measures advocating the importance of exercise, healthy diet, and smoking cessation (Puska, Vartiainen, Tuomilheto, Salomaa, & Nissinen, 1998). Attending early enough to the positive emotions and strengths of those who are genetically vulnerable to psychological problems or who live in neighborhoods that foster these difficulties could reduce their impact (e.g., by teaching skills to use strengths to cope with problems) and can have long-lasting beneficial effects on individuals and society. Similarly, investing in parent education in children's early years can prevent a number of physical as well as psychological problems in the children later on. Creating educational systems that promote the strengths-based well-being, happiness, and flourishing of students, and not necessarily imparting more cognitive knowledge, could pay future dividends. Unfortunately, most mental health resources are currently dedicated to treatment.

Research in prevention, albeit scarce, has demonstrated that positive emotions buffer individuals against depressive symptoms (Gillham & Reivich, 1999). Increased well-being has been identified as having a protective effect in terms of vulnerability to chronic and acute life stresses (Ryff & Singer, 2000). Several well-controlled studies have documented a clear link between frequent positive emotions and longevity. For example, in the Netherlands, Giltay and colleagues (Giltay, Geleijnse, Zitman, Hoekstra, & Schouten, 2004) studied 999 men and women (ages 65–85) and found that those who reported high levels of optimism had a 55% lower risk of death from all causes and a 23% lower risk of cardiovascular death than people who reported high levels of pessimism. Similar studies (e.g., Danner, Snowdon, & Friesen, 2001; Moskowitz, 2003; Ostir, Markides, Black, & Goodwin, 2000) have convinced us that identifying and then promoting positive emotions and strengths of nonclinical and at-risk individuals can provide effective prevention. In particular, a primary prevention that targets children and adolescents by promoting their strengths can act as a strong buffer against future psychopathology. Durlak (1995) has pointed out that only 8% of normal children go on to have serious adjustment problems as adults (as against 30% of clinically dysfunctional children). Thus, there is clearly a strong case for improving the lives of at-risk and normal individuals, as this will increase their vitality, capabilities, and skills, which in turn will act as a strong buffer against future psychopathology. After realizing that focusing on illness, disease, and physical symptoms does not address what it means to be truly healthy (Ryff & Singer, 1998, 2002), the medical field is gradually changing. From its emphasis on the treatment of disease, the focus first shifted to the prevention of disease and then to the promotion of physical well-being. Psychology needs to make a similar shift, because in its fascination with negatives, it has fallen short in identifying distal buffers such as positive emotions, individual strengths, and social connection, which could prevent psychopathology in the first place (Gable & Haidt, 2005). PPT, based on strengths, we believe, is well suited to provide effective prevention.

The notions of happiness, well-being, and fulfillment have not been invented by positive psychology or PPT. These notions, amid the great flurry of activity focused on symptoms, have been around for decades, although voiced quietly. In the following section we briefly review both the theoretical notions of happiness and interventions that have attempted to enhance happiness explicitly.

HAPPINESS: SOME THEORETICAL NOTIONS

For ages, philosophers and sages have pursued happiness—trying to define it and enumerating conditions that lead to it. Greek philosophers had differing notions of happiness. Socrates, Plato, and Aristotle essentially emphasized the pursuit of a virtuous and good life (eudemonic well-being) as necessary to attain happiness. Epictetus stressed suppressing desires and accepting fate as an essential condition of happiness, whereas Epicurus promoted the satisfaction of desire as necessary for happiness. Lord Byron thought that celebration of one's uniqueness and awareness of one's experience was happiness. For Jane Austin, virtues of constancy and amiability brought happiness, and Benjamin Franklin emphasized that industry, temperance, and cleanliness were essential for well-being. In *The Conquest of Happiness*, Bertrand Russell (1930) postulated that mental discipline or "hygiene of the nerve," which controls and counteract worrisome thoughts, and balance between work, family, and leisure achieved happiness. Psychologists have also explored happiness and related concepts. As early as 1894, Mark Baldwin and McKeen Cattell edited the *Psychological Review*, published by Macmillan & Company which included terms like *higher manifestations of mind, ideals and values and aesthetics* (Sloan, 1980). William James, the father of American psychology, observed in *Varieties of Religious Experience* (1902/1999) that courage, hope, and trust have conquering efficacy over doubt, fear, and worry. John Dewey's (1933) concept of optimal functioning was based on artistic-esthetic transactions between person and environment that fully absorb the individual. This resonates with Csikszentmihalyi's *Flow* (1990) (described later). Henry Murray (1938) deemed that the study of positive, joyful, and fruitful experiences of a person was essential to advance the course of psychology. Terman studied giftedness and marital happiness (Terman, 1939; Terman, Buttenweiser, Johnson, & Wilson, 1938). Jung (1934) explored the importance of individuation and meaning of life to attaining the fulfillment of the collective qualities of human beings. Thus, before World War II, well-being, optimal functioning, meaning, and happiness feature prominently in the psychological literature. In fact, Seligman and Csikszentmihalyi (2000) noted three clear missions of psychology before World War II: curing psychopathology, making the lives of all people more productive and fulfilling, and identifying and nurturing talent. However, immediately after the war, the assessment and treatment of psychopathology became the exclusive mission, largely owing to economic and political factors (Maddux, 2002). Yet humanistic psychology continued to advocate for positives in the therapeutic framework. Maslow felt that too little attention was given to subjects like creativity, healthy and normal personality, love, play, perspective in life, personal growth, and higher levels of consciousness. His books, such as *Towards a Psychology of Being* (1999), *Religions, Values and Peak Experiences* (1964) and *The Farther Reaches of Human Nature* (1971), represent seminal efforts to systematically study positive states and traits. Maslow believed that a healthy (self-actualizing) personality had a superior perception of reality, increased acceptance of self, others, and nature, increased spontaneity, increased problem centering, increased autonomy, resistance to enculturation, higher frequency of peak experiences, increased identification with human species, more democratic character structure, and increased creativity. Akin to the notion of *flow* (Csikszentmihalyi, 1990) in the contemporary movement of positive psychology (described later), Maslow (1971) described self-actualization as

> experiencing fully, vividly, selflessly, with full concentration and total absorption . . . this is the moment when the self is actualized itself. As individuals, we all experience such moments

occasionally. As counselors, we can help clients to experience them more often. We can encourage them to become totally absorbed in something and to forget their poses and their defenses and their shyness—to go at it "whole-hog." (pp. 45–50)

Maslow's contemporary, Rogers (1959), proposed that deep down, human beings strive to become all they can be. There is an inherent tendency of the organism to develop all its capacities in ways that enhance the organism. This is development toward autonomous determination, expansion and effectiveness, and constructive social behavior. Marie Jahoda (1958) wrote a provocative book, *Current Concepts of Positive Mental Health* (1958), that made a persuasive argument that well-being should be explicitly attended to in its own right. Jahoda extracted six processes that contribute to well-being: acceptance of oneself, growth/development/becoming, integration of personality, autonomy, accurate perception of reality, and environmental mastery. Similarly, Allport (1961) postulated that extension of the sense of self, warm relating of self to others, emotional security, realistic perception, insight, and humor are all hallmarks of a mature personality. More recently, Ryff and colleagues (Ryff & Singer, 1996, 1998) identified six components of psychological well-being that markedly overlap with Jahoda's notion of well-being. Rokeach (1973) and Schwartz (1994) also identified several factors, such as satisfaction of biological needs, coordination of social interaction, and facilitation of societal functioning, that are arguably "universal" requirements of fulfillment and survival. Ryan, Sheldon, Kasser, and Deci (1996) have postulated that well-being is based on three universal psychological needs, namely, autonomy, competence, and relatedness, and that the gratification of these needs is a key predictor of psychological well-being. These notions of happiness and well-being only dot the psychological literature, reflecting a minuscule minority of works as compared with the hundreds of thousands of volumes on psychopathology. Consequently, the holy grail of psychotherapy is rich, complex, and variegated in its efforts to cure psychopathology. Hundreds, if not thousands, of forms of psychotherapies are available to treat symptoms, but only a few have targeted happiness. We survey these few next.

Psychotherapies Targeting Happiness Explicitly

Fordyce (1977, 1983) was the first researcher to develop and test a "happiness" intervention. Fordyce focused on the characteristics of happy people to extract 14 strategies for increasing happiness, such as being active, socializing more, engaging in meaningful work, forming closer and deeper relationships with loved ones, lowering expectations, and prioritizing being happy. In order to assess level of happiness, Fordyce developed and tested the Fordyce Happiness Survey, a global measure of happiness that is still used widely. In a series of studies, Fordyce compared the happiness of students who had received detailed instructions on the 14 strategies to be happy, with a control group whose members had not received such instructions. He found that the students who had received detailed instructions were happier and showed fewer depressive symptoms at the end of the term than the members of the control group. In addition, Fordyce mailed a follow-up survey 9–18 months later to a small subset of participants and found that the gains in happiness and lack of depressive symptoms were maintained.

A well-being therapy (WBT) has been developed and tested in Italy (Fava 1999). It is based on Carol D. Ryff's multidimensional model of psychological well-being (Ryff & Singer, 1996, 1998), which converges closely with Jahoda's (1958) notions of positive mental health noted above. WBT focuses on building environmental mastery, personal growth, purpose in life, autonomy, self-acceptance, and positive relations with others. It uses various techniques to help clients focus on moments of well-being in their lives and keep a written record of them and encourages self-observation. The effectiveness of WBT in the residual phase of affective disorders was tested in a small controlled trial. Twenty patients with an affective disorder who successfully completed pharmacological or psychotherapeutic treatment were randomly assigned to WBT or cognitive-behavioral therapy (CBT) for residual symptoms. Both WBT and CBT were associated with a significant reduction of residual symptoms and an increase in personal well-being. However, a significant advantage of WBT over CBT was observed. In another validation study (Fava & Ruini, 2003) WBT was given to patients with recurrent major depression. All of these patients had been treated successfully with antidepressant medication. They were randomly assigned to either CBT plus WBT or a clinical management group. Participants who were exposed to CBT + WBT had a significantly lower rate of residual symptoms and a significantly lower relapse rate of 25% at a 2-year follow-up, as compared with members of the control group, who showed a relapse rate of 80%.

Integrating cognitive therapy with the ideas of positive psychology, Frisch has devised and empirically validated quality of life therapy (QOLT; Frisch 2006). Happiness in QOLT is conceived as the fulfillment of cherished goals, needs, and wishes in 16 valued areas of life, including health, spiritual life, work, play, learning, creativity, helping, love, friendship, and community. A bibliotherapy outcome study (Grant, Salcedo, Hynan, & Frisch, 1995) was conducted to assess the efficacy of QOLT in treating depression. Sixteen clinically depressed community volunteers who showed an aptitude for and interest in bibliotherapy, and were not suffering from other disorders, met weekly to discuss a manual on QOLT. All participants who completed treatment were reclassified as nondepressed and showed significant increases in quality of life and self-efficacy. All but one participant maintained these improvements at a follow-up assessment.

Instilling hope has been translated into formal treatment. Based on Snyder's (1994) theory of hope, Lopez and colleagues (2004) developed a program, Making Hope Happen, for seventh graders that aims to enhance hope through five weekly 45-mintue sessions. The children were taught about hope with the use of pictorial representations and narratives depicting characters with high hope, and were taught skills to distinguish between hopeful and unhopeful statements. Results showed that participants in the program had significantly higher levels of hope in comparison to their counterparts who did not participate in the program. Group and individual hope enhancement strategies for adults have also been developed and evaluated (Cheavens, Gum, Feldman, Michael, & Snyder, 2001). One such intervention, by Klausner, Snyder, and Cheavens (2000), has demonstrated that depressed older adults benefited from group therapy focused on goal setting, increasing the production of pathways and agency through actual work on reasonable goals, discussion of the process, and weekly homework assignments. Results indicated that hopelessness and anxiety decreased significantly, whereas hope increased reliably. Moreover, in comparison to members of a reminiscence therapy group, members of the hope-focused group experienced a more substantial decrease in depressive symptomatology.

These interventions have had a minimal impact on psychotherapy approaches and practice. Paradoxically, there are hundreds of self-help books, retreats, workshops, motivational talks, and camps and numerous similar television shows—most of which focus on positive affirmations, self-esteem uplifts, and freeing of spirit. These are delivered by armchair gurus and pop psychologists who often propose dramatic New Age solutions, which make the audience feel better temporarily but lack long-term curative effects. It is argued that distressed individuals seek these untested regimens because they seek happiness, which traditional therapy does not offer—at least not explicitly. We believe that by ignoring happiness, psychotherapy has missed happiness as a legitimate treatment goal. Its fascination with negatives, suffering, and pain has seen only "the half-empty glass." PPT brings the "half-full" part of the proverbial glass to the foreground. Next, we describe PPT in detail.

ASSUMPTIONS OF PPT

Human Nature Has an Inherent Capacity for Growth, Fulfillment, and Flourishing

Psychotherapies have existed throughout history and have always been rooted in philosophical views of human nature (Wachtel, 1997). Mainstream psychology views psychotherapy as a practice in which symptoms, usually leaking from the unconscious, are explored, or maladaptive behaviors strengthened by environmental reinforcement are unlearned, or irrational beliefs leading to problematic feelings and behaviors are correctly thought out, or troubled relationships are thoroughly explored. All of these therapeutic endeavors are rooted in beliefs about human nature. For example, the Freudian view, most prevalent in the popular culture, media, and academia, perceives human nature as motivated primarily by sexual and aggressive drives. Seligman (2002) calls it "rotten-to-the-core" (p. xiv), a dogmatic view of human nature that reduces the client to a mere slave of damaged habits and sexual drives. If this view is true, the function of therapy is essentially to keep aggressive and sexual drives in restraint. Maslow and Rogers, before Seligman, questioned this fundamental assumption of mainstream psychology and suggested that instead of tending toward destruction, human beings are motivated toward developing their full potential. Rogers observed:

> I have little sympathy with the rather prevalent concept that man is basically irrational, and thus his impulses, if not controlled, would lead to destruction of others and self. Man's behavior is exquisitely rational, moving with subtle and ordered complexity toward the goals his organism is endeavoring to achieve. (1969, p. 29)

PPT does not see a client as a mere slave of damaged habits, sexual drives, faulty thoughts, and troubled relationships. The client is not a passive actor whose behavior is reinforced by responses from the environment. Rather, the client has good and bad states and traits that influence each other. Unlike those who ascribe to the pathology-oriented model, we assume that psychopathology does not reside entirely within the client. Much like a client has a susceptibility to psychopathology, the client also has an inherent capacity for happiness. Indeed, it is the interaction between the client and the environment that generates psychopathology and happiness. In PPT we acknowledge that human beings in general, and clients seeking therapy in particular, are prone to attend to, perceive, analyze, and internalize negatives more sharply than positives. However, at the same time, we conceive human nature broadly, equipped with sophisticated executive centers, with the potential to rise above natural selection and consciously civilize actions and habits to alter genetic influences. A client's good and bad behaviors may be genetically influenced but not genetically determined. PPT assumes that a client's behavior is best understood on dimensions, not in categories. Dividing behavior into categories may confuse us as to reality. Alan Watts (1966) has stated, "However much we divide, count, sort, or classify [the world] into particular things and events, this is no more than a way of thinking about the world. It is never actually divided" (p. 54). In symptom- and disorder-oriented therapy, clients are generally viewed as passive victims of intrapsychic and biological forces who need help with their diseases and disorders *only*, not with their well-being. These victims are deemed to be a clinical population that forms a separate category from the nonclinical. Pointing to this artificial categorization, Bandura (1978) commented, "No one has ever undertaken the challenging task of studying how the tiny sample of clinic patrons differs from the huge population of troubled nonpatrons" (p. 94). Perhaps it is not a surprise that psychology has little to offer for nonclinical individuals who want to make their lives more fulfilling and happier. Psychology is not just a branch of medicine concerned with illness or health; it is much larger. It is about work, education, insight, love, growth, and play (Seligman & Csikszentmihalyi, 2000). But these larger aspects of psychology cannot be explained adequately when clients are viewed as victims of unconscious motivation or flawed thinking. Psychopathology appears not only because of unresolved conflicts and erroneous thinking, but when growth, fulfillment, and flourishing are thwarted. And clients are fully capable of growing, maturing to drop the old adjustment as outworn, like an old pair of shoes.

Positive Emotions and Traits Are as Authentic as Symptoms

As noted above, evolution and the psychological literature inform us that negatives command the attention of a psychotherapist more than positives. Clients seeking therapy are socialized to believe that therapy is a place to discuss and deal with troubles. They readily describe how negative emotions, negative actions, bad parents, and bad feedback impact their lives. Of course, they include the emotional impacts of relationship failures, traumas, sour interpersonal interactions, and setbacks at work, which outweigh the joy of their accomplishments, friendships, smiles, and giggles. They more vividly remember the pain of transgression than the pleasure of companionship. They want to discuss quickly formed and harder-to-change opinions about others. They share with the therapist the struggle they have because, despite trying, they cannot let go of painful experiences and keep on ruminating about them (Nolen-Hoeksema, Parker, & Larson, 1994). In the traditional, pathology-oriented model of psychotherapy, these negatives are perceived, analyzed, and further synthesized into personality structures with an underlying assumption that symptoms are authentic and central ingredients of therapy, whereas positives are seen as by-products of symptom relief, or at most, clinical peripheries that do not need exclusive attention. So steeped is this assumption in mainstream psychology that the *Diagnostic and Statistical Manual of Mental Disorders*, fourth edition (DSM-IV) calls affiliation, anticipation, altruism, and humor "defense mechanisms (American Psychiatric Association, 2000, p. 752). Altruistic behavior is considered as a defense, as noted by a psychodynamic theorist (McWilliams, 1994): "Depressive people often handle their unconscious dynamics by helping others, by philanthropic activity, or by contributions to social progress that have the effect of counteracting their guilt" (p. 238). Criticizing this view sharply, Seligman (1999) has asked:

> How has it happened that the social sciences view the human strengths and virtues—altruism, courage, honesty, duty, joy, health, responsibility and good cheer—as derivative, defensive or downright illusions, while weakness and negative motivations—anxiety, lust, selfishness, paranoia, anger, disorder and sadness—are viewed as authentic? (p. 559)

PPT regards positive emotions and strengths of clients as being as authentic as their weaknesses are, valued in their own right, contributing to happiness as weaknesses and symptoms contribute to psychological disorders. Moreover, we seriously question the assumption that strengths are psychological defenses. If true, was Mother Teresa's compassion for the poor of Calcutta a defense to deal with her anxiety? Was Princess Diana's struggle to rid the world of land mines anger against Prince Charles? Was Gandhi's civil disobedience movement an attempt to sublimate anger against his father? Was Eleanor Roosevelt's altruism a compensation for her mother's narcissism and her father's alcoholism? Was Martin Luther King Jr.'s struggle for civic rights an attempt to overcome his inferiority complex? Are the strivings of Aung San Suu Kyi of Burma, Ken SaroWiwa of Nigeria, and Shirin Ebadi of Iran mere defensive masks to hide their unconscious motives?

Human strengths are as real as human weaknesses, as old as time, and are valued in every culture (Lopez, Snyder, & Rasmussen, 2003; Peterson & Seligman, 2004). Some therapists may argue that it is difficult to assess positive emotions, because they tend to be fleeting, or strengths, which may not be as prominent as weaknesses. Furthermore, the social desirability of strengths may elude a valid assessment, as some clients, in order to seek the therapist's attention may overreport them, or to avoid a perception of vanity may underreport them. Our response is twofold. First, exclusive focus on psychopathology has yielded sophisticated ways to assess symptoms and disorders. We have four editions of the manual on insanities (DSM) and thousands of self-report, observational, and physiological measures of psychopathology. Yet the assessment of strengths has seriously lagged behind. Peterson and Seligman's *Character Strengths and Virtues* (2004) represents the first systematic effort in organizing core human strengths to complement the *Diagnostic and Statistical Manual* (DSM) of the American Psychiatric Association (2000). A number of measures have been developed and validated to assess positive emotions and strengths such as the Values in Action, an Inventory of Strengths (Peterson & Seligman, 2004), Hope Scale (Snyder et al., 1996), General Happiness Scale (Lyubomirsky & Lepper 1999), Satisfaction with Life Scale (Diener, Emmons, Larsen, & Griffin, 1985), Positive Affectivity and Negative Affect Schedule (PANAS; Watson, Clark, & Tellegen, 1988), Orientation to Happiness (Peterson, Park, & Seligman, 2005) and Scales for Psychological Well-being (Ryff & Singer, 1996). Second, we believe that the favorable or unfavorable self-representations of clients seeking to gain attention, are part of content, which should be not statistically controlled (Lopez et al., 2003). Positive emotions and strengths are authentic and should be valued in their own right.

Of course, negatives have adaptive value in our lives, but perhaps this has been taken to the extreme. The central point of this chapter is that human existence encompasses more then just resentment, deception, competition, jealousy, greed, worry, and anxiety— it also includes honesty, cooperation, gratitude, compassion, contentment, and serenity. Hence, our function in therapy is not only to put out fires, eliminate dangers, reduce hostility, or alleviate moral, social, and emotional malaise, it is also to restore and nurture courage, kindness, modesty, perseverance, and emotional and social intelligence. The former approach makes life less painful, but the latter makes it fulfilling. Therefore, psychotherapy—the most visible face of psychology to a layperson—should not address only human weaknesses and misery, but also strengths and happiness.

Discussing Positive Emotions and Strengths Is Curative

Most traditional therapy, especially before the drug revolution, was conducted by talking about troubles such as bad parenting, suppressed emotions and memories, faulty thinking patterns, and resentment in interpersonal relations. The portrayal of therapy in Hollywood films (e.g., *Prince of Tides, Good Will Hunting, A Clockwork Orange, One Flew over the Cuckoo's Nest*) and on television talk shows, mostly anchored by pop psychotherapists, have further reinforced the public perception that talking about troubles, ventilation of the "inner child," and exploring injuries to self-esteem are cathartic and thereby curative. Hence, clients have been socialized to believe that therapy entails talking about troubles. Some clients at the onset of therapy even tell their therapist that, courtesy of their "Goggle" search, they are convinced that they meet DSM criteria for a specific disorder. Most of those seeking treatment view themselves as deeply flawed, fragile victims of cruel environments or casualties of bad genes. Talking about troubles with an emphatic, warm, and genuine therapist is indeed a powerful cathartic experience, which is deemed necessary in any form of psychotherapy. Therefore, all major approaches to psychotherapy emphasize that the therapist–client interaction should be positive and that therapist should generally be empathetic, genuine, warm, and professional (Luborsky, McLellan, Woody, & O'Brien, 1985). Indeed, therapy outcome research has shown that this is one of the most robust curative factors (Orlinsky, Ronnestad, & Willutzki, 2004; Wampold, 2001). However, with this also comes the assumption, without much empirical evidence, that strong therapeutic relationships between clients and therapists are best built while discussing specific varieties of troubles, such as repressed emotions and memories, irrational and faulty thinking patterns or unhealthy relationships. So, in therapy, the therapist and client talk about occasions when parents ignored the client's needs, not when they fulfilled them; the therapist explores interpersonal conflicts, not the adaptive compromises that resolved them. Therapists discuss with clients the transgressions of others, not the occasions when clients were forgiven; therapists elicit the selfishness of others, not their or the clients' compassion. Clients are encouraged to discuss the times when they were insulted, not when they were admired, appreciated, and complimented. In PPT, however, we think that it is not an absolute *sine qua non* that only discussion of troubles builds a strong therapeutic relationship and leads to a cure. Of course, warmth and unconditional regard and emphatic listening to troubles builds a powerful therapeutic bond, but discussing deeply felt positive emotions, experiences that demonstrate character strengths, happy memories, and accounts of meaningful pursuits can do the same. Exploring the strengths that clients use to effectively deal with troubles leads to a very different discussion than pathology-oriented inquiry: "What weaknesses have led to your troubles?" However, the discussion of psychological pain and distress is not discouraged or undermined. Rather, such an expression is encouraged but is not necessarily elaborated needlessly. The client's attention is gently drawn to the discussion of positives. Acknowledging that positives may not be readily available or accessible to the consciousness and memory of troubled clients, we encourage clients, through systematic exercises, to recollect positive experiences. We believe that such a process will establish rapport from which a strong therapeutic relationship will naturally flow. Moreover, we hope that with this approach, the therapist no longer remains an authority figure with expertise in diagnosing the ills of clients, but becomes a witness of the clients' deepest and most authentic psychological assets.

Furthermore, curing mental illness purely through talk therapy and emotional ventilation seems to be a Western notion. Westerners tend to apply formal logic while reasoning about their emotional states. They prefer to verbalize their reasoning, to categorize things and experiences, and are likely to overlook the influence of context on their behavior. In contrast, Easterners are willing to entertain apparently contradictory propositions, reflect more, and are better able to see relationships between events (Nisbett, 2003). Talk therapy is an extension of the Western intellectual heritage of discussion and dialogue, whereas contemplation, reflection, and meditation are Eastern mechanisms used in dealing with problems. The habit of categorizing and judging experiences locks us into mechanical reactions, argues Jon Kabat-Zinn (1991). Clients seek therapy because negative feelings and thoughts are painful for them, and they find themselves reacting in ways that have maintained this pain. But if therapy becomes only an exercise of discussing these maintaining factors in minute detail, tracing the origin of childhood resentments or monitoring every distorted thought, the benefits of therapy may be compromised. In addition, locating the cause of resentments in unsupportive parents and significant others, or attributing problems to the environment, may be counterproductive for some clients, who may come out of therapy believing, "*It was not my fault anyway.*" It is an interesting paradox in much of Western therapy that the therapist is expected to give complete attention and unconditional positive regard to the client, but the client is expected to be more self-indulgent (Rogers, 1951). Eastern therapeutic traditions, instead of talking about troubles, suggest that healing begins by paying attention to what the mind is doing, how incessant negative thoughts and feelings drain mental energy. Rather than talking about troubles, a method of inquiry—not used much in Western therapies—meditation, is offered. Meditation does not necessarily change the contents of thoughts and feelings; rather, it increases the client's awareness of his or her relationship to thoughts and feelings. Its goal is for the client to become more aware of thoughts and feelings and to learn to relate to them from a wider, decentered perspective as "mental events" rather than aspects of the self or as necessarily accurate reflections of reality (Teasdale et al., 2000; Wallace & Shapiro, 2006). Similarly, we contend that the focus of therapy should not be limited to discussing negative feelings and thoughts, but should also direct the client's attention to positive feelings, thoughts, and experiences. For example, deep reflection on a positive experience that initially received insufficient appreciation, followed by a discussion with the therapist, can uplift a client's depressed mood. Similarly, recalling actions that brought joy, contentment, and satisfaction can undo negative feelings. Rewriting bad events through forgiveness can loosen the hold of anger and resentment. Therefore, talking about troubles and ventilation of anger may not be the only vehicles of cure, and we should be open to complementary possibilities such as the exploration of positive experiences in therapy. We now turn to explaining PPT, its content, and process.

THEORETICAL BACKGROUND OF PPT

Positive psychology, from which PPT evolved, is the scientific study of positive emotions, positive individual traits, and the institutions that facilitate their development. Its aim is to catalyze a change in the focus of psychology, from preoccupation only with repairing the worst things in life to also building positive qualities (Seligman & Csikszentmihalyi, 2000). PPT is positive psychology's therapeutic effort to broaden the scope of psychotherapy from the alleviation of suffering to systematically enhancing happiness. PPT views even the most distressed clients as more than the sum of damaged drives, childhood conflicts, dysfunctional habits, and dysregulated brains. It asks for a more serious consideration of these clients' intact faculties, ambitions, positive life experiences, and strengths of character and how these can be marshaled to treat and buffer against disorders. Our central hypothesis in PPT is that building positive emotions, building strengths, and finding meaning are efficacious in treating psychopathology. As noted previously, it is "building what's strong" by supplementing "fix what's wrong" (Duckworth et al., 2005). Positive emotions, strengths, and meaning serve us best not when life is easy, but when life is difficult. For example, when one is depressed, having and using such strengths as perspective, integrity, fairness, and loyalty may become more urgent than in good times, may shore up and enable positive institutions like strong family, peers, and social support to assume an added and immediate importance, and may cultivate positive emotions to counteract the negative emotions of depression. Therefore, through PPT, positive psychology may offer one of the best ways to treat and prevent psychopathologies including depression.

PPT is based primarily on Seligman's (2002) idea that the vague and fuzzy notion of "happiness" can be decomposed into three more scientifically measurable and manageable components: positive emotion (the pleasant life), engagement (the engaged life), and meaning (the meaningful life). Each exercise in PPT is designed to further one or more of these (see Table 11.1 for idealized session planning).

The Pleasant Life

The pleasant life successfully pursues positive emotions about the present, past, and future. The positive emotions about the past are satisfaction, contentment, and serenity. Optimism, hope, trust, faith, and confidence are future-oriented positive emotions. Positive emotions about the present are divided into two crucially different categories: pleasures and gratifications. Pleasures include bodily pleasures and higher pleasures. The bodily pleasures are momentary positive emotions that come through the senses: delicious tastes and smells, sexual feelings, moving your body well, delightful sights and sounds. The higher pleasures are also momentary, set off by events more complicated and more learned than sensory ones, and they are defined by the feelings they bring about: ecstasy, rapture, thrill, bliss, gladness, mirth, glee, fun, ebullience, comfort, amusement, relaxation, and the like. These are rock bottom subjective feelings. The final judge is "whoever lives inside a person's skin." Gratifications make up the other category of positive emotions about the present. Unlike pleasures, they are not feelings but activities one likes to engage in, such as reading, rock climbing, dancing, good conversation, baseball, and playing chess.

Positive emotions change people's mindsets, widening the scope of their attention (Fredrickson & Branigan, 2005; Chesney, Darbes, Hoerster, Taylor, & Chamber, 2005) and increasing intuition (Bolte, Goschke, & Kuhl, 2003). Positive emotions speed recovery from the cardiovascular aftereffects of negative effects (Fredrickson, Mancuso, Branigan, & Tugade, 2000), alter frontal brain asymmetry, and improve the immune system (Davidson et al., 2003). Similarly, Danner et al. (2001) found that positive emotions expressed at age 22 by women entering a Catholic convent predicted their longevity at age 75. Nuns with high levels of positive emotions in young adulthood lived, on average, more than 9 years longer than those with low levels of positive emotions in young adulthood. In general, positive states are linked closely with physical health (see, e.g., Ostir et al., 2000; also see Fredrickson, 1998, and Fredrickson & Losada, 2005, for a review).

The cognitive literature on depression documents a downward spiral in which depressed mood and narrowing thinking interact with each other, leading to a worsening of the clinical symptoms of depression (Beck, Rush, Shaw, & Emery, 1979; Peterson & Seligman, 1984). Conversely, Fredrickson's (2001) *broaden-and-build* model shows that positive emotions broaden the thought–action repertoire, leading individuals to increased well-being, which in turn builds their social and psychological resources, and in doing so increases their life satisfaction. Positive emotions likely serve as a buffer against depression and many other psychological problems. Tugade and Fredrickson (2004) have also

TABLE 11.1. Idealized Session-by-Session Description of Positive Psychotherapy

Session and theme	Description
1: Orientation	*Lack of positive resources maintains depression* The role played by absence or lack of positive emotions, character strengths, and meaning in maintaining depression and an empty life is discussed. The framework of PPT, therapist's role, and client's responsibilities are discussed. *HW:* Client writes a one-page (roughly 300-word) positive introduction, in which a concrete story illustrating his or her character strengths is narrated.
2: Engagement	*Identifying signature strengths* Signature strengths in the positive introduction are identified, and situations are discussed in which these signature strengths have helped previously. Three pathways to happiness (pleasure, engagement, and meaning) are discussed in light of PPTI results. *HW:* Client completes VIA-IS questionnaire online, which identifies his or her signature strengths.
3: Engagement/ pleasure	*Cultivation of signature strengths and positive emotions* Deployment of signature strengths is discussed. Client is coached to formulate specific, concrete, and achievable behaviors regarding cultivation of signature strengths. The role of positive emotion in well-being is discussed. *HW (ongoing):* Client starts a blessings journal in which three good things (big or small) that happened during the day are written.
4: Pleasure	*Good versus bad memories* The roles of good and bad memories are discussed in terms of maintenance of symptoms of depression. Client is encouraged to express feelings of anger and bitterness. Effects of holding onto anger and bitterness on depression and well-being are discussed. *HW:* Client writes three bad memories, anger associated with them, and their impact in maintaining depression.
5: Pleasure/ engagement	*Forgiveness* Forgiveness is introduced as a powerful tool that can transform anger and bitterness into feelings of neutrality or even, for some, into positive emotions. *HW:* Client writes a Forgiveness Letter describing a transgression and related emotions and pledges to forgive the transgressor (if appropriate), but may not deliver the letter.
6: Pleasure/ engagement	*Gratitude* Gratitude is discussed as enduring thankfulness, and the roles of good and bad memories are highlighted again with emphasis on gratitude. *HW:* Client writes and presents a letter of gratitude to someone he or she has never properly thanked.
7: Pleasure/ engagement	*Midtherapy check* Both forgiveness and gratitude homework are followed up. These assignments typically take more than 1 week. The importance of cultivating positive emotions is discussed. Client is encouraged to bring and discuss the effects of blessing journal. Goals regarding using signature strengths are reviewed. The process and progress are discussed in detail. Client's feedback on therapeutic gains is elicited and discussed.
8: Meaning/ engagement	*Satisficing instead of maximizing* Satisficing (good enough; Schwartz, Monterosso, Lyubomirsky, White, & Lehman, 2002), instead of maximizing in the context of the hedonic treadmill is discussed. Satisficing through engagement is encouraged instead of maximizing. *HW:* Client writes ways to increase satisficing and devises a personal satisficing plan.

(continued)

TABLE 11.1. *(continued)*

Session and theme	Description
9: Pleasure	*Optimism and hope* Client is guided to think of times when he or she lost out at something important, when a big plan collapsed, when he or she was rejected by someone. Then client is asked to consider that when one door closes, another one almost always opens. *HW:* Client identifies three doors that closed and three doors that then opened.
10: Engagement/ meaning	*Love and attachment* Active–constructive responding (Gable et al., 2004) is discussed. Client is invited to recognize signature strengths of significant other. *HW1 (ongoing):* Active–constructive feedback: Client is coached on how to respond actively and constructively to positive events reported by others. *HW2:* Client arranges a date that celebrates his or her signature strengths and those of her or his significant other.
11: Meaning	*Family tree of strengths* Significance of recognizing the signature strengths of family members is discussed. *HW:* Client asks family members to take VIA-IS online and then draws a tree that includes signature strengths of all members of the family, including children. A family gathering is to be arranged to discuss everyone's signature strengths.
12: Pleasure	*Savoring* Savoring is introduced as awareness of pleasure and a deliberate attempt to make it last. The hedonic treadmill is reiterated as a possible threat to savoring, along with discussion on how to safeguard against it. *HW:* Client plans pleasurable activities and carries them out as planned. Specific savoring techniques are provided.
13: Meaning	*Gift of time* Ways of using signature strengths to offer the gift of time in serving something much larger than the self are discussed. *HW:* Client is to give gift of time by doing something that requires a fair amount of time and whose creation calls on signature strengths, such as mentoring a child or doing community service.
14: Integration	*The full life* The concept of the full life, which integrates pleasure, engagement, and meaning, is discussed. Client completes PPTI and other measures before the final session. Therapeutic progress, gains, and maintenance are discussed.

Note. HW, homework.

shown empirically that resilient people use positive emotions to rebound from, and find positive meaning in, stressful encounters. Research has shown that gratitude and forgiveness exercises enhance positive memories and positive emotions (see, e.g., Seligman, Steen, Park, & Peterson, 2005; Lyubomirsky, Sheldon, & Schkade, 2005; Burton & King, 2004; Emmons & McCullough, 2003; McCullough, 2000). We believe that lack of positive emotion and pleasure is not just a symptom of psychopathology, especially depression, but may partly be the cause of depression. Therefore, enhancing the pleasant life can be a goal of psychotherapy for depression, and it should be appealing for patients in a way that exploring the details of childhood traumas, arguing against catastrophic cognitions, or taking medication with potential adverse side-effects, are not.

The Engaged Life

The second "happy" life in Seligman's theory is the engaged life, a life that pursues engagement, involvement and absorption in work, intimate relations, and leisure (Csikszentmihalyi, 1990). Engagement is synonymous with Csikszentmihalyi's *flow*, a psychological state that accompanies highly engaging activities. Time passes quickly. Attention is completely focused on the activity. Total absorption is experienced; even the sense of self is lost (Moneta & Csikszentmihalyi, 1996). PPT posits that not only does depression correlate with lack of engagement in the main areas of life, but that lack of engagement may cause depression. We think engagement is an important antidote to boredom, anxiety, and depression. Anhedonia, apathy, boredom, and restlessness—hallmarks of many psychological disorders—are largely functions of how attention is structured at a given time. When we are sad or bored, the low level of challenge relative to our skills allows attention to drift. When we are anxious, challenge is perceived to exceed our capacities. Negative states characterized by disruption of attention, disengagement, mood instability and inability to concentrate, which are typical features of several psychological disorders, can be effectively dealt with by cultivation of engagement that entails meaningful life challenges.

Seligman (2002) proposed that one way to enhance engagement is to identify peoples' salient character strengths and then help them to find opportunities to use these strengths more. He calls the highest strengths *signature strengths*. PPT contends that every client possesses several signature strengths. These are strengths of character that a client self-consciously owns and celebrates, of which he or she feels a sense of ownership and authenticity ("This is the real me"); the client feels excited while displaying these signature strengths, learns quickly as they are practiced, and continues to learn, feels more invigorated than exhausted when using them, and creates and pursues projects that revolve around them. PPT creates engagement by utilizing a client's signature strengths; therefore, we think that there is less likelihood that that a client will take such an exercise as just another have-to-do task.

Traditional therapy often focuses on conflict, with the assumption that once conflict has been worked through, happiness will take care of itself. The PPT approach is different; by utilizing signature strengths, it allows therapy to be an opportunity of growth based on a person's deepest psychological resources (signature strengths), with the assumption that when such growth occurs, happiness will take care of itself. Therapeutic interventions have been designed to transform daily negative experiences into more positive ones by increasing engagement (Massimini & Delle Fave, 2000; (Nakamura & Csikszentmihalyi, 2002). Moreover, these interventions have also been applied successfully in diverse cultural settings, including Nicaragua and Northern Somalia (Inghilleri, 1999). Adolescents who have more engagement and flow often develop more productive habits. They are happier and optimistic, have higher self-esteem, study more, are involved in active leisure more often, and spend more time with friends, irrespective of their income, their parents' education, or social status (Csikszentmihalyi, 2003).

PPT promotes the engaged life by encouraging clients to undertake intentional activities that use their signature strengths. Unlike activities that are short-cuts and rely on modern gadgets, these activities require a relatively substantial investment of time, such as rock climbing, chess, basketball, viewing works of art, composing music, reading, writing poetry or fiction, spiritual activities, social interactions, baking, playing with a child, making a slam dunk, dancing, helping others, and so forth. As compared with sensory pleasures that fade quickly, these activities last longer, involve quite a lot of thinking and interpretation, and do not cause habituation easily. These activities are essentially signature strengths in action. Consider this thought experiment by Robert Nozick (1997): If our brains were hooked to a machine that could give any kind of pleasure we desire, most of us would find this idea quite unattractive. The reason is that, in pursuing pleasure, we want to *do* certain things and *be* certain sorts of individuals. The goal here is to optimally use signature strengths to create engagement and happiness. Clients are coached to realize that happiness does not simply happen. It is something that they make happen, particularly when they are at their best, celebrating their signature strengths to feel authentic, fulfilled, and happy.

A key characteristic of engagement and flow is *interactionism* (Magnusson & Stattin, 1998). Rather than focusing on the self alone, which is often an accompanying feature of many psychological problems, engagement tends to involve the client in a dynamic system composed of the individual and the environment. Rock climbers, surgeons, writers, composers, and team sports players routinely find themselves deeply engaged. Moreover, a client can find engagement in virtually any interaction, even in the most trivial, depending on the strengths and skills that are brought to it and the challenge that can be identified in it (Csikszentmihalyi, 1996). Any activity that taps the client's signature strengths can be engaging. For example, a client with the signature strength of creativity may be encouraged to take a pottery, photography, sculpture, or painting class, or someone with the signature strength of curiosity may be encouraged to make a list of things he or she would like to know, identify ways to get such information, and meet someone who has successfully marshaled his or her curiosity to create engagement.

The following illustrations provided by Csikszentmihalyi (2003) give a flavor of these engagement-building activities.

- A lyrical description by a young man:

  The mystique of rock climbing is climbing; you get to the top of a rock glad it's over really wish it would go forever. The justification of climbing is climbing, like the justification of writing is writing . . . the act of writing justifies poetry. Climbing is the same: recognizing that you are in flow. The purpose of flow is to keep on flowing, not looking for a peak or utopia but staying in the flow. It is not a moving up but a continuous flowing; you move up only to keep the flow going. (p. 58)

- A 76-year-old woman who still farms in the Italian Alps describes her engagement and flow:

  It gives me a great satisfaction, to be outdoors, to talk with people, to be with my animals. . . . I talk to everybody—plants, birds, flowers, and animals. Everything in nature keeps you company, you see nature progress each day. You feel clean and happy. (p. 40)

- An African American teenager from the inner city who plays basketball reports:

  When the game is exciting, I don't seem to hear anything—the world seems to cut off from me and all there is [is] to think about my game. (p. 49)

When individuals are fully engaged, subjective states provide satisfaction and the motivation to continue. Despite distraction, they continuously adjust the ongoing relationship with the environment to find the optimal balance. Intrinsically rewarding and motivating engaging activities encourage clients to reproduce engagement. Thus, engagement can replace brooding and rumination. As people master challenges in an activity, they usually develop greater skills in using their signature strengths, and the activity may cease to be as involving as before. When such roadblocks occur, the therapist can help a client to identify increasingly complex challenges. As the process continues, the client realizes his or her full potential and sees that he or she is capable of creating his or her own happiness. The therapist can then discuss long-term engagement goals with the client. If the client reports that the present engagement is rewarding, then measures to maintain it are discussed. If it is less rewarding, as it may be in many cases, the deployment of other signature strengths or trying new pursuits is encouraged, because chance encounters may expose the client to new experiences. Thus, the whole process of using signature strengths to create engagement facilitates a client's growth and fulfillment.

The Meaningful Life

The third "happy" life in Seligman's theory is the pursuit of meaning. This consists of using one's signature strengths to belong to and to serve something that one believes is bigger than the self. Viktor Frankl (1963), a pioneer in the study of meaning, emphasized that happiness cannot be attainted by wanting to be happy—it must come as the unintended consequence of working for a goal greater than oneself. We want to make for ourselves a life that matters to the world and makes a difference for the better. People who successfully pursue activities that connect them to such larger matters achieve what we call the "meaningful life." There are a number of ways to achieve a meaningful life, such as those involving close interpersonal relationships, generativity, social activism or service, careers experienced as callings, and spirituality (see, e.g., Diener & Seligman, 2004; Larson, 2000; Pargament & Mahoney, 2002; Peterson & Stewart, 1993; Wrzesniewski, McCauley, Rozin, & Schwartz, 1997; McAdams, Diamond, de St. Aubin, & Mansfield, 1997). A necessary condition for meaning is an attachment and connection to something larger than oneself. Institutions such as a church, synagogue, mosque, or temple, a professional or leisure club, a nonprofit organization, or an environmental or humanitarian group offer opportunities to connect with something larger. Regardless of the particular way in which a person establishes a meaningful life, doing so produces a sense of satisfaction and the belief that he or she has lived well (Lyubomirsky, King, & Diener, 2005; Ackerman, Zuroff, & Mosokowitz, 2000; Debats, 1996; Myers, 1992). Lack of meaning, however, is linked with physical and psychological problems. Over the last 20 years more than a dozen large studies in the United States, Europe, and Japan have shown that people who are socially disconnected are two to five times more likely to die from all causes, as compared with matched individuals who have close ties to family, friends, and community (Berkman & Kawachi, 2000). Low levels of social support directly predict depression, even controlling for other risk factors (Sherbourne, Hays, & Wells, 1995), whereas social connections inhibit depression. Americans, like most Westerners, are preeminent individualists. Individualism, in terms of uniqueness and control, may be good, but we need balance between individuality and social identity, between personal control and community, between attachment and independence, as Seligman (1991) has noted that individualism need not lead to depression as long as we can fall back on larger institutions such as religion, country, and family. When you fail to reach some of your personal goals, as we all must, you can turn to these larger institutions for hope. However, for those standing alone without the buffer of larger beliefs, helplessness and failure can easily become hopelessness and despair. Individuals who are depressed because of cognitive distortions feel isolated, empty, bored, and hollow. A meta-analysis on the efficacy of volunteerism showed that volunteers, on average, are twice as likely to feel happy with themselves as nonvolunteers. Moreover, it showed that volunteering contributed to happiness by decreasing boredom and creating an increased sense of purpose in life (Cris-Houran, 1996). Life satisfaction was found to improve altruistic activities by 24% (William, Haber, & Freeman, 1998). PPT suggests that lack of meaning is not just a symptom, but a cause of depression and a number of other psychological disorders, and it follows that interventions that build meaning can relieve depression and host of other psychological problems. Through building the meaningful life, PPT helps clients to forge connections beyond themselves with others and communal institutions to deal with psychological problems.

The Full Life

The full life consists of experiencing positive emotions in the past, present, and future, savoring the positive feelings that come from pleasures, deriving abundant gratification through engagement, and creating meaning in life in the service of something larger than the self. We do not believe that the three "lives" noted above are either exclusive or exhaustive. Most engagement experiences have the potential for meaningfulness. Similarly, activities that produce gratification require considerable thinking and action and could become passion. A passion is usually sufficiently intense to engage an individual. Similarly, when an individual establishes and sustains engagement, the activity often evolves into a meaningful endeavor. The long-term careers of artists and scientists illustrate a sense of meaning emerging from an extended relationship with an activity that uses their highest abilities. Wrzesniewski and colleagues' (1997) study of people's relationship to their work provides an example of pleasure, engagement, and meaning found at work, which then translates into a career and, for some, into a calling. Individuals who view their work as a calling report both high work satisfaction and higher life satisfaction, in general, than those who view their work as a job or career. Similarly, Easterbrook (2004) has observed:

> that society is undergoing a fundamental shift from "material want" to "meaning want," with [an] ever larger number of people reasonably secure in terms of living standards, but feeling they lack significance in their lives. A transition from "material want" to "meaning want" is not a prediction that men and women will cease being materialistic; no social indicator points to such a possibility. It is a prediction that ever more millions will expect both pleasant living standards and a broad sense their lives possess purpose. (p. xix)

In short, a full life, we believe, entails pleasure, engagement, and meaning, through separate activities or through a single activity. In contrast, an empty life which lacks these elements, partly causes psychological problems.

VALIDATION STUDIES

RCT Pilot 1: Individual PPT with Unipolar Depressed Patients (Seligman, Rashid, & Parks, 2006)

Our individual PPT pilot was conducted at the Counseling and Psychological Services (CAPS), University of Pennsylvania, with clients diagnosed with major depressive disorder (MDD) and randomly assigned to PPT ($n = 11$), treatment as usual (TAU; $n = 9$) and TAU plus antidepressant medication (TAUMED; $n = 12$). PPT took place for up to 14 sessions over, at most, 12 weeks and was conducted by Rashid, who has a doctorate in clinical psychology. A manualized protocol (Rashid & Seligman, in press; see Table 11.1 for the session-by-session structure) was followed. TAU consisted of an integrative and eclectic approach administered by five doctoral-level licensed psychologists, two licensed social workers, and two graduate-level interns. Results indicated that on self-report measures, the Zung Self-Rating Scale (ZSRS; Zung, 1965) and the Outcome questionnaire (OQ; Lambert et al., 1996), PPT significantly exceeded TAUMED, with large effect sizes (d = 1.22 and 1.13, respectively). On clinician-rated measures, the Hamilton Rating Scale for Depression (HAM-D; Hamilton, 1960) and DSM-IV's Global Assessment of Functioning (GAF), rated by an independent clinician who was blind to treatment condition, PPT did significantly better than TAU, with large effect sizes (d = 1.41 and 1.16, respectively) as well. On well-being measures, the three groups did not differ significantly on the Satisfaction with Life scale, but PPT differed significantly from both TAU and TAUMED on our measure of happiness, the Positive Psychotherapy Inventory (PPTI), a 21-item PPT outcome measure we created and validated (Rashid, 2005), with large effect sizes (d = 1.26 and 1.03). Based on the fourfold remission criteria, seven of eleven clients (64%) in PPT, one of nine (11%) in TAU, and one of twelve (8%) in TAUMED remitted by the end of treatment ($\chi^2(2, n = 32) = 10.48, p < .005$).

RCT Pilot 2: Group PPT with Mild to Moderately Depressed Individuals (Seligman et al., 2006)

The participants in group PPT were 40 students at the University of Pennsylvania, randomly assigned to either group PPT (n = 19) or a no-treatment control group (n = 21). Outcome measures were the Beck Depression Inventory (BDI; Beck & Steer, 1992) and the Satisfaction with Life Scale (SWLS; Diener et al., 1985). Group PPT was conducted in two groups of eight to eleven participants, one led by a graduate student and the other by the Rashid, both trained extensively in PPT. In this trial, six PPT exercises were used, including Positive Introduction, Using Your Strengths, Three Good Things, Obituary/Biography, Active/Constructive Responding, and Savoring. Results indicate that participants who received group PPT experienced significant increases in life satisfaction (d = 0.30) and decreases in depressive symptoms over the course of the intervention (d = 0.48), and that these changes were maintained through a 1-year follow-up.

RCT Pilot 3: Group PPT with Middle School Students (Rashid, Anjum, & Lennox, 2006)

Our third randomized control pilot was with middle school students who were offered a group version of PPT. Group PPT included the following exercises: Positive Introduction, Using Signature Strengths, Three Blessings, Savoring, and Family Tree of Strengths. PPT was an 8-week, 1½ hour per week intervention administered in a group format, led by Rashid and Anjum. After the first orientation session, the children completed online the Values in Action Inventory of Strengths (VIA-IS) in a group format. Each was then asked to imagine him- or herself to be a better person at the end of the intervention by undertaking a signature strength project. In the following three sessions, the children were extensively coached about ways of using their signature strengths to devise a practical behavioral project. Legends, real-life narratives, and popular films such as *Pay It Forward*, *Billy Elliot*, *Forest Gump*, *Life Is Beautiful*, and *My Left Foot* illustrated the use of strengths. The 22 participants were students at the Westwood Middle School in Toronto,

Ontario, randomly assigned to an intervention group (n = 11) or a control group (n = 11). The mean age of participants was 11.77 years (SD = 0.69); 45% were Canadians, and 42% were females. We used three outcome measures. Depression was assessed by the Children's Depression Inventory (CDI; Helsel & Matson, 1984), happiness and well-being were assessed by a 7-item self-report Student's Life Satisfaction Scale (SLSS; Huebner, 1991) and an 18-item Positive Psychotherapy Inventory—Children's Version (PPTI; Rashid et al., 2006, Appendix 11.1). Results indicated that the two groups did not differ on a symptomatic measure (CDI). This was expected because pretest scores were in the nondepressive range. However, the two groups differed significantly on PPTI, but not on SLSS, with the intervention group demonstrating a significant increase, with a large effect size (d = 0.90). This is consistent with the results of the individualized PPT pilot. Both groups also differed significantly on weekly behavioral ratings completed the teachers. Our sample included a pair of identical twins, one randomly assigned to the intervention group, the other to the control group. Both scored similarly in the moderate depressive range on preintervention depressive symptoms. Although the postintervention score of the student in the intervention group dropped by 10 points, the score of the student in the control group increased by 2 points. Overall, group PPT worked well, as compared with the control. A substantial change in happiness was also noted.

RCT Pilot 4: Web-Based PPT (Seligman et al., 2005)

This RCT was completed before the individual and group PPT pilots. It addressed the issue of inexpensive dissemination of PPT, as well as the efficacy of the PPT exercises over the Internet, with no "human hands." This study was conducted via the Internet. Over the course of approximately 1 month, 577 adult participants were recruited, including 236 (41%) males. Participants did individual PPT exercises such as Three Good Things, Knowing Character Strengths, Using Character Strengths, and Gratitude Visit. The placebo group wrote childhood memories. Using character strengths and the Three Good Things exercise decreased depressive symptoms over 3–6 months, with effect sizes (Cohen's d) of 0.32 and 0.43, respectively. These two exercises also increased and sustained the level of happiness through 6 months, with an effect size of 0.32 for Three Good Things and 0.40 for Using Character Strengths. The Gratitude Visit, a third effective exercise, produced strong but short-term effects on depression and happiness. Other exercises (including the control exercise) created short-term effects in decreasing depressive symptoms and increasing happiness, but these effects were fleeting. Not surprisingly, we found that the degree to which participants actively continued their assigned exercise beyond the prescribed 1-week period mediated the lasting benefits.

PPT Exercises with Mental Health Professionals and College Students (Seligman, 2004)

Positive psychology exercises, from which PPT eventually was designed, were developed and piloted in non-clinical samples as well. This effort involved hundreds of participants, including undergraduates and depressed patients. One salient exercise was that in which Seligman trained more than 500 mental health professionals (clinical psychologists, life coaches, social workers, industrial and organizational psychologists, etc.) in four 48-hour, 6-month telephone and virtual courses. Each week the professionals were assigned one of the PPT exercises to carry out with their clients. A small portion of these professionals participated in an outcome study on exercises, which eventually formed PPT. As compared with a matched control group ($n = 83$), those who completed the course ($n = 102$), scored significantly low on a depression measure ($d = 0.31$) and significantly high on life satisfaction ($d = 0.33$). Depression was measured by the CES-D (Radloff, 1977) and life satisfaction by SWLS (Diener et al., 1985). In another study (Rashid, 2004) 24 character strengths classified by Peterson and Seligman (2004) were explicitly targeted through a positive psychology course. Intervention included readings, watching assigned films on character strengths, writing reaction papers weekly, classroom discussions and out-of-class exercises. Results indicated that the intervention group ($n = 35$), as compared with the control group ($n = 30$), demonstrated significant increases in character strengths with medium effect size ($d = 0.37$). In addition, significant pre- to postintervention changes were found in vitality, social intelligence, humor and playfulness, open-mindedness, bravery, hope, and fairness. Similarly, Peterson and Seligman (2004) have found that college students ($n = 20$) enrolled in an undergraduate course at the University of Pennsylvania showed reliable increases in the strengths of love, prudence, gratitude, perspective, and spirituality. All of these strengths were targeted in classroom discussion and out-of-class exercises.

Summary of Preliminary Studies

In summarizing these studies, we found that individual PPT with severely depressed clients led to more symptomatic improvement and to more remission from depressive disorders than TAU and TAUMED. It also enhanced happiness. Group PPT given to mild to moderately depressed college students led to significantly greater symptom reduction and greater increases in life satisfaction than shown in the no-treatment control group. This improvement, moreover, lasted for at least 1 year after treatment. Group PPT with middle school children increased their well-being, with a large effect size. Web-based study and studies with mental health professionals and students, which initially validated individual PPT exercises, yielded reliable changes in strengths and well-being, with medium effect sizes.

HOW PPT WORKS?

Table 11.1 presents an idealized session-by-session description of PPT. Consistent with the theory described above, themes of pleasure, engagement, and meaning are integrated throughout the course of therapy. PPT, right from the outset, encourages clients to explore their strengths—in comparison with their weaknesses. It builds a congenial and positive relationship by asking clients to introduce themselves through real-life stories that show them at their best. This is followed by clients identifying their signature strengths and the therapist coaching them to find practical ways of using them more often in work, love, play, friendship, and parenting. The clients set goals for using and enhancing their signature strengths through real-life exercises. A substantial amount of time is spent in coaching clients to re-educate their memory and attention to what is good in their lives, with the goal of providing them a more balanced context in which to place their problems. Although some problem solving and discussion of troubles does occur in PPT, the goal is to keep the positive aspects of the clients' lives at the forefront of their minds, to teach behaviors that bring positive feedback from others, and to strengthen already existing positive aspects, rather than teaching the reinterpretation of negative aspects. When clients report negative emotions or troubles, however, they are empathically attended to. This balanced process enables the therapist to become a witness to the client's deepest positive characteristics rather than just an authority figure who highlights faulty thinking, negative emotions, and maladjusted relationships. Usually, there are already plenty of such critical individuals in a client's life, and this can be the very reason the client seeks therapy. We advocate that PPT be custom-tailored to meet clients' immediate clinical needs (e.g., addressing conflict with significant others, romantic breakup, or career-related issues), and the order of the exercises can be varied according to each client's circumstances and the feasibility of completing the exercises. Likewise, homework assignments are selected from the pool of potential exercises presented in Table 11.1 and the exercises that are tailored to the individual clients.

PPT Is Not Mere Positives

PPT is not just about positives, although it is understandable that the name may imply that to some. Nor do we assume that other psychotherapies are negative. It is utopian to conceive of a life without negative experiences. Therefore, PPT does not deny distressing, unpleasant, and negative states and experiences, nor is its aim to help clients see the world with wishful thinking and rose-colored glasses. It fully validates clients' negative experiences originating from physical disorders and psychopathologies, dysfunctional families, or ineffective social institutions (Gable & Haidt, 2005). PPT is a systematic therapeutic effort to treat symptoms by explicitly building positive emotions, character strengths, and meaning. In doing so, it fully appreciates that human strengths cannot be fully understood without comprehending human weaknesses. We believe that a viable way of undoing negative states is to accentuate positive states and traits. Folkman and Moskowitz (2000) have shown that positive reappraisal (focusing on the good in what is happening or what has happened) and creating positive events can help in dealing with negative emotions and experiences. Indeed, looking for the bright side of negative experiences enhances adjustment (Affleck & Tennen, 1996).

PPT also draws heavily on clients' signature strengths and suggests undertaking endeavors that best use these strengths. However, even in utilizing signature strengths, clients are coached on the use of practical wisdom, as suggested by Schwartz and Sharpe (2006). Specifically, clients are taught about three issues: first, *relevance* (does a particular situation requires a signature strength or some other strength?); second, *conflict* (should one be honest or kind?) and *specificity* (translating signature strengths into concrete actions, as real-life situations rarely come labeled with the need to exercise a particular signature strength).

Although it seems counterintuitive to believe that clients can experience positive emotions in the midst of significant acute or chronic pain, in a review on this topic, Calhoun and Tedeschi (1998) highlighted the fact that there are positive aspects to stress (such as growth and personal transformation, which have been reported) that can no longer be ignored. Furthermore, instructing people to find the positives in traumatic life events can lead to health benefits as well as growth (King & Miner, 2000). Therefore, the role of the therapist in PPT is also to help the client to turn adversity to advantage, keeping the client attuned to positives and leading him or her, through systematic and sustained efforts, to create positive experiences. Amid the warmth, understanding, and goodwill created in the therapeutic milieu, the PPT therapist aids the client in learning ways to encounter negative states and traits by keeping genuine positives in the foreground. The PPT therapist works diligently and deeply to articulate the genuine and authentic positives of the client. He or she does not create an epitome of happiness or a caricature of positive thinking, like Dr. Pangloss and Pollyanna. Nor does the therapist minimize or mask as positives the negative events and experiences of life, such as abuse, neglect, and threats to the safety of the client and others. Therefore, such issues are dealt with within the standard clinical protocols.

Negatives Are Never Dismissed

Because clients have long been socialized to believe that therapy entails talking about troubles, any perceived failure to take their troubles seriously violates their expectations and can undermine good rapport. Therefore, PPT adopts a flexible approach. Although the focus is on helping clients explore their positives, it is inevitable that a client will discuss, or in some cases, display negative emotions and experiences. In PPT, an expression of negative emotions is never dismissed, nor are such emotions superficially replaced with positive ones. Rather, the aim is to explore the role of negative emotions. One PPT exercise explicitly asks clients to write down their bad and bitter memories or resentments and then discuss in therapy the effects of holding onto them. This allows the easing of cognitive and emotional constrictions associated with such memories. Moreover, in some cases, negative emotions may have adaptive functions, albeit not explored by the client. For example, fear, sadness, or anger may have prompted a client to utilize his or her support system. Drawing on the vital strength of the personal emotional intelligence of the client, PPT helps the client to allocate his or her emotional resources. That is, the client is encouraged to undertake activities at the appropriate time and in proper proportion. In doing so, PPT follows Seligman (2002)'s advice: "Choose your venue and design your mood to fit the task at hand" (p. 39). Clients are taught that positive emotions are best utilized in seeking out and establishing new social ties, attempting difficult tasks, undertaking tasks that call for creative, generous, and tolerant thinking, finding ways to increase the amount of love in life, pondering a new career, thinking about hobbies and noncompetitive sports, and creative writing. Because negative emotions activate critical thinking (Alloy & Abramson, 1979; Norem & Chang, 2002), clients who are faced with making decisions in regard to taking important exams, calculating income taxes, determining whom to fire, where to move, dealing with repeated romantic rejections, copyediting, or making important judgments in competitive endeavors, are advised to undertake them when they feel slightly gloomy.

POTENTIAL MECHANISM OF CHANGE

Reeducating Attention, Memory, and Expectations

Human beings are naturally biased toward remembering the negative, attending to the negative, and expecting the worst. Negative emotion is most proximally driven by negative memories, attention, and expectations, and depressed individuals exaggerate this natural tendency. They strongly gravitate toward attending to and remembering the most negative aspects of their lives, and several of our exercises aim to reeducate attention, memory, and expectations, directing them away from the negative and the catastrophic toward the positive and the hopeful. For example, when a client does the Three Good Things exercise ("Before you go to sleep, write down three things that went well today and why they went well"), the depressive bias toward ruminating only about what has gone wrong is counteracted. The client is more likely to end the day remembering positive events and completions, rather than his or her troubles and unfinished business. The Gratitude Visit exercise, similarly, may shift memory away from the embittering aspects of a client's past relationships to savoring the good things that friends and family members have done for him or her. This reeducation of attention, memory, and expectation is not done only orally. PPT relies on written narratives that help the client to articulate positives coherently and deeply. There is considerable evidence for the physical and psychological benefits of writing about traumas and adversities (Bauer & McAdams, 2004; Pennebaker, 1993); the benefits of writing about positive experiences are just beginning to emerge (see, e.g., Burton & King, 2004). PPT starts by asking clients to introduce themselves by writing a story about when they were at their best. This is followed by writing three bad memories, a forgiveness letter, a gratitude letter, and logging constructive-active responding.

Broadening and Building by Positive Emotions

A number of PPT exercises explicitly aim to create more positive emotions (e.g., the Three Good Things Exercise, Savoring, the Gratitude Letter and the Gratitude Visit, Three Doors Closed; Three Doors Opened the Active-Constructive Responding Exercise). Building positive emotions does not necessarily restrict the client to a specific action, like negative emotions do. Positive emotions seem to broaden a client's repertoires of things he or she likes to pursue. As noted earlier, the cultivation of positive emotions helps individuals to flourish (Fredrickson & Losada, 2005). Over the course of therapy, through a number of exercises, clients gradually broaden their thinking beyond their regular baseline, and regular discussions of this cognitive broadening allows clients to discover and learn new things. It likely fuels self-transformation and allows them to identify their negative thinking patterns. Moreover, PPT exercises attempt to create positive emotions in a number of domains of life—noticing positive emotions in the present through the Savoring and the Three Blessings exercises, remembering a good deed of someone in the past, providing constructive and active feedback to a loved one—thus allowing the client to generalize the role of positive emotions across situations. In addition, positive emotions that stem from the Gratitude Letter and Gratitude Visit, and the Active-Constructive Responding Exercise, essentially strengthen close interpersonal relations and help clients to notice and value positive things in their lives rather than brooding over negative aspects.

Intentional Activities

The mechanisms of other PPT exercises are likely more external and behavioral. For example, increasing clients' awareness of their signature strengths likely encourages them to more effectively apply themselves at work by approaching tasks in a way that better uses their abilities. Having more flow at work and doing better work can lead to an upward spiral of engagement and positive emotion. Similarly, teaching clients to respond in an active and constructive manner to good news from coworkers, friends, and family members teaches a social skill that likely improves most relationships (Gable, Reis, Impett, & Asher, 2004).

Another possible mechanism is PPT's sustained emphasis on the use of strengths as a way to have more engagement and meaning in life. Throughout therapy, PPT clients are encouraged and assisted in identifying their signature strengths: Near the outset of the therapy, clients are asked to introduce themselves through real-life stories about their highest character strengths. Then they take the Values in Action Inventory of Strengths (VIA-IS; Peterson & Seligman, 2004; *www.authentichappiness.org*), a well-validated test that identifies clients' signature strengths. The therapist and client collaboratively devise new ways of using the client's signature strengths at work and in love, friendship, parenting, and leisure. Furthermore, we ask clients to recount detailed and rich narratives about what they have been good at. Although we do not ignore clients' concerns about their "deficiencies," lest we seem unfeeling and unsympathetic about their troubles, we emphasize identifying, attending to, remembering, and using more often the core positive traits that they already possess. This may produce "end-runs" around their perceived faults, faults they know all too well. A newspaper article headlined this approach as "You already have a life, now use it." In addition, we emphasize using signature strengths to solve problems.

In addition to increasing their general awareness of strengths, we coach clients on how to explicitly employ their signature strengths to counter depression. For example, in our individual PPT pilot with severely depressed clients, one client devised several new, specific ways of using her signature strength of appreciation of beauty to manage negative moods. She rearranged her room in way that she found to be most aesthetically pleasing and decorated a wall with a print by her favorite artist, so that she woke up to beauty. She had always wanted to write poetry but had never had time for it, and now she was able to find a poetry club. For one week, she wrote three experiences of beauty every day in her journal. Among her entries were watching the sunset at the Schuylkill River near Fairmount Park, noticing beauty in the face of a child, seeing how happy and beautiful her dog looked while they were playing. She also loved hiking, so she took a hiking trip and climbed Mount Washington.

Another client used his signature strength of love to undo his depression: His girlfriend was away in Europe for the spring semester, and he was quite depressed on Valentine's Day. He decided to arrange a long-distance Valentine dinner. He and his girlfriend each independently acquired their favorite foods and talked via Internet phone as they ate together, listened to their favorite songs together, and talked about their appreciation of each other's character strengths. Then, during spring break, he traveled to Europe, took her to a surprise dinner at her favorite restaurant and read his Gratitude Letter. At the end of the therapy, their relationship, which had been on the brink of breakup, was flourishing.

Balance between Possessions, Pleasures, and Engaging Pursuits

PPT helps clients to expand the notion of happiness. Influenced by a negativity bias, the academic zeitgeist, and the media's fascination with bad and evil, clients may initially see happiness as undefined, immeasurable, fleeting, illusionary, relative, and hence impractical (Smart & Williams, 1973). Moreover, some clients may come with the stereotypic notion that hedonic pleasures such as Aspen ski vacations, first-class travel, a deluxe mobile home, a designer wardrobe, or a luxury SUV with heated leather seats may bring them unlimited happiness. PPT educates clients to see that happiness is measurable, diverse, practical, and can last. Without negating the need for hedonic pleasures, PPT tells clients that beyond basic needs, additional material possessions have in fact very little impact on our happiness. Because people are phenomenally adaptable, and incremental increases in material possessions fail to produce sustained increments in happiness within a year, both lottery winners and those who become paraplegic as a result of spinal cord injuries quickly adapt to their baseline of happiness (Brickman, Coates, & Janoff-

Bulman, 1978; Schulz & Decker, 1985; Suh, Diener, & Fujita, 1996). As we adapt, especially after acquiring material resources, our expectations about what will make us happy increase. We compare our situations to where we want to be, and ourselves to other people. As we attain our goals, we change our comparisons. We do not just become habituated, we recalibrate. We create for ourselves a world of targets, and each time one is hit, another replaces it (Haidt, 2006). Nesse and Williams (1994) note, "We all compare [ourselves] with those who are the best in the world" (p. 220). One implication of this is that depression stems from self-perceived failures resulting from erroneous comparisons between our own lives and the glamorously depicted lives on television. "Retail therapy" (Faber, 2004) is another notion explored in PPT. Like substance abuse, self-cutting, sexual promiscuity, and other high-risk behaviors, "retail therapy" and obsessive acquisition are maladaptive ways to cope with unpleasant, empty, or anxious feelings. The Satisficing Instead of Maximizing Exercise, which is based on Schwarz et al. (2002), encourages clients to settle down for good enough.

PPT also educates clients to understand the engaging in intense experiences that produce ecstasy is not the cornerstone of a happy life. Research informs us that people who seek ecstasy much of the time are likely to be disappointed. Even worse, they may move from one job or relationship to another, seeking intense levels of happiness (Diener, Sandvik, & Pavot, 1991). Furthermore, highly pleasurable experiences may have the disadvantage of serving as contrast points against which other positive experiences are measured, thus making these events less pleasurable (Parducci, 1995). Therefore, a client's notion of happiness is carefully expanded, emphasizing that these findings are descriptive, derived from decades of rigorous research that is not readily available to the public nor significantly influences public policy.

The Therapeutic Relationship Is Important

We believe that when PPT is effectively delivered with the basic therapeutic essentials—warmth, empathy, and genuineness—exploring and promoting positives establishes an authentic therapeutic relationship. This relationship, we posit, is equally authentic and genuine as the one in which a therapist attends only to the negatives. In PPT, the therapist is asked to care more for the therapeutic alliance than adherence to the treatment protocol. For example, tensions and misunderstandings may arise when a client wishes only symptom relief but the therapist is convinced that the client will benefit from the active promotion of happiness. In addition, a stressed client may be more inclined to do pleasure-based exercises and not the engagement and meaning-making exercises. Furthermore, in some cases, because of their initial emotional distress some clients may not immediately appreciate the benefits of engaging and connecting with others. It is therefore suggested that the therapist focus on establishing a strong therapeutic alliance initially, as it is from this relationship that adherence to the treatment protocol may naturally flow.

CAVEATS

Descriptive Not Prescriptive

A daunting task for the PPT therapist is to ensure that what he or she purports as "positive" is not perceived by the client as prescriptive. PPT is a descriptive therapeutic approach based on convergent research findings that clearly document the benefits of positive emotions, character strengths, and making meaning. Just as medical research shows that eating vegetables and exercising is "good" for us, we believe that PPT can and should encourage people to adopt behaviors and mental habits that are "good" for them (Gable & Haidt, 2005). PPT recognizes that in an increasingly diverse clientele, contextual and cultural factors must be considered. For example, a client brought up in a typical European American culture may think of happiness as a personal hedonic state, whereas, a client from another culture may see happiness as relating to others and fulfilling obligations. PPT needs to delivered with sensitivity and flexibility to accommodate individual and cultural differences, and a fixed moral vision that sees happiness as the yardstick of a good life should be avoided.

Motivation for Change

The PPT therapist must be sensitive and appreciative of the complexities of human beings. How positive states and traits interact within a client may differ markedly from one person to another. Clients also differ in their motivation to change long-standing behavioral and emotional patterns. In addition, each client's motivation fluctuates as a result of dynamic changes within the environment. Therefore, the therapist must not adopt a "one size fits all" approach, as it may not work with all clients. Having a clear understanding of the basic assumptions of PPT and the basic skills needed in establishing a solid therapeutic relationship with the client can help the therapist tremendously. In regard to the structure and sequence of the exercises, the therapist should be flexible enough to adapt them to accommodate the uniqueness of each client. At the same time, we would not want a therapist to think that for fear of being perceived as "prescriptive," he or she should hold back and accept a client's interpretations regarding his or her reluctance to own positive emotions and strengths readily. Most clients are unaware of their strengths and that of others. However, the challenge for a therapist is to help clients to articulate and internalize their strengths deeply.

It should be noted that telling clients that happiness is possible by adopting the precepts of PPT comes with the risk of advising clients. No matter how many scientific facts are stacked in the consulting room, proving that enhancing engagement and meaning yields lasting happiness, clients may not resist negative thinking and feelings and coping with them through shortcuts, because, these possibilities are readily available to them. Contemporary Western culture encourages indulgence, accumulation of possessions, and shortcuts. It may be an uphill task for a PPT therapist to motivate a client to resist mainstream cultural trends.

Pilot Studies

Although PPT led to clinically and statistically significant decreases in depression and increases in happiness in our controlled trials, these results are preliminary and caution is warranted on several grounds. First, our face-to-face therapy was done with small samples. Second, the clients in these trials were college and high school students and mental health professionals. This may well limit the generalizability of PPT to other populations that vary in age, ethnicity, socioeconomic status, and IQ. Third, we did not study therapist effect and so we do not know if the results can be attributed to "talented therapist" effects. Hence, the mechanisms by which PPT operates, including the moderating role of therapists and the commonalities of PPT and other therapeutic approaches, are matters of further research.

FUTURE DIRECTIONS

Benjamin Franklin said that wasted strengths are like sundials in the shade. Psychotherapy has not utilized vital therapeutic assets within the symptom and disorder-based model. We have tapped these resources in a systematic and planned therapy, and we are encouraged by the potency of the positive psychology exercises, by the congeniality of the approach to depressed clients, by how long the benefits lasted after treatment ended, and by the sheer effect size of PPT when delivered by a skilled therapist. Should these results replicate well, we speculate that future therapy for depression may combine talking about troubles with understanding and building positive emotion, engagement, and meaning. Nevertheless, we suspect that the effects of PPT are specific to depression, and we expect that increasing positive emotion, engagement, and meaning promote highly general ways of buffering against a variety of disorders and troubles. With the proliferation of research in positive psychology in the last few years, therapies based on notions of happiness, growth, and well-being are gaining momentum in both theory and application (e.g., Lent, 2004; Joseph & Linley, 2005). Currently, Lisa Lewis and her colleagues at the Menninger Clinic are comparing PPT with a traditional psychotherapy with a larger inpatient sample ($n = 100$). We hope such endeavors will help us to unearth important questions regarding PPT's generalizability, specificity, and response rate. Moreover, the scope of positive emotions and strengths is increasingly rapidly. Courses in positive psychology are becoming common in universities and high schools. The popularity of the Positive Psychology course at Harvard (855 undergraduates enrolled in spring 2006; Goldberg, 2006) is likely related to the impact of this material on the lives of students. We believe this appeal will further refine the therapeutic potential of positive emotions and strengths. Furthermore, in order to justify interventions based on happiness and well-being in mainstream clinical practice, PPT may need to demonstrate with more rigorous research that not only the presence of symptoms but also the lack of happiness and well-being is a causal factor in psychopathology, which can demonstrate change in outcome measures that directly related with treatment outcome. Through longitudinal and prospective studies, treatments like PPT should be given to at-risk populations to demonstrate their potential as effective preventive strategies. In short, making life happier and more fulfilling, not just less sad and miserable, should be more appealing for Emma, and PPT provides her a systematic and planned opportunity for doing so.

ACKNOWLEDGMENTS

We acknowledge the work of Martin E. P. Seligman, Illene Rosentein, William Alexander, Acacia Parks, Carolyn Lennox, Ruth Baumal, Peter Chang, Anna Epitrpou, Charles May, Christopher Brown, and Anneli Jaevel.

REFERENCES

Ackerman, S., Zuroff, D. C., & Moskowitz, D. S. (2000). Generativity in midlife and young adults: Links to agency, communion, and subjective well-being. *International Journal of Aging and Human Development, 50,* 17–41.

Affleck, G., & Tennen, H. (1996). Construing benefits from adversity: Adaptational significance and dispositional underpinnings. *Journal of Personality, 64,* 899–922.

Alloy, L. B., & Abramson, L. Y. (1979). Judgment of contingency in depressed and nondepressed students: Sadder but wiser. *Journal of Experimental Psychology: General, 108,* 441–485.

Allport, G. (1961). *Patterns and growth in personality*. New York: Holt, Rinehart & Winston.

American Psychiatric Association. (2000). *Diagnostic and statistical manual of mental disorders* (4th ed., text rev.). Washington, DC: Author.

Bandura, A. (1978). On paradigms and recycled ideologies. *Cognitive Therapy and Research, 2,* 79–103.

Barrett, P. M., & Ollendick, T. H. (Eds.). (2004). *Handbook of interventions that work with children and adolescents: Prevention and treatment*. West Sussex, UK: Wiley.

Baumeister, R. F., Bratslavsky, E., Finkenauer, C., & Vohs, K. D. (2001). Bad is stronger than good. *Review of General Psychology, 5,* 323–370.

Beck, A. T., Rush, A. J., Shaw, B. F., & Emery, G. (1979). *Cognitive therapy of depression*. New York: Guilford Press.

Beck, A. T., & Steer, R. A. (1992). *Beck Anxiety Inventory manual*. San Antonio: The Psychological Corporation.

Berkman, L. F., & Kawachi, I. (2000). *Social epidemiology*. New York: Oxford University Press.

Bolte, A., Goschke, T., & Kuhl, J. (2003). Emotion and intuition: Effects of positive and negative mood on implicit judgments of semantic coherence. *Psychological Science, 14,* 416–421.

Brickman, P., Coates, D., & Janoff-Bulman, R. (1978). Lottery winners and accident victims: Is happiness relative? *Journal of Personality and Social Psychology, 36,* 917–927.

Burton, C. M., & King, L. A. (2004). The health benefits of writing about intensely positive experiences. *Journal of Research in Personality, 38,* 150–163.

Buss, D. M. (2000). The evolution of happiness. *American Psychologist, 55,* 15–23.

Calhoun, L. G., & Tedeschi, R. G. (1998). Posttraumatic growth: Future directions. In R. Tedeschi & L. Calhoun (Eds.), *Posttraumatic growth: Positive changes in the aftermath of crisis* (pp. 215–240). Mahwah, NJ: Erlbaum.

Cheavens, J., Gum, A., Feldman, D. B., Michael, S. T., & Snyder, C. R. (2001, August). *A group intervention to increase hope in community sample*. Poster presented at the annual convention of the American Psychological Association, San Francisco.

Chesney, M. A., Darbes, L. A., Hoerster, K., Taylor, J. M., & Chamber, D. B. (2005). Positive emotions: Exploring the other hemisphere in behavioral medicine. *International Journal of Behavioral Medicine, 12,* 50–58.

Cottrell, C. A., & Neuberg, S. L. (2005). Different emotional reactions to different groups: A sociofunctional threat-based approach to "prejudice." *Journal of Personality and Social Psychology, 88,* 770–789.

Cris-Houran, M. (1996). Efficacy of volunteerism. *Psychological Reports, 79,* 736–738.

Csikszentmihalyi, M. (1990). *Flow: The psychology of optimal experience*. New York: HarperCollins.

Csikszentmihalyi, M. (1996). *Flow and the psychology of discovery and intervention*. New York: HarperCollins.

Csikszentmihalyi, M. (2003). *Good business*. New York: Viking Press.

Danner, D., Snowdon, D., & Friesen, W. (2001). Positive emotions in early life and longevity: Findings from the nun study. *Journal of Personality and Social Psychology, 80,* 804–813.

Davidson, R. J., Kabat-Zinn, J., Schumacher, J., Rosenkranz, M., Muller, D., Santorelli, S. F., et al. (2003). Alterations in brain and immune function produced by mindfulness meditation. *Psychosomatic Medicine, 65,* 564–570.

Debats, D. L. (1996). Meaning in Life: Clinical relevance and predictive power. *British Journal of Clinical Psychology, 35,* 503–516.

Dewey, J. (1933). *How we think: A restatement of the relation of reflective thinking to the educative process*. Boston: Heath.

Diener, E., Emmons, R. A., Larsen, R. J., & Griffin, S. (1985). The Satisfaction with Life Scale. *Journal of Personality Assessment, 49,* 71–75.

Diener, E., & Oishi, S. (2000) Money and happiness: Income and subjective well-being across nations. In E. Diener & E. M. Suh (Eds.), *Subjective well-being across cultures* (pp. 185–218). Cambridge, MA: MIT Press.

Diener, E., Sandvik, E., & Pavot, W. (1991). Happiness is the frequency, not the intensity of positive versus negative affects. In F. Strack, M. Argyle, & N. Schwarz (Eds.), *Subjective well-being: An interdisciplinary perspective* (pp. 119–139). New York: Pergamon Press.

Diener, E., & Seligman, M. E. P. (2004). Beyond money: Towards an economy of well-being. *Psychological Science in Public Interest, 5*, 31–62.

Duckworth, A. L., Steen, T. A., & Seligman, M. E. P. (2005). Positive psychology in clinical practice. *Annual Review of Clinical Psychology, 1*, 629–651.

Durlak, C. (1995). *School based prevention programmes for children and adolescents.* London: Sage.

Easterbrook, G. (2004). *The progress paradox: How life gets better while people feel worse.* New York: Random House.

Emmons, R. A., & McCullough, M. E. (2003). Counting blessings versus burdens: Experimental studies of gratitude and subjective well-being in daily life. *Journal of Personality and Social Psychology, 84*, 377–389.

Faber, R. J. (2004). Self-control and compulsive buying. In T. Kasser & A. D. Kanner (Eds.), *Psychology and consumer culture: The struggle for a good life in a materialistic world* (pp. 169–187). Washington, DC: American Psychological Association.

Fava, G. A. (1996). The concept of recovery in affective disorders. *Psychotherapy and Psychosomatics, 65*, 2–13.

Fava, G. (1999). Well-being therapy: Conceptual and technical issues. *Psychotherapy and Psychosomatics, 68*, 171–179.

Fava, G. A., & Ruini, C. (2003). Development and characteristics of a well-being enhancing psychotherapeutic strategy: Well-being therapy. *Journal of Behavior Therapy and Experimental Psychiatry, 34*, 45–63.

Folkman, S., & Moskowitz, J. T. (2000). Stress, positive emotion, and coping. *Current Directions in Psychological Science, 9*, 115–118.

Fordyce, M. W. (1977). Development of a program to increase personal happiness. *Journal of Counseling Psychology, 24*, 511–520.

Fordyce, M. W. (1983). A program to increase happiness: Further studies. *Journal of Consulting Psychology, 30*, 483–498.

Frankl, V. E. (1963). *Man's search for meaning: An introduction to logotherapy.* New York: Washington Square Press.

Fredrickson, B. L. (1998). What good are positive emotions? *Review of General Psychology, 2*, 300–319.

Fredrickson, B. L. (2001). The role of positive emotions in positive psychology: The broaden-and-build theory of positive emotions. *American Psychologist, 56*, 218–226.

Fredrickson, B. L., & Branigan, C. (2005). Positive emotions broaden the scope of attention and thought–action repertoires. *Cognition and Emotion, 19*, 313–332.

Fredrickson, B. L., & Losada, M. (2005). Positive affect and the complex dynamics of human flourishing. *American Psychologist, 60*, 678–686.

Fredrickson, B. L., Mancuso, R. A., Branigan, C., & Tugade, M. M. (2000). The undoing effects of positive emotions. *Motivation and Emotion, 24*, 237–258.

Freud, S. (1995). Civilization and its discontent. In P. Gay (Ed.), *The Freud reader.* London: Vintage.

Freud, S. (1996). NUMBER: 23091. In R. Andrews, M. Biggs, & M. Seidel (Eds.), *Columbia world of quotations* (Letter dated October 9, 1918, "Psycho-analysis and faith: The letters of Sigmund Freud and Oskar Pfister," no. 59, from the International Psycho-Analytical Library in 1963, New York: Columbia University Press).

Frisch, M. B. (2006). *Quality of life therapy: Applying a life satisfaction approach to positive psychology and cognitive therapy.* Hoboken, NJ: Wiley.

Frisch, M. B., Cornell, J., Villanueva, M. & Retzlaff, P. J. (1992). Clinical validation of the Quality of Life Inventory: A measure of life satisfaction for use in treatment planning and outcome assessment. *Psychological Assessment, 4*, 92–101.

Gable, S. L., & Haidt, J. (2005). What (and why) is positive psychology? *Review of General Psychology, 9,* 103–110.

Gable, S. L., Reis, H. T., Impett, E. A., & Asher, E. R. (2004). What do you do when things go right?: The intrapersonal and interpersonal benefits of sharing positive events. *Journal of Personality and Social Psychology, 87,* 228–245.

Gillham, J. E., & Reivich, K. J. (1999). Prevention of depressive symptoms in school children: A research update. *Psychological Science, 10,* 461–462.

Giltay, E. J., Geleijnse, J. M., Zitman, F. G., Hoekstra, T., & Schouten, E. G. (2004). Dispositional optimism and all-cause and cardiovascular mortality in a prospective cohort of elderly Dutch men and women. *Archives of General Psychiatry, 61,* 1126–1135.

Gladis, M. M., Gosch, E. A., Dishuk, N. M., & Crits-Christoph, P. (1999). Quality of life: Expanding the scope of clinical significance. *Journal of Consulting and Clinical Psychology, 67,* 320–331.

Goldberg, C. (2006, March 10). Harvard's crowded course to happiness: "Positive psychology" draws students in droves, *The Boston Globe.* Retrieved March 21, 2006, from *www.boston.com/news/local/articles/2006/03/10/harvards_crowded_course_to_happiness/.*

Grant, G., Salcedo, V., Hynan, L., & Frisch, M. B. (1995). Effectiveness of quality of life therapy for depression. *Psychological Reports, 76,* 1203–1208.

Haidt, J. (2006). *The happiness hypothesis: Finding modern truth in ancient wisdom.* New York: Basic Books.

Hamilton, M. (1960). A rating scale for depression. *Journal of Neurology, Neurosurgery, and Psychiatry, 23,* 56–62.

Helsel, W. J., & Matson, J. L. (1984). The assessment of depression in children: The internal structure of the Children's Depression Inventory (CDI). *Behavior Research and Therapy, 22,* 289–298.

Hoorens, V. (1996). Consequences of unrealistic optimism for positive and negative events. *International Journal of Psychology, 31,* 184–185.

Huebner, E. S. (1991). Initial development of the Student's Life Satisfaction Scale. *School Psychology International, 12,* 231–240.

Inghilleri, P. (1999). *From subjective experience to cultural change.* New York: Cambridge University Press.

Ito, T. A., Larsen, J. T., Smith, N. K., & Cacioppo, J. T. (1998). Negative information weighs more heavily on the brain: The negativity bias in evaluative categorizations. *Journal of Personality and Social Psychology, 75,* 887–900.

Jahoda, M. (1958). *Current concepts of positive mental health.* New York: Basic Books.

James, W. (1999). *The varieties of religious experience: A study in human nature.* New York: Modern Library. (Original work published 1902)

Joseph, S., & Linley, A. P. (2005). Positive psychological approaches to therapy. *Counseling and Psychotherapy Research, 5,* 5–10.

Jung, C. G. (1934). The integration of the personality. New York: Harcourt, Brace & World.

Kabat-Zin, J. (1991). *Full catastrophe living: Using the wisdom of your body and mind to face stress, pain, and illness.* New York: Dell.

Kahneman, D., & Tversky, A. (1984). Choices, values, and frames. *American Psychologist, 39,* 341–350.

Kazdin, A. E., & Weisz, J. R. (Eds.). (2003). Evidence-based psychotherapies for children and adolescents. New York: Guilford Press.

Keyes, C. L. M. (2003). Complete mental health: An agenda for the 21st century. In C. L. M. Keys & J. Haidt (Eds.), *Flourishing: Positive psychology and the life well-lived* (pp. 293–312). Washington, DC: American Psychological Association.

Keyes, C., & Lopez, S. (2002). Toward a science of mental health: Positive directions in diagnosis and interventions. In C. Snyder & S. Lopez (Eds.), *Handbook of positive psychology* (pp. 45–62). New York: Oxford University Press.

King, L., & Miner, K. (2000). Writing about the perceived benefits of traumatic events: Implications for physical health. *Personality and Social Psychology Bulletin, 26*, 220–230.

Klausner, E., Snyder, C. R., & Cheavens, J. (2000). A hope-based group treatment for depressed older adult outpatients. In G. M. Williamson, D. R. Shaffer, & P. A. Parmelee (Eds.), *Physical illness and depression in older adults: A handbook of theory, research, and practice* (pp. 295–310). New York: Plenum Press.

Lambert, M. J., Hansen, N. B., Umphress, V., Lunnen, K., Okiishi, J., Burlingame, G. M., et al. (1996). *Administration and scoring manual for the Outcome Questionnaire (OQ-45.2)*. Stevenson, MD: American Professional Credentialing Services.

Lambert, M. J., Whipple, J. L., Hawkins, E. J., Vermeersch, D. A., Nielsen, S. L., & Smart, D. W. (2003). Is it time for clinicians to routinely track patient outcome?: A meta-analysis. *Clinical Psychology: Science and Practice, 10*, 288–301.

Larson, R. W. (2000). Toward a psychology of positive youth development. *American Psychologist, 55*, 170–183.

Lent, R. W. (2004). Towards a unifying theoretical and practical perspective on well-being and psychosocial adjustment. *Journal of Counseling Psychology, 5*, 482–509.

Lopez, S. J., Snyder, C. R., Magyar-Moe, J. L., Edwards, L. M., Pedrotti, J. T., Janowski, K., et al. (2004). Strategies for accentuating hope. In P. A. Linley & S. Joseph (Eds.), *Positive psychology in practice* (pp. 388–404). Hoboken, NJ: Wiley.

Lopez, S. J., Snyder, C. R., & Rasmussen, N. H. (2003). Striking a vital balance: Developing a complementary focus on human weakness and strength through positive psychological assessment. In S. J. Lopez & C. R. Snyder (Eds.), *Positive psychological assessment: A handbook of models and measures* (pp. 3–20). Washington, DC: American Psychological Association.

Luborsky, L., McLellan, A. T., Woody, G., & O'Brien, C. (1985). Therapist success and its determinants. *Archives of General Psychiatry, 42*, 602–611.

Luu, P., Collins, P., & Tucker, D. M. (2000). Mood, personality, and self-monitoring: Negative affect and emotionality in relation to frontal lobe mechanisms of error monitoring. *Journal of Experimental Psychology: General, 129*, 43–60.

Lyubomirsky, S., King, L. A., & Diener, E. (2005). The benefits of frequent positive affect. *Psychological Bulletin, 131*, 803–855.

Lyubomirsky, S., & Lepper, H. S. (1999). A measure of subjective happiness: Preliminary reliability and construct validation. *Social Indicators Research, 46*, 137–155.

Lyubomirsky, S., Sheldon, K. M., & Schkade, D. (2005). Pursuing happiness: The architecture of sustainable change. *Review of General Psychology, 9*, 111–131.

Maddux, J. E. (2002). Stopping the "madness": Positive psychology and the deconstruction of illness ideology and the DSM. In C. R. Snyder & S. J. Lopez (Eds.), *Handbook of positive psychology* (pp. 13–25). New York: Oxford University Press.

Magnusson, D., & Stattin, H. (1998). Person–context interaction theories. In R. M. Lerner (Ed.), *Handbook of child psychology: Vol. 1. Theoretical models of human development* (5th ed., pp. 685–759). New York: Wiley.

Maslow, A. H. (1964). *Religions, values, and peak experiences.* New York: Penguin.

Maslow, A. H. (1971). *The farther reaches of human nature.* New York: Penguin.

Maslow, A. H. (1999). *Towards a psychology of being* (3rd ed.). New York: Wiley. (Original work published 1968)

Massimini, F., & Delle Fave, A. (2000). Individual development in a bio-cultural perspective. *American Psychologist, 55*, 24–33.

McAdams, D. P., Diamond, A., de St. Aubin, E., & Mansfield, E. (1997). Stories of commitment: The psychological construction of generative lives. *Journal of Personality and Social Psychology, 72*, 678–694.

McCullough, M. E. (2000). Forgiveness as a human strength: Conceptualization, measurement, and links to well-being. *Journal of Social and Clinical Psychology, 19*, 43–55.

McWilliams, N. (1994). *Psychoanalytic diagnosis.* New York: Guilford Press.

Moneta, G. B., & Csikszentmihalyi, M. (1996). The effect of perceived challenges and skills on the quality of subjective experience. *Journal of Personality, 64,* 275–310.

Moskowitz, J. T. (2003). Positive affect predicts lower risk of AIDS mortality. *Psychosomatic Medicine, 65,* 620–626.

Murray, H. A. (1938). *Explorations in personality.* Hoboken, NJ: Wiley.

Myers, D. G. (1992). *The pursuit of happiness: Who is happy—and why.* New York: William Morrow.

Nakamura, J., & Csikszentmihalyi, M. (2002). The concept of flow. In C. R. Snyder & S. J. Lopez (Eds.), *Handbook of positive psychology* (pp. 89–105). New York: Oxford University Press.

Nesse, R. M. (1991). What good is feeling bad? *The Sciences, 31,* 30–37.

Nesse, R. M., & Williams, G. C. (1994). *Why we get sick.* New York: New York Times Books.

Nisbett, R. E. (2003). *The geography of thought: How Asians and Westerners think differently . . . and why?* New York: Free Press.

Nolen-Hoeksema, S., Parker, L. E., & Larson, J. (1994). Ruminative coping with depressed mood following loss. *Journal of Personality and Social Psychology, 67,* 92–104.

Norem, J., & Chang, E. (2002). The positive psychology of negative thinking. *Journal of Clinical Psychology, 58,* 993–1001.

Nozik, R. (1997). Value and pleasure. In T. L. Carson & P. L. Moser (Eds.), *Morality and the good life* (pp. 135–144). New York: Oxford University Press.

Orlinsky, D. E., Ronnestad, M. H., & Willutzki, U. (2004). Fifty years of psychotherapy process–outcome research: Continuity and change. In M. J. Lambert (Ed.), *Bergin and Garfield's handbook of psychotherapy and behavior change* (5th ed., pp. 307–389). New York: Wiley.

Ostir, G. V., Markides, K. S., Black, S. A., & Goodwin, J. S. (2000). Emotional well-being predicts subsequent functional independence and survival. *Journal of the American Geriatrics Society, 48,* 473–478.

Parducci, A. (1995). *Happiness, pleasure and judgment: The contextual theory and its implications.* Mahwah, NJ: Erlbaum.

Pargament, K. I., & Mahoney, A. (2002). Spirituality: Discovering and conserving the sacred. In C. R. Snyder & S. J. Lopez (Eds.), *Handbook of positive psychology* (pp. 646–659). New York: Oxford University Press.

Pennebaker, J. W. (1993). Putting stress into words: Health, linguistic, and therapeutic implications. *Behavioral Research and Therapy, 31,* 539–548.

Peterson, B. E., & Stewart, A. J. (1993). Generativity and social motives in young adults. *Journal of Personality and Social Psychology, 65,* 186–198.

Peterson, C., Park, N., & Seligman, M. E. P. (2005). Orientations to happiness and life satisfaction: The full life versus the empty life. *Journal of Happiness Studies, 6,* 25–41.

Peterson, C., & Seligman, M. E. P. (1984). Causal explanations as a risk factor for depression: Theory and evidence. *Psychological Review, 91,* 347–374.

Peterson, C., & Seligman, M. E. P. (2004). *Character strengths and virtues: A handbook and classification.* Washington, DC: American Psychological Association.

Plante, T. G. (2005). *Contemporary clinical psychology* (2nd ed.). Hoboken, NJ: Wiley.

Puska, P., Vartiainen, E., Tuomilehto, J., Salomaa, V., & Nissinen, A. (1998). Changes in premature deaths in Finland: Successful long-term prevention of cardiovascular diseases. *Bulletin of the World Health Organization, 76,* 419–425.

Radloff, L. S. (1977). The CES-D scale: A self-report depression scale for research in the general population. *Applied Psychological Measurement, 1,* 385–401.

Rashid, T. (2004). Enhancing strengths through the teaching of positive psychology. *Dissertation Abstracts International, 64,* 6339.

Rashid, T. (2005). *Positive Psychotherapy Inventory.* Unpublished manuscript, University of Pennsylvania, Philadelphia.

Rashid, T., Anjum, A., & Lennox, C. (2006). *Positive psychotherapy for middle school children.* Unpublished manuscript, Toronto District School Board.

Rashid, T., & Seligman, M. E. P. (in press). *Positive psychotherapy: A treatment manual.* New York: Oxford University Press.

Rogers, C. R. (1951). *Client-centered therapy: Its current practice, implications, and theory.* Boston: Houghton Mifflin.

Rogers, C. R. (1959). A theory of therapy, personality and interpersonal relationships, as developed in the client-centered framework. In S. Koch (Ed.), *Psychology: A study of a science: Vol. 3. Foundations of the person and the social context* (pp. 184–256). New York: McGraw-Hill.

Rogers, C. (1969). *Freedom to learn.* Columbus, OH: Merrill.

Rokeach, M. (1973). *The nature of human values.* New York: Free Press.

Rozin, P., & Royzman, E. B. (2001). Negativity bias, negativity dominance, and contagion. *Personality and Social Psychology Review, 5,* 296–320.

Russell, B. (1930). *The conquest of happiness.* New York: Liveright.

Ryan, R. M., Sheldon, K. M., Kasser, T., & Deci, E. L. (1996). All goals are not created equal: An organismic perspective on the nature of goals and their regulation. In P. M. Gollwitzer & J. A. Bargh (Eds.), *The psychology of action: Linking cognition and motivation to behavior* (pp. 7–47). New York: Guilford Press.

Ryff, C. D., & Keyes, C. L. M. (1995). The structure of psychological well-being revisited. *Journal of Personality and Social Psychology, 69,* 719–727.

Ryff, C. D., & Singer, B. (1996). Psychological well-being: Meaning, measurement, and implications for psychotherapy research. *Psychotherapy and Psychosomatics, 65,* 14–23.

Ryff, C. D., & Singer, B. (1998). Contours of positive human health. *Psychological Inquiry, 9,* 1–28.

Ryff, C. D., & Singer, B. (2000). Interpersonal flourishing: A positive health agenda for the new millennium. *Personality and Social Psychology Review, 4,* 30–44.

Ryff, C. D., & Singer, B. (2002). From social structure to biology: Integrative science in pursuit of human health and well-being. In C. R. Snyder & S. J. Lopez (Eds.), *Handbook of positive psychology* (pp. 541–555). New York: Oxford University Press.

Schulz, R., & Decker, D. (1985). Long-term adjustment to physical disability: The role of social support, perceived control, and self-blame. *Journal of Personality and Social Psychology, 48,* 1162–1172.

Schwartz, B., Monterosso, J., Lyubomirsky, S., White, K., & Lehman, D. R. (2002). Maximizing versus satisficing: Happiness is a matter of choice. *Journal of Personality and Social Psychology, 83,* 1178–1197.

Schwartz, B., & Sharpe, K. E. (2006). Practical wisdom: Aristotle meets positive psychology. *Journal of Happiness Studies, 7,* 377–395.

Schwartz, S. H. (1994). Are there universal aspects in the structure and account of human values? *Journal of Social Issues, 50*(4), 19–45.

Seligman, M. E. P. (1991). *Learned optimism.* New York: Knopf.

Seligman, M. E. P. (1995). The effectiveness of psychotherapy: The *Consumer Reports* study. *American Psychologist, 50,* 965–974.

Seligman, M. E. P. (1999). The president's address. *American Psychologist, 54,* 559–562.

Seligman, M. E. P. (2002). *Authentic happiness: Using the new positive psychology to realize your potential for lasting fulfillment.* New York: Free Press.

Seligman, M. E. P. (2004, September). Positive interventions: More evidence of effectiveness. *Authentic Happiness Newsletter.* Retrieved January 9, 2007, from *www.authentichappiness. sas.upenn.edu/newsletter.aspx?id=45.*

Seligman, M. E. P., & Csikszentmihalyi, M. (2000). Positive psychology: An introduction. *American Psychologist, 55,* 5–14.

Seligman, M. E. P., Rashid, T., & Parks, A. C. (2006). Positive psychotherapy. *American Psychologist, 61,* 774–788.

Seligman, M. E. P., Steen, T. A., Park, N., & Peterson, C. (2005). Positive psychology progress: Empirical validation of interventions. *American Psychologist, 60,* 410–421.

Shadish, W. R., Navarro, A. M., Matt, G. E., & Phillips, G. (2000). The effects of psychological therapies under clinically representative conditions: A meta-analysis. *Psychological Bulletin, 126*, 512–529.

Sherbourne, C. D., Hays, R. D., & Wells, K. B. (1995). Personal and psychosocial risk factors for physical and mental health outcomes and course of depression among depressed patients. *Journal of Consulting and Clinical Psychology, 63*, 345–355.

Sloan, D. (1980). Teaching of ethics in the American undergraduate curriculum, 1876–1976. In D. Callahan & S. Bok (Eds.), *Ethics teaching in higher education* (pp. 2–37). New York: Plenum Press.

Smart, J. J. C., & Williams, B. A. O. (1973). *Utilitarianism: For and against.* London: Cambridge University Press.

Snyder, C. R. (1994). *The psychology of hope: You can get there from the here.* New York: Free Press.

Snyder, C. R., Sympson, S. C., Ybasco, F. C., Borders, T. F., Babyak, M. A., & Higgins, R. L. (1996). Development and validation of the State Hope Scale. *Journal of Personality and Social Psychology, 2*, 321–335.

Suh, E., Diener, E., & Fujita, F. (1996). Events and subjective well-being: Only recent events matter. *Journal of Personality and Social Psychology, 70*, 1091–1102.

Teasdale, J. D., Segal, Z. V., William, J. M., Ridgeway, V. A., Soulsby, J. M., & Lou, M. A. (2000). Prevention of relapse/recurrence in major depression by mindfulness-based cognitive therapy. *Journal of Consulting and Clinical Psychology, 68*, 615–623.

Terman, L. (1939). The gifted student and his academic environment. *School and Society, 49*, 65–73.

Terman, L., Buttenweiser, P., Johnson, W., & Wilson, D. (1938). *Psychological factors in marital happiness.* New York: McGraw-Hill.

Tolstoy, L. (1999). *Anna Karenina.* New York: Modern Library. (Original work published 1877)

Tugade, M. M., & Fredrickson, B. L. (2004). Resilient individuals use positive emotions to bounce back from negative emotional experiences. *Journal of Personality and Social Psychology, 86*, 320–333.

Wachtel, P. L. (1977). *Psychoanalysis and behavior therapy and the relational world.* Washington, DC: American Psychological Association.

Wallace, A. B., & Shapiro, S. L. (2006). Mental balance and well-being: Building bridges between Buddhism and Western psychology. *American Psychologist, 61*, 690–701.

Wampold, B. E. (2001). *The great psychotherapy debate: Models, methods, and findings.* Mahwah, NJ: Erlbaum.

Watson, D., Clark, L. A., & Tellegen, A. (1988). Development and validation of a brief measure of positive and negative affect: The PANAS scales. *Journal of Personality and Social Psychology, 54*, 1063–1070.

Watts, A. (1966). *The book: On the taboo against knowing who you are.* New York: Vintage.

Weinberger, J. (1995). Common factors aren't so common: The common factors dilemma. *Clinical Psychology: Science and Practice, 2*, 45–69.

William, A., Haber, D., Weaver, G., & Freeman, J. (1998). Altruistic activity. *Activities, Adaptation and Aging, 22*, 31–43.

Wright, B. A. (1988). Attitudes and the fundamental negative bias. In H. E. Yuker (Ed.), *Attitudes toward persons with disabilities* (pp. 3–21). New York: Springer.

Wrzesniewski, A., McCauley, C., Rozin, P., & Schwartz, B. (1997). Jobs, careers, and callings: People's relations to their work. *Journal of Research in Personality, 31*, 21–33.

Zung, W. W. K. (1965). A self-rating depression scale. *Archives of General Psychiatry, 12*, 63–70.

APPENDIX 11.1. Positive Psychotherapy Inventory—Children's Version

Please read each group of statements carefully. Then pick the one statement in each group that best describes the way you have been feeling for the past two weeks, including today. Be sure to read all of the statements in each group before making your choice.

Some questions are regarding strengths. Strengths are actions, behaviors, habits, thoughts, and feelings that are good to you and others. Examples of strengths are being kind, hopeful, cooperative, cheerful, gentle, honest, curious, creative, open minded, playful, fair, nice, organized, thoughtful, graceful, responsible, thankful, and flexible.

	Theme	Item			
1.	Pleasure	I am cheerful.	Often	Sometimes	Never
2.	Engagement	I know what are my strengths.	Often	Sometimes	Never
3.	Meaning	What I do benefits others.	Often	Sometimes	Never
4.	Pleasure	Others say I look happy.	Often	Sometimes	Never
5.	Engagement	I look for creative ways to use my strengths.	Often	Sometimes	Never
6.	Meaning	I am close to my loved ones.	Often	Sometimes	Never
7.	Pleasure	I am thankful for many good things in my life.	Often	Sometimes	Never
8.	Engagement	I solve problems using my strengths.	Often	Sometimes	Never
9.	Meaning	I pray or participate in religious/spiritual activities.	Often	Sometimes	Never
10.	Pleasure	I feel relaxed.	Often	Sometimes	Never
11.	Engagement	My concentration is very good in tasks and activities that use my strengths.	Often	Sometimes	Never
12.	Meaning	I participate in volunteer activities in my school and neighborhood.	Often	Sometimes	Never
13.	Pleasure	I slow down to enjoy things that bring me pleasure.	Often	Sometimes	Never
14.	Engagement	Time passes quickly when I am busy in tasks and activities that use my strengths.	Often	Sometimes	Never
15.	Meaning	I know strengths of my loves ones.	Often	Sometimes	Never
16.	Pleasure	I laugh and smile.	Often	Sometimes	Never
17.	Engagement	I complete tasks and activities, which use my strengths despite hurdles.	Often	Sometimes	Never
18.	Meaning	I use my strengths to help others.	Often	Sometimes	Never

Note. Scoring: Never = 0; Sometimes = 1; Often = 2.
Copyright by Tayyab Rashid. This inventory can be used for research or clinical purposes without contacting the author. For psychometric details, e-mail *tayyab@psych.upenn.edu*.

12 Interpersonal Psychotherapy for Treatment and Prevention of Adolescent Depression

Jami F. Young and Laura Mufson

Adolescent depression is a serious mental health concern. Although estimates vary across studies, approximately 15% of adolescents experience a major depressive episode during their lifetimes (Kessler & Walters, 1998). Depression in adolescence is associated with significant impairment (Puig-Antich et al., 1993) and an increased risk for developing a future major depressive episode (Lewinsohn, Rohde, Klein, & Seeley, 1999). Unfortunately, community studies indicate that many adolescents who meet criteria for a depressive disorder do not receive an adequate course of treatment (e.g., Lewinsohn & Clarke, 1999). This points to the need for treatments that can be delivered in schools and other community settings, where children and adolescents are most likely to receive services (Hoagwood, Burns, Kiser, Ringeisen, & Schoenwald, 2001; Hoagwood & Olin, 2002; Weisz & Jensen, 2001), and the need for preventive interventions that can reach a larger portion of the population. We believe that interpersonal psychotherapy (IPT) can help address this need.

In this chapter, we discuss the treatment and prevention of adolescent depression using IPT. First, we provide a discussion of the theoretical underpinnings of IPT. Next, we discuss the adolescent adaptation of IPT, interpersonal psychotherapy for depressed adolescents (IPT-A; Mufson, Dorta, Moreau, & Weissman, 2004), providing detailed information about the structure and techniques of this treatment. We also summarize the empirical findings. Finally, we outline interpersonal psychotherapy–adolescent skills training (IPT-AST), an adaptation of IPT-A that was developed as a preventive intervention (Young & Mufson, 2003). We also present preliminary efficacy data supporting its use as an indicated and universal preventive intervention for depression.

THEORETICAL BACKGROUND OF IPT

IPT is a brief treatment that was developed for depressed adults (Weissman, Markowitz, & Klerman, 2000) and has been shown to be efficacious in numerous studies (e.g., Elkin et al., 1989; Frank, Kupfer, Wagner, McEachran, & Cornes, 1991; Sloane, Stapes, & Schneider, 1985; Weissman et al., 1979). IPT is based on the premise that depression occurs in an interpersonal context. Regardless of the etiology, depression affects our relationships and our relationships affect our mood. Thus, the focus of treatment is on patients' depressive symptoms and the interpersonal context in which these symptoms occur. The theoretical roots of IPT stem from the work of interpersonal theorists, who argued that interpersonal interactions form the basis of personality. For instance, Meyer (1957) argued that you need to understand the individual's current interpersonal experiences to understand his or her psychiatric illness. Sullivan (1953) believed that psychiatric problems stem from and are perpetuated by poor communication with others. As such, treatment needs to address the individual's interpersonal interactions, as well as his or her symptoms and behaviors.

Research supports an interpersonal approach to the conceptualization and treatment of depression (Hammen, 1999; Joiner, Coyne, & Blalock, 1999). Depression, even at subthreshold levels, has been found to be associated with significant interpersonal problems in community and clinical samples of adults and adolescents (e.g., Lewinsohn et al., 1994; Puig-Antich et al., 1993; Sheeber, Hops, Alpert, Davis, & Andrews, 1997; Stader & Hokanson, 1998). Research has documented that interpersonal experiences are often precipitants of the onset of depression (Hammen, 1999). Once depressed, individuals engage with others in ways that cause them to lose interpersonal support and can lead to a loss of or difficulties in relationships, further exacerbating their depression (Coyne, 1976; Weissman & Paykel, 1974). These findings point to the importance of focusing on interpersonal events and interpersonal skills when treating depression.

IPT conceptualizes depression as composed of three elements—symptom formation, social functioning, and personality—and focuses mainly on the first two. The central goals of IPT are to decrease depressive symptoms and to improve interpersonal functioning. To accomplish these goals, the therapist and patient identify a specific problem area, discuss relevant communication and problem-solving techniques for that problem area, and practice these skills in session, with the patient applying them outside sessions in the context of significant relationships.

IPT-A FOR TREATMENT OF ADOLESCENT DEPRESSION

Based on the success of IPT with adults, the interpersonal literature discussed above, and the similarities between adolescent and adult depression (Ryan et al., 1987), IPT has been adapted to treat adolescent depression. IPT-A is developmentally relevant for adolescents who are becoming increasingly focused on their relationships. IPT-A addresses developmental issues that are pertinent to adolescence, including the development of romantic relationships, separation from parents, experiencing the death of a loved one, and negotiating peer relationships. By focusing on increasing adolescents' independence and negotiating their interdependence on others, IPT-A is very relevant and appealing to teens. The treatment is structured, active, and emphasizes psychoeducation. In treatment, the adolescent is encouraged to take an active role in applying new strategies to the identified problem area. In this way, IPT-A is developmentally appropriate to the changes in problem-solving strategies that adolescents experience (Marx & Schulze, 1991).

Several specific changes have been made to adapt IPT for adolescent depression. A separate discussion has been added to the problem area of role transitions to deal with transitions related to family changes, such as divorce. These transitions pose significant interpersonal difficulties and have been shown to be associated with depressive symptoms in adolescents (Hetherington, Bridges, & Insabella, 1998). A second change is the inclusion of parents in the treatment. Although we recommend their attendance at each phase of treatment, the involvement of parents in IPT-A is flexible. The degree of parental involvement is discussed and negotiated between the therapist and the adolescent during the course of treatment, with the support and cooperation of the parents.

The treatment techniques and strategies have been modified as well, to address the developmental level of the adolescents. Techniques employed specifically with adolescents include giving them a scale from 1 to 10 to rate their depressed mood to help monitor changes from week to week; doing more basic social skills work; teaching perspective-taking skills to counteract adolescent black-and-white thinking about problems; and helping them to negotiate parent–child tensions. Additional techniques can be used to deal with issues that can affect the treatment of adolescents, such as suicidality, abuse, school refusal, and the involvement of child protective services.

IPT-A is an outpatient treatment designed for adolescents with nonpsychotic, unipolar depression. It is not indicated for adolescents who are currently in crisis, actively suicidal or homicidal, psychotic, bipolar, or mentally retarded. If an evaluation reveals that an adolescent is using alcohol or drugs, the clinician needs to make a decision about whether the substance use is severe enough to warrant substance abuse treatment before addressing the depression. In general, IPT-A is not recommended for adolescents who are actively abusing substances. Among teens with unipolar depression, our clinical experience has shown us that those who are motivated to be in treatment derive the most benefit from IPT-A. Because the adolescent and clinician regularly review the adolescent's depressive symptoms and link these symptoms to interpersonal events, it is important that the adolescent be able to acknowledge that he or she is depressed and to agree with the therapist that at least one interpersonal problem exists. Experience also suggests that adolescents whose families are supportive of treatment are more likely to have positive treatment outcomes, although family involvement is not a requirement for treatment.

Course of IPT-A

IPT-A is a time-limited treatment. It is designed as a once weekly, 12-session treatment. Treatment can be extended to 16 sessions if it is clinically indicated, but this should be determined at the beginning of treatment. In certain settings, a more flexible schedule may be necessary. For instance, in the school effectiveness study conducted by Mufson and colleagues (Mufson, Dorta, Wickramaratne, et al., 2004), adolescents received IPT-A for 8 consecutive weeks. The remaining 4 sessions were more flexible, depending on the individual patient's need or school schedule and were conducted over an additional 8-week time period.

IPT-A is divided into three phases: (1) the initial phase, (2) the middle phase, and (3) the termination phase. At the beginning of each session, regardless of the phase of treatment, the clinician assesses the adolescent's depressive symptoms, noting any changes that occurred over the course of the week, and links changes in symptoms to interpersonal events. Following the review of symptoms, the session progresses to the tasks particular to the phase of treatment—for instance, conducting the interpersonal inventory, role playing an interpersonal interaction, or discussing the adolescent's warning signs of depression. This structure ensures that the treatment focuses on issues related to the identified problem area. Throughout treatment, both the therapist and the adolescent play an active role in the sessions. The therapist assesses depressive symptoms, inquires about interpersonal relationships, links the symptoms to interpersonal functioning, and guides the work on the interpersonal problem area. The adolescent is expected to discuss his or her interpersonal relationships, work to find solutions to the interpersonal problem, and practice new interpersonal techniques.

Initial Phase of Treatment

The initial phase of IPT-A typically consists of the first four sessions. We recommend that the parent(s) participate in one session during the initial phase of treatment, most typically the first session. There are several objectives for this phase of treatment:

1. Confirm the depression diagnosis.
2. Educate the adolescent and family about depression and assign the adolescent the "limited sick role."
3. Introduce the principles of IPT-A and the structure of treatment.
4. Conduct the interpersonal inventory to identify an interpersonal problem area.
5. Make a treatment contract.

CONFIRMING THE DEPRESSION DIAGNOSIS

Although the diagnostic assessment is typically conducted before beginning IPT-A, it is important to confirm the depression diagnosis in the first session. The clinician should assess the adolescent's current depressive symptoms, history of depression, and other symptoms, such as mania, psychosis, or substance abuse, that might make IPT-A an inappropriate treatment. As discussed earlier, in the remaining sessions, the therapist conducts a brief review of the adolescent's symptoms to monitor weekly changes in mood and other depression symptoms.

EDUCATION ABOUT DEPRESSION AND ASSIGNING THE "LIMITED SICK ROLE"

Educating the adolescent and the parents about depression is an important objective in the first session. This follows directly from the review of symptoms and involves educating the adolescent and parents about the symptoms and behaviors associated with depression. This provides a context for depression symptoms that may not have been understood. For instance, parents and adolescents may not be aware that the recent increase in arguments may be attributable to the adolescent's irritability, a core symptom of depression. Part of the education component is likening depression to a medical illness that can be treated. This medical model of depression helps decrease the stigma associated with depression, takes the blame off the adolescent or others for causing the depression, and provides an optimistic prognosis. The therapist should communicate to the adolescent and parents that the likelihood of recovery from depression is relatively high and that other treatments for depression exist if IPT-A is not effective for that individual.

Next, the therapist assigns the adolescent the limited sick role. This involves discussing with the adolescent and parents that, similar to someone with a medical illness, an adolescent with symptoms of depression may not be able to do things as well as before the depression. It is important to balance encouraging understanding of decreased functioning while also communicating that the adolescent should continue to attend school and fulfill family and academic responsibilities. The adolescent should also be encouraged to socialize with family and friends. The purpose of the limited sick role is to help the family to be more understanding and to shift the blame from the adolescent to the disorder while also encouraging involvement in normal daily activities. This differs from adult IPT, in which the patient is given the sick role (i.e., not the limited sick role) and is encouraged to scale back on activities until he or she feels better. The reason for this difference is that, developmentally, it is important to get the adolescent back to regular school attendance as soon as possible.

INTRODUCING THE PRINCIPLES AND STRUCTURE OF IPT-A

At the beginning of treatment, the therapist explains the structure and context of the treatment to the adolescent and parents, including the time-limited nature of IPT-A, the roles of the therapist, adolescent, and parents, and the theory behind IPT-A. The discussion of the theory and structure of the therapy makes the course of treatment predictable and decreases the likelihood of dropout. In addition, this discussion helps to enlist the parents as collaborative agents in treating the adolescent's depression. The therapist should explain that the therapy will target the depressive symptoms and relationship problems most relevant to the depression itself. The therapist and adolescent will work together to identify important interpersonal strategies and to practice them to improve certain relationships, and thus his or her mood. In the majority of the sessions, only the adolescent will be present, but the parents may be invited to one or two sessions during the middle phase if the therapist and the adolescent feel that it would be helpful.

CONDUCTING THE INTERPERSONAL INVENTORY TO IDENTIFY AN INTERPERSONAL PROBLEM AREA

Much of what is described above occurs in the first session. The rest of the initial phase of treatment is focused on conducting the interpersonal inventory, which is an assessment of the important relationships in the adolescent's life. Similar to placing an emphasis on the assessment of the adolescent's symptoms, IPT-A also emphasizes the assessment of the adolescent's interpersonal functioning. The inventory is similar to a diagnostic instrument in that it is intended to help the therapist to gain a better understanding of the adolescent's interpersonal world. The goal of the interpersonal inventory is to identify those interpersonal issues that are most closely related to the onset and/or persistence of the depression. Although the primary informant for the interpersonal inventory is the adolescent, parents can also provide information about the adolescent's relationships.

During the interpersonal inventory, the therapist asks the adolescent to identify important people in his or her life. The therapist then asks detailed questions about these relationships to obtain an idea of the adolescent's daily life and to determine which relationships might be the focus of the therapy. The information collected should include the positive and negative aspects of the relationships, how the relationships have changed over time, the context and frequency of interactions within the relationships, and goals for changing the relationships during treatment. In addition, the therapist asks about significant past relationships and important interpersonal events that may be connected to the onset of the disorder.

On the basis of the interpersonal inventory, the therapist identifies common themes or problems in the various relationships (e.g., the adolescent does not discuss things that are bothering him or her until he or she explodes in anger). The adolescent and therapist choose one of the four interpersonal problem areas that will be the focus of treatment: grief, role disputes, role transitions, or interpersonal deficits. The therapist should explain to the adolescent the connection between the depressive symptoms and his or her interpersonal difficulties and how that fits into the framework of the identified problem area. Although it is most common to identify one interpersonal problem area to address in treatment, there are times when two problem areas are identified. In this case, part of the treatment contract (see below) will involve discussing how the two problem areas will be addressed during the rest of treatment—for instance, by addressing the most pressing problem first and then discussing the generalization of strategies from the primary to the secondary problem area.

MAKING THE TREATMENT CONTRACT

Following the identification of the interpersonal problem area, the adolescent and therapist establish a verbal treatment contract. In this contract, the adolescent's and parents' roles in treatment are specified, the identified problem area is highlighted, and practical details regarding the treatment are reviewed. While discussing the treatment contract, the therapist stresses to the adolescent that, for treatment to be most helpful, he or she will need to provide information about interactions that occurred in his or her relationships. In addition, the adolescent is informed that his or her parents may be invited to sessions to work on the identified problem area. The structure of treatment is also reviewed at this time. It is useful to highlight the number of sessions that have elapsed and the number of sessions that remain. The therapist emphasizes the importance of the adolescent coming to treatment on time and calling to cancel if necessary. Finally, the goals of the treatment for the individual teen are explained. These goals should be attainable and should emphasize reduction of depressive symptoms and improvement of interpersonal functioning. This contract is helpful for the treatment and serves as a model of clearly communicating expectations.

Middle Phase of Treatment

The middle phase of treatment is made up of sessions five through nine. During this phase there are three important treatment goals:

1. Further clarification of the identified problem area.
2. Identification of strategies for effectively targeting the problem.
3. Implementation of interventions to resolve the problem.

In this phase of treatment, the therapist continues to monitor the depression symptoms and considers adjunctive therapy, such as pharmacotherapy, if symptoms are worsening or failing to improve. The therapist should guide the discussion so that the focus remains on the problem area, helping the adolescent to link his or her feelings to interpersonal events and to express these feelings appropriately. The therapist educates the adolescent about interpersonal strategies and encourages the adolescent to identify strategies on his or her own. The therapist and adolescent may practice these strategies in session using role plays, and the adolescent is asked to apply these techniques outside the session. In addition, as the adolescent shares and discusses interpersonal difficulties and improvements, the therapist helps elucidate the connection between the adolescent's mood or symptom level and the interpersonal events. Finally, the therapist maintains contact with the adolescents' parents so that they can be involved in the treatment as the therapist sees necessary.

Although some of the techniques vary, depending on the problem area being addressed, several techniques are used across all of the problem areas. These general techniques are discussed in more detail before outlining the strategies and techniques that are particular to the specific problem areas.

LINKING AFFECT TO INTERPERSONAL EVENTS

An important technique in IPT-A is linking affect with interpersonal events. This is done both in the beginning of the session, when reviewing symptoms, and during the rest of the session. There are typically two types of adolescents: those who discuss events that have occurred without any discussion of feelings and those who report feeling a certain way but do not know what caused the feeling. For both types of adolescents, it is beneficial to link interpersonal events with their moods. If an adolescent comes in and reports increased irritability, it is important to link that change to any events that occurred in the past week. It may be necessary to review the week in great detail to uncover what event(s) may have been responsible for the change in mood. Conversely, if an adolescent comes in and reports a fight with her boyfriend, it is important for the therapist to ask how this event made her feel and whether or not the event affected her depressive symptoms. This approach serves to educate an adolescent about the link between interpersonal events and his or her mood, as well as making the young person more comfortable with and adept at identifying and communicating feelings.

COMMUNICATION ANALYSIS

Communication analysis is an important technique in the middle phase of treatment. When the adolescent presents an interpersonal event that occurred during the week, it is helpful to analyze the communication as it occurred. The goals of communication analysis are to help the adolescent recognize the impact of his or her words on others, the feelings he or she conveyed verbally and nonverbally, the feelings generated by the communication, and how modifying the communication may impact both the outcome of the interaction and the adolescent's associated feelings. This involves getting detailed information about the conversation such as, How did the discussion start? What exactly did the adolescent say? Is that what he or she wanted to say? What did the person say back? How did that make the adolescent feel? What happened next? Is that the outcome the adolescent wanted?

Once the therapist has a clear understanding of the communication, it is useful to discuss how altering the communication at various points may have led to a different outcome. The therapist should ask the adolescent if he or she has any ideas about what could have been said differently. For instance, starting the conversation calmly or letting the other person know you understand his or her point of view may have made the other person more willing to listen. After the therapist and adolescent identify more adaptive communication strategies, it is helpful to role-play the communication using these techniques.

DECISION ANALYSIS

Once the adolescent and therapist have a better understanding of the interpersonal problem, including any communication issues, it is useful to conduct a decision analysis to determine the best course of action. Decision analysis closely resembles problem-solving techniques in other therapies but focuses on addressing interpersonal problems. Decision analysis includes selecting an interpersonal situation that is causing a problem, encouraging the adolescent to generate solutions, evaluating the pros and cons of each solution, selecting a solution to try first, and role-playing the interaction needed for the chosen solution. In the following session, the therapist and adolescent should review the interaction, examining possible reasons for its success or failure. It is important to start with a topic that is manageable and has a high likelihood of success. This can generate hope in adolescents that these strategies can help facilitate change in their relationships.

ROLE PLAYING

Role playing follows directly from both communication analysis and decision analysis. It is helpful to role-play the interpersonal interaction for the adolescent to feel more comfortable utilizing the strategies in real life. For instance, following a decision analysis, if an adolescent decides to talk to his parent about going out with friends, the therapist and adolescent would role-play this discussion. When doing a role play, it is important to act out the conversation, not just talk about it. Adolescents may be initially uncomfortable with role plays. To make an adolescent more comfortable, it is helpful if the role play is structured so that he or she knows what to expect. In addition, an adolescent may be more willing to role-play if allowed to choose which role to play first. Before the role play, the therapist and adolescent can discuss how the adolescent could start the conversation and how the other person might respond. In this way, the adolescent is prepared for the role play. It is important to role-play ideal outcomes, as well as less successful interactions, to prepare the adolescent to handle any type of response that may occur when the strategies are practiced outside the session.

WORK AT HOME

Homework is considered a natural extension of the work done in the session and is based on the assumption that treatment will be more effective when the adolescent addresses difficulties in outside relationships by practicing skills between sessions. In IPT-A, we have characterized homework as interpersonal "work at home," to reflect the fact that these assignments typically follow the interpersonal work conducted in treatment sessions. We have found that calling the activities "work at home" decreases the possible resistance of adolescents who associate homework with academic assignments. In our experience, the metaphor of an interpersonal experiment is useful for engaging adolescents. As in a lab experiment, in which one needs to figure out the right combination of chemicals, these interpersonal experiments can help the adolescent determine the best combination of strategies for dealing with important people or problems in his or her life. The therapist emphasizes that the adolescent is experimenting with new strategies and collecting data to bring back to the therapist about how useful the strategies are for the identified problem, thereby decreasing the notion of failing an assignment.

Although the aforementioned techniques apply across multiple problem areas, the middle phase of treatment also utilizes techniques specific to the identified problem area. A brief description of each problem area is provided below, as well as goals and techniques of the middle phase. More detailed information is available in the IPT-A manual (Mufson, Dorta, Moreau, et al., 2004).

GRIEF

Grief is identified as the problem area when the adolescent has experienced a loss through death that is associated with the onset of depressive symptoms. The depression does not need to follow the death immediately. It can be identified in adolescents who are suffering from an extended grieving period as well as those experiencing a more typical bereavement. IPT-A helps the adolescent mourn the loss of a loved one, while encouraging him or her to develop other relationships that can help fill some of the voids left by the death.

According to IPT-A, it is important for the adolescent to discuss the loss in significant detail, including his or her relationship with the deceased. During this process, the therapist encourages the adolescent to identify and express feelings associated with the relationship and the loss. In addition, the therapist helps the adolescent find a way to honor the memory of the deceased while engaging in other relationships. This includes creating a more realistic memory of the deceased person and the relationship. As treatment progresses, the therapist encourages the adolescent to develop new relationships or to further develop established relationships to help replace the support and the roles that were lost. This involves exploring the adolescent's fears about developing new relationships and rehearsing the skills needed to develop relationships or to engage in new activities.

INTERPERSONAL DISPUTES

Interpersonal role disputes often arise within a family or a peer relationship. This is the problem area that should be selected when the interpersonal difficulties precipitating the depression stem mainly from disagreements over what the adolescent's expected role is within the relationship. Such diverging expectations often lead to conflicts over issues such as money, sexuality, autonomy, and intimacy. Disputes do not necessarily lead to adolescent depression. However, when these disputes become chronic and unmanageable, they become more stressful and can act as precipitants of depression. Conversely, adolescents who are experiencing depression may become more irritable or may have other symptoms that make them ill equipped to manage interpersonal conflict. In such cases, the dispute may exacerbate the adolescent's depression.

When an adolescent presents with an interpersonal dispute, the therapist should help the adolescent clarify the dispute and any differences in expectations that may be contributing to the disagreement. The therapist works with the adolescent and the other person, if possible, to modify maladaptive communication patterns and any unrealistic expectations about the relationship. When a conflict involves a parent, he or she is invited to treatment to help address the problem. However, this problem area can be addressed with an adolescent alone when necessary. If a resolution seems impossible, the therapist works with the adolescent to develop strategies for coping with a relationship that cannot be changed. For instance, the therapist points out that decreasing the frequency of conflict can result in improved mood, even if the relationship cannot be changed completely. The therapist also encourages the adolescent to seek out other adaptive relationships that may address the adolescent's emotional needs more effectively.

ROLE TRANSITIONS

Role transitions occur when an adolescent progresses from one social role to another. When the adolescent is unable to adapt to such a change in circumstance, it may lead to depression. Such a shift may be particularly stressful when it happens quickly and without warning, if the adolescent experiences the change as a loss, or if other stressors arise concurrently. As discussed earlier, family structural changes, such as divorce, are especially common among adolescents. Other role transitions include starting high school, moving to a new town, and adjusting to increasing responsibilities associated with adolescence.

Treatment of this problem area begins by identifying and defining the role transition, followed by a discussion about what the transition means to the adolescent, demands associated with this change, and gains and losses associated with the transition. In addition, the therapist helps the adolescent learn skills that are necessary to manage the new role. If the role transition involves the adolescent's parents, they should be involved in some of the middle phase sessions whenever possible. For instance, if parents are not allowing their child to socialize with peers, then treatment attempts to address these difficulties in the context of a developmental transition.

INTERPERSONAL DEFICITS

Interpersonal deficits are the identified problem area when an adolescent lacks the social skills needed to have positive relationships with family members and friends owing to prolonged social isolation. Adolescents with problems in this area often experience loneliness and decreased self-confidence and self-esteem, which can lead to or exacerbate feelings of depression. The goal of treatment is to help the adolescent develop the skills needed to have more satisfying interpersonal relationships.

Treatment of interpersonal deficits involves reviewing past significant relationships, with a focus on problematic patterns in these relationships. The therapist helps the adolescent recognize the relationship between these interpersonal problems and his or her depression. For instance, when working with an adolescent who has difficulty in interacting with peers, the therapist might point out that the adolescent's social isolation leads to an increase in depressive symptoms, which in turn leads to an increase in social isolation. Next, the therapist introduces new strategies for handling interpersonal relationships, and then the adolescent and therapist practice these strategies in role plays. For example, a middle session may involve having the adolescent practice asking a friend to do something or telling a parent how he or she feels. The adolescent is then encouraged to try these strategies outside the session and to report on what happened the following week. Family members may be involved in treatment, particularly to help support the adolescent as he or she develops and practices these skills.

Termination Phase of Treatment

Sessions ten through twelve constitute the termination phase of IPT-A. During these sessions, the therapist and adolescent review the adolescent's progress, especially in regard to the identified problem area. Changes in interpersonal functioning and relationships are linked to improved mood and decreased symptoms. The therapist and adolescent identify the strategies that have been most helpful and discuss the importance of continuing to implement these strategies after termination. The therapist and adolescent should also discuss areas that still need improvement or may benefit from additional treatment. Because depression is a recurrent illness, it is important to discuss the adolescent's warning signs of depression and what he or she can do to address these symptoms if they return. In addition, the conclusion of the relationship with the therapist needs to be addressed during the final sessions.

The therapist should also meet with the parents for a termination session, if possible. Depending on the situation and the wishes of the adolescent, the therapist might meet with the parents separately or have a session with the adolescent and parents together. It is important for parents to hear about the progress made, the skills and strategies that were learned, and the warning signs of a possible relapse. Some adolescents may not be fully recovered at the end of treatment. These adolescents may still be experiencing symptoms or may be suffering from an additional disorder. If the therapist believes this is the case, he or she should discuss the possibility of continuing treatment with the adolescent and parents and the treatment options they might consider.

Efficacy and Effectiveness Research in IPT-A

Research has shown IPT-A to be an efficacious treatment for adolescent depression. Several randomized controlled clinical trials of IPT-A have been conducted, and two separate investigator teams have demonstrated its effects. In an open clinical trial, 12- to 18-year-olds with depressive symptoms who were referred to a hospital outpatient clinic were treated with IPT-A. After treatment, none of the subjects met the *Diagnostic and Statistical Manual of Mental Disorders*, third edition, revised (DSM-III-R) criteria for depression. The subjects were functioning at a higher level in school and at home and showed a significant decrease in psychological distress and depressive symptoms (Mufson et al., 1994).

In a controlled trial, conducted by Mufson and colleagues (Mufson, Weissman, Moreau, & Garfinkel, 1999), depressed adolescents who had been referred to a hospital-based clinic were randomized to receive either IPT-A or clinical monitoring for 12 weeks. At the end of treatment, significantly more adolescents receiving IPT-A met the recovery criteria for major depression than adolescents receiving clinical monitoring. Adolescents receiving IPT-A also had a significant decrease in depressive symptoms and increased social functioning and problem-solving skills.

Rosselló and Bernal (1999) compared a different adaptation of IPT, designed specifically for depressed adolescents in Puerto Rico, with cognitive-behavioral therapy (CBT) and those assigned to a waiting list condition. They showed that depressed adolescents receiving IPT or CBT experienced a greater reduction in symptoms, greater increase in self-esteem, and more improvement in social functioning than those in the waiting list condition. Furthermore, 52% of those receiving CBT versus 82% of those receiving IPT met the recovery criteria.

Mufson and colleagues recently investigated the effectiveness of IPT-A in community settings (Mufson, Dorta, Wickramaratne, et al., 2004). Clinicians in several school-based health clinics were trained to deliver IPT-A. Adolescents with major depression, dysthymia, depression disorder not otherwise specified, or adjustment disorder with depressed mood were randomized to receive either treatment as usual (supportive, individual counseling) or IPT-A. Both treatments were delivered by school-based clinicians. Adolescents with comorbid anxiety disorders, attention-deficit/hyperactivity disorder (ADHD), and oppositional defiant disorder (ODD) were allowed to participate in the study. The results showed that subjects receiving IPT-A, as compared with treatment as usual, demonstrated a greater decrease in depression symptoms and depression severity, greater overall functioning, and significantly better social functioning. These findings support IPT-A as an effective treatment when delivered by community clinicians.

Mufson and colleagues (Mufson, Gallagher, Dorta, & Young, 2004) recently developed a group model of IPT-A (IPT-AG). A pilot controlled clinical trial of this group adaptation was conducted in a mental health specialty clinic, comparing IPT-A to IPT-AG in treating depressed adolescents. Data from this preliminary study found no significant differences between the treatment conditions, indicating that IPT-AG may be an efficacious treatment for depression in adolescents. Currently, a randomized controlled clinical trial is under way, studying the effectiveness of IPT-AG in comparison to treatment as usual as delivered by clinicians in school-based health clinics.

IPT-AST FOR PREVENTION OF ADOLESCENT DEPRESSION

Community studies indicate that many adolescents who meet the criteria for a depressive disorder do not receive an adequate course of treatment (e.g., Lewinsohn & Clarke, 1999). Thus, although many adolescents become depressed, few receive services and those who do receive services may not improve. This suggests the need for additional services that can augment traditional treatment approaches. Preventive interventions targeting adolescents who are at risk for developing a depressive disorder are one option. If efficacious, these interventions can prevent the onset of a depressive episode and its associated risks and impairments.

Preventive interventions are classified as universal, selective, and indicated (Gordon, 1983). Both selective and indicated interventions target individuals who are considered at risk for developing a disorder. One of the most salient risk factors for developing a depressive disorder is elevated depressive symptoms (Horwath, Johnson, Klerman, & Weissman, 1992; Lewinsohn et al., 1994; Pine, Cohen, Cohen, & Brook, 1999). Adolescents with depressive symptoms have a two- to threefold greater risk for developing a major depressive disorder in adulthood (Pine et al., 1999). In addition, the elevated depressive symptoms are persistent over time (Garrison, Jackson, Marsteller, McKeown, & Addy, 1990) and are associated with considerable psychosocial impairment (Gotlib, Lewinsohn, & Seeley, 1995; Judd, Paulus, Wells, & Rapaport, 1996; Lewinsohn, Solomon, Seeley, & Zeiss, 2000). In recognition of the considerable risk and impairment associated with depressive symptoms in adolescence, there has been a call for an increase in indicated preventive intervention research, targeting adolescents who report symptoms of depression but who do not meet the diagnostic criteria for a depressive disorder (Mrazek & Haggerty, 1994; U.S. Public Health Service, 2000).

We chose to adapt IPT-A as a preventive intervention for several reasons. First, IPT-A is an effective treatment for adolescent depression (Mufson et al., 1999; Mufson, Dorta, Wickramaratne, et al., 2004; Rosselló & Bernal, 1999). Second, IPT-A addresses conflict and interpersonal deficits, which have been shown to increase the risk for depression (e.g., Lewinsohn et al., 1994; Reinherz et al., 1989), and enhances communication and positive relationships, factors that protect against the development of depression (Carbonell, Reinherz, & Giaconia, 1998). The development of depression may be prevented by directly targeting these risk and protective factors. Third, IPT-A emphasizes psychoeducation and skill development, which are both relevant to prevention. Finally, IPT-A, with its focus on interpersonal issues, addresses the kinds of difficulties adolescents encounter on a day-to-day basis.

Course of IPT-AST

IPT-AST, known to the adolescents as "Teen Talk," was initially designed as an indicated preventive intervention for adolescent depression for adolescents in 7th to 10th grades. In its original format, IPT-AST involves two initial individual sessions and eight weekly 90-minute group sessions (Young & Mufson, 2003). The ideal group size is four to six adolescents of similar age (i.e., 7th and 8th graders). A group is led by one therapist or by cotherapists. Recently, IPT-AST was used as a universal intervention with 9th graders in rural Tennessee (Horowitz, Garber, Young, & Mufson, 2005). In this study, it was not feasible to include the initial individual sessions, given the large number of adolescents in each group (between 8 and 15 adolescents). Materials typically covered during the individual sessions were incorporated into the first group session. The remaining sessions followed the format provided below.

The group focuses on psychoeducation and general skill building that can be applied to various relationships within the framework of three interpersonal problem areas: interpersonal role disputes, role transitions, and interpersonal deficits. IPT-AST follows a modification of the group IPT-A manual (Mufson, Gallagher, Dorta, & Young, 2004). The primary modifications include decreasing the number of group sessions from 12 to 8; adding games and activities to illustrate the link between what we say and how others respond; and teaching the interpersonal techniques to group members, using fictional scenarios before applying them to real-life situations.

In the initial studies of IPT-AST discussed below, there was no parent involvement. Currently, we are examining the impact of involving parents in the intervention. In this iteration, parents are asked to join one of the individual pregroup sessions to receive psychoeducation about depression and to learn about the focus and structure of IPT-AST. The group leader has a second meeting with each set of parents and adolescents following group session five. This dyadic session provides an opportunity to update the parents on the adolescent's progress and provides a setting for the adolescent to practice the new techniques in a real-life situation, with the therapist present to act as coach. After the completion of the group, the parents and adolescent meet again with one of the group leaders to review what has been accomplished and to assess the need for additional services.

Pregroup Sessions

In the two individual pregroup sessions, the therapist meets with the adolescent to review his or her depression symptoms, to provide psychoeducation about depression and prevention, to explain the purpose of the group, and to conduct an abbreviated interpersonal inventory. The adolescent is told that the purpose of the group is to help prevent him or her from developing depression. Just as people brush their teeth to help prevent cavities, the hope is that participating in the group will help prevent the adolescent from becoming depressed. The therapist explains that although problems with peers or family members are not necessarily the cause of depression, they can make these problems worse. By teaching adolescents new skills to help them deal better with the people in their lives, we hope to prevent them from developing more serious depression.

In the rest of the pregroup sessions, the therapist completes an abbreviated interpersonal inventory with the adolescent, asking the types of questions indicated earlier. At the completion of the inventory, the therapist and adolescent outline goals for the group sessions. These goals may be focused on particular relationships, such as arguing less with parents, or may be more general, such as the adolescent's talking more to people about how he or she feels. We do not assign a particular problem area after the inventory, because it is unknown whether the adolescent's current relationship difficulties will be associated with the onset of a future depressive episode. Therefore, we choose to focus on interpersonal skill building that applies across problem areas with the hope that this will increase the potential preventive effects of the intervention.

Initial Phase

The initial phase of the intervention includes group sessions one through three. The goals of the initial phase are to:

1. Establish group rules.
2. Educate group members about depression.
3. Illustrate the impact of communication on others.
4. Introduce interpersonal strategies that will be used in the remaining group sessions.

EDUCATION ABOUT DEPRESSION

As in IPT-A, much time in IPT-AST is spent in the beginning of group educating adolescents about the symptoms of depression and the difference between having symptoms of depression and being depressed. The therapist describes a number of adolescents with various levels of depression and asks the group members to identify the symptoms and discuss the differences in severity. In addition, in all group sessions, each group member is given a binder that includes a weekly depression checklist and mood rating. The adolescents complete a depression checklist and a mood rating so that they quickly become familiar with the symptoms of depression.

ILLUSTRATING THE IMPACT OF COMMUNICATION ON OTHERS

Much of the initial phase of the group focuses on how what we say and how we say it impacts others. This is done primarily through the consideration of various scenarios and group activities. First, the therapist provides an example of an adolescent who is having an argument with her mother and says things out of anger, which she later regrets. The group discusses how the interaction might end and how the adolescent and mother may end up feeling. Next, the adolescents are given a piece of paper that asks them to make a statement in a certain way. For instance it may ask them to say, looking down, in a quiet voice, "I'm fine, really I'm fine." Each adolescent is asked to act out his or her statement, and then the group discusses how the person may be feeling and what conveyed that feeling. This leads to a discussion of verbal and nonverbal cues and how words can mean different things depending on how they are said.

In the second activity, group members are asked to role-play different scenarios to illustrate how communicating in a certain way influences another person's response. Examples of scenarios include wanting to ask your parent if you can go out with friends or talking to a friend who is spending all of his time with his girlfriend. Following each role play, the group discusses what was said and how each of the people felt during the exchange, highlighting moments when the conversation took on a positive or negative tone. In this way, the group leaders model communication analysis, which will be used more formally in the middle phase of treatment.

INTRODUCING INTERPERSONAL STRATEGIES

During group session three, the therapist introduces group members to several interpersonal strategies that they will be encouraged to use in their own relationships. Because this is a group intervention focused on prevention, we felt that it was important to have an explicit language for these techniques to increase the long-term use of these skills. Each strategy is listed on a cue card that is included in the group members' binders and has an associated label to help them to remember the strategy, such as "Strike while the iron is cold." Examples of the techniques include letting the other person know you understand his or her point of view and being specific when talking about a problem. Adolescents are taught each of these techniques and then practice using them by role-playing various scenarios.

Middle Phase

The middle phase of the group includes sessions four through six and closely follows the middle phase of IPT-A. Throughout the middle phase, the therapist helps the group members to link changes in their moods with interpersonal events. Adolescents are encouraged to identify interpersonal interactions that occurred during the previous week and to work on them in the group. This involves having an adolescent explain what happened, conducting a communication analysis, talking about what interpersonal techniques may be particularly relevant to the problem, engaging in decision analysis when needed, and practicing the revised interaction using role plays. The other group members are encouraged to help the adolescent identify interpersonal strategies and possible solutions and then act as coaches during the role plays. They are also asked to think about how the problem being discussed may be similar to what they have experienced and how the techniques may apply to their own interpersonal relationships. Group members are given work-at-home assignments to try these techniques at home and then report back to the group on how they went.

Termination Phase

The termination phase includes sessions seven and eight. During these sessions, the therapist and adolescents review the techniques that worked and practice the techniques that were more difficult. The group also discusses how these strategies may be useful in future stressful situations. This helps to emphasize the need to continue working on one's relationships after the group ends. Time is also spent in talking about other sources of support for an adolescent if problems arise and discussing characteristics of other group members that made them particularly supportive. The group leader hopes to identify for each adolescent people in his or her life who can act as a support system, as well as to outline characteristics that group members should look for when forming new relationships. Finally, the therapist reviews the symptoms of depression and discusses the importance of paying attention to warning signs of depression, so that if symptoms worsen, the adolescent can seek help.

Efficacy Research in IPT-AST

In a pilot randomized controlled trial, 41 adolescents with elevated depression symptoms were randomized to receive either IPT-AST or treatment as usual (TAU) as delivered by school guidance counselors and social workers (Young, Mufson, & Davies, 2006). Adolescents in the two intervention conditions were compared, as to depression symptoms, overall functioning, and depression diagnoses, postintervention and at 3-month and 6-month follow-ups. Adolescents who received IPT-AST had significantly fewer depression symptoms and better overall functioning postintervention and at follow-up assessments. Adolescents in IPT-AST also had fewer depression diagnoses than adolescents in usual care (Young et al., 2006). These results point to the promise of IPT-AST as an intervention for adolescents with subthreshold depression.

A universal prevention study (Horowitz et al., 2005) evaluated the efficacy of two programs in preventing depressive symptoms in adolescents. Participants were 380 high school students randomly assigned to a cognitive-behavioral therapy (CBT) program, to IPT-AST, or to a no-intervention, assessment-only control group. Both interventions involved eight 90-minute weekly sessions held during 9th grade wellness classes. At postintervention, students in both the CBT and IPT-AST groups reported significantly lower levels of depressive symptoms than did those in the no-intervention group, controlling for baseline scores; the two intervention groups did not differ significantly from each other. At 6-month follow-up there were no significant differences between the three conditions. Approximately 15% of the sample could not be located to complete the 6-month follow-up assessment. It is possible that the group effects found at postintervention would have been maintained at follow-up had these participants remained in the study. However, it is also possible that as a universal intervention with a larger group size and no pregroup sessions, IPT-AST does not have sustained preventive effects.

Both of the aforementioned studies implemented IPT-AST in schools without formal mental health services. School administrators appreciated having these projects in the schools, recognizing that adolescents who receive needed services are better able to engage in school and complete academic tasks. In the studies described above, the group leaders were outside clinicians who were trained to deliver IPT-AST. If future studies continue to support the efficacy of IPT-AST delivered by outside clinicians, the goal will be to train school guidance counselors to implement this intervention so that this model can be sustained in schools.

CONCLUSIONS

IPT-A is a short-term, manualized treatment for adolescent depression that has been shown to be efficacious in three randomized clinical trials (Mufson et al., 1999; Mufson, Dorta, Wickramaratne, et al., 2004; Rosselló & Bernal, 1999). The treatment focuses on alleviating depressive symptoms and improving interpersonal functioning. IPT-A is divided into three treatment phases: initial, middle, and termination. By the conclusion of the initial phase, the therapist identifies an interpersonal problem area that is related to the adolescent's depression. This serves as the focus of treatment and determines the treatment goals and relevant strategies. The therapist plays an active and directive role in the treatment. The adolescent also is expected to be increasingly active over the course of the treatment. Whenever possible, parents or guardians are involved in the treatment periodically to receive psychoeducation about depression, to learn and practice effective communication skills, and to support the adolescent's gains in treatment.

IPT-AST is a group preventive intervention based on IPT-A, which has been studied as both an indicated intervention with adolescents with elevated depression symptoms and a universal intervention. The intervention focuses on psychoeducation and interpersonal skill building that can be applied to various relationships in the adolescents' lives. Adolescents are taught communication analysis and interpersonal techniques through role plays and activities and are then encouraged to apply these techniques to address current interpersonal problems. To date, parents have not been involved in IPT-AST, but a study under way is including parents in the three phases of the intervention to determine if this enhances outcomes.

The development and research of IPT-AST is still in the preliminary phase. If it is found to be efficacious as a prevention intervention, we will have efficacious interpersonal psychotherapy models for both the prevention and treatment of adolescent depression. This continuum of care would allow us to intervene with adolescents with different levels of depression severity. This two-stage model would be particularly useful in schools or other community settings. By screening adolescents for depression, one could allocate adolescents to either IPT-A or IPT-AST, thereby addressing current depression as well as decreasing the risk for future depressive episodes. Training clinicians who work in these community settings to systematically identify adolescents and to treat them with the appropriate IPT model would afford the opportunity for sustainability of the prevention and treatment of adolescent depression in these settings.

REFERENCES

Carbonell, D. M., Reinherz, H. Z., & Giaconia, R. M. (1998). Risk and resilience in late adolescence. *Child and Adolescent Social Work Journal, 15,* 251–272.

Coyne, J. (1976). Toward an interactional description of depression. *Psychiatry, 39,* 28–40.

Elkin, I., Shea, M. T., Watkins, J. T., Imber, S. D., Sotsky, S. M., Collins, J. F., et al. (1989). National Institute of Mental Health Treatment of Depression Collaborative Research Program: General effectiveness of treatments. *Archives of General Psychiatry, 46,* 971–983.

Frank, E., Kupfer, D. J., Wagner, E. E., McEachran, A. B., & Cornes, C. (1991). Efficacy of interpersonal psychotherapy as a maintenance treatment of recurrent depression: Contributing factors. *Archives of General Psychiatry, 48,* 1053–1059.

Garrison, C. Z., Jackson, K. L., Marsteller, F., McKeown, R., & Addy, C. (1990). A longitudinal study of depressive symptomatology in young adolescents. *Journal of the American Academy of Child and Adolescent Psychiatry, 29,* 581–585.

Gordon, R. S. (1983). An operational classification of disease prevention. *Public Health Reports, 98,* 107–109.

Gotlib, I. H., Lewinsohn, P. M., & Seeley, J. R. (1995). Symptoms versus a diagnosis of depression: Differences in psychosocial functioning. *Journal of Consulting and Clinical Psychology, 63,* 90–100.

Hammen, C. (1999). The emergence of an interpersonal approach to depression. In T. Joiner & J. Coyne (Eds.), *The interactional nature of depression: Advances in interpersonal approaches* (pp. 22–36). Washington, DC: American Psychological Association.

Hetherington, E. M., Bridges, M., & Insabella, G. M. (1998). What matters? What does not? Five perspectives on the association between marital transitions and children's adjustment. *American Psychologist, 53,* 167–184.

Hoagwood, K., Burns, B. J., Kiser, L., Ringeisen, H., & Schoenwald, S. K. (2001). Evidence-based practice in child and adolescent mental health services. *Psychiatric Services, 52,* 1179–1189.

Hoagwood, K., & Olin, S. S. (2002). The NIMH Blueprint for Change Report: Research priorities in child and adolescent mental health. *Journal of the American Academy of Child and Adolescent Psychiatry, 41,* 760–767.

Horowitz, J. L., Garber, J., Young, J. F., & Mufson, L. (2005, November). *Prevention of depressive symptoms: A comparison of cognitive-behavioral and interpersonal intervention programs.* Paper presented at the annual meeting of the Association for Behavioral and Cognitive Therapies, Washington, DC.

Horwath, E., Johnson, J., Klerman, G. L., & Weissman, M. M. (1992). Depressive symptoms as relative and attributable risk factors for first-onset major depression. *Archives of General Psychiatry, 49,* 817–823.

Joiner, T., Coyne, J., & Blalock, J. (1999). On the interpersonal nature of depression: Overview and synthesis. In T. Joiner & J. Coyne (Eds.), *The interactional nature of depression: Advances in interpersonal approaches* (pp. 3–20). Washington, DC: American Psychological Association.

Judd, L. L., Paulus, M. P., Wells, K. B., & Rapaport, M. H. (1996). Socioeconomic burden of subsyndromal depressive symptoms and major depression in a sample of the general population. *American Journal of Psychiatry, 153,* 1411–1417.

Kessler, R. C., & Walters, E. E. (1998). Epidemiology of DSM-III-R major depression and minor depression among adolescents and young adults in the National Comorbidity Survey. *Depression and Anxiety, 7,* 3–14.

Lewinsohn, P. M., & Clarke, G. N. (1999). Psychosocial treatments for adolescent depression. *Clinical Psychology Review, 19,* 329–342.

Lewinsohn, P. M., Roberts, R. E., Seeley, J. R., Rohde, P., Gotlib, I. H., & Hops, H. (1994). Adolescent psychopathology: II. Psychosocial risk factors for depression. *Journal of Abnormal Psychology, 103,* 302–315.

Lewinsohn, P. M., Rohde, P., Klein, D., & Seeley, J. R. (1999). Natural course of adolescent major depressive disorder: I. Continuity into young adulthood. *Journal of the American Academy of Child and Adolescent Psychiatry, 38,* 56–63.

Lewinsohn, P. M., Solomon, A., Seeley, J. R., & Zeiss, A. (2000). Clinical implications of "subthreshold" depressive symptoms. *Journal of Abnormal Psychology, 109,* 345–351.

Marx, E. M., & Schulze, C. C. (1991). Interpersonal problem-solving in depressed students. *Journal of Clinical Psychology, 47,* 361–370.

Meyer, A. (1957). *Psychobiology: A science of man.* Springfield, IL: Charles C. Thomas.

Mufson, L., Dorta, K. P., Moreau, D., & Weissman, M. M. (2004). *Interpersonal psychotherapy for depressed adolescents* (2nd ed.). New York: Guilford Press.

Mufson, L., Dorta, K. P., Wickramaratne, P., Nomura, Y., Olfson, M., & Weissman, M. M. (2004). A randomized effectiveness trial of interpersonal psychotherapy for depressed adolescents. *Archives of General Psychiatry, 63,* 577–584.

Mufson, L., Gallagher, T., Dorta, K. P., & Young, J. F. (2004). Interpersonal psychotherapy for adolescent depression: Adaptation for group therapy. *American Journal of Psychotherapy, 58,* 220–237.

Mufson, L., Moreau, D., Weissman, M. M., Wickramaratne, P., Martin, J., & Samoilov, A. (1994). The modification of interpersonal psychotherapy with depressed adolescents IPT-A: Phase I and Phase II studies. *Journal of the American Academy of Child and Adolescent Psychiatry, 33,* 695–705.

Mufson, L., Weissman, M. M., Moreau, D., & Garfinkel, R. (1999). Efficacy of interpersonal psychotherapy for depressed adolescents. *Archives of General Psychiatry, 56,* 573–579.

Mrazek, P. J., & Haggerty, R. J. (1994). *Reducing risks for mental disorders: Frontiers for preventive intervention research.* Washington, DC: National Academy Press.

Pine, D. S., Cohen, E., Cohen, P., & Brook, J. (1999). Adolescent depressive symptoms as predictors of adult depression: Moodiness or mood disorder? *American Journal of Psychiatry, 156,* 133–135.

Puig-Antich, J., Kaufman, J., Ryan, N. D., Williamson, D. E., Dahl, R. E., Lukens, E., et al. (1993).

The psychosocial functioning and family environment of depressed adolescents. *Journal of the American Academy of Child and Adolescent Psychiatry, 32,* 244–253.

Reinherz, H. Z., Stewart-Berghauer, G., Pakiz, B., Frost, A. B., Moeykens, B. A., & Holmes, W. M. (1989). The relationship of early risk and current mediators to depressive symptomatology in adolescence. *Journal of the American Academy of Child and Adolescent Psychiatry, 28,* 942–947.

Rosselló, J., & Bernal, G. (1999). The efficacy of cognitive-behavioral and interpersonal treatments for depression in Puerto Rican adolescents. *Journal of Consulting and Clinical Psychology, 67,* 734–745.

Ryan, N. D., Puig-Antich, J., Ambrosini, P., Rabinovich, H., Robinson, D., Nelson, B., et al. (1987). The clinical picture of major depression in children and adolescents. *Archives of General Psychiatry, 44,* 854–861.

Sheeber, L., Hops, H., Alpert, A., Davis, B., & Andrews, J. (1997). Family support and conflict: Prospective relations to adolescent depression. *Journal of Abnormal Child Psychology, 25,* 333–344.

Sloane, R. B., Stapes, F. R., & Schneider, L. S. (1985). Interpersonal therapy versus nortriptyline for depression in the elderly. In G. D. Burrow, T. R. Norman, & L. Dennerstein (Eds.), *Clinical and pharmacological studies in psychiatric disorders* (pp. 344–346). London: Libbey.

Stader, S., & Hokanson, J. (1998). Psychological antecedents of depressive symptoms: An evaluation using daily experiences methodology. *Journal of Abnormal Psychology, 107,* 17–26.

Sullivan, H. S. (1953). *The interpersonal theory of psychiatry.* New York: Norton.

U.S. Public Health Service. (2000). *Report of the Surgeon General's conference on children's mental health: A national action agenda.* Washington, DC: U.S. Public Health Service.

Weissman, M. M., Markowitz, J. C., & Klerman, G. L. (2000). *Comprehensive guide to interpersonal psychotherapy.* New York: Basic Books.

Weissman, M. M., & Paykel, E. S. (1974). *The depressed woman: A study of social relationships.* Chicago: University of Chicago Press.

Weissman, M. M., Prusoff, B. A., DiMascio, A., Neu, C., Goklaney, M., & Klerman, G. L. (1979). The efficacy of drugs and psychotherapy in the treatment of acute depressive episodes. *American Journal of Psychiatry, 136,* 555–558.

Weisz, J. R., & Jensen, A. L. (2001). Child and adolescent psychotherapy in research and practice contexts: Review of the evidence and suggestions for improving the field. *European Child and Adolescent Psychiatry, 10*(Suppl. 1), 12–18.

Young, J. F., Mufson, L., & Davies, M. (2006). Efficacy of interpersonal psychotherapy adolescent skills training: An indicated preventive intervention for depression. *Journal of Child Psychology and Psychiatry, 47,* 1254–1262.

Young, J. F., & Mufson, L. (2003). *Manual for interpersonal psychotherapy–adolescent skills training (IPT-AST).* [Unpublished manual].

IV PREVENTION OF DEPRESSION

13 Preventing Depression in Early Adolescence

The Penn Resiliency Program

Jane E. Gillham, Steven M. Brunwasser, and Derek R. Freres

Depression is one of the most prevalent psychological disorders and, as such, it is an important target for prevention efforts. It is associated with considerable suffering, impairments in interpersonal relationships, work, and achievement, and increased mortality through the exacerbation of health problems and increased risk for suicide (American Psychiatric Association, 2000). Recent research has identified several risk factors for depression, including genetic vulnerabilities, family conflict, traumatic life experiences, maladaptive cognitive styles, and elevated depressive symptoms, which has paved the way for the development of a wide range of prevention programs. During the past decade several prevention programs have been designed to prevent depressive symptoms and disorders in adults and children. Most of these interventions are based on cognitive-behavioral theories and treatments of depression, although this is starting to change as researchers begin to explore interpersonal, family, and other models of prevention.

In this chapter we focus on the Penn Resiliency Program (PRP; Gillham, Jaycox, Reivich, Seligman, & Silver, 1990), an intervention designed to target cognitive and behavioral risk factors, to promote resilience, and to prevent symptoms of depression in early adolescence. We begin with a discussion of definitional issues. Next, we provide a brief overview of the theoretical and empirical background to PRP. We then describe the PRP intervention and review existing research on PRP's effectiveness. We close with a discussion of current work in progress and directions for future research.

DEFINITIONAL ISSUES

We conceptualize "depression" as including depressive symptoms as well as clinical depression. Although there is some debate about whether depressive symptoms and clinical depression exist on a continuum of severity or reflect qualitatively different experiences, recent reviews provide more evidence for the continuum model of depression (Hankin & Abela, 2005). High levels of depressive symptoms increase risk for depressive disorders. There is also evidence that individuals with elevated (but subclinical) levels of depressive symptoms have similar levels of interpersonal difficulties as those meeting diagnostic criteria for depressive disorders (Gotlib, Lewinsohn, & Seeley, 1995). Thus, we believe that it is important for prevention efforts to focus on depressive symptoms as well as diagnosable depressive disorders.

For the purposes of this chapter, we conceptualize prevention broadly as involving (1) the delivery of an intervention to individuals without the target disorder (or problem) and (2) a reduction of risk through a period of time. In previous writing we suggested that prevention of depression involves the prevention of the development of depressive episodes or *increases* in symptoms over time (Gillham, Shatté, & Freres, 2000). Although we think that this criterion could prove useful in future research, we have not used it in this chapter because it is often difficult to evaluate on the basis of published findings alone. Most depression prevention studies examine effects on average levels of depressive symptoms and do not examine effects on depressive disorders or high levels of symptoms. The typical pattern of findings for effective interventions is a reduction in average depressive symptoms in the intervention group and little change in depressive symptoms in the control group, a pattern resembling treatment more than prevention (Horowitz & Garber, 2006). Analyses that examine the onset of clinical levels of symptoms or effects in subgroups of participants may demonstrate the prevention of increases in symptoms, but these are rarely reported.

BACKGROUND

The Importance of Early Adolescence

The Penn Resiliency Program (PRP) was inspired by cognitive-behavioral theories and treatments of depression, as well as by research on adolescent development. Adolescence may be a particularly important period for depression prevention efforts. Rates of depression increase dramatically during adolescence, beginning at about age 15 (Hankin, Abramson, Moffitt, Silva, & McGee, 1998). In addition, recent research indicates that depression is often recurrent, with first episodes of depression occurring most often during adolescence (Kim-Cohen et al., 2003). Thus, prevention of depression during adolescence may help to prevent suffering across the lifespan.

PRP was designed for children between the ages of 10 and 14. By targeting the early adolescent developmental period, we hoped to prevent the steep increase in depression that occurs just a few years later. Early adolescence is also an important developmental period. Young adolescents deal with a number of physical, cognitive, social, and environmental changes that often occur together and may increase their risk for emotional and behavioral problems (Eccles et al., 1993). Most children go through puberty at this time. Social relationships become far more complex. Peer relationships become more important, and students' vulnerability to peer pressure increases (Hill & Holmbeck, 1986). The transition from elementary to middle school is marked by increased academic demands and often by a decrease in the individualized attention students receive from their teachers as they rotate through many classrooms each school day. These changes may increase risk for a variety of difficulties, including eating disorders, conduct problems, substance use, and underachievement, as well as depression (Cicchetti & Rogosch, 2002). At the same time, early adolescents also make important cognitive gains that may enable them to learn cognitive and problem-solving skills that can increase their resilience. During early adolescence, abstract reasoning and perspective-taking abilities increase. As compared with younger children, early adolescents are better able to reflect on their beliefs and to engage in hypothesis testing by examining evidence and considering alternatives (Inhelder & Piaget, 1958). These metacognitive skills are at the heart of cognitive-behavioral therapy, currently one of the most widely researched and empirically supported therapies for depression.

Cognitive-Behavioral Theories of Depression

Several cognitive risk factors are implicated in depression, including negative self-schemas, stringent standards or dysfunctional attitudes, information-processing biases, and negative interpretive styles (Abramson, Metalsky, & Alloy, 1989; Abramson, Seligman, & Teasdale, 1978; Beck, 1967; Ellis, 1962). An interpretive style that has received a great deal of research attention is a pessimistic explanatory style, which is marked by the tendency to attribute negative events to internal, stable, and global causes (Abramson et al., 1978). Behavioral factors that have been implicated in depression include problem-solving, coping, and response styles. In adults and adolescents, depression is linked to greater reliance on passive, unassertive, and ruminative styles and less engagement in distraction and problem solving (Abela, Vanderbilt, & Rochon, 2004; Chaplin & Cole, 2005; Nolen-Hoeksema, 1991). Maladaptive cognitive and behavioral risk factors can exacerbate each other, creating negative downward spirals. For example, negative cognitive styles can lead to maladaptive behaviors. In turn, maladaptive coping strategies can worsen problems and create new stressors that reinforce negative cognitive styles.

Most cognitive-behavioral models of depression are vulnerability–stress models. Individuals with cognitive vulnerabilities or maladaptive coping styles are particularly susceptible to depression when confronted by negative life events. In support of this premise, several studies have found that depression is predicted by an interaction between negative life events and explanatory style (Hankin & Abela, 2005).

As children enter adolescence, cognitive models of depression appear to become increasingly relevant. Negative life events appear to increase (Hankin & Abela, 2005), and there is some evidence that cognitive styles become more stable (McCauley, Mitchell, Burke, & Moss, 1988) and more closely linked to depressive symptoms (Nolen-Hoeksema, Girgus, & Seligman, 1992). Children's self-concepts become more complex and abstract (Damon & Hart, 1982). As self-perceptions rely more on abstract personality dimensions and less on concrete, observable behaviors, children may become increasingly vulnerable to cognitive distortions related to depression. It may become more difficult to evaluate the accuracy of such self-perceptions.

Cognitive-Behavioral Interventions for Depression

Cognitive-behavioral therapy (CBT) is an efficacious treatment for depression in adults (Butler, Chapman, Forman, & Beck, 2006) and shows promise in treating depression in children and adolescents (Reinecke & Ginsburg, Chapter 8, this volume; see also Weisz, McCarty, & Valeri, 2006). Depressed adults who are treated with CBT are less likely to relapse than those treated with medication, perhaps because CBT teaches them cognitive and problem-solving skills that can be used to cope with stressful events and feelings of sadness long after the treatment has ended (Hollon et al., 2005). Since the mid-1990s several research teams have developed and evaluated depression prevention programs based on CBT. Several of these interventions have prevented depressive symptoms or disorders in children and adults (for recent reviews see Dozois & Dobson, 2004; Horowitz & Garber, 2006; Merry, McDowell, Hetrick, Bir, & Muller, 2004).

THE PENN RESILIENCY PROGRAM

The PRP (Gillham et al., 1990) is a prevention program that is largely based on cognitive-behavioral therapy and designed for early adolescents. PRP comprises twelve 90- to 120-minute group sessions. It is most often delivered by teachers and counselors in schools, but can also be delivered in clinic or other community settings. A group leader's manual provides detailed outlines for each lesson and step-by-step instructions for each activity. Students receive an illustrated notebook with in-class activities and homework assignments for each lesson. PRP is structured in a manner intended to make abstract cognitive-behavioral concepts both accessible and relevant to children between the ages of about 10 and 14.

PRP's pedagogic approach involves three major steps. The first step is to establish a conceptual framework for each skill. This is typically accomplished using skits, role plays, short stories, or cartoons that illustrate the underlying concepts on a basic level. Once the children have a firm grasp of the key concepts, the group tackles hypothetical examples that demonstrate how the skill is germane to real-world experiences. Finally, students apply the skills in their own lives. The children are encouraged to share personal examples of times when they used, or could have used, the skill in question. Weekly homework activities encourage students to use the skills in real-life situations.

PRP includes two major components: a cognitive component and a social-problem-solving component. These sections are by no means disparate. Cognitive techniques are the foundation of the program and are pervasive throughout. When teaching problem-solving skills, the program encourages students to consider beliefs and expectations that can hinder or facilitate the implementation of these skills. In addition, effective problem-solving techniques can provide evidence that helps to challenge negative assumptions or hopeless expectations.

The Cognitive Component

Skill 1: The ABC Model

The goal of the initial PRP lessons is to establish the most fundamental concept of cognitive theories of depression: that our emotions and behaviors are not a direct consequence of the events that happen to us, but rather are a consequence of how we interpret these events. To illustrate this concept, the program introduces Ellis's (1962) ABC model. There is an Activating event or Adversity, which prompts an automatic Belief or an interpretation of the situation, which in turn leads to an emotional and/or behavioral Consequence. This model states that the Belief mediates the relationship between the activating event and the resulting emotion or behavior. The first PRP lesson focuses on the components of the model—adversities, beliefs, and emotions. Once the students have a firm grasp of these components, the group begins to examine the relationship between them.

ADVERSITIES (OR PROBLEMS)

The group leader facilitates a discussion of Adversities that adolescents commonly face. The students generate an extensive list of problems they encounter on a regular basis. Students typically cite a wide range of challenges, including difficulties with academics and achievement, interpersonal relationships with family members, friends, and peers, and even community problems such as crime and poverty. The goal of this discussion is two-fold: to help students think about adversities that can be addressed in the program and to demonstrate that problems are common occurrences and a normal part of life.

BELIEFS

The next step is to establish the role of Beliefs, or cognitions, in the ABC model. The group leader introduces the concept of internal dialogue, or "self-talk." Students perform several skits that illustrate self-talk as characters confront adversities that are common during early adolescence. Students learn that each adversity elicits thoughts or beliefs. Although self-talk occurs instantaneously and usually goes undetected, it has a great influence on how we respond when problems arise. The goal of this step is to help students understand self-talk as a normal process and to encourage them to be aware of their underlying cognitions.

EMOTIONS

The third step is to ensure that students are able to label and describe emotional experiences—one type of "C" in the ABC model. The group leader prompts the students to describe the experiencing of common emotions as if they were explaining the experiences to an alien. Students describe the bodily sensations and actions that typically accompany each emotion. Initially, the conversation focuses on the most basic emotions—happiness, sadness, and anger—and then progresses to more complex emotions such as shame and guilt. The group leader also encourages students to think about emotional intensity by asking students to share instances in which they felt each emotion and to describe how intense the experience was, using a scale of 1 (a little) to 10 (extremely intense). Students later learn that cognitions not only determine the type of emotional experience, but also the intensity of the experience.

THE LINK BETWEEN BELIEFS AND EMOTIONS

To establish the causal influence of cognitions, the group leader first uses a role play to demonstrate that people often experience different emotions in response to the same activating event. The group leader pretends to be a volatile sports coach who berates a team's performance. Students are instructed to visualize the situation and to imagine that it is actually happening. Each student then describes his or her feelings during the role play and the intensity of this emotional experience. Invariably, students report a variety of emotions such as shame, sadness, anger, or anxiety. Group members are encouraged to consider the sources of the different emotional reactions.

The group leader then asks the students to describe their internal dialogues during the role play. In doing so, it becomes apparent that there is a pattern in which specific thoughts elicit specific emotions. For example, a child who believes that the coach's behavior is excessive and unjustified ("He has no right to yell at me like that") experiences anger, whereas a child who expects negative consequences ("I'm going to get kicked off the team") experiences anxiety. In contrast, a child who attributes the coach's display of anger to a personal flaw or failing ("I must have really messed up to make the coach so angry") experiences sadness. The group leader draws attention to these patterns between beliefs (B) and consequential emotions (C), stressing that it is the belief—not the adversity—that causes an emotion.

Skill 2: Recognizing Cognitive ("Thinking") Styles

Students learn about "thinking styles," such as a pessimistic explanatory style, that can precipitate and perpetuate negative emotions. For several reasons, PRP focuses primarily on the stable (or permanent) dimension of explanatory style for negative events. Stable and global attributions appear to be more closely linked to depression than internal attributions (Abramson et al., 1989). In addition, internal attributions appear to be maladaptive primarily when they occur in the context of an explanatory style that is also stable and global. Internal attributions that are unstable and specific are often adaptive, because they encourage behavioral change and self-improvement. In contrast, external explanatory styles can increase anger and aggression and prevent people from recognizing the ways in which they contribute to the problems in their lives. An early pilot of PRP, however, indicated that children had difficulty understanding the global dimension of explanatory style. As a result, PRP devotes this section to improving the stable dimension of explanatory style.

Skits are used to portray and contrast different thinking styles. For example, a character named "Gloomy Greg" demonstrates a pessimistic thinking style. When a friend encourages Greg to try out for the school basketball team, Greg cites several personal and stable deficiencies. He convinces his friend that trying out for the team would be fruitless and that it is not worth the effort to practice. In a parallel skit, "Hopeful Holly" encounters the same situation but responds with an optimistic thinking style. Although she recognizes that making the team will be difficult, she concludes that she has a good chance if she practices before the tryouts. The group members discuss the emotional and behavioral consequences of both cognitive styles. Greg's behavior is used to demonstrate the notion of "self-fulfilling prophecy." The group leader points out that Greg's actions (not practicing) are likely to bring about the very outcome he fears and wants to avoid (not making the team).

Perhaps the most important component of the thinking styles section is the discussion of accuracy. The group discusses the likelihood that Greg's permanent negative beliefs (e.g., "I can't do anything right"; "I mess everything up") are accurate. Students learn that, in addition to making them feel bad, permanent negative beliefs are typically erroneous and counterproductive. In contrast, optimistic thinking styles promote emotional well-being and more effective coping strategies. The group leader also cautions students that the goal of the program is not blind optimism, nor is it to eradicate negative emotions. The students learn that over optimistic beliefs can hinder effective coping and prevent people from taking action to avert negative consequences. This conversation reinforces the main goal of the program: resilience through accurate thinking.

Skill 3: Cognitive Restructuring

Students learn to actively dispute negative cognitions by generating alternatives and examining evidence. To demonstrate the importance of hypothesis testing, the group leader reads a short story describing two detectives, one good and one bad. The good detective makes a list of possible suspects and looks for clues before drawing any conclusions, whereas the bad detective simply blames the first suspect that comes to mind. The group leader then makes the point that, when faced with real-world problems, people often behave just like the bad detective by accepting their initial beliefs without considering alternatives or looking for evidence. The group leader then prompts the students to share situations in which they jumped to conclusions erroneously.

Students practice searching for evidence with a hands-on activity called the "File Game." The group leader distributes file folders containing documents with information pertaining to fictional but realistic adolescent characters. The files contain a variety of materials: report cards, graded tests, awards, various diary entries, and notes from teachers, friends and family members. The first document in each file is a diary entry in which the character writes about a problem he or she is experiencing, along with several pessimistic beliefs. The students work in small groups and peruse the contents of the file to find evidence that supports or refutes the character's beliefs. For homework, students practice generating alternatives and examining evidence for pessimistic beliefs that seem to be operating in their own lives.

Skill 4: Decatastrophizing—Put It in Perspective

The program introduces the concept of catastrophic thinking (Ellis, 1962), or the tendency to exaggerate and distort the implications of negative events. The group leader recounts the well-known parable "Chicken Little," to make the concept of catastrophic thinking highly accessible and to provide a point of reference for future discussions. Students learn that when faced with an adversity, people often focus exclusively on the most negative contingencies at the expense of accurate appraisal. Such beliefs are likely to initiate a spiral of negative thoughts that can result in intense anxiety or sadness. For example, a child who witnesses an argument between his parents might report the following chain of thoughts: My parents are fighting → they're never going to stop fighting → they're going to get divorced → my dad will leave → I'll never see my dad again.

The Putting It in Perspective (PIIP) skill is designed to counter this spiral. Students learn to consider the worst, best, and most likely outcomes of problematic situations. Whereas it is easy for most students to envision the worst-case scenario (e.g., the child does not get to see his father again), students often have difficulty providing an equally improbable positive outcome. When discussing the best-case scenario, the group leader encourages the students to imagine outlandishly positive outcomes—the parents never fight again, and to celebrate, they plan a long vacation in Hawaii for the entire family. The group leader then addresses the probability of the worst and best possible outcomes coming to fruition, stressing that they are equally unlikely, yet we are more likely to believe the worst-case scenario. PIIP provides a frame of reference for the implausibility of catastrophic beliefs by embellishing the best possible outcome and equating it with the worst possible outcome.

Once the group establishes that focusing on either the worst or best possible outcome is counterproductive, students begin discussing a problem's most likely outcome. Students apply skills from previous lessons to generate alternative scenarios and gather evidence that supports and refutes the plausibility of each outcome. In the marital conflict example, students generally conclude that most parents fight from time to time and a single argument is unlikely to end in divorce. The final step is to develop an active strategy for coping with the situation and the most likely outcome if it is negative. Following this discussion, students apply the PIIP skill to situations in which they find themselves catastrophizing.

A crucial component of this section is to acknowledge that, occasionally, the students will be faced with significant negative events and experiences (e.g., severe illness, a divorce, or the death of a family member). It is vital that students do not feel as though the program is minimizing the importance of such events. On the contrary, the program stresses that the experience of strong negative emotions is appropriate in these circumstances. However, even in extreme situations, it is important that students maintain a realistic outlook and use coping skills to improve the situation or to help themselves feel better if the situation is uncontrollable.

Skill 5: Hot Seat

The "Hot Seat" (or "Rapid-Fire Disputation") is a skill for challenging negative thoughts rapidly in situations that do not allow for extensive deliberation. The Hot Seat combines several skills—searching for evidence, generating alternatives, and putting the situation in perspective—that can be used to fight back against negative thoughts in the moment as they occur. Each student is presented with hypothetical adversities that require immediate refutation of negative beliefs. For example, a student is asked to imagine that she is taking a difficult math test and begins having negative thoughts that interfere with her performance. The group leader provides the student's internal dialogue by stating negative thoughts ("I'm going to fail this test . . . I'll never be able to pass this class . . . I'm stupid"). The student's task is to refute these negative beliefs by providing credible counter-evidence, generating more realistic alternative thoughts, or by providing a more accurate appraisal of the adversity and its ramifications. The group leader ensures that the students are providing plausible refutations and not simply minimizing the problem ("Who cares about a stupid math test?") or denying their personal contributions to the problem ("It's the teacher's fault that I don't know the material"). Students practice using the Hot Seat with their own experiences several times during the rest of the program.

The Social-Problem-Solving Component

The goal of the social-problem-solving component is to provide students with a variety of skills for handling difficult interpersonal situations and circumstances that elicit overwhelming emotions. These skills build on and reinforce the cognitive skills that are taught in the first six PRP sessions. Here, we briefly describe three of the major skills covered within this component: assertiveness, relaxation, and problem solving.

Skill 6: Assertiveness

In this part of the program, students learn to identify three behavioral approaches to interpersonal conflict—aggressiveness, passiveness, and assertiveness—and the consequences of each. Students enact three skits involving an interaction between a child and a friend who repeatedly cancels plans at the last minute. The three skits illustrate aggressive, passive, and assertive responses to this situation. Students discuss the advantages and disadvantages of the different styles, including the likelihood that both aggressive and passive responses will fail to solve the problem. With the deficiencies of the aggressive and passive approaches apparent, assertiveness is introduced as an alternate and prescriptive model. PRP's assertiveness model has four steps, denoted by the acronym DEAL, and is partly based on the work of Bower and Bower (1977). This method emphasizes approaching the other person in a manner that is clear, yet respectful and nonconfrontational. The first step is to Describe the problem objectively—"The last few times we made plans, you canceled at the last minute." The second step is to Express how the problem makes the student feel without blaming the other person for these emotions—"When this happens, I feel that you don't really want to spend time with me." In the third step, the person Asks for a specific change—"In the future, will you please try to let me know further in advance if you have to cancel plans?" This must be a reasonable request, and the requester must also be willing to change an aspect of his or her own behavior if the situation calls for it—"Maybe I could call you the day before to confirm our plans." Finally, the person Lists how these changes would improve the situation— "This would make me feel a lot better about making plans to get together again." The group leader works with students to identify situations in their own lives in which the DEAL model could be helpful. Students then role-play the skill during the session in anticipation of applying the skill in their lives.

Acting assertively can be difficult, even for adults. An important part of teaching assertiveness is to discuss the kinds of cognitions that deter assertive behavior in favor of a passive approach (e.g., "It's not nice to be assertive") or an aggressive approach ("People won't take me seriously"). It is also important that the group leader acknowledges that assertiveness will not always bring about the desired outcome. Occasionally, the students will encounter a situation in which they and the other person do not agree on how to resolve the dilemma. Students learn an approach to negotiation that can be helpful in these instances.

Skill 7: Relaxation

PRP teaches students a variety of relaxation skills, including deep breathing, progressive muscle relaxation, and positive imagery. These strategies can be used to cope with strong negative emotions and uncontrollable stressors, such as family conflict, that often inhibit effective coping processes like cognitive restructuring. The goal of relaxation techniques is not to alter the type of emotion experienced (sadness or anxiety is often an appropriate emotion in these situations), but rather to assuage the emotional intensity. Once the emotion is manageable, the child can use cognitive skills to evaluate the situation accurately and develop an adaptive coping strategy.

Relaxation skills are designed to counteract the body's sympathetic response to stress (muscle tension, increased heart rate, rapid breathing, etc.), which can contribute to and exacerbate negative cognitions and emotional states (see, e.g., Clark, 1986). The first step is to make participants aware of situations in which relaxation techniques are useful and appropriate. The group leader asks participants to visualize a time when they witnessed their parents or family members having an argument, in order to simulate a situation in which these techniques may be helpful. This example is ideal not only because family conflict tends to elicit strong emotions, but also because the child typically has little or no control over the situation. During the visualization exercise, students attempt to recall the thoughts, emotions, and bodily sensations they experienced during the argument. The PRP group leader then demonstrates several relaxation exercises and has students practice as a group. When demonstrating deep breathing, the group leader ensures that the students focus on taking deep, slow breaths. The group leader counts out loud while the students inhale and exhale to help them monitor the rate of their breathing. During the muscle relaxation task, students learn to tense, and then release, each of the major muscle groups in the body—starting with the toes and progressively working up to the face. The third technique, positive imagery, involves visualizing a pleasant place or activity. To demonstrate this skill, the group leader has the students close their eyes as he or she reads a vivid passage. Students are encouraged to imagine they are at the beach and to imagine all of the sights, sounds, smells, and other sensations described in the passage. Students then write down their own examples of a relaxing image that they can visualize when feeling overwhelmed by emotion.

Skill 8: Problem Solving

The final skill taught in PRP is a five-step approach to problem solving that is based largely on Dodge and Crick's (1990) social-information-processing model and is similar to techniques used in other problem-solving interventions (Lochman, Coie, Underwood, & Terry, 1993). This skill incorporates many of the cognitive and behavioral skills from previous lessons. When confronted with problems, students learn to (1) stop and think, and make sure they are interpreting the problem situation and others' perspectives accurately; (2) identify their goals; (3) brainstorm to create a list of possible solutions, and to put assertiveness and other skills they have learned on this list as appropriate; (4) make a decision by considering the likely outcomes and listing the pros and cons of different solutions; and (5) enact a solution. Following these five steps, students are encouraged to evaluate the outcome and to return to the five-step process (often starting with step 3) if the solution they tried was not successful. Students first learn to apply this process to several hypothetical but common situations, typically related to achievement or interpersonal issues, and then apply the skill to situations in their own lives. This problem-solving technique was originally included in PRP to help reduce behavioral problems that are often comorbid with depression in children (Garber, Quiggle, Panak, & Dodge, 1991). The skill may also reduce hopelessness by conveying that there are several pathways for solving many of the problems that students encounter.

RESEARCH ON PRP

Table 13.1 lists the empirical evaluations of PRP. The first controlled study of PRP (study 1; see Table 13.1) included fifth and sixth graders who were identified as being at risk for depression based on elevated depressive symptoms and/or reports of family conflict. PRP groups were led by the three lead authors of the curriculum, who were graduate students in clinical psychology at the time. Findings from this first study suggested that PRP improved explanatory style. The positive effects on explanatory style endured through the final assessment point, 3 years after the intervention ended (Gillham & Reivich, 1999). PRP participants also reported fewer symptoms of depression through the 2-year (but not the 3-year) follow-up. PRP significantly prevented moderate to severe levels of depression. At the 2-year follow-up, PRP participants were only half as likely as controls to report moderate to severe levels of depressive symptoms (Gillham, Reivich, Jaycox, & Seligman, 1995). Although these findings were encouraging, the study had several methodological limits, most notably the lack of random assignment.

TABLE 13.1. Empirical Evaluations of the Penn Resiliency Program

Evaluation and empirical paper citation(s)	Setting and sample	Design and length of follow-up	Significant improvement/prevention of depression symptoms?	Effect size at postintervention	Effect size at follow-up closest to 6 months	Avg. effect size across study follow-up	Range of effect sizes (smallest to largest)
1. Initial evaluation (Jaycox, Reivich, Gillham, & Seligman, 1994; Gillham, 1994; Study 1; Gillham et al., 1995; Reivich 1996; Gillham & Reivich, 1999; Zubernis, Cassidy, Gillham, Reivich, & Jaycox, 1999)	• Targeted[a] • School • N = 143 • 5th and 6th graders	• PRP (3 versions) vs. control • Matched control design • 36-month follow-up	Yes	0.25	0.36 (6-month)	0.33	0.16 (30-month) to 0.46 (12-, 24-month)
2. First parent program pilot (Gillham, 1994; Study 2)	• Universal • School • N = 108 • 5th and 6th graders	• PRP vs. PRP + parent component vs. control • Random assignment by school • 6-month follow-up reported for cohort 1 sample	PRP vs. control—Yes PRP + parent vs. control—No	0.35 0.08	0.30 (6-month) −0.09 (6-month)	0.49 0.06	0.30 (6-month) to 0.81 (2-month) −0.09 (6-month) to 0.20 (2-month)
3. Effectiveness and specificity study (Reivich, 1996; Shatté, 1997)	• Universal • School • N = 152 • 6th–8th graders	• PRP vs. alternate intervention vs. control • RCT[b] • 12-month follow-up	Yes	0.04	0.24 (4-month) 0.39 (8-month)	0.20	0.04 (postintervention) to 0.39 (8-month)
4. Incarcerated adolescents study (Miller, 1999)	• Targeted • Juvenile detention center • N = 56 • 14- to 18-year-olds, predominantly male	• PRP vs. control • Randomized within one of the two juvenile detention centers. In second center, all participants were assigned to the control condition. • Postintervention	No	Standard deviations unavailable	Standard deviations unavailable	NA	NA

(continued)

319

TABLE 13.1. (continued)

Evaluation and empirical paper citation(s)	Setting and sample	Design and length of follow-up	Significant improvement/prevention of depression symptoms?	Effect size at postintervention	Effect size at follow-up closest to 6 months	Avg. effect size across study follow-up	Range of effect sizes (smallest to largest)
5. First Australian study (Pattison & Lynd-Stevenson, 2001)	• Universal • School • N = 66 5th and 6th graders	• PRP vs. reverse PRP vs. attention control vs. control • Most participants randomly assigned, but control condition also included participants not randomized to condition. • 8-month follow-up	No	0.09	0.50 (8-month)	0.30	0.09 (postintervention) to 0.50 (8-month)
6. Australian girls' school study (Quayle, Dziurawiec, Roberts, Kane, & Ebsworthy, 2001)	• Universal • School • N = 47 7th-grade girls	• PRP vs. control • RCT • 6-month follow-up	Mixed • No at postintervention • Yes at 6-month follow-up	−0.62	0.62 (6-month)	0.00	−0.62 (postintervention) to 0.62 (6-month)
7. Inner-city study[c] (Cardemil, Reivich, & Seligman, 2002; Cardemil, Reivich, Beevers, Seligman, & James, 2007)	• Universal • School • N = 168 5th & 6th graders	• PRP vs. control • RCT • 24-month follow-up	Mixed • moderation by race/ethnicity • Yes for Latino sample • No for African American sample	0.27	0.26 (6-month)	0.18	0.10 (3-, 24-month) to 0.27 (postintervention)
8. PRP in Beijing, China (Yu & Seligman, 2002)	• Targeted • School • N = 220 8- to 15-year-olds	• PRP vs. control • RCT • 6-month follow-up	Yes	0.23	0.39 (6-month)	0.31	0.23 (postintervention) to 0.39 (6-month)
9. Rural Australian study (Roberts, Kane, Thompson, Bishop, & Hart, 2003; Roberts, Kane, Bishop, Matthews, & Thompson, 2004)	• Targeted • School • N = 189 11- to 13-year-olds	• School-based evaluation • PRP vs. control • Schools randomized to condition • 30-month follow-up	No	0.05	0.07 (6-month)	0.04	−0.12 (12-month) to 0.15 (30-month)

Study	Sample	Design[b]	Moderation[c]			
10. All girls vs. co-ed PRP study (Chaplin et al., 2006)	• Universal • School • N = 208 • 6th to 8th graders	• PRP vs. control (Boys randomized to coed PRP vs. control; Girls randomized to coed PRP vs. all-girls PRP vs. control) • RCT • Postintervention; 12-month follow-up attempted but very low response limited analyses	Yes	0.40	NA	0.40	Large attrition rates preclude meaningful analyses beyond postintervention assessment

11. Primary care study (Gillham, Hamilton, Freres, Patton, & Gallop, 2006)	• Targeted
	• Clinic
	• N = 271
	• 11- to 12-year-olds
		• PRP vs. usual care control
		• RCT
		• 24-month follow-up
			Mixed
			• No for full sample
			• Moderation by gender
			  • Yes for girls.
			  • No for boys.
				-0.02	0.22
					(6-month)
						0.13	-0.02
							(postintervention)
							to
							0.22
							(6-, 12-month)

12. Large universal effectiveness study (Cutuli, 2004; Cutuli et al., 2006; Gillham et al., 2007)	• Universal
	• School
	• N = 697
	• 6th to 8th graders
		• PRP vs. alternate intervention vs. control
		• RCT
		• 36-month follow-up
			Mixed
			• No for full sample
			• Moderation by school
			  • Yes in two schools
			  • No in third school
				0.05	0.06
					(6-month)
						0.12	-0.01
							(36-month)
							to
							0.22
							(30-month)

13. Evaluation of PRP + parent component (Gillham, Reivich, et al., 2006)	• Targeted • School • N = 44 • 6th and 7th graders	• PRP + parent component vs. control • RCT • 12-month follow-up	Yes	0.08	0.59 (6-month)	0.35	0.08 (postintervention) to 0.59 (6-month)

Note. The table includes published studies as well as unpublished dissertation studies.

[a] For the purposes of this table, "targeted" refers to samples selected because they had elevated depressive symptoms, family conflict, or other risk factors assessed at the individual level.

[b] RCT, randomized controlled trial, with individuals randomized to condition.

[c] Elsewhere in the literature (e.g., Cardemil et al., 2002; Gillham, Hamilton, Freres, Patton, & Gallop, 2006; Horowitz & Garber, 2006), this study has been divided into two studies (with study 1 including the Latino sample study and study 2 including the African American sample study). We list this study as a single study (following Cardemil et al., 2007) because it was originally planned and implemented as a single study and divided into two studies when race/ethnicity emerged as a moderator. Estimates of effect sizes for this evaluation are based on intent-to-treat data provided by Dr. Esteban Cardemil.

During the past 10 years, our research group and others have conducted several additional studies examining the efficacy of PRP. To our knowledge, there are 13 published, in press, and unpublished dissertation studies of PRP, making PRP one of the most widely researched depression prevention programs. All of these studies examine PRP's effect on depressive symptoms by comparing intervention and control groups. Most used randomized controlled designs. Together, they included more than 2,000 children and adolescents. In most studies, samples were predominantly European American and from middle-class suburban communities, but PRP has also been evaluated with children of African and Latino descent, with children living in China and Australia, and in inner-city, suburban, and rural communities. About half of the studies investigated PRP with targeted samples that included children at risk for depression because of elevated depressive symptoms or family conflict. The other half investigated PRP when delivered to all children who signed up for the project regardless of risk status. PRP group leaders have included the PRP intervention developers, graduate students, and researchers, as well as teachers, psychologists, and counselors in school and other community settings.

Table 13.1 summarizes these 13 studies, including information about the significance of intervention effects on depressive symptoms as measured by the Children's Depression Inventory (Kovacs, 2001). Effect sizes were estimated by dividing the difference between experimental and control group means by the standard deviation of the control group, following procedures used by Smith, Glass, and Miller (1980) and in recent meta-analyses of depression prevention and treatment programs for children and adolescents (Horowitz & Garber, 2006; Weisz et al., 2006). This effect size is one variation of Cohen's d (Cohen, 1988), which can also be calculated using the pooled standard deviation. A major advantage of using experimental and control group means and the control group standard deviation is that this information is typically reported in research reports and therefore allows for a standard procedure across studies. It is important to note, however, that the effect size estimates generated by this approach sometimes differ from the effect sizes reported in research papers. Discrepancies can reflect several issues, including (1) the use of raw scores rather than transformed scores, (2) the use of raw means rather than means controlling for baseline symptoms and baseline differences on other variables, and (3) the underestimation of effect sizes when the pooled standard deviation is lower than the control group standard deviation (as in study 1, for example).

For each study, we report the range of effect sizes from postintervention through the final follow-up. Like Horowitz and Garber (2006), we also report effect sizes at the postintervention assessment and for the assessment closest to 6 months postintervention. Estimates were calculated so that positive values represent a benefit of the intervention relative to the control group. For studies that compared PRP with both a no-intervention control and an alternate intervention or attention control group (3, 5, and 12), we report effect sizes for the PRP versus no-intervention control comparisons. In studies that evaluated two different versions of the PRP children's program (1, 5, and 10), we pooled the means of the two different PRP conditions and calculated one effect size comparing the combined PRP groups with those in the control condition. For the study (2) that included PRP, PRP combined with a parent intervention, and a no-intervention control, we report the comparison of each intervention condition to the control condition.

Effects on Depression

Taken together, the existing studies suggest that PRP reduces and prevents symptoms of depression, although some studies have failed to find positive effects. An examination of statistical significance indicates that five studies report significant effects on depressive symptoms. Five studies report mixed results such as significant effects at one of two assessments (study 6), for one of two subgroups of participants (7, 11, and 12) or for one of two PRP conditions (2). Three studies report no significant intervention effects on depressive symptoms. The lack of significant findings in two of these (4 and 5) may in part reflect limited statistical power due to small sample size. The dissertation study by Miller (4) should probably be discounted, as it was limited by several serious methodological constraints, including a nonrandomized design, baseline differences between intervention and control participants, and participants who were in mid- to late adolescence, well above the recommended age range for PRP.

An examination of effect sizes indicates that intervention effects vary across studies and across assessments within studies. The average study intervention effect size across studies is approximately 0.09 at postintervention and 0.32 at the 6-month follow-up. These effect sizes are approximately 0.12 and 0.22, respectively, when weighted for sample size. A few studies find moderate effect sizes ($d > 0.40$) at some assessments. In comparison, a recent meta-analysis of depression prevention studies with children and adolescents reported average effect sizes of 0.16 at postintervention and 0.11 at the 6-month follow-up (Horowitz & Garber, 2006).

Effects on Other Outcomes

In theory, PRP works because it teaches cognitive restructuring and a variety of problem-solving skills that students can use to effectively manage negative emotions and challenging or stressful events in their lives. Consistent with this view, a few studies have found that PRP reduces children's negative automatic thoughts and hopelessness, and improves explanatory style (e.g., studies 1, 7, 8, and 10).

Depressive symptoms and disorders are associated with a variety of other problems during childhood and adolescence, particularly anxiety and behavioral problems. A few studies have looked at PRP's effects on these outcomes. Three studies (5, 9, and 13) examined PRP's effects on anxiety symptoms and two (9 and 13) found significant intervention effects. An evaluation of PRP that included a parent intervention component (study 13) found significant and substantial prevention of anxiety symptoms through 1 year of follow-up. More specifically, during the year following the intervention, 30% of controls, but only about 5% of PRP participants, reported very high levels of anxiety symptoms. Interestingly, in the evaluation by Roberts and colleagues (study 9), PRP reduced anxiety symptoms at most assessment points but did not significantly affect depressive symptoms. Although there was no direct effect of PRP on depression, the researchers reported that PRP's effects on anxiety appeared to mediate effects on depressive symptoms.

There is some evidence that PRP reduces and prevents behavioral problems. In the initial evaluation, PRP reduced externalizing symptoms through the 6-month follow-up (the last assessment point at which these symptoms were examined; study 1). An evaluation of PRP in Australia found significant reductions in externalizing symptoms relative to control at postintervention, but not at later follow-up assessments (study 9). A recently completed evaluation of PRP found significant prevention of externalizing symptoms over a 30-month follow-up period (study 12; Cutuli, 2004). This study also found that PRP's effects on depression were particularly strong for children who exhibited behavioral problems at the start of the study (study 12; Cutuli, Chaplin, Gillham, Reivich, & Seligman, 2006).

To our knowledge, only one completed study has examined PRP's effect on psychological disorders. In that study (11), PRP was delivered by mental health professionals working in a primary care setting. The researchers tracked children's diagnoses of depression, anxiety, and adjustment disorders that included depressed or anxious mood for 2 years postintervention. No overall prevention effect was found. At the same time, there was a significant interaction of intervention condition with initial symptom level, such that PRP prevented disorders in children with high (but not low) levels of depressive symptoms at baseline. Among the high symptom group, 56% of controls, as compared with 36% of PRP participants, were diagnosed with depression, anxiety, or adjustment disorders during the follow-up period. Our research group is currently conducting a large school-based evaluation of PRP that will also examine whether PRP prevents depression and anxiety disorders.

These research findings are encouraging. They suggest that PRP has beneficial effects on depression, anxiety, and behavioral symptoms in children and adolescents. In some studies, these effects are long-lasting, enduring for 2 or more years after the intervention (e.g., studies 1, Gillham, 1995; 7, Cardemil, Reivich, Beevers, Seligman, & James, 2007; 12, Gillham et al., 2007). As is clear in Table 13.1, however, there is considerable variability in PRP's effects across studies and even within studies. PRP's effects sometimes vary by gender (studies 1, Reivich, 1996; and 11), by race or ethnicity (7), by school (7, 12, Gillham et al., 2007) or by participants' initial levels of depression (11) or behavioral symptoms (12, Cutuli, Chaplin, Gillham, Reivich, & Seligman, 2006). We are unable to detect a clear, consistent pattern to such moderators. Most studies of PRP do not find or do not examine moderators. Among studies that report moderator effects, the direction of these effects often varies. For example, although the initial evaluation of PRP found stronger effects for boys than for girls, the opposite pattern was observed in the study of PRP in a primary care setting (11). To some degree, the inconsistencies across studies reflect variations in methods, including sample size (statistical power), condition assignment (group equivalence), and statistical analyses.

Recently, we have become concerned about the possibility that the inconsistency in findings reflects, in part, a drop-off in effects as evaluations of PRP move along the continuum from efficacy to effectiveness to dissemination. Our observations are speculative at this point because the number of studies is quite small. With that caveat in mind, we report some preliminary findings. Of the four studies (1, 2, 7, and 13) in which groups were led by PRP developers and others close to the research team, three (1, 2, and 13) found significant effects on depression and one (7) produced mixed results. The average of the postintervention and 6-month effect sizes for these studies is about 0.27, unweighted, and 0.26, weighted for sample size. (Average effect sizes were similar when calculated excluding data from PRP interventions that included a parent component.) Of the five studies (3, 8, 10, 11, and 12) in which group leaders were real-world providers trained and supervised by the PRP research team, three (3, 8, and 10) found significant effects and two yielded mixed results. The average of the postintervention and 6-month effect sizes for these studies is about 0.19, unweighted, and 0.16, weighted for sample size. Of the three studies in which group leaders received some initial training but not ongoing supervision from the PRP research team, one (6) yielded mixed results and the others (5 and 9) found no significant effects of PRP on depression. The average of postintervention and 6-month effect sizes for these studies is about 0.12, unweighted, and 0.09, weighted for sample size. (The findings of Miller (1999) would also fit into this third category inasmuch as the groups were led by an individual with some previous PRP training, but no supervision from the PRP research team while implementing the intervention. Effect sizes could not be estimated for that study because standard deviations were not reported.)

The apparent drop-off in effectiveness is similar to that reported for the Resourceful Adolescent Program (another cognitive-behavioral depression prevention program) when group leaders were school staff rather than members of the research team (Harnett & Dadds, 2004; Shochet et al., 2001). This parallels the observations by Weisz and others that psychotherapies found to be efficacious in university-based studies often fail to have dramatic effects in the real world (Weisz, Donenberg, Han, & Weiss, 1995). There are many possible explanations for this difference, including differences in the intervention participants, intervention providers, and institutional environments and supports (Schoenwald & Hoagwood, 2001; Weisz & Jensen, 2001; Weisz & Kazdin, 2003).

Research on PRP is only beginning to explore the process of intervention dissemination. The reduction in findings as contact with the PRP research team diminishes suggests that intervention integrity (the degree to which leaders cover the PRP material) is a key factor in the success of PRP. In support of this possibility, the evaluation of PRP in the primary care setting found that intervention integrity was related to PRP's effects on depressive symptoms. PRP prevented depressive symptoms among participants in high, but not low, integrity groups (Gillham, Hamilton, Freres, Patton, & Gallop, 2006). Clearly, it will be important to address intervention integrity and other factors affecting dissemination if PRP is to live up to its initial promise and benefit a large number of children in real-world settings.

CURRENT AND FUTURE DIRECTIONS

Most of the current work on PRP explores three related questions:

1. How does PRP work when it is effective?
2. How can PRP's effects be enhanced?
3. How can we facilitate effective real-world implementation and dissemination?

In theory, PRP works by teaching cognitive-restructuring, coping, and problem-solving skills that help participants to counter pessimistic attributions and expectancies and manage life stressors more effectively. Previous studies have often found beneficial effects of PRP on automatic thoughts, explanatory style, hopelessness, and self-esteem (e.g., studies 1, 7, 8, and 11), and some research suggests that changes in such cognitions partially mediate PRP's effects on depressive symptoms (e.g., studies 1 and 8). To date, there is little research examining whether PRP improves children's coping and problem-solving skills. Recent research suggests that much of cognitive-behavioral therapy's effect is a function of the behavioral component (Jacobson et al., 1996). Research is under way that examines PRP's effect on children's use of the coping and problem-solving techniques such as assertiveness, negotiation, relaxation, and decision making, and whether increases in these skills mediate PRP's effects on depression and anxiety. Through understanding the mechanisms by which PRP works, we hope to further refine the intervention so that it produces more powerful and more consistent effects.

Another way in which we are trying to boost PRP's effects is by including parents in the intervention. Research suggests that children internalize their parents' explanatory styles and adopt the coping strategies that their parents habitually use when confronting stressors in their lives (Garber & Flynn, 1998). Thus, interventions with parents may provide a powerful pathway to prevention. Over the past few years, our research team has developed and begun to evaluate a group intervention designed to teach parents to use the cognitive and problem-solving skills of PRP in their own lives. We hope that this intervention will boost PRP's effects by facilitating parents' abilities to model effective coping strategies and support their children's use of these strategies.

In a recently completed pilot study, the combined PRP and parent intervention (study 13) significantly reduced symptoms of depression and anxiety relative to a control condition over a 12-month follow-up period. A large longitudinal study, currently in progress, is investigating whether the combination of the PRP and parent interventions is superior to PRP alone. In this study, children and parents are also participating in booster sessions that are designed to help them apply the PRP skills to stressors and challenges they face during the first 2 years following the intervention, as the children make the transition from middle to high school. All students and parents participating in the intervention conditions attend booster sessions, so this study will not directly examine the efficacy of the booster sessions. We will examine whether the addition of a parent intervention component strengthens PRP's effects on children's cognitions related to depression, coping and problem-solving skills, and depression and anxiety symptoms. We will also examine the effects of the parent intervention on parents' explanatory styles and depressive symptoms and whether changes in these outcomes mediate PRP's effects on children's well-being.

We are also collaborating on research that integrates PRP with interventions that more directly target parent and family factors. Children whose parents suffer from clinical depression are at particularly high risk for depression (Beardslee, 2002; Goodman & Tully, Chapter 17, this volume). In addition, childhood depression is associated with family conflict and with parenting characterized by low levels of care and high levels of criticism or intrusiveness (Diamond, Serrano, Dickey, & Sonis, 1996). These different parent and family risk factors often co-occur, so that parents who are depressed are more likely to exhibit parenting characterized by low levels of care and high levels of criticism. Their marriages are characterized by higher levels of conflict (Downey & Coyne, 1990). Many of the PRP skills can be applied to children's responses to family turmoil and parental depression. For example, PRP specifically teaches children to challenge negative beliefs (particularly self-blame and catastrophic predictions) associated with parental conflict and to cope more effectively with the strong emotions that often result from such conflict. However, interventions that combine and integrate cognitive-behavioral and family approaches may more powerfully address the family factors that increase children's risk for depression. To that end, we are collaborating with a research group that is developing an intervention that blends PRP skills with Attachment-Based Family Therapy (Boyd, Diamond, & Bourjolly, 2006).

PRP's effects may also be enhanced by tailoring it to subgroups of children at elevated risk for depression. Given the gender difference in depression that emerges in adolescence, one subgroup of particular interest is girls. In most studies, PRP groups include both boys and girls. However, there are several reasons to expect that early adolescent girls would benefit from an all-girls format. Educational research suggests that in coed environments, girls may receive less attention than boys (Bailey, 1993). Over the years, several group leaders in our PRP studies have expressed concern about this issue, reporting that they devote more energy into engaging boys—perhaps at the expense of girls—because boys are more likely to call out and be disruptive during sessions. Most important, girls experience different stressors than boys during early adolescence. For example, the physical changes associated with puberty are viewed more negatively by girls than by boys. These concerns about body image appear to be closely connected to the rise in depressive symptoms that begins in early adolescence (Petersen, Sarigiani, & Kennedy, 1991). Many girls feel more comfortable discussing these and other concerns in an all-girls rather than coed setting.

A recent study evaluated PRP's effectiveness when delivered in an all-girls format (study 10). Girls were randomly assigned to coed PRP, all-girls PRP, or control conditions. Both PRP conditions covered the same content, and both significantly reduced depressive symptoms relative to control. There was some evidence for greater benefits in all-girls PRP. At the end of the intervention, girls in the all-girls PRP condition reported significantly lower levels of hopelessness than girls in the coed PRP and control groups. In addition, girls' attendance was higher in the all-girls PRP group than in the coed PRP group, suggesting a preference for that intervention format.

Moving PRP to an all-girls format was a fairly simple change. PRP's effects could be enhanced further by taking advantage of the all-girls format to target more explicitly such risk factors as body image concerns, sociocontextual factors, and response styles (such as rumination), which are particularly relevant to girls during the transition from childhood to adolescence. We recently developed a new intervention, the Girls in Transition (GT) program, which attempts to do just this. GT includes many of the PRP concepts and skills, but also includes new lessons that focus on additional concepts and skills that may be particularly important to girls as they navigate the challenges of early adolescence. In GT, the application of cognitive skills is extended as the girls are encouraged to examine deeper beliefs, such as underlying assumptions (e.g., "It's very important to be popular or physically attractive") and stringent standards (e.g., "Good people are liked by everyone"; "Good students do well at everything") that may be common during the middle school years. The girls are encouraged to apply the cognitive restructuring techniques to these kinds of dysfunctional beliefs and to the negative thoughts they generate, as well as to media and societal messages about the importance of attractiveness and gender stereotypes that can be harmful to girls. In the assertiveness and problem-solving lessons, the girls learn the approaches covered in PRP, but these skills are applied more explicitly to relational aggression (Crick & Grotpeter, 1995). In addition, there is more emphasis on examining beliefs that can make it difficult for girls and women to express anger or to act assertively. Anger expression is a particularly important issue to address, inasmuch as recent research suggests that girls and women who restrict anger expression may be at increased risk for depression (Chaplin & Cole, 2005). In an expanded section on coping with emotions, the girls discuss rumination and other response styles and learn specific strategies for managing sadness and anxiety and for breaking the cycle of rumination. The final sections of GT encourage the girls to think critically about societal and media messages that seem to place limits on women's abilities or great importance on unrealistic ideals for physical appearance. The girls are encouraged to put these messages in perspective by (1) thinking about the qualities that are important in their lives, particularly in their close relationships, (2) reflecting on their own goals, and (3) identifying positive role models (see, e.g., Wilgosh, 2002). A small pilot of this intervention is currently under way.

Although research on PRP is encouraging, the inconsistency in findings across studies (and within some studies) reminds us of the importance of keeping dissemination at the forefront as research on PRP moves into the future. Members of our research team are working to develop and integrate new intervention components, such as videos and a computer program based on PRP that can provide a standardized wide-scale delivery of the intervention or can be used to supplement the in-person PRP curriculum. Our primary focus is on developing and refining training procedures to help ensure successful delivery of the PRP intervention as it is delivered in schools, after-school programs, clinics, and other real-world community settings that serve children and their families.

Schools offer great promise for wide-scale prevention. The majority of adolescents in this country attend public or private schools, and schools are major providers of mental health services. Most schools are ill-equipped to take on the challenges and opportunities posed by prevention, however, as they are not adequately staffed to treat children's mental health problems, let alone prevent them (Doll, 1996; Gutkin, 1995; Pfeiffer & Reddy, 1998; Reeder et al., 1997). In addition, recent surveys of school psychologists suggest that most do not have the training needed to deliver cognitive-behavioral interventions like PRP (Miller, DuPaul, & Lutz, 2002).

To better prepare school staff to deliver interventions like PRP, we are refining our procedures for group leader training and supervision. In our current trainings, as in the past, we teach prospective group leaders about the cognitive-behavioral models of depression that underlie the PRP skill set and we coach leaders and provide extensive feedback as they practice delivering the intervention. But our current training also teaches prospective leaders to use and apply the PRP concepts and skills in their own lives. We hope that this personal, deeper knowledge of the cognitive-behavioral concepts and skills will increase group leaders' competence and effectiveness as they help their students apply the PRP skills to the day-to-day experiences and challenges of early adolescence.

CONCLUSIONS

Adolescence appears to be a crucial time in the etiology of depression and an important opportunity for prevention efforts. Interventions that teach cognitive and problem-solving skills may prevent depression by helping students to navigate the challenges of adolescence more successfully. Several group cognitive-behavioral interventions, including PRP, show promise in preventing depression and appear to improve other outcomes, such as in anxiety and conduct problems, that often co-occur with depression in youth. However, findings across and within studies are inconsistent, underscoring the need to determine when and how interventions like PRP work and how to boost their effectiveness as they are implemented in real-world settings. Depression prevention research will live up to its promise if interventions like PRP can be successfully implemented by schools, clinics, and other community settings. It is one thing to show that depression can be prevented and quite another to actually achieve wide-scale prevention. The challenge ahead is to bridge this gap (Weisz et al., 1995).

ACKNOWLEDGMENTS

We are grateful to the children, parents, teachers, counselors, and clinicians who have participated in PRP research over the years and to the National Institute of Mental Health, Kaiser Foundation Research Institute, University of Pennsylvania, and Swarthmore College for funding previous research on PRP. A special thank you is extended to Dr. Esteban Cardemil for providing data from the inner-city evaluation of PRP.

The Penn Resiliency Program is available for use in research. For more information, contact Jane Gillham at *jgillha1@swarthmore.edu* or *jgillham@psych.upenn.edu* or the Penn Resiliency Program research team at *info@pennproject.org*.

REFERENCES

Entries followed by an asterisk denote empirical evaluations of PRP.

Abela, J. R. Z., Vanderbilt, E., & Rochon, A. (2004). A test of the integration of response styles and social support theories of depression in third- and seventh-grade children. *Journal of Social and Clinical Psychology, 23,* 653–674.

Abramson, L. Y., Metalsky, G. I., & Alloy, L. B. (1989). Hopelessness depression: A theory-based subtype of depression. *Psychological Review, 96,* 358–372.

Abramson, L. Y., Seligman, M. E. P., & Teasdale, J. E. (1978). Learned helplessness in humans: Critique and reformulation. *Journal of Abnormal Psychology, 87,* 49–74.

American Psychiatric Association. (2000). *Diagnostic and statistical manual of mental disorders* (4th ed., text rev.). Washington, DC: Author.

Bailey, S. M. (1993). The current status of gender equity research in American schools. *Educational Psychologist, 28,* 321–339.

Beardslee, W. R. (2002). *Out of the darkened room: When a parent is depressed: Protecting the children and strengthening the family.* Boston: Little, Brown.

Beck, A. T. (1967). *Depression: Clinical, experimental, and theoretical aspects.* New York: Harper & Row.

Bower, S. A., & Bower, G. H. (1977). *Asserting yourself: A practical guide for positive change.* Cambridge, MA: Addison-Wesley.

Boyd, R. C., Diamond, G. S., & Bourjolly, J. (2006). Developing a family-based depression prevention program in urban community mental health clinics: A qualitative investigation. *Family Process, 45,* 187–203.

Butler, A. C., Chapman, J. E., Forman, E. M., & Beck, A. T. (2006). The empirical status of cognitive-behavioral therapy: A review of meta-analyses. *Clinical Psychology Review, 26,* 17–31.

Cardemil, E. V., Reivich, K. J., Beevers, C. J., Seligman, M. E. P., & James, J. (2007). The prevention of depressive symptoms in low-income, minority children: Two-year follow-up. *Behaviour Research and Therapy, 45,* 313–327.*

Cardemil, E. V., Reivich, K. J., & Seligman, M. E. P. (2002). The prevention of depressive symptoms in low-income minority middle school students. *Prevention and Treatment, 5.*

Chaplin, T. M., & Cole, P. M. (2005). The role of emotion regulation in the development of psychopathology. In B. L. Hankin & J. R. Z. Abela (Eds.), *Development of psychopathology: A vulnerability–stress perspective* (pp. 49–74). Thousand Oaks, CA: Sage.

Chaplin, T. M., Gillham, J. E., Reivich, K., Elkon, A. G. L., Samuels, B., Freres, D. R., et al. (2006). Depression prevention for early adolescent girls: A pilot study of all-girls versus co-ed groups. *Journal of Early Adolescence, 26,* 110–126.*

Cicchetti, D., & Rogosch, F. A. (2002). A developmental psychopathology perspective on adolescence. *Journal of Consulting and Clinical Psychology, 70,* 6–20.

Clark, D. (1986). A cognitive approach to panic. *Behaviour Research and Therapy, 24,* 461–470.

Cohen, J. (1988). *Statistical power analysis for the behavioral sciences* (2nd ed.). Hillsdale, NJ: Erlbaum.

Crick, N. R., & Grotpeter, J. K. (1995). Relational aggression, gender and social-psychological adjustment. *Child Development, 66,* 710–722.

Cutuli, J. J. (2004). *Preventing externalizing symptoms and related features in adolescence.* Unpublished honors thesis, University of Pennsylvania, Philadelphia.*

Cutuli, J. J., Chaplin, T. M., Gillham, J. E., Reivich, K. R., & Seligman, M. E. P. (2006). Preventing co-occurring depression symptoms in adolescents with conduct problems: The Penn Resiliency Program. *Annals of the New York Academy of Sciences, 1094,* 282–286.*

Damon, W., & Hart, D. (1982). The development of self-understanding from infancy through adolescence. *Child Development, 53,* 841–864.

Diamond, G. S., Serrano, A. C., Dickey, M., & Sonis, W. A. (1996). Current status of family-based outcome and process research. *Journal of the American Academy of Child and Adolescent Psychiatry, 35,* 6–16.

Dodge, K. A., & Crick, N. R. (1990). Social information-processing bases of aggressive behavior in children. *Personality and Social Psychology Bulletin, 16,* 8–22.

Doll, B. (1996). Prevalence of psychiatric disorders in children and youth: An agenda for advocacy by school psychology. *School Psychology Quarterly, 11,* 20–47.

Downey, G., & Coyne, J. C. (1990). Children of depressed parents: An integrative review. *Psychological Bulletin, 108,* 50–76.

Dozois, D. J. A., & Dobson, K. S. (Eds.). (2004). *The prevention of anxiety and depression: Theory, research and practice.* Washington, DC: American Psychological Association.

Eccles, J. S., Midgley, C., Wigfield, A., Buchanan, C. M., Reuman, D., Flanagan, C., et al. (1993). Development during adolescence: The impact of stage–environment fit on young adolescents' experiences in schools and in families. *American Psychologist, 48,* 90–101.

Ellis, A. (1962). *Reason and emotion in psychotherapy.* New York: Lyle Stuart.

Garber, J., & Flynn, C. (1998). Origins of depressive cognitive style. In D. K. Routh & R. J. DeRubeis (Eds.), *The science of clinical psychology: Accomplishments and future directions* (pp. 53–93). Washington, DC: American Psychological Association.

Garber, J., Quiggle, N. L., Panak, W., & Dodge, K. A. (1991). Aggression and depression in children: Comorbidity, specificity, and social cognitive processing. In D. Cicchetti & S. L. Toth (Eds.), *Internalizing and externalizing expressions of dysfunction* (pp. 225–264). Hillsdale, NJ: Erlbaum.

Gillham, J. E. (1994). *Preventing depressive symptoms in school children.* Unpublished doctoral dissertation, University of Pennsylvania, Philadelphia.*

Gillham, J. E., Hamilton, J., Freres, D. R., Patton, K., & Gallop, R. (2006). Preventing depression among early adolescents in the primary care setting. A randomized controlled study of the Penn Resiliency Program. *Journal of Abnormal Child Psychology, 34,* 203–219.*

Gillham, J. E., Jaycox, L. H., Reivich, K. J., Seligman, M. E. P., & Silver, T. (1990). *The Penn Resiliency Program.* Unpublished manual, University of Pennsylvania, Philadelphia.

Gillham, J. E., & Reivich, K. J. (1999). Prevention of depressive symptoms in school children: A research update. *Psychological Science, 10,* 461–462.*

Gillham, J. E., Reivich, K. J., Freres, D. R., Chaplin, T. M., Shatté, A. J., Samuels, B., et al. (2007). School-based prevention of depressive symptoms: Effectiveness and specificity of the Penn Resiliency Program. *Journal of Consulting and Clinical Psychology, 75,* 9–19.*

Gillham, J. E., Reivich, K. J., Freres, D. R., Lascher, M., Litzinger, S., Shatté, A., et al. (2006). School-based prevention of depression and anxiety symptoms in early adolescence: A pilot of a parent intervention component. *School Psychology Quarterly, 21,* 323–348.*

Gillham, J. E., Reivich, K. J., Jaycox, L. H., & Seligman, M. E. P. (1995). Preventing depressive symptoms in schoolchildren: Two year follow-up. *Psychological Science, 6,* 343–351.*

Gillham, J. E., Shatté, A. J., & Freres, D. R. (2000). Depression prevention: A review of cognitive-behavioral and family interventions. *Applied and Preventive Psychology, 9,* 63–88.

Gotlib, I. H., Lewinsohn, P. M., & Seeley, J. R. (1995). Symptoms versus a diagnosis of depression: Differences in psychosocial functioning. *Journal of Consulting and Clinical Psychology, 63,* 90–100.

Gutkin, T. B. (1995). School psychology and health care: Moving service delivery into the twenty-first century. *School Psychology Quarterly, 10,* 235–246.

Hankin, B. L., & Abela, J. R. Z. (2005). Depression from childhood through adolescence and adulthood: A developmental vulnerability and stress perspective. In B. L. Hankin & J. R. Z. Abela (Eds.), *Development of psychopathology: A vulnerability–stress perspective* (pp. 245–288). Thousand Oaks, CA: Sage.

Hankin, B. L., Abramson, L. Y., Moffitt, T. E., Silva, P. A., & McGee, R. (1998). Development of depression from preadolescence to young adulthood: Emerging gender differences in a 10-year longitudinal study. *Journal of Abnormal Psychology, 107,* 128–140.

Harnett, P. H., & Dadds, M. R. (2004). Training school personnel to implement a universal school-based prevention of depression program under real-world conditions. *Journal of School Psychology, 42,* 343–357.

Hill, J. P., & Holmbeck, G. N. (1986). Attachment and autonomy during adolescence. In G. Whitehurst (Ed.), *Annals of child development* (Vol. 3., pp. 145–189). Greenwich, CT: JAI Press.

Hollon, S. D., DeRubeis, R. J., Shelton, R. C., Amsterdam, J. D., Salomon, R. M., O'Reardon, J. P., et al. (2005). Prevention of relapse following cognitive therapy vs. medication in moderate to severe depression. *Archives of General Psychiatry, 62*, 417–422.

Horowitz, J. L., & Garber, J. (2006). The prevention of depressive symptoms in children and adolescents: A meta-analytic review. *Journal of Consulting and Clinical Psychology, 74*, 401–415.

Inhelder, B., & Piaget, J. (1958). *The growth of logical thinking from childhood to adolescence.* New York: Basic Books.

Jacobson, N. S., Dobson, K. S., Truax, P. A., Addis, M. E., Koerner, K., Gollan, J. K., et al. (1996). A component analysis of cognitive-behavioral treatment for depression. *Journal of Consulting and Clinical Psychology, 64*, 295–304.

Jaycox, L. H., Reivich, K. J., Gillham, J., & Seligman, M. E. P. (1994). Prevention of depressive symptoms in school children. *Behaviour Research and Therapy, 32*, 801–816.*

Kim-Cohen, J., Caspi, A., Moffitt, T. E., Harrington, H., Milne, B. J., & Poulton, R. (2003). Prior juvenile diagnoses in adults with mental disorder: Developmental follow-back of a prospective-longitudinal cohort. *Archives of General Psychiatry, 60*, 709–717.

Kovacs, M. (2001). *Children's Depression Inventory manual.* North Tonawanda, NY: Multi-Health Systems.

Lochman, J. E., Coie, J. D., Underwood, M. K., & Terry, M. (1993). Effectiveness of a social relations intervention program for aggressive and nonaggressive, rejected children. *Journal of Consulting and Clinical Psychology, 61*, 1053–1058.

McCauley, E., Mitchell, J. R., Burke, P., & Moss, S. (1988). Cognitive attributes of depression in children and adolescents. *Journal of Consulting and Clinical Psychology, 56*, 903–908.

Merry, S., McDowell, H., Hetrick, S., Bir, J., & Muller, N. (2004). Psychological and/or educational interventions for the prevention of depression in children and adolescents. *The Cochrane Database of Systematic Reviews, 2.* Art No.: CD003380. D01: 10.1002/14651858.CD003380.pub2.

Miller, D. N., DuPaul, G. J., & Lutz, J. G. (2002). School-based psychosocial interventions for childhood depression: Acceptability of treatments among school psychologists. *School Psychology Quarterly, 17*, 78–99.

Miller, J. B. (1999). *The effect of a cognitive-behavioral group intervention on depressive symptoms in an incarcerated adolescent delinquent population (juvenile delinquents).* Unpublished doctoral dissertation, University of Pennsylvania, Philadelphia.*

Nolen-Hoeksema, S. (1991). Responses to depression and their effects on the duration of depressive episodes. *Journal of Abnormal Psychology, 100*, 569–582.

Nolen-Hoeksema, S., Girgus, J. S., & Seligman, M. E. P. (1992). Predictors and consequences of childhood depressive symptoms: A 5-year longitudinal study. *Journal of Abnormal Psychology, 101*, 405–422.

Pattison, C., & Lynd-Stevenson, R. M. (2001). The prevention of depressive symptoms in children: The immediate and long-term outcomes of a school based program. *Behaviour Change, 18*, 92–102.*

Petersen, A. C., Sarigiani, P. A., & Kennedy, R. E. (1991). Adolescent depression: Why more girls? *Journal of Youth and Adolescence, 20*, 247–271.

Pfeiffer, S. I., & Reddy, L. A. (1998). School-based mental health programs in the United States: Present status and a blueprint for the future. *School Psychology Review, 27*, 84–96.

Quayle, D., Dziurawiec, S., Roberts, C., Kane, R., & Ebsworthy, G. (2001). The effect of an optimism and lifeskills program on depressive symptoms in preadolescence. *Behaviour Change, 18*, 194–203.*

Reeder, G. D., Maccow, G. C., Shaw, S. R., Swerdlik, M. E., Horton, C. B., & Foster, P. (1997). School psychologists and full-service schools: Partnerships with medical, mental health, and social services. *School Psychology Review, 26*, 603–621.

Reivich, K. J. (1996). *The prevention of depressive symptoms in adolescents.* Unpublished doctoral dissertation, University of Pennsylvania, Philadelphia.*

Roberts, C., Kane, R., Bishop, B., Matthews, H., & Thompson, H. (2004). The prevention of depressive symptoms in rural children: A follow-up study. *International Journal of Mental Health Promotion, 6,* 4–16.*

Roberts, C., Kane, R., Thomson, H., Bishop, B., & Hart, B. (2003). The prevention of depressive symptoms in rural school children: A randomized controlled trial. *Journal of Consulting and Clinical Psychology, 71,* 622–628.*

Schoenwald, S. K., & Hoagwood, K. (2001). Effectiveness, transportability, and dissemination of interventions: What matters when? *Psychiatric Services, 52,* 1190–1197.

Shatté, A. J. (1997). *The prevention of depressive symptoms in adolescents: Issues of dissemination and mechanisms of change.* Unpublished doctoral dissertation, University of Pennsylvania, Philadelphia.*

Shochet, I. M., Dadds, M. R., Holland, D., Whitefield, K., Harnett, P. H., & Osgarby, S. M. (2001). The efficacy of a universal school-based program to prevent adolescent depression. *Journal of Clinical Child Psychology, 30,* 303–315.

Smith, M. L., Glass, G. V., & Miller, T. L. (1980). *The benefits of psychotherapy.* Baltimore: Johns Hopkins University Press.

Weisz, J. R., Donenberg, G. R., Han, S. S., & Weiss, B. (1995). Bridging the gap between laboratory and clinic in child and adolescent psychotherapy. *Journal of Consulting and Clinical Psychology, 63,* 688–701.

Weisz, J. R., & Jensen, A. L. (2001). Child and adolescent psychotherapy in research and practice contexts: Review of the evidence and suggestions for improving the field. *European Child and Adolescent Psychiatry, 10,* 112–118.

Weisz, J. R., & Kazdin, A. E. (2003). Concluding thoughts: Present and future of evidence-based psychotherapies for children and adolescents. In A. E. Kazdin & J. R. Weisz (Eds.), *Evidence-based psychotherapies for children and adolescents* (pp. 439–451). New York: Guilford Press.

Weisz, J. R., McCarty, C. A., & Valeri, S. M. (2006). Effects of psychotherapy in children and adolescents: A meta-analysis. *Psychological Bulletin, 132,* 132–149.

Wilgosh, L. (2002). Examining gender images, expectations, and competence as perceived impediments to personal, academic and career development. *International Journal for the Advancement of Counselling, 24,* 239–260.

Yu, D. L., & Seligman, M. E. P. (2002). Preventing depressive symptoms in Chinese children. *Prevention and Treatment, 5.*

Zubernis, L. S., Cassidy, K. W., Gillham, J. E., Reivich, K. J., & Jaycox, L. H. (1999). Prevention of depressive symptoms in preadolescent children of divorce. *Journal of Divorce and Remarriage, 30,* 11–36.*

14 Integrating Individual and Whole-School Change Approaches in the Prevention of Depression in Adolescents

Susan H. Spence

To date, most approaches to the prevention of depression in children and adolescents have emerged from theories that propose that intrinsic cognitive and behavioral characteristics of the individual can influence the impact of life stress events or biological predisposition, and/or have a direct effect upon the development of depression (Abramson et al., 1999; Clark, Beck, & Alford, 1999; Lewinsohn, Clarke, Hops, & Andrews, 1990; Stark, Rouse, & Livingston, 1991; Vostanis & Harrington, 1994). There has been a good deal of overlap in the content of depression prevention programs, with most aiming to enhance individual attributes such as social skills, coping skills, self-regulation, optimistic and adaptive cognitive style, and problem-solving skills. In some instances prevention programs have been implemented with whole populations of young people, irrespective of risk status (universal prevention). In others, the intervention has been restricted to individuals who are already experiencing elevated but subclinical symptoms (indicated prevention) or who are judged to be at increased risk of developing a disorder as a consequence of some specific feature within the individual or environment, such as the offspring of parents with an affective disorder, children with a pessimistic cognitive style, or children who have experienced abuse, family conflict, parental divorce, or death of a parent (selected prevention) (Mrazek & Haggerty, 1994).

The focus of this chapter is on school-based, universal approaches to prevention, rather than approaches that are restricted to individuals at specific risk or who already show elevated symptoms of depression. Universal, indicated, and selected approaches to prevention are proposed to have relative advantages and disadvantages (Offord, Kraemer, Kazdin, Jensen, & Harrington, 1998). The proponents of universal approaches suggest that the advantages of universal prevention over selected or indicated programs include (1) avoidance of labeling effects associated with being selected as being "at risk," (2) better participation rates, and (3) ability to target a wide range of risk factors simultaneously (Shochet & Ham, 2004). The population health approach of universal prevention aims to reduce the overall burden of depressive disorders in the community by changing the distribution of one or more risk or protective factors in a population. A relatively small reduction in a risk factor at a whole-population level may produce a greater reduction in the number of clinical cases of a disorder than a large reduction in that same risk factor for a relatively small number of individuals with initially high levels of that risk factor (Mason, Scott, Chapman, & Shihfen, 2000; Rose, 1992). The major disadvantages of universal programs are the fiscal and logistical costs involved and the inability to provide in-depth, individualized intervention.

THE EVIDENCE

Research into the efficacy and effectiveness of interventions to prevent depression in young people is still in its early stages. Although studies have been conducted in this area, they have suffered from a range of methodological design problems that severely limit the conclusions that can be drawn (Merry, McDowell, Hetrick, Bir, & Muller, 2004). These problems include small sample sizes, low participation rates and poor retention rates (raising issues of representativeness of the sample), inadequate durations of follow-up, lack of attention to placebo control conditions, insufficient training of staff, absence of independent confirmation of quality and fidelity in program delivery, and reliance on self-report of depressive symptoms. Most research has also failed to examine whether a program was successful in changing the cognitive or behavioral skills that it aimed to improve and whether such changes played a mediating role in reducing or preventing depression. In a recent Cochrane meta-analysis, Merry, McDowell, Hetrick, et al. (2004) concluded that "psychological interventions were effective compared with nonintervention immediately after the programmes were delivered with a significant reduction in scores on depression rating scales for targeted (standardized mean difference [SMD] of −0.26 and a 95% confidence interval (CI) of −0.40 to −0.13) but not universal interventions (SMD −0.21, 95% CI −0.48, 0.06)." Effect sizes were minimal when long-term effects of universal interventions for depression prevention were considered. Merry et al. concluded that there was currently insufficient evidence to justify widespread dissemination of psychological approaches to depression prevention.

Although additional studies have been published since the Merry, McDowell, Hetrick, et al. (2004), meta-analysis, the results relating to universal prevention for depression continue to be conflicting. For example, Pössel, Horn, Groen, and Hautzinger (2004) examined the effects of a school-based intervention that included cognitive restructuring and assertiveness and social competence training. An experienced trainer and cotrainer led each session, with single-sex groups, over 10 weeks. Trainers received thorough training, which included observation of all sessions led by another trainer, followed by regular supervision of videotaped sessions. The results indicated a significantly different pattern of results for students at different levels of risk. Those with minimal levels of depressive symptoms at pretest showed significantly lower rates of increase in depression symptoms following participation in the intervention, as compared with no-intervention controls over the 6-month follow-up period. Students who initially reported subsyndromal depression scores showed a significant decrease in depression scores over time, whereas the control group continued to show elevated levels of depression. Of those who initially had depression scores in the clinical range, only the no-intervention control group showed a significant reduction in depression. A subsequent article reporting on the same study noted that, contrary to expectations, students who were low in self-efficacy benefited more from the program than high self-efficacy students (Pössel, Baldus, Horn, Groen, & Hautzinger, 2005).

Shochet et al. (2001) reported small, but significant preventive effects in an evaluation of the Resourceful Adolescent Program (RAP), although this benefit was evident in only one of the two depression measures. The study was also limited by the lack of random assignment to conditions. Two subsequent evaluations of RAP have also been reported. In the first study, no short-term or long-term effects were found for RAP in comparison to no intervention when it was implemented by teachers (Harnett & Dadds, 2004). In the second study, the RAP approach was compared with a placebo intervention, with log-transformed data for depression scores, averaged over time to 18-month follow-up, showing significantly greater effects for the active intervention group on one out of two depression measures (Merry, McDowell, Wild, Bir, & Cunliffe, 2004). However, the effect sizes between intervention and attention placebo control groups at each follow-up were minimal. It was noted that the placebo intervention included elements that had the potential to influence depressive symptoms, including identification of pleasant activities, group problem solving, and body language. Thus, we cannot discount the possibility that the placebo condition may also have had an active effect on student well-being. Moreover, the study did not include a no-intervention control group, making it difficult to draw conclusions about the impact of RAP.

In their Cochrane meta-analysis, Merry, McDowell, Hetrick, et al. (2004) noted that most follow-up periods were limited to less than 1 year and little evidence existed regarding long-term outcomes. Spence, Sheffield, and Donovan (2005) reported the 2-, 3-, and 4-year follow-up results of a universal preventive intervention. The study involved a randomized controlled trial of the Problem Solving for Life program, a teacher-administered, classroom-based, universal intervention that aimed to teach a range of problem-solving and cognitive coping skills to assist grade 8 students to deal successfully with challenging life situations. Sixteen schools were randomly assigned to either the intervention or control group. In an earlier article, the authors reported positive short-term preventive effects (Spence, Sheffield, & Donovan, 2003). From pre- to posttest, high-symptom students in the intervention group showed a significantly greater decrease in depressive symptoms and increase in problem-solving skills than high-symptom students in the control group. For students with low levels of baseline depression symptoms, the control group demonstrated a short-term increase in depression scores and a decrease in problem-solving skills, whereas those in the intervention condition demonstrated a slight decrease in depression scores and an increase in problem-solving ability immediately following the intervention. For students in general, those who reported greater reductions in depression following the intervention tended to be those who reported greater improvements in problem-solving skills, supporting the mediational role of problem-solving skills in preventing depressive symptoms. Although the short-term results were encouraging, at 12-month follow-up the intervention effects were no longer present.

Spence, Sheffield, and Donovan (2005) suggested that although benefits were not evident at 12-month follow-up, positive effects would be likely to emerge over subsequent years, as the students encountered the stressful life events related to adolescence. However, no significant differences were found between the intervention and control conditions in the trajectories of depressive symptoms over the 4-year follow-up period. Similarly, there were no long-term differences between groups in the level of problem-solving skills or attributional style.

A study reported by Sheffield et al. (2006) also failed to find positive outcomes for the Problem Solving for Life program, even at posttest. This was a complex study comparing the outcomes of universal, indicated, and combined universal plus indicated approaches to the prevention of depression among adolescents with elevated symptoms of depression. The rationale for the study was based on the premise that universal, classroom-based preventive programs may be insufficient to produce lasting protective effects for at-risk youth. It was proposed that the addition of a small-group, intensive indicated intervention, implemented by highly trained health professionals, for students with elevated depression symptoms can produce stronger and more durable benefits than a universal approach alone. Two separate state teams implemented the study so as to provide built-in replication of results. All students in grade 9 (ages 13–15 years) of 36 high schools were approached to participate. Approximately 50% provided consent and were then screened with the use of two self-report questionnaires on depressive symptoms. Students scoring in the top 20% on the composite scores of the Children's Depression Inventory (CDI) and the Center for Epidemiologic Studies Depression Scale (CES-D) were followed-up over the intervention period and at 12-month follow-up. Schools were matched across a range of demographic variables relating to socioeconomic status, gender mix of school, public/private status, and rural/urban location and randomly assigned to a universal, indicated, combined universal + indicated, or control condition. The universal program was the Problem Solving for Life curriculum (discussed above), implemented by teachers, with whole classrooms of students, which was conducted for one classroom session (45–50 minutes) per week over 8 weeks. In this condition, the high-symptom students completed the sessions along with the rest of their classmates. The indicated intervention, Adolescent Coping with Emotions (Kowalenko et al., 2002), was conducted in small groups of 8–10 students by a trained health professional or school counselor and was designed specifically to build resilience and reduce depressive symptoms in students who reported initial elevated but subclinical levels of depression. It included extended session duration (eight, 90-minute, weekly sessions) and an intensive focus on social skills training, self-reward skills, conflict resolution, and assertiveness, in addition to cognitive restructuring and life-problem-solving skills training. Students in the combined approach received the universal program first, followed by the intensive indicated program.

The 12-month follow-up commenced at the end of the combined intervention. Contrary to hypotheses, there were no significant differences in depression trajectories between any of the intervention approaches and the no-intervention control condition for either self-reported depressive symptoms or incidence of depressive episodes, as measured by clinical interview, for the high-symptom students. Also contrary to predictions, the combined universal plus indicated program did not produce superior results to either intervention alone. Irrespective of experimental condition, students with high initial levels of depressive symptoms reported a steady decline in depressive symptoms over time. There were also no significant differences between groups in terms of changes in anxiety, hopelessness, thinking style, coping skills, or social adjustment. An important finding was that the outcomes were the same at the two intervention sites. There was no evidence of differential outcomes for boys and girls, nor according to severity of initial depressive symptoms. The sample size was large (455 high-symptom students), which was sufficient to detect even a small intervention effect. The attrition rate was relatively low, with 86% of the students being available at 12-month follow-up. In addition, there were no significant differences in demographic or pretest mental health variables between those who remained in the study and those who were not available at follow-up.

Of particular relevance to this chapter were the findings for the universal versus no-intervention control conditions. The universal condition included all children within the classroom, irrespective of level of depressive symptoms. This component of the study compared students in the nine intervention schools with those in the nine no-intervention control condition. No significant differences between the intervention and control students were found in terms of changes in depression, anxiety, coping skills, or social adjustment over time from baseline to postintervention and 12-month follow-up. Both conditions showed a small but significant decrease in depression scores over time.

The Sheffield et al. (2006) study has some important methodological strengths; thus, these findings should be taken seriously. Two independent research teams conducted the evaluation, and equivalent results were found at the two sites. The sample size was large, the attrition rate was relatively low, and the schools were broadly representative of the general population. Its weaknesses include reliance on student self-reports and a relatively low participation rate. Moreover, the 6 hours of teacher training may not have been sufficient to ensure adequate skill in program delivery, and fidelity checks relied on teacher reports rather than direct observation. Nevertheless, the study clearly brings into question the effectiveness of cognitive-behavioral, school-based interventions in preventing depression in adolescents.

WHAT HAVE WE LEARNED?

In response to the relatively poor results, we considered various possible explanations and ways in which we could strengthen the efficacy and effectiveness of school-based interventions for depression prevention. A valid test of efficacy requires that we can demonstrate that the intervention has been administered with fidelity. As noted above, studies to date have typically relied on staff members' self-reports of their quality and rigor in implementation, rather than independent evaluation, leaving open the question of reporter bias. Most studies have involved teachers or graduate students in implementation of the programs, and it remains to be demonstrated that they have the skills, knowledge and expertise in mental health and cognitive-behavior therapy to enable high-quality administration.

A second possible explanation for the poor results is the relatively short length of intervention. The vast majority of studies to date have evaluated interventions of about 8–20 weeks duration, usually involving rather brief sessions of 30–90 minutes. It may be unrealistic to expect such a low dosage to be sufficient to teach the skills necessary to alter the developmental pathways of children at high risk for depression. Those studies that examined whether intervention produced significant and durable learning of targeted skills have yielded mixed results. For example, short-term positive changes in response to intervention have been reported for negative automatic thoughts (Cardemil, Reivich, & Seligman, 2002) and negative problem-solving orientation (Spence et al., 2003). In both studies, these skills were found to mediate short-term changes in depressive symptoms, although Spence et al. (2003) did not find maintenance of problem-solving skills by 1-year follow-up. Other researchers have failed to find positive changes in targeted skills, including explanatory style, negative automatic thoughts, coping skills, and social skills (Cardemil et al., 2002; Harnett & Dadds, 2004; Pattison & Lynd Stevenson, 2001; Pössel et al., 2004; Quayle, Dziurawiec, Roberts, Kane, & Ebsworthy, 2001). Thus, one of the explanations for the relatively poor effects on depression may be the failure of the interventions to produce significant improvements in the skills they purport to teach.

A third potential reason for the poor results is the tendency for interventions to focus on changing the characteristics of the young people in the absence of efforts to change environmental factors that influence emotional well-being. Ecological models of mental health emphasize the causal influence of the environment and suggest that a focus purely on individual change is unlikely to be sufficient to promote emotional well-being (Bronfenbrenner, 1979; Lerner, 1986). It is well recognized that family and social factors, including parent psychopathology, marital discord, parent–child relationships, and low parental support, are implicated as risk factors for depression in young people (Reinecke & Simons, 2005; Spence & Reinecke, 2003). Similarly, children's experience of school, such as being exposed to bullying, and the quality of relationships with peers and teachers have an important influence on emotional well-being (Bond, Carlin, Thomas, Rubin, & Patton, 2001; Roeger, Allison, Martin, Dadds, & Keeves, 2001). To date, efforts to involve families in programs to prevent depression have mainly involved children at risk as the result of a bereavement, trauma, or parental separation/divorce (Beardslee, Versage, Wright, & Salt, 1997; Sandler et al., 2003; Wolchik et al., 2002). Very few studies involving universal approaches have attempted to involve parents. The one notable study that tried to do so found a low rate of parental attendance at sessions (Shochet et al., 2001), and it is likely that parents of students most at risk were those least likely to attend.

There has also been little attempt to change school environments in an effort to reduce the development of depression. However, the increasing awareness of the impact of the school experience on emotional development has resulted in a shift toward school-based policies that promote mental health in young people, consistent with recommendations in the World Health Organization's Global School Health Initiative (World Health Organization, 1998). In Australia, these include the MindMatters whole-school change initiative (Wyn, Cahill, Holdsworth, Rowling, & Carson, 2000) and the National Safe Schools Framework (Curriculum Corporation, 2003). Consistent with these approaches, the Gatehouse Project, described by Patton, Bond, Thomas, and Toumbourou (1998), attempted to promote the emotional and behavioral well-being of youth in secondary schools through an intervention that targeted both individual and school-level factors. The project demonstrated a significant impact on young people's substance use, although contrary to expectations, it had no impact on depressive symptoms (Bond et al., 2004).

The beyondblue Schools Research Initiative

The *beyondblue* schools research initiative is a new approach that aims to overcome many of the limitations in previous approaches to the prevention of depression in young people. It was developed in response to the increasing awareness of the need for preventive interventions for depression in young people, while recognizing the relatively poor outcomes resulting from approaches that focus solely on individual skill acquisition. It was funded by *beyondblue*, the national depression initiative, which was established by the Australian commonwealth government to reduce the prevalence, risks for, and impact of depressive disorders within the Australian community. The ongoing evaluation is now funded by the National Health and Medical Research Council of Australia. The initiative involves the development and evaluation of a school-based, universal approach to the prevention of depression in adolescents that aims to enhance both individual and environmental protective factors.

Rationale and Content

Although evaluation is still in progress and outcomes are yet to be determined, the program is described here as it illustrates the type of intervention that we need to develop and evaluate in order to further our knowledge regarding the prevention of depression in young people. The following sections focus on the practical aspects of the intervention, rather than the research methodology of the study.

As noted above, the *beyondblue* schools research initiative recognizes the importance of enhancing protective factors within the adolescent's environment, in addition to developing individual resiliency skills. The elements of the program draw upon evidence relating to causal factors for depression, both intrinsic and extrinsic to the young person, and upon knowledge of organizational change processes. The conceptual framework that underpins the intervention is shown in Figure 14.1. It notes that although many adolescents experience adverse and stressful life situations, individuals vary in their psychological response to these events. The model conceptualizes resilience as a dynamic process involving individual and environmental factors that reduce the effects of adverse or stressful life experiences, in line with attachment, stress-coping, and social support theories of adjustment (Garmezy, 1991; Rutter, 1987). Factors influencing emotional well-being may be innate (e.g., temperament, gender, genetics), acquired (e.g., coping styles, interpersonal skills, help-seeking behavior), or present in the immediate environment (e.g., supportive family, peer relationships, social or school environments, access to professional help). Figure 14.1 highlights those protective factors that are targeted within the *beyondblue* schools research initiative. These relate, first, to individual cognitive and behavioral competencies, qualities, and skills, and, second, to factors within the young person's environment (school, family, friends, social networks, and the community; Spence, Burns, et al., 2005).

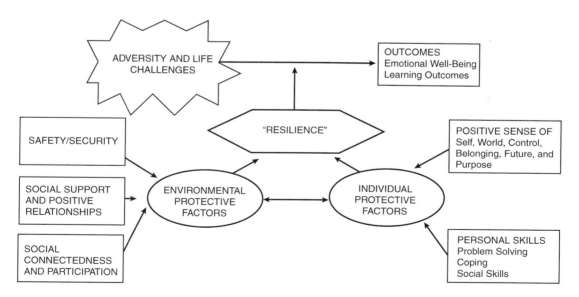

FIGURE 14.1. Conceptual framework. From Spence, Burns, et al. (2005). Copyright 2005 by Blackwell. Reprinted by permission.

Building Cognitive and Behavioral Strengths in the Young Person

Evidence suggests that individuals with strong problem-solving and social skills, and who attempt to deal with difficult situations in a constructive, rather than highly emotional or avoidant way, are less likely to experience depression in the face of adverse life events (Adams & Adams, 1996; Goodman, Gravitt, & Kaslow, 1995; Herman Stahl & Petersen, 1996; Muris, Schmidt, Lambrichs, & Meesters, 2001; Spence, Sheffield, & Donovan, 2002). There is also a good deal of evidence that a rational and optimistic thinking style acts as a protective factor against the adverse psychological impacts of negative life situations in young people (Abramson et al., 1999; Nolen-Hoeksema & Girgus, 1995; Spence et al., 2002).

Drawing on this literature, the *beyondblue* schools research initiative aims to enhance the protective skills of problem solving, coping, emotional regulation, stress reduction, social skills, conflict resolution, assertiveness, and methods of building social support. These skills are taught through a classroom program that is delivered sequentially each year over a 3-year period, from grade 8 through grade 10. Elements also focus on enhancing adaptive cognitive styles, such as increasing positive, but realistic, expectancies and constructive views of the self, the world, and the future, building self-efficacy and self-awareness, and facilitating the understanding of mental health issues and readiness and capacity to seek help for the self and others.

In terms of cognitive style, it emphasizes six dimensions that are proposed to protect against the development of depression, drawing on the empirical literature (Abramson et al., 1999; Beck, Rush, Shaw, & Emery, 1979; Seligman, Reivich, Jaycox, & Gillham, 1995). These concepts are communicated to students as the six "senses," which relate to the way individuals think about themselves, the world in general, their ability to control aspects of their world, their sense of belonging, sense of future, and sense of purpose in life. Individuals who tend to expect bad outcomes to occur in the future, blame themselves for bad events, focus on negative characteristics of themselves, and the world, or who lack a sense of belonging or purpose in life, and feel that there is little they can do to change things, are proposed to be at risk for the development of depression. In contrast, individuals who generate more realistic explanations for negative events, expect more positive things from the future, focus more on the positive attributes of themselves and the world, feel a sense of attachment and belonging within their social environments (family, peer group, or school), and have a strong sense of personal control and purpose in life, are suggested to cope more adaptively in the face of difficult situations. Table 14.1 summarizes the core skills that the program aims to develop at each grade level.

In each of the 3 years, the students participate in 10 weekly classroom sessions, of 30–45 minutes duration. The grades 9 and 10 curriculum materials include videotaped examples and dramatized stories that illustrate target skills. Each year, students complete a practical assessment task relating to their acquired knowledge. Program delivery uses a range of interactive methods, including small-group exercises and discussions, role plays, deep-learning tasks, and quizzes. It is guided by key *principles of effective practice*, including:

- The skills taught have high face validity for staff and students (are acceptable and relevant) and are developmentally appropriate.
- Students understand not just *what* skills are important in dealing with relationship issues, but *why* they are important.

TABLE 14.1. Cognitive and Behavioral Skills Taught at Each Year Level

Core skill/ component	Year 8: Getting to know yourself	Year 9: Building positive and supportive relationships	Year 10: Building strengths for the future
1. Emotional literacy and regulation	• Identifying emotions • Distinguishing thoughts and feelings • Recognizing link between thoughts and feelings • Managing negative emotions • Increasing positive mood	• Further work on the link between thoughts and feelings • Recognizing emotions in self and others	• Consolidating emotional recognition and management skills
2. Stress reduction	• Identifying stress and the physical, emotional, psychological, and behavioral responses to stress • Techniques for coping with stress • Reducing negative emotions	• Identifying relationship issues and coping methods	• Techniques for managing stress to cope with challenging situations—relaxation, thought challenging, self-soothing • Time management and planning skills
3. Social skills	• Basic skills for group work	• Developing and maintaining relationships—conversation and listening skills, assertion, negotiation, conflict resolution skills • Perspective-taking skills	• Communication skills • Conflict resolution skills • Perspective-taking skills
4. Life problem solving	• Identifying challenging situations	• Positive problem orientation • Steps and skills of interpersonal problem solving	• Solving interpersonal and life problems in a variety of contexts
5. Cognitive skills—building rationale and constructive thinking styles. Enhancing the six senses—positive sense of self/ world/ future/ belonging/ control/ meaning	• Basic emotional education—links between thoughts and feelings • Helpful self-talk • Changing unhelpful thoughts • Building positive sense of self	• Cognitive components of problem solving—predicting consequences, evaluating options, selecting responses • Links between thoughts and feelings • Self-reflection • Helpful self-talk • Changing unhelpful thoughts	• Role of self-talk • Identifying automatic thoughts • Challenging automatic thoughts and unhelpful beliefs • Realistic thinking • Realistic expectations • Developing a realistic sense of control • Building a sense of humor • Setting goals and developing a positive sense of future
6. Building social supports and connectedness	Identifying sources of support	• Introduction to relationships—types of relationships, types of support • The value of relationships • Building support networks • Evaluating the usefulness of sources of support	• Value of belonging (family, friends, sporting groups, cultures) • Identifying social connections • Identifying and building sources of support

(continued)

TABLE 14.1. *(continued)*

Core skill/component	Year 8: Getting to know yourself	Year 9: Building positive and supportive relationships	Year 10: Building strengths for the future
7. Participation in pleasant events	Identifying personal pleasant events		• Importance of participation in pleasant activities • Programming for pleasant events • The value of laughter
8. Awareness of mental health issues and help seeking	• Awareness of concept of resiliency • Introducing help-seeking behavior	• Understanding health and well-being (including emotional well-being) • Skills to identify and access available health resources and services within the school and community • Skills for seeking help for self and others • Evaluating the usefulness of sources of support	• Knowing how and when to access help for mental health issues • Skills for seeking help for self and others

- Skills need to be taught in a hierarchical manner, ensuring that one skill is well established before moving on to the next skill.
- Skills need to be clear and specific (e.g., using eye contact or monitoring facial expression) and not vague/general (e.g., appearing cooperative).
- Students have opportunities to practice the skills (the more practice, the greater the skill acquisition).
- Practice of skills needs to take place in a variety of different realistic contexts, as this will make it more likely that the skills will be used in these real-world settings in the future.
- Students need an opportunity to receive feedback from practice attempts.
- Role plays that are tailored to include real-life cues are an effective means of practicing skills and increase the likelihood that skills will be used in real situations.
- Based on the evidence about skill acquisition, the program needs to include relevant and interesting examples/demonstrations of the use of the skills by models with whom the students can identify.
- Skills taught should be likely to lead to positive outcomes in real-life situations, so that their use is rewarded and reinforced.

Each year of the curriculum addresses the contexts and situations faced by adolescents of that particular age, using teaching methods appropriate to that level of cognitive and emotional development. The program builds each year on the skills and knowledge taught previously, in a hierarchical manner. Prior to the development of materials and program content, students and teachers participated in focus groups and interviews to ensure the validity and relevance of the curriculum. The content was also influenced by concepts of diversity, being respectful of student differences in culture, gender, sexuality, abilities, and life circumstances. The curriculum is taught within the context of a whole-school-climate approach that aims to support the acquisition and maintenance of individual protective skills.

Building a Protective School Environment

Rationale

There is convincing evidence that factors within the school environment may have a significant impact on students' emotional development. As noted in the conceptual framework (Figure 14.1), factors associated with school *security and safety, social support and positive relationships with teachers and peers*, and *sense of connectedness and participation (belonging)* have all been identified as protective factors within the school environment (Spence, Burns, et al., 2005). For example, student perceptions of school as a safe and nonthreatening environment are associated with emotional well-being, and the experience of being bullied, victimized, or feeling threatened in school is linked with poor mental health outcomes (Bond et al., 2001). As a consequence, many school systems are emphasizing policies and practices that promote a safe, supportive learning environment and that, in particular, aim to reduce bullying, harassment, and victimization (e.g., the Australian National Safe Schools Framework; Curriculum Corporation, 2003). Similarly, the quality of *social support and positive social relationships* with teachers, peers, and family members are well-established factors that protect against the development of depression in adolescents (Brendgen, Vitaro, Turgeon, & Poulin, 2002; Dumont & Provost, 1999; Puig-Antich et al., 1985).

Clear links have also been shown between psychological adjustment in adolescents and the level of attachment, social connectedness, belonging, and participation with respect to family, peer groups, and school (Kobak, Sudler, & Gamble, 1991; McGee & Williams, 1991; Nada Raja, McGee, & Stanton, 1992; Resnick et al., 1997; Sargent, Williams, Hagerty, Lynch-Sauer, & Hoyle, 2002). An important element of the concept of school connectedness concerns the degree of participation and active engagement in school activities (Patton, Bond, Butler, & Glover, 2003).

Drawing on this literature, the intervention emphasizes the need to enhance factors within the school environment that are proposed to have a protective effect against the development of depression and to support emotional well-being. As such, the supportive environments component of the *beyondblue* schools research initiative aims to build a school environment that is safe and that promotes positive, supportive social relationships within the school community. It also attempts to increase students' sense of connectedness and belonging in school by increasing the opportunities and encouragement for students to participate in all aspects of the school experience. This not only aims to increase student participation in the social, recreational, and sporting aspects of school, but also encourages them to play an active role in policy development and decision making relating to the classroom, schoolyard, recreational activities, and all other aspects of their school's operations. Copies of the program materials can be found at *www.beyondblue.org.au/index.aspx?link_id=4.64.*

The Whole-School Change Process

In an attempt to achieve these goals in terms of a protective school environment, the change process in each school is led by a *school action team*, consisting of three to nine staff members (average, five) in partnership with a *beyondblue* research team member (the facilitator). Action team members are generally guidance officers, school counselors, deputy principals or principals, pastors, year coordinators, heads of departments, or teachers with specific interests and expertise in student well-being. Facilitators come from a range of professional backgrounds relating to psychology and education. The role of the school action team is to develop and implement an *action plan* for whole-school change, informed by feedback from an audit of school health promotion activities and student and staff survey data. Given that whole-school change is a long-term process, this component of the intervention occurs over a 3-year period. It aims to build policies, procedures, structures, and frameworks within each school that will lead to sustained organizational change once the research team withdraws. During the 3 years of the intervention, the facilitator meets with the school action team approximately monthly, supported by weekly telephone contact.

The first year of the "whole-school change" component focuses on training of school action team members, conducting an audit of mental health-promoting activities that the school is already undertaking, and collecting baseline data that informs the development of the school action plan. A progress chart (Figure 14.2) is used by school facilitators as a planning and reporting tool in the implementation of the first year of the whole-school change process.

We recognize that most schools are already doing a great deal to provide a safe and supportive school environment and to develop individual resiliency skills. The audit highlights the school's strengths and areas in which the school can focus its efforts to enhance the supportive qualities of the school environment. This process involves mapping the current structures, policies, programs, and practices relating to the enhancement of student participation, relationships, and pathways to support for those in need of assistance. The schools' activities in these areas are then critically analyzed and rated against a list of *principles of effective practice* for three levels of activity, namely, the classroom, the whole school, and the local community. Figure 14.3 provides an example of the audit tool used for assessment of programs, policies, and practices at the whole-school level in relation to the principles of effective practice. The same process is then used for classroom and community aspects of school activities.

Drawing on the outcomes of the audit and the data provided by teacher and student questionnaires, the action team develops its action plan, specifying goals, objectives, strategies, required resources, person responsible for each action, and time frames. The resource book (*beyondblue* Schools Research Initiative, 2006) and training for school action teams provide information and examples of whole-school change approaches to enhancing participation and student support. Action teams are also encouraged to examine the literature and empirical evidence concerning outcomes of school programs in order to develop an evidence-based approach to whole-school change.

During the first year, and in each of the following 2 years, students and teachers in each school complete a battery of questionnaires. For students, these questionnaires relate to social support, depression, anxiety, emotional and behavioral problems, risk-taking behavior, experience of victimization, social skills, thinking styles, interpersonal problem-solving and coping skills, stressful life events, mental health literacy, perceptions of school climate (supportive relationships, safety, and participation) and help-seeking behavior. For teachers, the questionnaires relate to emotional well-being, school climate and environment, work stress and job satisfaction, and methods of dealing with challenging student issues. The school principal (or in some instances, the deputy principal) also completes these measures, in addition to questions concerning leadership style and school structure, policies, and operations.

The data obtained from these questionnaires is then used to provide feedback to the school action team to inform the development of the action plan. The data are provided in a group-mean format for each school, so that schools can compare their own values with the overall mean for comparison schools in the same state. The feedback includes

Tool 1: Progress Chart	Completed	Well established	Partly established	Not at all
Stage 1—Engage school communities				
• Involvement in *beyondblue* schools research initiative (bbsri) acknowledged & supported by school administration				
• School staff consulted about involvement in bbsri				
• Involvement in bbsri acknowledged & supported by school staff				
• Parent bodies consulted about involvement in bbsri				
• Involvement in bbsri acknowledged & supported by parent bodies				
• Student bodies consulted about involvement in bbsri				
• Involvement in bbsri acknowledged & supported by student bodies				
• Facilitator from beyondblue met with school staff to support setting up of school team				
Stage 2—Establish local infrastructure				
• Set up school's *beyondblue* Action Team representative of the school community				
• Appointed a leader/co-ordinator				
• Clarified role & goals of the team				
• Clarified role & goals of individual members				
• Established a meeting schedule				
• Decided how meetings would be conducted				
• Established a process for record keeping, particularly in relation to what action is to be taken when, and by whom				
• Established processes for reporting to and consulting with the school community				
Stage 3—Gather information				
• Examined policies, programs, and practices using audit tools				
• Consulted with relevant sectors of the school community				
• Conducted student survey				
• Conducted teacher survey				
Stage 4—Planning				
• Identified & prioritized goals				
• Identified objectives & strategies for achieving them				
• Consulted broadly with school community on action plan				
• Finalized action plan				
• Identified & planned training needs of staff and broader school community				
Stage 5—Training & implementation				
• Undertook training				
• Implemented strategies				
Stage 6—Evaluate & monitor				
• Completed monitoring/evaluation process				
• Reported to members of the school community				
• Made recommendations based on experience				

FIGURE 14.2. Tool 1: Progress chart for action team in first year of the intervention. Reprinted with permission of *beyondblue* schools research initiative.

	Tool 2: Review of Current Activities				
	B. Critical analysis of current structures, policies, programs, and practices				
	Whole School				
		How well do our structures, policies, programs, and practices uphold PEPS?			
	Principles of Effective Practice (PEPS)	Not really	A little	Well	Very well
Participation	1. Make it meaningful, authentic, and fun 2. Provide adequate resources, skills, and support 3. Put decision making about teaching, learning, and curriculum on the agenda 4. Encourage students to be active researchers of issues 5. Build collaborative and inclusive learning communities of adults and young people 6. Promote creative risk taking and innovation 7. Provide processes for reflection, feedback, and review 8. Explore and share understandings of attitudes, barriers, and enabling factors 9. Have genuine support and endorsement from school leadership 10. Acknowledge and celebrate contributions				
Relationships	1. Promote an ethos of care and support 2. Develop and maintain safe and secure environments 3. Develop physical environments that promote interaction and collaboration 4. Promote autonomy and empowerment 5. Provide opportunities for learning and practicing social skills 6. Build respectful communication processes and practices 7. Foster connectedness, belonging, and inclusivity 8. Negotiate clear and consistent definitions of roles and expectations 9. Develop processes for negotiating and resolving conflict 10. Celebrate and share milestones and achievements				
Pathways	1. Clearly identify roles, responsibilities and partnerships for supporting mental health and well-being 2. Respect and include differences in language, culture, faith, gender, sexuality, abilities, and life circumstances 3. Develop strategies to meet group and individual needs within a comprehensive whole-school approach 4. Assess and manage situations from both an individual and an environmental perspective 5. Comply with privacy principles, while meeting mandated safety requirements and legal issues of consent 6. Promote effective help-seeking (people, information, and services) for mental health and well-being 7. Provide flexible access to learning to meet varied and changing student needs 8. Promote effective links with school-based services 9. Promote effective links with community-based services 10. Promote positive connections between school, family, and community				

FIGURE 14.3. Tool 2: Review of current activities—Section relating to whole-school activities. Reprinted with permission of *beyondblue* schools research initiative.

data concerning student perceptions of social support, participation, level and types of victimization, acceptance and belonging, and help-seeking behavior. Information is also provided regarding staff perceptions of the learning environment, student participation, quality of relationships, and level of collaboration between staff members. These variables are chosen for feedback purposes, as they represent those factors that are the targets for change within schools and that are proposed to mediate changes in depression and mental health. Data concerning indicators of mental health per se are not provided to schools in the feedback process.

Action teams review the implementation and outcomes of their action plans at 6-month intervals. Then, at the end of each of the 3 years, the action teams from the various schools meet to present their activities and describe their progress. Schools engage in a broad range of activities designed to build supportive environments. Examples are listed in Table 14.2

Building Pathways for Care and Support

Young people with depression frequently fail to seek or receive help from professional services. The incidence of depression can be reduced if young people can identify and articulate protective and risk factors, learn to self-manage these to minimize harm and promote well-being, and act early to identify and access relevant professional and other assistance for themselves and others. The severity, persistence, and adverse educational and social outcomes associated with depression can be significantly minimized if depression can be identified and treated early. The "pathways" element of the *beyondblue* schools research initiative facilitates young people's access to educational, health, and community support and professional services at school and within the wider community. It also provides information and training for education personnel to increase their awareness of students in need of alternate learning programs and school-based support, and ways in which they can facilitate young people's access to appropriate pathways to help for themselves and others. This process involves the enhancement of partnerships between families, school staff, education support/welfare personnel, and community-based health professionals. School staff members and students are provided with a range of resources (many of which are complied on a CD ROM and included on the school website) that outline information about mental health issues, help and support services, and methods of referral. Teacher training sessions are presented that examine the roles and responsibilities of educators in relation to mental health promotion and prevention and early intervention for problems, and provide details regarding health care planning protocols to support the learning and well-being of individuals with identified needs for care related to depression and other health issues.

In addition, students are encouraged to develop their own local resource materials, as an activity within the *beyondblue* schools curriculum or within the supportive environments component. Schools are also asked to build on and update the foundation materials they are provided with, in order to develop a more extensive resource relating to pathways for student care and support. One focus in this work involves building the capacity of peers to respond to requests for help in a manner that recognizes that they cannot be expected to be the sole support for their friends; strategies for encouraging their friends to disclose their problems to adult professionals are explored.

A key activity that schools engage in is the development of a mental health charter and interagency protocols for ensuring that students, staff members, and families can access education, health, and other community services in a timely manner. Schools are

TABLE 14.2. Some Examples of Whole-School Change Activities

Classroom
- Increase group and team work within class
- Use "home class" teachers and reduce number of teachers working with each class
- Ensure physical environment encourages interaction and communication between students and teachers (e.g., setup of tables/desks)
- Review curriculum to increase opportunities for interaction and communication
- Increase use of positive behavior management approaches (use of praise, attention, rewards), rather than punitive
- Create a constructive, encouraging, and participative classroom environment
- Personal skills development programs (e.g., anger management, stress management, conflict resolution, social skills)
- Active recognition of student efforts and achievements
- Encouragement and recognition of successes relative to individual's abilities
- Provision of feedback (re: academic and behavioral performance) in a constructive rather than critical manner
- Showcase student work and successes
- Create opportunities for all students to succeed at their own levels
- Invite student input to planning of class activities
- Professional development activities for teachers in communication skills and classroom management
- Involve students in the development of classroom policies and practices to enhance safety, confidentiality, respect, and communication

School
- Mentoring/coaching/buddy programs (within and across age groups)
- Peer mediation/peer support programs
- Increase number of student counseling and support staff
- Establish home group structure
- Enhance activities of "house" groups
- Train all staff members in awareness of mental health issues
- Create a welcoming atmosphere for parents and visitors to the school
- Enhance parent and community participation in school activities, including decision making
- Increase opportunities to participate in school activities and decision making (student councils, student representatives)
- Enhance communication content in school newsletters
- Seek feedback from parents and caregivers (surveys and focus groups)
- Increase supervision at free-time periods, particularly in high-risk areas
- Establish confidential reporting systems for dealing with bullying
- Develop and publicize school policies and practices regarding bullying in line with international best practice
- Establish confidential systems to facilitate student help-seeking behaviors
- Increase staff and student awareness of and ease of access to support services within the school and the wider community
- Establish a school mental health charter that recognizes and respects the needs and rights of students and teachers

Wider community
- Develop transition programs with elementary schools, colleges, and universities
- Increase involvement by community organizations (e.g., Rotary Clubs, sports groups, volunteer groups) and support services within the school (e.g., health, mental health, family services, police)
- Strengthen referral systems between schools
- Encourage students' participation in voluntary activities outside school and as part of their studies
- Increase links with local media organizations regarding school and student activities and achievements

provided with a process and guidelines for student and staff input into the development of a charter that specifies the vision, purpose, values/principles, rights, responsibilities, actions, and roles of school members in relation to the mental health of the school community. Professional development gives guidance in the establishment of local community service agreements to support interagency service models that are realistic within each school's community.

Community Forums

Toward the end of the first year, or early in the second year, school action teams organize a community forum in partnership with the local community. Each forum aims to enhance community awareness of the nature and prevalence of mental health issues among school students, risk and protective factors, and help-seeking strategies for students, family members, and friends. The format of the forum is negotiated with the local community members, service providers, teachers, students, and parents. Personnel from the *beyondblue* schools research initiative work with schools and organizations such as local health and welfare agencies, Rotary Clubs, and sporting clubs, to achieve high levels of community participation.

Evaluation

Outcomes of the intervention will be assessed through the end of 2007 to determine whether this integrated approach to prevention is effective in reducing the development of depression among adolescents. The evaluation examines not only mental health outcomes (in terms of depression, anxiety, and emotional well-being), but also the impact of the intervention on the skills and competencies it aims to develop. Thus, it examines the impact on social skills, problem-solving and coping skills, cognitive style, and interpersonal relationships. In addition, it explores whether the intervention is associated with changes in school environment factors, such as quality of supportive relationships, levels of bullying and safety, opportunities for participation, and sense of belonging from the perspective of both students and staff. The evaluation compares outcomes of the 25 intervention schools with 25 matched comparison schools, which were initially randomized to either intervention or no-intervention conditions. Students and staff are to provide annual assessments over the 3 years of the intervention and for the 2 subsequent years until the students leave school.

In addition to quantitative outcomes, the study is conducting extensive process evaluations in order to determine the level of program adherence and the difficulties/issues in implementation. We will also be able to examine the level of sustainability once the research teams withdraw, to determine whether intervention schools continue to implement the activities without external support and prompting. The process data will also enable examination of the full cost of implementation in order to conduct cost–benefit analyses at a later stage.

SUMMARY

This chapter aimed to provide a brief history of research into school-based interventions for the prevention of depression in adolescents. It concluded that the outcomes for programs that focus purely on building skills within the young person have been weak, particularly for universal rather than selected approaches to prevention. A case was then made to propose that further efforts are required to build protective environments, in addition to using individual skill-development approaches. School represents one such environment in which young people spend a good deal of their time, and the quality of which has been shown to influence emotional well-being. The *beyondblue* schools research initiative was described, which represents an attempt to integrate individual and whole-school change approaches. This is the type of intervention that needs to be evaluated in order to inform school and mental health policy. However, whole-school change is a process that takes place over several years, and it remains to be determined whether such approaches are effective in preventing depression in adolescents.

REFERENCES

Abramson, L. Y., Alloy, L. B., Hogan, M. E., Whitehouse, W. G., Donovan, P., Rose, D. T., et al. (1999). Cognitive vulnerability to depression: Theory and evidence. *Journal of Cognitive Psychotherapy, 13*(1), 5–20.

Adams, J., & Adams, M. (1996). The association among negative life events, perceived problem solving alternatives, depression, and suicidal ideation in adolescent psychiatric patients. *Journal of Child Psychology and Psychiatry and Allied Disciplines, 37*(6), 715–720.

Beardslee, W. R., Versage, E. M., Wright, E. J., & Salt, P. (1997). Examination of preventive interventions for families with depression: Evidence of change. *Development and Psychopathology, 9,* 109–130.

Beck, A. T., Rush, A. J., Shaw, B. F., & Emery, G. (1979). *Cognitive therapy of depression.* New York: Wiley.

beyondblue Schools Research Initiative. (2006). The *beyondblue* schools research initiative resource pack. Melbourne: *beyondblue*—The national depression initiative.

Bond, L., Carlin, J. B., Thomas, L., Rubin, K., & Patton, G. (2001). Does bullying cause emotional problems? A prospective study of young teenagers. *British Medical Journal, 323*(7311), 480–484.

Bond, L., Patton, G., Glover, S., Carlin, J. B., Butler, H., Thomas, L., et al. (2004). The Gatehouse Project: Can a multi-level school intervention affect emotional well being and health risk behaviours? *Journal of Epidemiology and Community Health, 58,* 997–1003.

Brendgen, M., Vitaro, F., Turgeon, L., & Poulin, F. (2002). Assessing aggressive and depressed children's social relations with classmates and friends: A matter of perspective. *Journal of Abnormal Child Psychology, 30*(6), 609–616.

Bronfenbrenner, U. (1979). *The ecology of human development: Experiments by nature and design.* Cambridge, MA: Harvard University Press.

Cardemil, E. V., Reivich, K. J., & Seligman, M. E. P. (2002). The prevention of depressive symptoms in low-income minority middle school students. *Prevention and Treatment, 5*(Article 8). *www.journals.apa.org/prevention/volume2005/pre005500008a.html.*

Clark, D. A., Beck, A. T., & Alford, B. A. (1999). *Scientific foundations of cognitive theory and therapy of depression.* New York: Wiley.

Curriculum Corporation. (2003). *National Safe Schools Framework.* Carlton South, Australia: Ministerial Council on Education, Employment, Training and Youth Affairs.

Dumont, M., & Provost, M. A. (1999). Resilience in adolescents: Protective role of social support, coping strategies, self-esteem, and social activities on experience of stress and depression. *Journal of Youth and Adolescence, 28*(3), 343–363.

Garmezy, N. (1991). Resiliency and vulnerability to adverse developmental outcomes associated with poverty. *American Behavioral Sciences, 34,* 416–430.

Goodman, S. H., Gravitt, G. W., & Kaslow, N. J. (1995). Social problem solving: A moderator of the relation between negative life stress and depression symptoms in children. *Journal of Abnormal Child Psychology, 23,* 473–485.

Harnett, P. H., & Dadds, M. R. (2004). Training school personnel to implement a universal school-based prevention of depression program under real-world conditions. *Journal of School Psychology, 42*(5), 343–357.

Herman Stahl, M., & Petersen, A. C. (1996). The protective role of coping and social resources for depressive symptoms among young adolescents. *Journal of Youth and Adolescence, 25*(6), 733–753.

Kobak, R. R., Sudler, N., & Gamble, W. (1991). Attachment and depressive symptoms during adolescence: A developmental pathways analysis. *Development and Psychopathology, 3*(4), 461–474.

Kowalenko, N., Wignall, A., Rapee, R. M., Simmons, J., Whitefield, K., & Stonehouse, R. (2002). The ACE program: Working with schools to promote emotional health and prevent depression. *Youth Studies Australia, 21*(2), 23–30.

Lerner, R. M. (1986). *Concepts and themes of human development* (2nd ed.). New York: Random House.

Lewinsohn, P. M., Clarke, G. N., Hops, H., & Andrews, J. A. (1990). Cognitive-behavioral treatment for depressed adolescents. *Behavior Therapy, 21*(4), 385–401.

Mason, C. A., Scott, K. G., Chapman, D. A., & Shihfen, T. (2000). A review of some individual- and community-level effect size indices for the study of risk factors for child and adolescent development. *Educational and Psychological Measurement, 60*(3), 385–410.

McGee, R., & Williams, S. (1991). Social competence in adolescence: Preliminary findings from a longitudinal study of New Zealand 15-yr-olds. *Psychiatry: Journal for the Study of Interpersonal Processes, 54*(3), 281–291.

Merry, S., McDowell, H., Hetrick, S., Bir, J., & Muller, N. (2004). Psychological and/or educational interventions for the prevention of depression in children and adolescents (Cochrane Review). *The Cochrane library* (Issue 2). Chichester, UK: Wiley.

Merry, S., McDowell, H., Wild, C. J., Bir, J., & Cunliffe, R. (2004). A randomized placebo-controlled trial of a school-based depression prevention program. *Journal of the American Academy of Child and Adolescent Psychiatry, 43*(5), 538–547.

Mrazek, P. J., & Haggerty, R. J. (Eds.). (1994). *Reducing the risks for mental disorders: Frontiers for preventive intervention research.* Washington, DC: National Academy Press.

Muris, P., Schmidt, H., Lambrichs, R., & Meesters, C. (2001). Protective and vulnerability factors of depression in normal adolescents. *Behaviour Research and Therapy, 39,* 555–565.

Nada Raja, S., McGee, R., & Stanton, W. R. (1992). Perceived attachments to parents and peers and psychological well-being in adolescence. *Journal of Youth and Adolescence, 21*(4), 471–485.

Nolen-Hoeksema, S., & Girgus, J. S. (1995). Explanatory style and achievement, depression, and gender differences in childhood and early adolescence. In G. M. Buchanan & M. E. P. Seligman (Eds.), *Explanatory style* (pp. 57–70). Hillsdale, NJ: Erlbaum.

Offord, D. R., Kraemer, H. C., Kazdin, A. E., Jensen, P. S., & Harrington, R. (1998). Lowering the burden of suffering from child psychiatric disorder: Trade-offs among clinical, targeted, and universal interventions. *Journal of the American Academy of Child and Adolescent Psychiatry, 37*(7), 686–694.

Pattison, C., & Lynd Stevenson, R. M. (2001). The prevention of depressive symptoms in children: The immediate and long-term outcomes of a school based program. *Behaviour Change, 18*(2), 92–102.

Patton, G., Bond, L., Butler, H., & Glover, S. (2003). Changing schools, changing health? Design and implementation of the Gatehouse Project. *Journal of Adolescent Health, 33*(4), 231–239.

Patton, G., Bond, L., Thomas, L., & Toumbourou, J. (1998, December). *Adolescent health and well being survey: Phase 1 report.* Melbourne, Australia: Centre for Adolescent Health.

Pössel, P., Baldus, C., Horn, A. B., Groen, G., & Hautzinger, M. (2005). Influence of general self-efficacy on the effects of a school-based universal primary prevention program of depressive symptoms in adolescents: A randomized and controlled follow-up study. *Journal of Child Psychology and Psychiatry, 46*(9), 982–994.

Pössel, P., Horn, A. B., Groen, G., & Hautzinger, M. (2004). School-based prevention of depressive symptoms in adolescents: A 6-month follow-up. *Journal of the American Academy of Child and Adolescent Psychiatry, 43*(8), 1003–1010.

Puig-Antich, J., Lukens, E., Davies, M., Goetz, D., Brennan-Quattrock, J., & Todak, G. (1985). Psychosocial functioning in prepubertal major depressive disorders: I. Interpersonal relationships during the depressive episode. *Archives of General Psychiatry, 42*, 500–507.

Quayle, D., Dziurawiec, S., Roberts, C., Kane, R., & Ebsworthy, G. (2001). The effect of an optimism and lifeskills program on depressive symptoms in preadolescence. *Behavior Change, 18*(4), 194–203.

Reinecke, M. A., & Simons, A. (2005). Vulnerability to depression among adolescents: Implications for cognitive-behavioral treatment. *Cognitive and Behavioral Practice, 12*(2), 166–176.

Resnick, M., Bearman, P., Blum, R., Bauman, K. E., Harris, K. M., Jones, J., et al. (1997). Protecting adolescents from harm: Findings from the National Longitudinal Study on Adolescent Health. *Journal of the American Medical Association, 278*(10), 823–832.

Roeger, L., Allison, S., Martin, G., Dadds, V., & Keeves, J. (2001). Adolescent depressive symptomatology: Improve schools or help students? *Australian Journal of Psychology, 53*(3), 134–139.

Rose, G. (1992). *The strategy of preventative medicine.* Oxford, UK: Oxford University Press.

Rutter, M. (1987). Psychosocial resilience and protective mechanisms. *American Journal of Orthopsychiatry, 57*, 316–331.

Sandler, I. N., Ayers, T. S., Wolchik, S. A., Tein, J.-Y., Kwok, O.-M., Haine, R. A., et al. (2003). The Family Bereavement Program: Efficacy evaluation of a theory-based prevention program for parentally bereaved children and adolescents. *Journal of Consulting and Clinical Psychology, 71*(3), 587–600.

Sargent, J., Williams, R. A., Hagerty, B. M., Lynch-Sauer, J., & Hoyle, K. (2002). Sense of belonging as a buffer against depressive symptoms. *Journal of the American Psychiatric Nurses Association, 8*(4), 120–129.

Seligman, M. E. P., Reivich, K., Jaycox, L., & Gillham, J. (1995). *The optimistic child.* Boston: Houghton Mifflin.

Sheffield, J., Spence, S. H., Rapee, R. M., Kowalenko, N., Wignall, A., Davis, A., et al. (2006). Comparison of universal, indicated, and combined universal plus indicated approaches to the prevention of depression among adolescents. *Journal of Consulting and Clinical Psychology, 74*(1), 66–79.

Shochet, I. M., Dadds, M. R., Holland, D., Whitefield, K., Harnett, P. H., & Osgarby, S. M. (2001). The efficacy of a universal school-based program to prevent adolescent depression. *Journal of Clinical Child Psychology, 30*(3), 303–315.

Shochet, I. M., & Ham, D. (2004). Universal school-based approaches to preventing adolescent depression: Past findings and future directions of the resourceful adolescent program. *International Journal of Mental Health Promotion, 6*(3), 17–25.

Spence, S. H., Burns, J., Boucher, S., Glover, S., Graetz, B., Kay, D., et al. (2005). The *beyondblue* schools research initiative: Conceptual framework and intervention. *Australasian Psychiatry, 13*(2), 159–164.

Spence, S. H., & Reinecke, M. A. (2003). Cognitive approaches to understanding, preventing and treating child and adolescent depression. In M. A. Reinecke & D. A. Clark (Eds.), *Cognitive therapy over the lifespan: Theory, research and practice* (pp. 358–395). Cambridge, UK: Cambridge University Press.

Spence, S. H., Sheffield, J., & Donovan, C. (2002). Problem-solving orientation and attributional style: Moderators of the impact of negative life events on the development of depressive symptoms in adolescence? *Journal of Clinical Child and Adolescent Psychology, 31*(2), 219–229.

Spence, S. H., Sheffield, J. K., & Donovan, C. L. (2003). Preventing adolescent depression: An evaluation of the Problem Solving for Life program. *Journal of Consulting and Clinical Psychology*, *71*(1), 3–13.

Spence, S. H., Sheffield, J., & Donovan, C. L. (2005). Long-term outcome of a school-based universal approach to prevention of depression in adolescents. *Journal of Consulting and Clinical Psychology*, *73*(1), 160–167.

Stark, K. D., Rouse, L. W., & Livingston, R. (1991). Treatment of depression during childhood and adolescence: Cognitive-behavioral procedures for the individual and family. In P. C. Kendal (Ed.), *Child and adolescent therapy: Cognitive-behavioral procedures* (pp. 165–208). New York: Guilford Press.

Vostanis, P., & Harrington, R. (1994). Cognitive-behavioural treatment of depressive disorder in child psychiatric patients: Rationale and description of a treatment package. *European Child and Adolescent Psychiatry*, *3*(2), 111–123.

Wolchik, S. A., Sandler, I. N., Millsap, R. E., Plummer, B. A., Greene, S. M., Anderson, E. R., et al. (2002). Six-year follow-up of preventive interventions for children of divorce: A randomized controlled trial. *Journal of the American Medical Association*, *288*(15), 1874–1881.

World Health Organization. (1998). WHO's global school health initiative: Helping schools to become "health-promoting schools." *Fact Sheet No 92.* Retrieved February5, 2003, from *www.who.int/inf-fs/en/fact092.html.*

Wyn, J., Cahill, H., Holdsworth, R., Rowling, L., & Carson, S. (2000). MindMatters, a whole-school approach promoting mental health and wellbeing. *Australian and New Zealand Journal of Psychiatry*, *34*, 596–601.

15 Positive Youth Development Programs

*An Alternative Approach
to the Prevention of Depression
in Children and Adolescents*

Chad McWhinnie, John R. Z. Abela, Nora Hilmy,
and Ilyan Ferrer

The goal of this chapter is to present positive youth development programs as a possible mode of intervention/prevention for depression in youth. We begin by briefly reviewing the current state of positive youth development (PYD) programs, specifically examining the findings of comprehensive reviews conducted by Roth, Brooks-Gunn, Murray, and Foster (1998), Catalano, Berglund, Ryan, Lonczak, and Hawkins (2002). We also review the current state of depression prevention programs, specifically examining the findings of two meta-analytic reviews of such programs by Merry, McDowell, Hetrick, Bir, and Muller (2004) and Horowitz and Garber (2006). We highlight and discuss the differences found in the PYD and prevention literatures, focusing on the implications of the overlap and discrepancies of their respective intervention approaches to depression prevention efficacy. We examine the overall resulting outcomes of PYD and depression prevention programs with respect to their differing program goals. We present and discuss a focused review of PYD programs that embody alternative approaches to depression prevention among children and adolescents, as well as findings from studies examining the effectiveness of these programs. We conclude with a summary and suggestions concerning the advancement of knowledge in the area of positive youth development approaches to preventing depression.

CENTRAL QUESTION

Can depression be prevented? People have typically sought the answer to this question by examining the efficacy of prevention programs designed to reduce cognitive, interpersonal, and emotional deficits in order to prevent future incidence of depressive episodes. In this chapter, we propose that there are alternative approaches to depression prevention other than deficit-based approaches. Thus, in order to determine whether depression can be prevented, the investigative scope must be widened to include these alternative programs and methods (i.e., PYD programs that utilize competency enhancement techniques). Thus, the central question of this chapter is: Can a strength-based program designed to enhance competencies produce developmental outcomes similar to those of deficit-based programs designed to prevent or reduce depression?

WHAT IS PYD?

Youth development programs are defined as "developmentally appropriate programs designed to prepare children and adolescents for productive adulthood by providing opportunities and supports to help them gain the competencies and knowledge needed to meet the increasing challenges they will face as they mature" (Roth et al., 1998). In addition to focusing on the reduction of disorders and problem behaviors, youth development programs recognize the need to build the strengths and competencies of children and adolescents (Benson, 1997). *Competence* refers to "adaptational success in the developmental tasks expected of individuals of a given age" (Masten et al., 1995). Competence is a complex, multifaceted construct that can exist singularly as domain-specific abilities or skills (e.g., cognitive, social, emotional, academic) or in aggregate with multiple constructs underlying a "pattern of effective adaptation in the environment" (Masten & Coatsworth, 1998; Haggerty, Sherrod, Garmezy, & Rutter, 1994). Youth development programs tend to emphasize the development of competencies to counteract risk factors and to enhance protective factors in order to increase the likelihood of positive outcomes (Roth et al., 1998). Enhancement of competencies may not remove environmental risk factors, but may mitigate the detrimental influence of persistent risk factors.

In the early 1990s, the term *positive youth development* emerged as a reiteration of the strength-based approach to youth development programs. The focus of PYD is a child's strengths, interests, and talents (Damon, 2004; Seligman et al., 2005). Central to PYD is the notion that children possess an innate capacity for resiliency. Thriving among youth can occur not only as a result of this resiliency, but in combination with protective factors found within various socializing institutions. Encouraging such personal and environmental assets can help children make full use of their potential (Seligman et al., 2005). The goal of PYD is to tap into the potential that lies within each young person, helping to build and to strengthen assets that enable youth to grow and flourish throughout life (Catalano, Hawkins, Berglund, Pollard, & Arthur, 2002; Damon, 2004; Park, 2004).

PYD programs, by their nature, do not intentionally target depression or depressive symptoms. However, many of the attitudinal (i.e., self-concept, self-efficacy, prosocial beliefs, etc.) and behavioral (i.e., problem solving, decision making, conflict resolution, etc.) targets of such programs are implicated in the etiology and maintenance of depression. That is, deficits in such cognitive, emotional, and interpersonal constructs are associated with depressive disorders (see Abela & Hankin, Chapter 1, and Rudolph, Flynn, &

Abaied, Chapter 4, this volume). At the same time, strengths in such constructs are associated with higher levels of psychological well-being (Seligman et al., 2005).

The term *positive youth development* gained prominence in the lexicon with the rise of the positive psychology movement. Proponents of positive psychology adopted youth development programs and described such programs in a manner that intimated their place as nested within the larger movement. The strength-based approaches conceptualized by youth development and PYD researchers can be considered synonymous because both program classifications primarily seek to promote positive development through competency enhancement. The most comprehensive definitions of youth development and PYD offered to date are those of Roth and Brooks-Gunn (2003) and Catalano and colleagues (Catalano, Berglund, et al., 2002), respectively.

Roth and Brooks-Gunn (2003) view youth development programs as consisting of three aspects: goals, atmosphere, and activities. In terms of goals, acknowledging the national youth policy contributions of Lerner, Fisher, and Weinberg (2000), Roth and Brooks-Gunn identify five constructs (the five C's) as specific youth development program goals: (1) building academic, social, and vocational *competence*, (2) building *confidence*, (3) strengthening *connection* to family, community, and peers, (4) building *character*, and (5) strengthening *caring and compassion*. With respect to environment, Roth and Brooks-Gunn propose five essential qualities for an effective program: (1) supportive relationships between program participants and staff, (2) empowerment through autonomy and agency among participants, (3) expectations for success and positive behavior, (4) recognition and/or reward of positive behaviors, and (5) sufficient duration (at least 9 months). In terms of activities, Roth and Brooks-Gunn note that program activities should consist of those that provide opportunities for participants to build skills, to engage in genuinely challenging tasks and exercises, and to broaden their horizons. According to the authors, these program characteristics cumulatively help to distinguish youth development programs from other youth programs that do not seek to promote the positive development of participants.

Catalano and colleagues (Catalano, Berglund, et al., 2002) formulated an operational definition of positive youth development after conducting an extensive literature search of youth development programs and consulting with national authorities and researchers in youth development and mental health. Catalano et al. (Catalano, Berglund, et al., 2002) assert that programs seek to (1) promote bonding, (2) foster resilience, (3) promote social competence, (4) promote emotional competence, (5) promote cognitive competence, (6) promote behavioral competence, (7) promote moral competence, (8) foster self-determination, (9) foster spirituality, (10) foster self-efficacy, (11) foster clear and positive identity, (12) foster belief in the future, (13) provide recognition for positive behavior, (14) provide opportunities for prosocial involvement, and (15) foster prosocial norms. According to the authors, programs that aim to accomplish one or more of the above constructs are considered PYD programs.

PYD PROGRAMS: IN GENERAL, ARE THEY EFFECTIVE?

Recently, PYD researchers have attempted to examine whether programs conducted to date have been successful in producing positive developmental outcomes (i.e., academic competency, enhanced problem-solving skills, increased community involvement, etc.) More specifically, two comprehensive literature reviews have been conducted to date aimed at (1) characterizing components of effective PYD programs (Catalano, Berglund, et al., 2002) and (2) demonstrating the effectiveness of relevant youth development programs in terms of achieving their stated goals (Roth et al., 1998). At this point, no formal meta-analysis of PYD programs has been conducted to substantiate the prevailing assumption maintained by researchers in the field that, in general, PYD programs produce positive developmental outcomes for participating youth. The lack of systematic reviews precludes any definitive representation of the effectiveness of PYD. However, an investigation of relevant reviews, which have conducted thorough literature searches and critical appraisals of available PYD or equivalent programs, is a step in the right direction toward properly assessing the impact of PYD programs.

In order to examine the characteristics of effective PYD programs, Catalano and colleagues (Catalano, Berglund, et al., 2002) selected 77 programs with participants between the ages of 6 and 20 that aimed to fulfill at least one of their 15 PYD definitional constructs via a research design that utilized control or comparison groups and used youth behavioral outcome measures for evaluative purposes. A program was excluded if the content was treatment or action taken in response to a disorder, if there was a lack of rigorous scientific evaluation of the program, or if there was a lack of evidence of its effectiveness (Catalano, Berglund, et al., 2002). Ultimately, 25 programs were identified that met these three criteria. Of the 25 evaluated programs, the majority utilized random assignment to conditions (64%), employed a consistent curriculum of program activities (96%), used skills-based strategies (96%), and were implemented for at least 9 months (80%). The evaluated programs demonstrated positive changes in youth behavior (76%) and showed significant improvement in problem behaviors (96%). Positive changes included improved interpersonal skills, quality of peer and adult relationships, self-control, problem solving, cognitive competencies, self-efficacy, and commitment to school and academic achievement. Reduced problem behaviors included drug and alcohol use, school misbehavior, aggression, violence, truancy, risky sexual behavior, and smoking.

The importance of the Catalano, Berglund, et al. (2002) review is that it was among the first to suggest that PYD programs may be effective in achieving their stated goals. In addition, it was among the first to identify common core components of effective PYD interventions. At the same time, the authors' conclusions should be interpreted with caution. More specifically, the authors failed to evaluate both effective and ineffective programs. Thus, the review was unable to provide an adequate assessment of the overall efficacy of PYD programs. In addition, the authors failed to compare characteristics of effective and ineffective programs, precluding an enriched understanding of program characteristics specific to effective programs. Finally, as the reviewed programs had different intended goals, the authors were unable to identify program characteristics unique to achieving any specific goal (e.g., prevention of depressive symptoms, increased prosocial behavior, enhanced interpersonal competency, etc.).

Roth et al. (1998) conducted another program analysis, in which the authors identified and evaluated the efficacy of 15 youth programs that satisfied their definitional and research design criteria. Included studies implemented either an experimental or a quasi-experimental design to evaluate the efficacy of programs that targeted youth populations with no manifest deficits. The authors categorized the programs into three groups according to the goals of the intervention: (1) positive-behavior-focused competency/asset-enhancing programs, (2) problem behavior-focused competency/asset-enhancing programs, and (3) resistance skills-based prevention programs. Participants in the positive-behavior-focused competency programs exhibited enhanced competencies (e.g., improved school behavior, improved academic achievement, higher academic self-efficacy) and reduced deficits (e.g., less involvement in the criminal justice system, substance use, violent behavior). Such promising findings were tempered by no significant gains on several cognitive and behavioral measures of interest (e.g., self-esteem; depression; alcohol, tobacco, and drug use; aggression). Problem behavior-focused competency/asset-enhancing programs reported short-term, but not long-term, enhanced competencies (e.g., community service, drug resistance skills, commitment to school). Further, problem behavior-focused competency/asset-enhancing programs showed no effect on problem behavior (school dropout, drug use). Resistance skills-based prevention programs reported positive results in their ability to invoke enhanced competencies (e.g., alcohol-resistant skills) or reduced deficits and problem behavior (e.g., alcohol use).

Roth and colleagues (1998) observed the emergence of two trends in the programs' ability to generate effective outcomes: substantial adult–youth relationships and sustained program duration. With respect to adult–youth relationships, in a structured and supportive environment the formation and nurturance of warm adult–youth relationships (e.g., mentors–mentees) was associated with positive outcomes. With respect to program duration, sustained interventions, which included increased contact with participants, were associated with more positive outcomes as compared with short-term interventions. Roth et al. also found support for aggregated effects produced by longer-term programs. For example, the authors cited an instance in which control and intervention groups did not differ significantly after 1 year in a program, but positive effects occurred after 2 years for the intervention group.

The importance of the review conducted by Roth and colleagues is that it not only demonstrated the overall efficacy of the reviewed PYD programs in attaining their stated goals, but it also identified characteristics of programs that likely contribute to their success (i.e., program length and mentoring relationships). At the same time, two limitations of this review should be noted. First, the authors were unable to systematically determine the efficacy of the reviewed PYD programs because of inadequate information gained from individual studies. Second, although Roth and colleagues demonstrated at a generic level that the reviewed programs can result in positive developmental outcomes, little can be said about any specific outcome examined, as the assessment protocols of the included studies varied widely (i.e., only one study assessed depressive symptoms).

Despite the limitations of the Catalano, Berglund, et al. (2002) and Roth et al. (1998) reviews, combined findings related to PYD program outcomes reveal the potentially effective nature of strength-based interventions. Findings included increases in factors thought to buffer against depression such as interpersonal skills, quality of peer and parent relationships, self-control, problem solving, cognitive competencies, self-efficacy, commitment to schooling, and academic achievement (see Spence, Sheffield, & Donovan, 2003). In addition, there were reductions in factors typically thought to be associated with depression, such as substance use (see, e.g., Rohde, Lewinsohn, & Seely, 1991), aggressive behavior (see, e.g., Capaldi, 1991, 1992), and smoking (see, e.g., Beardslee & Gladstone, 2001).

At this point it may be useful to reconsider the central question of this chapter: Can the strength-based approach of PYD programs, which seeks to enhance competencies, generate similar outcomes in depression prevention as traditional depression prevention programs and their utilization of deficit-reduction strategies? Unfortunately, and of central relevance to this chapter, the assessment of depression and depressive symptoms has not been a typical feature of research examining the efficacy of PYD programs. Such measures are more commonly administered in research examining the efficacy of prevention programs, specifically depression prevention programs. Thus, at this point in time, this question cannot be adequately answered. At the same time, as PYD programs have been found to enhance competencies thought to buffer against depression as well as to reduce factors thought to confer risk for depression, a logical assumption is that farther along the developmental trajectory these effects may be translated into the prevention of depression. Future research, of course, is needed in directly examining this possibility.

If PYD researchers ultimately hope to uncover whether a promotive approach represents an alternative path to outcomes similar to those obtained by deficit-based approaches, a brief review of outcomes obtained to date by such prevention programs is needed.

PREVENTION PROGRAMS

Prevention programs are intentional interventions to prevent or to reduce the future incidence of mental disorders or problem behavior. Prevention programs are characterized by the manner in which populations are selected for intervention (Durlak & Wells, 1997). *Universal* prevention (referred to as primary prevention in previous literature) refers to an intervention that targets the general public or normal populations in whom there is no identifiable risk. *Selective* (secondary) prevention targets at-risk (imminent or lifetime) subgroups or individuals who have yet to present with a symptomatic profile. *Indicated* (tertiary) prevention pertains to individuals manifesting prodromal symptoms or subclinical features of a mental disorder.

The overall findings from two comprehensive prevention program reviews substantiate the effectiveness of such programs in reducing the future incidence of problem behaviors or symptoms. First, in assessing the effects of universal prevention programs, Durlak and Wells (1997) created three categories characterizing the level of program intervention (environment-centered, transition, and person-centered programs) and demonstrated that these programs were generally effective at ameliorating internalizing disorders, although the effects varied in magnitude. Second, building on the findings of Durlak and Wells (1997), Greenberg, Domitrovich, and Bumbarger (2001) found support for the effectiveness of universal and targeted prevention programs, as findings indicated that such programs have both short- and long-term effectiveness in the reduction of symptomatology related to mental disorders and associated maladaptive behaviors.

Although both the Durlak and Wells (1997) and Greenberg et al. (2001) reviews convey the effectiveness of prevention programs, the support is at a generic level, which prohibits any conclusions about the effectiveness of prevention programs specifically targeting depression. The findings of two depression prevention program meta-analytic reviews (Horowitz & Garber, 2006; Merry, McDowell, Hetrick, et al., 2004) are therefore instrumental in (1) enriching the general understanding of prevention programs imparted by these reviews and (2) advancing pertinent information on the efficacy of prevention programs that specifically target the reduction and/or prevention of depression.

Merry, McDowell, Hetrick, et al. (2004) evaluated universal and targeted (selective and indicated) depression prevention programs. The findings of this meta-analysis reveal that universal programs were not effective at preventing depression, whereas targeted programs, specifically those with an indicated approach, effectively reduced depressive symptoms immediately following the intervention, although there was no maintenance of gains in subsequent assessments. In other words, according to the analysis of Merry, McDowell, Hetrick, et al. (2004), universal and selective programs (directed at nonclinical populations, which are representative of PYD target populations) are not successful in meeting their first-order goal of depression prevention. The unfavorable results should reasonably elicit questions about the value of developing and implementing such interventions.

Interestingly, significant second-order effects were seen in depression-related constructs among universal and selective programs. Adolescents showed fewer negative automatic thoughts, lower levels of hopelessness, and better self-esteem immediately after intervention and at 6-months follow-up (Cardemil et al., 2002). Some universal programs were able to improve functioning (Clarke et al., 1995) and decrease levels of state and, trait anger expression at the end of intervention (Hains & Ellman, 1994). One study showed a significant effect for self-worth, as measured by the Self Perception Profile, with adolescents showing a higher sense of self-worth at 6-months follow-up (Quayle, Dzuirawiec, Roberts, Kane, & Ebsworthy, 2001). An additional study (Spence et al., 2003) showed a significant increase in problem-solving skills and a reduction in negative/avoidant problem solving for adolescents who were at high risk for depression. Despite these second-order effects, the overall findings reported by Merry, McDowell, Hetrick, et al. (2004) demonstrate that although the indicated depression prevention programs were effective at reducing depressive symptoms in the short term, depression prevention programs with universal and selected populations showed nominal effects.

Results of a meta-analysis conducted by Horowitz and Garber (2006) essentially echo the depression prevention program findings reported in Merry, McDowell, Hetrick, et al. (2004). Using an approach similar to that of Merry, McDowell, Hetrick, et al. (2004), Horowitz and Garber (2006) found that, in regard to reduction of depressive symptoms, selective prevention programs were effective immediately following the intervention, and selective and indicated programs were effective at follow-up. Regarding the universal approach, depression scores in control and intervention groups remained static over time, which precluded any determination of prevention effect. Whereas Merry, McDowell, Hetrick, et al. (2004) reported second-order effects of depression prevention programs, Horowitz and Garber (2006) focused exclusively on the programs' influence on depressive symptoms. These authors offered conclusions similar to those of Merry, McDowell, Hetrick, et al. (2004) on the practicality of implementing universal prevention programs, by suggesting that the benefits of targeting populations with no identifiable risk need to be weighed with the cost of doing so. Although the findings on depression prevention are meager, Horowitz and Garber (2006) present impressive in-depth guidelines to consider when investigating depression prevention in youth. Interestingly, these authors acknowledge that depression can be the result of multiple, diverse factors and recommend that more than one construct (e.g., negative thoughts, relationships, and coping strategies) should be targeted to effectively prevent depression.

The findings from both the Merry, McDowell, Hetrick, et al. (2004) and Horowitz and Garber (2006) meta-analytic reviews imply that for more normative populations, a narrow focus on specific symptoms or problem behavior may not necessarily result in a successful intervention. However, it is important to note that some specific universal depression prevention programs have demonstrated an ability to reduce depressive symptoms immediately following the intervention (Cardemil et al., 2002; Spence et al., 2003; Yu & Seligman, 2002), as well as at subsequent follow-ups (Shochet et al., 2001; Merry, McDowell, Wild, Bir, & Cunliffe, 2004). Thus, researchers should not discard universal depression prevention programs completely. Elucidating the mechanisms contributing to the effectiveness of these specific programs (see Gillham, Brunwasser, & Freres, Chapter 13, this volume) may hold, in part, the key to the future success of universal approaches.

There are suggestions that the disappointing findings in regard to depression may be at least partly attributable to certain program characteristics and implementation.

School-based programs are sometimes delivered by trained classroom teachers, which may impede the potential effects of the program content, as compared with programs delivered by more skilled practitioners (Merry, McDowell, Hetrick, et al., 2004). The duration of many of the programs may be inadequate to engender significant effects among intervention participants (Sheffield et al., 2006). In addition to the limited number of sessions, exposure to the intervention may be insufficient in many programs, as sessions typically last between 45 and 90 minutes. Immediate postintervention effects are often the only findings reported because of a lack of long-term follow-up assessments (Horowitz & Garber, 2006; Merry, McDowell, Hetrick, et al., 2004). Many of the acknowledged limitations of depression prevention programs correspond to the utilization of treatment-based models and techniques as the basis for prevention interventions. The results of universal and selective depression prevention programs reflect this derivative nature, as the effects of such programs are better classified as treatment effects, rather than prevention effects (Horowitz & Garber, 2006).

PREVENTION VERSUS PROMOTION

The structure of depression prevention programs is often uniform. Depression prevention programs explicitly target one problem, are frequently implemented in one domain (school-based), focus solely on the participant, and are conducted for a contracted number (8–12) of brief (40–120 minutes) sessions over an abbreviated length of time (2–3 months) (Merry, McDowell, Hetrick, et al., 2004). Researchers have surmised that such brief interventions may be insufficient in facilitating the acquisition of protective skills that may result in positive outcomes (Sheffield et al., 2006).

The framework of PYD interventions naturally addresses many of these shortcomings. First, in contrast to the directed focus of past deficit reduction programs, PYD programs focus on multiple targets. Such a multidimensional approach has been found to be associated with more positive outcomes at both the broad-based (Roth et al., 1998) and depression-specific (Felner et al., 1993; Vinokur, Schul, Vuori, & Price, 2000; Kellam, Rebok, Mayer, Ialongo, & Kalodner, 1994) levels, especially in universal populations. Second, whereas past deficit-based programs have typically operated in one domain (i.e., school setting), the majority of PYD programs operate in multiple domains, including family, community, and school settings. Operating in multiple domains is argued to be associated with greater program efficacy (Catalano, Berglund, et al., 2002). Third, expanding on past deficit-based programs, the majority of PYD programs aim to directly effectuate change not only at the individual level but also at the group (i.e., family, community) level. Finally, in contrast to the typically limited duration of past deficit-based interventions, PYD programs tend to be conducted over several months if not years. Programs conducted over many hours for extended periods of time have been shown to lead to greater positive outcomes than short interventions (Evans et al., 2005). As previously mentioned, Catalano, Berglund, et al. (2002) identified 80% of effective programs as lasting 9 months or more.

PYD INTERVENTIONS

The pool of PYD programs is composed of heterogeneous interventions that utilize a diverse array of cognitive, interpersonal, and environmental techniques in a multitude of domains to effect change in youth. A full discussion of all relevant interventions is beyond the scope of this chapter, but to illustrate the diverse approaches of PYD programs, a discussion of exemplar interventions follows. The selected interventions capture the resourceful nature of the strength-based approach and present the multitude of methods implemented to positively influence a wide array of outcome variables. In addition, an examination of the results from studies examining the efficacy of the selected interventions (see Tables 15.1–15.4) illustrates that these programs have demonstrated effectiveness in invoking change in many constructs thought to play a role in either the development of or resistance to depression (i.e., perceived competence, quality of interpersonal relations, problem solving, etc.).

Adventure programs are programs that utilize the natural environment (often wilderness) to create realistic situations in which the employment of decision-making and problem-solving strategies, as well as effective interpersonal skills, is necessary to successfully overcome the obstacles and challenges encountered and to achieve the intended goals of the activity. The interpretation of environmental cues and the actions undertaken to cope with challenging situations provide learning opportunities (Hans, 2000). In turn, the learning opportunities can facilitate the development and strengthening of cognitive and interpersonal skills that may generalize beyond the realm of the adventure program.

Adventure programs have not been developed with any particular theoretical framework. Rather, there have been attempts to place the mechanisms at work in adventure programs within some theoretical context. The most notable of these theories is Walsh and Golins' (1976) adventure education process model. This model identifies the constituent parts that comprise the adventure program experience and attempts to describe, with some predictive validity, the interrelationships between the elements that ultimately defines participant development. Sibthorp (2003) provides a description of the model:

> A motivated program participant is placed into a prescribed social and physical environment where he or she masters specific problem solving tasks. The course instructor acts as a guide to ensure that the tasks are both authentic and manageable and provides the necessary feedback to aid mastery, which, in turn leads to participant development.

Hattie, Marsh, Neill, and Richards (1997) describe common features of adventure programs, including wilderness or backcountry settings; small groups (generally fewer than 16 participants); mentally or physically challenging objectives; group interactions centered on tasks that involve group problem solving and decision making; autonomy-supportive, trained leader; and program duration of 2–4 weeks.

In a meta-meta-analysis comparing adventure-based with classroom-based programs, Hattie (1987, 1992, 1993) found that the benefits in achievement and affective outcomes of adventure programs exceed the levels of similar outcomes of classroom-based educational interventions. Hattie et al. (1997) conducted a meta-analysis examining the effects of adventure-based programs and determined that the initial effects of the program were maintained and increased over the typical follow-up period (5.5 months). The additive nature of program effects denotes that the effects of adventure-based programs persist and increase over time, which distinguishes them from classroom-based programs.

A key determinant of the effectiveness of adventure programs is duration. The mean length of reviewed adventure programs was 24 days (*SD* = 16). Programs longer than 20 days showed greater effect sizes immediately following a program as well as during the follow-up period, as compared with programs categorized as short (less than 9 days) and medium (10–19 days) in duration.

Hattie et al. (1997) identified 40 categories, which were collapsed into six dimensions that capture the outcome measures: leadership (e.g., decision-making ability), academic (e.g., problem-solving ability), self-concept, personality, interpersonal, and adventuresome. In general, the effect size of each dimension was high immediately following the program, and the positive effects were maintained throughout the follow-up period, with the exception of adventuresome (see Table 15.1 for a summary of results).

Leadership, conceptualized as interpersonal competence by the authors, included measures on decision-making, conscientiousness, general and teamwork leadership, organizational ability, time management, values, and goals. On all measures, with the exception of goals and values, there are substantial effect sizes. Decision-making ability shows the greatest effect size for the immediate and follow-up intervals.

Most adventure programs do not have an explicit academic achievement target with designs for improving cognitive functioning. However, an interpretation of findings from

TABLE 15.1. Characteristics of Adventure Programs

Program name
Adventure programs (e.g., Outward Bound)

Sample
Children through adults

Description of intervention
• Mental and physical challenges in wilderness or backcountry settings
• Small groups (less than 16)
• Interactions centered on tasks that involve group problem solving and decision making
• Duration: 2–4 weeks

Measures of interest
• Leadership
• Self-concept
• Academic
• Personality
• Interpersonal
• Adventuresome

Outcomes
• Leadership, self-concept, academic, personality, and interpersonal all significantly increased immediately following the program
• Greatest effects were shown for independence, confidence, self-efficacy, self-understanding, assertiveness, internal locus of control, and decision making
• Leadership (mean ES = 0.38; range = 0.05–0.71); highest significant effect on decision-making ability for immediate (mean ES = 0.47) and follow-up intervals (mean ES = 0.64)
• Academic (mean ES = 0.46; range = 0.23–0.70); general academic proficiencies (mean ES = 0.45) increase among participants in broad-focused adventure programs
• Self-concept (mean ES = 0.28; range = 0.07–0.47); significant effect on independence (mean ES = 0.47), confidence (mean ES = 0.33), self-efficacy (mean ES = 0.31), and self-understanding (mean ES = 0.31)
• Personality (mean ES = 0.37; range = 0.10–0.65); reduced aggressive behavior (mean ES = 0.33), increased assertiveness (mean ES = 0.42), cultivated an internal locus of control (mean ES = 0.30), and enhanced emotional stability (mean ES = 0.49)
• Interpersonal (mean ES = 0.32; range = 0.00–0.64); cooperation (mean ES = 0.34) and social competence (mean ES = 0.34)
• Adventuresome; no significant effect

the meta-analysis illustrates that general academic proficiencies increase among participants in broad-focused adventure programs. The nature of activities in such programs fosters problem-solving abilities, including enhancement of identification, resolution, and implementation strategies (Ewert, 1989), which are skills integral to general academic competence.

Historically, the impact of self-concept and its various components has been the most studied outcome of adventure-based programs (Hattie, 1987, 1992). Specifically, Hattie et al. (1997) identified a number of components that are thought to at least partly relate to independence, physical ability, peer relations, general self-concept, physical appearance, academic competence, confidence, self-efficacy, family relations, self-understanding, and well-being. Findings in the meta-analysis reveal that the greatest effect immediately following the program occurred in the areas of independence, confidence, self-efficacy, and self-understanding.

Personality was associated with behavioral constructs, specifically aggressive behavior, as well as assertiveness, locus of control, and emotion regulation. Adventure programs exhibited the beneficial effects of reduced aggressive behavior, increased assertiveness, cultivation of an internal locus of control, and enhanced emotional stability.

The challenging activities and tasks performed by adventure program participants are normally done in small groups, requiring reciprocal communication and efforts to accomplish certain goals. Thus, strengthening interpersonal skills can be considered a focal point of adventure programs. According to Hattie et al. (1997), the social aspects of the programs contributed to substantial effect sizes immediately following a program and throughout the follow-up period. The interpersonal skills associated with the greatest effect are cooperation and social competence. Table 15.1 presents a summary of the characteristics of adventure programs, including results from studies examining the efficacy of such programs.

Across Ages is a year-long, multidomain prevention program that combines mentoring with community service, a classroom-based life skills curriculum, and parent workshops. The program is intended to reduce the incidence of substance use among adolescents, as well as to benefit the older mentors and deconstruct myths regarding age (LoSciuto, Rajala, Townsend, & Taylor, 1996; Taylor, LoSciuto, Fox, Hilbert, & Sonkowsky, 1999). The theoretical models in which Across Ages operates include positive youth development, Erikson's (1960) concept of generativity, youth identity development, the social developmental model, and social problem solving (Catalano, Berglund, et. al., 2002).

Program participants were divided into three groups at the inception of the program: no intervention, program, and mentoring. In addition to the community service, classroom-based life skills curriculum, and parent workshops, in which both intervention groups participated, the mentoring group participated in the mentoring component. The authors hypothesized that the participants engaged in all four program components would have significantly more positive outcomes than those who did not participate in any of the program components. A second hypothesis posited that the mentoring group would show greater positive outcomes on the evaluation battery than the program group.

Mentoring in Across Ages involves meeting with an elder twice a week, for a minimum of 4 hours a week. The community service component includes biweekly nursing home visits and a neighborhood environmental project. The students keep a journal and discuss their experiences at the nursing home in their class. The life skills curriculum is a 26-session positive youth development curriculum (PYDC) made up of a social problem-solving model and a substance abuse prevention curriculum taught for 45 minutes twice a week. The PYDC is implemented through didactic teaching, classroom discussions, videos, journal keeping, role plays in small groups, and homework assignments. The highly structured social-problem-solving model addresses six areas: stress management, self-esteem, problem solving, substance knowledge, health information, and social networks. Parent workshops provide opportunities for positive parent–youth interaction with the aim of strengthening the bonds between parents and children. The workshops provide awareness of school resources available to students and provide teachers with an understanding of the risk factors to which the students are exposed. Parents learn about subjects such as adolescent sexuality and engage in activities such as talent shows and story-telling. (LoSciuto et al., 1996; Taylor et al., 1999).

Five hundred sixty-two sixth-grade students completed both the pre- and posttest measures for the evaluation of Across Ages. Of the youth involved, 53% were female; 52% identified as African American, 16% as European American, 9% as Asian American, 9% as Hispanic, and 14% as other. The majority were living in poor, high-crime neighborhoods. Only a minority (15–20%) reach or surpass the national average on standardized achievement tests (LoSciuto et al., 1996; Taylor et al., 1999).

The results demonstrated that mentoring led to positive effects, above and beyond participation in the three other program components. The authors conjectured that the success of the mentoring was largely attributable to the mentor's ability to plan collaboratively, to listen, and to respect the mentee's pace in disclosing information and building trust with the mentor (LoSciuto et al., 1996; Taylor et al., 1999). Table 15.2 presents a summary of characteristics of Across Ages, including results from studies examining the efficacy of the program.

The *Big Brothers and Big Sisters Program* uses mentoring relationships independently, seeking to provide social, cultural and recreational enrichment to its mentees (Tierney, Grossman, & Resch, 2000). Eight Big Brother/Big Sister (BB/BS) networks were followed to determine whether this mentoring relationship would lead to positive outcomes—specifically, reductions in problem behavior and improvements in competencies and overall well-being. From these networks, 1,138 Little Brothers and Little Sisters (LB/LS) were selected to participate in the 17-month study. Within this sample, 62.4% were boys, 56.8% were visible minorities, and 90% were living with only one parent. The mean age of the participants was 12 years.

Participants were randomly placed in one of two conditions: with a mentor who was matched according to shared interest, reasonable geographical proximity, and preference for same-race, or on a waiting list for future placement with a mentor. On average, mentors interacted with their mentees three times a month (4 hours each time) for 12 months. Outcome evaluation was based on participant and parent surveys and interviews conducted at initial and follow-up assessments.

Six outcome areas were considered in Tierney and colleagues' (2000) evaluation of the Big Brother/Big Sister program: (1) antisocial activities, (2) academic performance, attitudes and behaviors, (3) relationships with family, (4) relationships with friends, (5) self-concept, and (6) social and cultural enrichment. Overall, the relationships established between the mentors and the mentees produced positive outcomes. Tierney et al. (2000) noted that beneficial relationships were likely a function of BB/BS's matching ability as well as the sustained nature (1 year minimum, or 144 hours) of the program (see Table 15.3 for a summary of results). Table 15.3 presents a summary of characteristics of BB/BS, including results from studies examining the efficacy of the program.

The *School Transitional Environment Project* (STEP; Felner & Adan, 1988; Felner et al., 1993; Felner, Ginter, & Primavera, 1982) is a school-based universal prevention pro-

TABLE 15.2. Characteristics of Across Ages

Program name

Across Ages

Sample

- 562 sixth-grade students
- Participants divided into:
  - Mentoring group
  - Program group
  - Control group
- Low socioeconomic status

Description of intervention

- Classroom intervention
  - 45 minutes
  - 2 times/week
- Parent workshops
  - Biweekly
  - 1-hour visits
- Community service
  - 1 hour/week
  - Nursing home visits
- Mentoring
  - 2 times/week
  - 4 hours

Measures of interest

Evaluation battery assessing:

- Ability to deal with peer pressure
- Frequency of adaptive behavior to stress and anxiety
- Self-perceptions
- Perceived competency and self-worth
- Frequency of specific substance abuse
- Knowledge about aging and older people
- Mood and emotional state
- Efficacy of problem-solving skills
- Knowledge about the effects of various drugs
- Attitudes about alcohol, drugs, elders, school, and community

Outcomes

- Participants in the *mentor group in combination with the program* showed positive effects in:
  - Ability to react to situations involving drug use
  - Attitudes toward school
  - Attitudes toward elders
  - Attitudes toward community service issues
  - Attitudes toward the future
- Participants in the *mentor group* showed a significant decrease in frequency of specific substance abuse over a 2-month period
- Participants in the *mentor group* were significantly less absent from school
- Participants in the *exceptional mentor group* showed significant improvement on all 11 outcome measures

TABLE 15.3. Characteristics of Big Brothers/Big Sisters

Program name

Big Brothers/Big Sisters

Sample

- 1,138 youths
- 487 in treatment group
- 472 in control group
- Mean age = 12 years
- Low socioeconomic status

Description of intervention

- Interaction with mentors 3 times a month for a minimum of 4 hours over the course of a year

Measures of interest

- Antisocial activities (initiation of drug abuse, initiation of alcohol abuse, hitting someone, stealing, or destroying property)
- Academic performance, attitudes, behavior
- Relationships with family
- Relationships with friends
- Self-concept
- Social and cultural enrichment

Outcomes

- Youths in the treatment group were less likely to initiate drug and alcohol abuse and less likely to hit others
- No differences in stealing / property damage
- Increased quality of relationship with primary caregiver
- Positive impact in treatment group on academic competence, GPA, classes/school days skipped
- Emotional support increased among youths in treatment group; and increase in intimacy in communication
- No differences in self-concept, social, or cultural enrichment

gram designed to modify the school environment to ease transitioning students, in hope of preventing or reducing the associated negative outcomes, including psychopathology. STEP directly addresses contextual factors in the school setting to create a supportive atmosphere to reduce the stress associated with the normative transition of middle or high school matriculation.

Theoretically, STEP operates within the transactional-ecological/transitional life-events model, which states that normal changes can increase the risk of maladaptive outcomes. The risk associated with transitions from one school to another is a result of "heightened complexity and developmental demands of the new school setting" (Felner et al., 1993, p. 110) and the inherent difficulty schools may have in accommodating students with the support necessary for a positive transitional outcome. Risk reduction occurs when additional resources are provided to address the specific needs of transitioning students.

Strategies central to the program include an emphasis on broadening the capacities of homeroom teachers to deal closely with the transitional issues of the students. The responsibilities accorded homeroom teachers establish a stabilizing source from which students can seek information and advice about school-related matters, and are similar to the duties of a guidance counselor. The expanded role of homeroom teachers includes increased contact with the families and teachers of the students, which ensures a healthy interchange between students, teachers, and families. The result is increased awareness of maladaptive behavior and assistance in identifying potential problems to be targeted with supplemental support. A "cohort" was established, intended to provide a stable, familiar social unit that would attend homeroom and core classes together. Class size was lowered to produce smaller, more advantageous "learning communities." The modifications to the school environment were intended to diminish the potential risk of transitioning and to enhance the peer and faculty support systems by creating a stable, predictable school environment.

Multiple studies examining the impact of STEP implementation have been conducted in middle and high schools, which have produced an extensive body of findings supporting environmental modification to facilitate school transitions for students. Longitudinal data have indicated that, as compared with control groups, STEP participants demonstrated higher levels of academic (e.g., grades, commitment to school) and behavioral (e.g., regarding delinquency, substance abuse) functioning (Felner et al., 2001). Specific to psychosocial outcomes, STEP has demonstrated a significant effect in the reduction of depressive symptoms. In a large study ($n = 1,965$) of students transitioning to middle school, measures of stress, anxiety, depression, self-esteem, and problem behavior were administered to students to determine their transitional adjustment. As compared with the control group, students in the intervention group showed higher levels of adaptive adjustment, as indicated by lower levels of depression and anxiety symptoms, higher ratings of self-esteem, and less problematic behavior (Felner et al., 1993). A summary of characteristics of the STEP program, including results from studies examining its efficacy, is presented in Table 15.4.

CONCLUSION

In closing, it is essential to return again to our central question of whether strength-based programs designed to enhance competencies can produce developmental outcomes similar to those of deficit-based programs designed to prevent or reduce depression. A complete answer to this question must both (1) identify the developmental outcomes produced by deficit-focused depression programs and (2) examine whether PYD programs produce similar effects. Recent reviews of the depression prevention literature (Horowitz & Garber, 2006; Merry, McDowell, Hetrick, et al., 2004) have demonstrated that although certain specific programs have shown some effectiveness in preventing (i.e., Jaycox, Reivich, Gillham, & Seligman, 1994) or reducing (i.e., Clarke et al., 2001) depression, the majority of others have been ineffective (i.e., Spence et al., 2003; Quayle et al., 2001), particularly those programs utilizing a universal approach. Given that past deficit reduction programs have in many instances not fully obtained their intended effects (Horowitz & Garber, 2006; Merry, McDowell, Hetrick, et al., 2004), the question with respect to PYD programs becomes whether they demonstrate greater, rather then equal, success in achieving such effects. On a surface level, PYD programs address many of the design shortcomings attributed to past deficit reduction programs, suggesting that PYD programs may represent a valuable alternative approach. Further, our review of the available literature suggests that PYD programs are likely to be effective in invoking change in many psychosocial variables implicated in the development of and resistance to depression (see Catalano, Berglund, et al., 2002). Such a conclusion, however, must be

TABLE 15.4. Characteristics of School Transitional Environment Project (STEP)

Program name

School Transitional Environment Project (STEP)

Sample

- 1,204 sixth-grade students in treatment group
- 761 sixth-grade students in control group

Description of intervention

- Partial reorganization of social/school system:
  - Treatment groups were assigned to classes so their core academic subjects were taken only with other treatment students
- Redefinition of homeroom teacher by giving more responsibility (e.g., contacting parents when adolescent is absent)

Measures of interest

- School Transitions Index
- Children's Depression Inventory
- Revised Children's Manifest Anxiety Scale
- Self-Evaluation Outcome
- Delinquency Scale of the Youth Self-Report
- Teacher–Child Rating Scale

Outcomes

- STEP students reported significantly lower levels of school transitional stress and better adjustment on measures of:
  - Anxiety
  - Depression
  - Self-esteem
  - Delinquent behavior
- Teacher ratings of class behavior were also significantly better for STEP participants than for controls
- Grades and attendance were better among treatment group

tempered, owing to flaws in both the studies and the literature reviews on which such conclusions are based. Further, the assertion that positive changes in such vulnerability and resiliency factors necessarily result in the prevention of depression, although intuitive, has yet to be empirically examined.

One beneficial feature of PYD programs that bolsters their capacity to serve as an alternative approach to traditional deficit-based programs is their use of a broadly targeted approach that emphasizes competence enhancement, generally within the context of normative development. The promotive goals of PYD lessen the stigma associated with participation in a depression prevention program and increase the relevancy of PYD interventions to children and adolescents. The result is an intervention with content that is more identifiable to youth, as well as program goals that are more likely to be embraced by participants and potential participants.

When beginning to unravel how PYD programs appeal to youth and are able to generate positive outcomes, it may be constructive to consider the theory of developmental intentionality (Walker, Marczak, Blyth, & Borden, 2005). The theory posits three precepts that drive the development and implementation of youth programs. The first is a strong focus on long-term developmental outcomes within all facets of the program. In other words, the program has a well-defined set of developmental goals and every aspect of the program is crafted to increase the likelihood of participants being able to attain such goals. In line with this precept, preliminary results from multiyear follow-up studies suggest that the acquisition of skills that benefit participants in multiple domains positively impact long-term developmental outcomes (see Catalano, Berglund, et al., 2002). The second precept is active engagement by participants in the learning opportunities provided by the program. In other words, the success of PYD programs relies on collaboration between participating youth and program facilitators, which is often enhanced by parental and community involvement. Finally, the third precept states that engagement is facilitated by a good fit between the youth and the program. A good fit can occur as a result of multiple factors, including program content and activities, program delivery style, facilitator–participant congruency, and interparticipant identification. The value that PYD places on normative developmental processes and outcomes inherently fosters a good fit between participant and program.

An area of the PYD literature that has received scant attention to date is the development of coherent, systematic theoretical frameworks that guide program design and implementation. That is, these programs are often interventions in search of a theory. An incomplete theoretical framework for PYD programs is implicated in nonoptimal program development and implementation and, ultimately, hindrance of evaluation efforts. The active proliferation of programs designed and implemented within the promising but not-quite-sound PYD framework raises concerns of replicability and exposes a weakness in the dissemination of PYD programs. Without necessarily understanding the mechanisms that underlie the effectiveness of PYD programs, efforts to modify programs to improve ecological validity may be ill-informed.

There are a limited number of well-defined models devised explicitly for PYD programs. A notable one is the Search Institute's developmental assets model (Benson, 1997), which posits that internal and external developmental assets are imperative for positive youth development. The authors identify 40 assets, which are defined as building blocks that are crucial for the promotion of healthy youth development and well-being (Benson, Leffert, Scales, & Blyth, 1998). The assets are grouped in seven categories, which include both external and internal assets. Whereas external assets consist of support, boundaries and expectations, empowerment, and constructive use of time, internal assets consist of commitment to learning, positive values, and social competence. Leffert, Benson, Sharma, Drake, & Blyth (1998) demonstrated that programs that foster a greater number of developmental assets tend to produce higher levels of positive outcomes as well as lower levels of negative outcomes among secondary school students.

Finally, the suggestion that PYD interventions provide a promising alternative to depression prevention is not a call to replace depression prevention programs. Depression prevention programs have demonstrated success in treating, and in a limited number of instances, preventing depression (Horowitz & Garber, 2006; Merry, McDowell, Hetrick, et al., 2004). Much of the success has occurred in targeted populations in which participants either are at risk of developing depression or exhibit prodromal symptoms. Perhaps depression prevention strategies are able to effectively identify and target clear-cut risk groups with well-established processes. PYD interventions may be able to capitalize on the differential effectiveness among prevention programs and provide the content and environment needed to successfully target youth populations for whom depression prevention programs are not the best option. As there are many ways to prevent depression, the future of the field may ultimately lie in identifying the intrapersonal and environmental variables that predict the greatest response to specific prevention approaches.

REFERENCES

Beardslee, W. R., & Gladstone, T. R. G. (2001). Prevention of childhood depression: Recent findings and future prospects. *Society of Biological Psychiatry, 49,* 1101–1110.

Benson, P. L. (1997). *All kids are our kids: What communities must do to raise responsible and caring children and adolescents.* San Francisco: Jossey-Bass.

Benson, P. L., Leffert, N., Scales, P. C., & Blyth, D. A. (1998). Beyond the "village" rhetoric: Creating healthy communities for children and adolescents. *Applied Developmental Science, 2*(3), 138–158.

Capaldi, D. M. (1991). Co-occurrence of conduct disorder and depressive symptoms in early adolescent boys: I. Familial factors and general adjustment at grade 6. *Development and Psychopathology, 3,* 277–300.

Capaldi, D. M. (1992). Co-occurrence of conduct disorder and depressive symptoms in early adolescent boys: II. A 2-year follow-up at grade 8. *Development and Psychopathology, 4,* 125–144.

Cardemil, E. V., Reivich, K. J., & Seligman, M. E. P. (2002). The prevention of depressive symptoms in low-income minority middle school students. *Prevention and Treatment, 5.* Retrieved January 15, 2006, from *journals.apa.org/prevention/volume5/pre/5/1/8a.html.*

Catalano, R. F., Berglund, M. L., Ryan, J. A. M., Lonczak, H. S., & Hawkins, J. D. (2002). Positive youth development in the United States: Research findings on evaluations of positive youth development programs. *Prevention and Treatment, 5*(15). Retrieved January 15, 2006, from *content2.apa.org/journals/pre/5/1/15a.html.*

Catalano, R. F., Hawkins, J. D., Berglund, M. L., Pollard, J. A., & Arthur, M. W. (2002). Prevention science and positive youth development: Competitive or cooperative frameworks. *Journal of Adolescent Health, 31,* 230–239.

Clarke, G. N., Hawkins, W., Murphy, M., Sheeber, L. B., Lewinsohn, P. M., & Seeley, J. R. (1995). Targeted prevention of unipolar depressive disorder in an at-risk sample of high school adolescents: A randomized trial of a group cognitive intervention. *Journal of the American Academy of Child and Adolescent Psychiatry, 34,* 312–321.

Clarke, G. N., Hornbrook, M., Lynch, F., Polen, M., Gale, J., Beardslee, W., et al. (2001). A randomized trial of a group cognitive intervention for preventing depression in adolescent offspring of depressed parents. *Archives of General Psychiatry, 58,* 1127–1134.

Damon, W. (2004). What is positive youth development? *The Annals of the American Academy of Political and Social Science, 591*(1), 13–24.

Durlak, J. A., & Wells, A. M. (1997). Primary prevention mental-health programs for children and adolescents: A meta-analytic review. *American Journal of Community Psychology, 25*(2), 115–152.

Erikson, E. (1959). *Identity and the life cycle.* New York: International Universities Press.

Evans, D. L., Foa, E. B., Gur, R. E., Hendin, H., O'Brien, C. P., Seligman, M. E. P., et al. (Eds.). (2005). *Treating and preventing adolescent mental health disorders: What we know and what we don't know.* Oxford, UK: Oxford University Press.

Ewert, A. (1989). *Outdoor adventure pursuits: Foundations, models, and theories.* Columbus, OH: Publishing Horizons.

Felner, R. D., & Adan, A. M. (1988). The school transitional project: An ecological intervention and evaluation. In R. H. Price, E. L. Cowen, R. P. Lorion, & J. Ramos-McKay (Eds.), *14 ounces of prevention: A casebook for practitioners* (pp. 111–122). Washington, DC: American Psychological Association.

Felner, R. D., Brand, S., Adan, A. M., Mulhall, P. F., Flowers, N., Sartain, B., et al. (1993). Restructuring the ecology of the school as an approach to prevention during school transitions: Longitudinal follow-ups and extensions of the School Transitional Environment Project (STEP). *Prevention in Human Services, 10,* 103–136.

Felner, R. D., Favazza, A., Shim, M., Brand, S., Gu, K., & Noonan, N. (2001). Whole school improvement and restructuring as prevention and promotion: Lessons from STEP and Project on Performance Learning Communities. *Journal of School Psychology, 39*(2), 177–202.

Felner, R. D., Ginter, M., & Primavera, J. (1982). Primary prevention during school transitions: Social support and environmental structure. *American Journal of Community Psychology, 10,* 277–290.

Greenberg, M. T., Domitrovich, C., & Bumbarger, B. (2001). The prevention of mental disorders in school-aged children: Current state of the field. *Prevention and Treatment, 4*(1). Retrieved January 15, 2006, from *content2.apa.org/journals/pre/4/1/1a.html.*

Haggerty, R. J., Sherrod, L. R., Garmezy, N., & Rutter, M. (1994). *Stress, risk, and resilience in children and adolescents: Processes, mechanisms, and interventions.* New York: Cambridge University Press.

Hains, A. A., & Ellman, S. W. (1994). Stress inoculation training as a preventative intervention for high school youths. *Journal of Cognitive Psychotherapy, 8,* 219–232.

Hans, T. A. (2000). A meta-analysis of the effects of adventure programming on locus of control. *Journal of Contemporary Psychotherapy, 30,* 33–60.

Hattie, J. A. (1987). Identifying the salient facets of schooling: A synthesis of meta-analyses. *International Journal of Educational Research, 11,* 187–212.

Hattie, J. A. (1992). Towards a model of schooling: A synthesis of meta-analyses. *Australian Journal of Education, 36,* 5–13.

Hattie, J. A. (1993). Measuring the effects of schooling. *SET, 2,* 1–4.

Hattie, J., Marsh, H. W., Neill, J. T., & Richards, G. E. (1997). Adventure education and Outward Bound: Out-of-class experiences that make a lasting difference. *Review of Educational Research, 67,* 43–87.

Horowitz, J. L., & Garber, J. (2006). The prevention of depressive symptoms in children and adolescents: A meta-analytic review. *Journal of Consulting and Clinical Psychology, 74,* 401–415.

Jaycox, L. H., Reivich, K. J., Gillham, J., & Seligman, M. E. P. (1994). Prevention of depressive symptoms in school children. *Behavior Research and Therapy, 32,* 801–816.

Kellam, S. G., Rebok, G. W., Mayer, L. S., Ialongo, N., & Kalodner, C. R. (1994). Depressive symptoms over first grade and their response to a developmental epidemiologically based preventive trial aimed at improving achievement. *Developmental Psychopathology, 6,* 463–481.

Leffert, N., Benson, P. L., Sharma, A. R., Drake, D. R., & Blyth, D. A. (1998). Developmental assets: Measurement and prediction of risk behaviors among adolescents. *Applied Developmental Science, 2*(4), 209–230.

Lerner, R. M., Fisher, C. B., & Weinberg, R. A. (2000). Toward a science for the people: Promoting civil society through the application of developmental science. *Child Development, 71,* 11–20.

LoSciuto, L., Rajala, A. K., Townsend, T. N., & Taylor, A. S. (1996). An outcome evaluation of Across Ages: An intergenerational mentoring approach to drug prevention. *Journal of Adolescent Research, 11*(1), 116–129.

Masten, A. S., & Coatsworth, J. D. (1998). The development of competence in favorable and unfavorable environments: Lessons from research on successful children. *American Psychologist, 53,* 205–220.

Masten, A. S., Coatsworth, J. D., Neemann, J., Gest, S. D., Tellegen, A., & Garmezy, N. (1995). The structure and coherence of competence from childhood through adolescence. *Child Development, 66,* 1635–1659.

Merry, S., McDowell, H., Hetrick, S., Bir, J., & Muller, N. (2004). Psychological and/or educational interventions for the prevention of depression in children and adolescents (Review). *The Cochrane Library, 4,* 1–124.

Merry, S., McDowell, H., Wild, C. J., Bir, J., & Cunliffe, R. (2004). A randomized placebo controlled trial of a school-based depression prevention program. *Journal of the American Academy of Child and Adolescent Psychiatry, 43,* 538–547.

Park, N. (2004). Character strengths and positive youth development. *The Annals of the American Academy of Political and Social Science, 591*(1), 40–54.

Quayle, D., Dzuirawiec, S., Roberts, C., Kane, R., & Ebsworthy, G. (2001). The effect of an optimism and life skills program on depressive symptoms in preadolescence. *Behaviour Change,* *18,* 194–203.

Rohde, P., Lewinsohn, P. M., & Seely, J. R. (1991). Comorbidity of unipolar depression: II. Comorbidity with other mental disorders in adolescents and adults. *Journal of Abnormal Psychology,* *100,* 214–222.

Roth, J. L., & Brooks-Gunn, J. (2003). Youth development programs: Risk, prevention and policy. *Journal of Adolescent Health, 32*(3), 170–182.

Roth, J. L., Brooks-Gunn, J., Murray, L., & Foster, W. (1998). Promoting healthy adolescents: Synthesis of youth development program evaluations. *Journal of Research on Adolescence, 8*(4), 423–459.

Seligman, M. E. P., Berkowitz, M. W., Catalano, R. F., Damon, W., Eccles, J. S., Gillham, J. E., et al. (2005). The positive perspective on youth development. In D. L. Evans, E. B. Foa, R. E. Gur, H. Hendin, C. P. O'Brien, M. E. P. Seligman, et al. (Eds.), *Treating and preventing adolescent mental health disorders: What we know and what we don't know* (pp. 498–527). Oxford, UK: Oxford University Press.

Sheffield, J. K., Spence, S. H., Rapee, R. M., Kowalenko, N., Wignall, A., & Davis, A., (2006). Evaluation of universal, indicated, and combined cognitive-behavioral approaches to the prevention of depression among adolescents. *Journal of Consulting and Clinical Psychology,* *74*(1), 66–79.

Shochet, I. M., Dadds, M. R., Holland, D., Whitefield, K., Harnett, P. H., & Osgarby, S. M. (2001). The efficacy of a universal school-based program to prevent adolescent depression. *Journal of Clinical Child Psychology, 30,* 303–315.

Sibthorp, J. (2003). An empirical look at Walsh and Golins' adventure education process model: Relationships between antecedent factors, perceptions of characteristics of an adventure education experience, and changes in self-efficacy. *Journal of Leisure Research, 35,* 80–106.

Spence, S. H., Sheffield, J. K., & Donovan, C. L. (2003). Preventing adolescent depression: An evaluation of the Problem Solving for Life program. *Journal of Consulting and Clinical Psychology, 71,* 3–13.

Taylor, A. S., LoSciuto, L., Fox, M., Hilbert, S. M., & Sonkowsky, M. (1999). The mentoring factor: Evaluation of the Across Ages' intergenerational approach to drug abuse prevention. *Child and Youth Services, 20,* 77–99.

Tierney, J. P., Grossman, J. B., & Resch, N. L. (2000). *Making a difference: An impact study of Big Brothers Big Sisters.* Philadelphia: Public/Private Ventures.

Vinokur, A. D., Schul, Y., Vuori, J., & Price, R. H. (2000). Two years after a job loss: Long-term impact of the JOBS program on reemployment and mental health. *Journal of Occupational Health Psychology, 5,* 32–47.

Walker, J., Marczak, M., Blyth, D., & Borden, L. (2005). Designing youth development programs: Toward a theory of developmental intentionality. In J. L. Mahoney, R. W. Larson, & J. S. Eccles (Eds.), *Organized activities as contexts of development: Extracurricular activities, afterschool and community programs* (pp. 399–418). Mahwah, NJ: Erlbaum.

Walsh, V., & Golins, G. (1976). *The exploration of the Outward Bound process.* Denver: Outward Bound.

Yu, D. L., & Seligman, M. E. P. (2002). Preventing depressive symptoms in Chinese children. *Prevention and Treatment, 5*(9). Retrieved January 15, 2006, from *content2.apa.org/journals/pre/5/1/9a.html.*

V SPECIAL POPULATIONS

16 Sex Differences in Child and Adolescent Depression

A Developmental Psychopathological Approach

Benjamin L. Hankin, Emily Wetter,
and Catherine Cheely

One of the most consistent findings in the literature on depression is the sex difference in prevalence rates: Twice as many women are depressed as men, starting sometime around menarche during adolescence and lasting throughout most of adulthood (Hankin & Abramson, 1999; Mazure & Keita, 2006; Nolen-Hoeksema, 1990, 2002). Understanding why this sex differences exists, why it begins around puberty, how it unfolds over development, and how it affects normal and abnormal development are some of the most captivating and least understood phenomena in developmental psychopathology.

Given the focus of this edited volume, this chapter concentrates on sex differences in depression during childhood and adolescence and reviews what is known about sex differences in rates and manifestation of depression, its etiology, treatment, and prevention among youth. In particular, we cover five main areas. First, we review briefly the extensive literature concerning typical sex differences in normal development during childhood and adolescence. Next, we summarize the developmental epidemiological findings to explicate when the sex difference in depression emerges. Third, we consider etiological explanations for the sex difference in depression, with a particular emphasis on the few integrative, coherent developmentally sensitive conceptual theories. Fourth, we evaluate whether and how sex affects interventions (treatment and prevention) in youth depression. Finally, we suggest future directions and discuss broad issues facing the field.

We take a developmental psychopathological perspective in covering these topics (see Cicchetti, 2006; Cicchetti & Rogosch, 2002), drawing attention to a few points here and throughout the chapter (see also Crick & Zahn-Waxler, 2003; Rutter, Caspi, & Moffitt, 2003; Zahn-Waxler, Crick, Shirtcliff, & Woods, 2006). First, it is important to study and consider both normal and abnormal factors and processes together, as both are important and inform each other. Most of the writing in the area of sex differences broadly focuses on either normal (e.g., emotions, social relationships, parental socialization) or abnormal (e.g., clinical depression, conduct disorder) development. We review the literature on sex differences from both normal and abnormal development perspectives. Second, we consider theory and empirical findings pertaining to the infant, child, and adolescent periods in order to promote a developmental pathways and lifespan perspective. We do not cover adulthood, as doing so would be beyond the scope of this chapter and sex differences in adult depression are reviewed elsewhere (e.g., Hankin & Abramson, 1999; Keyes & Goodman, 2006; Kuehner, 2003; Mazure & Keita, 2006; Nolen-Hoeksema, 2002). Most of the earlier literature has focused largely on adolescence, which is sensible, given that the sex difference in depression is most pronounced during this developmental period. Yet this means that less attention has been paid to sex differences in childhood and the potential developmental precursors contributing to the emergence of the sex difference in depression (but see Crick & Zahn-Waxler, 2003; Keenan & Hipwell, 2005, for notable exceptions). Third, we examine the role of developmental pathways in the emergence of sex differences in depression. Specifically, we consider homotypic and heterotypic continuity in the manifestation of depressive symptoms in boys and girls over time. *Homotypic continuity* refers to stability in both the manifestation and underlying processes of depression (i.e., the presentation of depression in boys and girls is similarly stable over time, as are the latent processes contributing to the manifestation of the symptoms), whereas *heterotypic continuity* denotes that there is stability over time in the underlying processes or latent construct of depression, but the observable and measurable manifestation of depressive symptoms may change over time. We also consider the etiological processes contributing to the rise in depression by sex over time and discuss equifinality and multifinality. Equifinality, in which different pathways lead to the same outcome, may make boys and girls similar to each other at one developmental point. Multifinality, in which different pathways emanate from a similar starting point, may make boys and girls follow different developmental trajectories with varying risk and protective factors at later stages. Finally, we emphasize an integrative approach involving multiple levels of analysis (e.g., genetics, hormones, cognition, relationships, emotions, etc.) to understand why more girls exhibit depression starting in adolescence. To date, there is no truly integrative theory of the emergence of the sex difference in depression that aptly includes all levels of analysis, including developmental and contextual influences. The few extant integrative models (e.g., Cyranowski, Frank, Young, & Shear, 2000; Hankin & Abramson, 2001; Keenan & Hipwell, 2005; Zahn-Waxler, 2000) have emphasized and integrated certain factors and levels of analysis to the relative exclusion of other potential influences.

TYPICAL SEX DIFFERENCES IN NORMAL DEVELOPMENT

Biological Factors

At the simplest level, there are genetic differences between boys and girls that begin at birth and have developmental significance throughout life. Males have one X and one Y chromosome, whereas females have two X chromosomes. Apart from these basic genetic differences having clear functional significance (e.g., X-linked mutations like color blindness), they also affect later biological factors, such as hormones, that may influence the ontogeny of the sex difference in depression (Steiner, Dunn, & Born, 2003).

Hormones regulate and influence gene expression. Androgenic hormones directly contribute to the processes that make a male's brain masculine and less feminine, depending on the amount of hormone present *in utero*. These neuroendocrine effects on brain and behavior are affected by later developmental events at puberty and throughout adolescence (McEwen, 1992). During puberty, testosterone levels rise dramatically for boys, and estradiol levels increase for girls (Hayward, 2003). Despite these clear changes in sex hormones, the effects they have on mood, emotion, and behavior are subtle, complex, and depend on an individual's developmental stage and other biosocial influences (McEwen & Alves, 1999; Steiner et al., 2003; Udry, 2000).

In addition, gonadal steroids can moderate the functional role of other hormones for girls, as compared with boys. The hypothamalamic–pituitary–adrenal (HPA) axis, which is important for managing the body's response to stress, interacts with gonadal steroids: Testosterone suppresses and estrogen enhances HPA axis activity (Rhodes & Rubin, 1999). Thus, girls may respond more to the long-term consequences of stress. Moreover, girls' response to stress differs from boys' because oxytocin (a hormone that enhances caregiving and relaxation and reduces fearfulness and sympathetic activity) and endogenous opioids appear to be fundamental to females' response to stress, whereas vasopressin (a hormone involved in aggressive social behavior) is more indicative of males' stress response (Insel & Fernald, 2004; Rhodes & Rubin, 1999; Taylor et al., 2000). Estrogen also enhances girls' more typical social/affiliative response to stress (i.e., tend-and-befriend), whereas testosterone decreases this response (Taylor, Dickerson, & Klein, 2002).

There are also sex differences in most neurotransmitter levels and activity. For example, females respond less to serotonin (5-HT), 5-HT receptors are down-regulated more in girls than boys, 5-HT binds more in males, and there are sex differences in the way in which sex hormones regulate 5-HT (McEwen, 2001; McEwen & Alves, 1999).

Emotional Development and Temperament

Starting as early as infancy and toddlerhood, there are sex differences in the display of basic emotions. Boys tend to exhibit more irritability and anger, whereas girls show more fearfulness (Brody, 1999; Ruble & Martin, 1998; Ruble, Martin, & Berebaum, 2006). By age 2, girls show greater levels of empathy (Zahn-Waxler, Robinson, & Emde, 1992). Also early in life, girls are more socially aware and sensitive to others' affective states (Brody, 1985). In contrast, boys exhibit more frustration, anger, and emotional dysregulation than girls starting by preschool and persisting thereafter (Zahn-Waxler, Schmitz, Fulker, Robinson, & Emde, 1996). By adolescence, boys tend to deny their sadness and seek to hide internalizing and submissive forms of negative emotions, especially sadness and anxiety, whereas girls report higher levels and more intense degrees of sadness, shame, and guilt (Brody & Hall, 2000; Zahn-Waxler, 2000; Zeman & Shipman, 1997). It has been suggested that these differences may be due to temperamental factors or parental socialization factors, as discussed in greater detail next.

Generally consistent with these findings from individual studies of emotion, a recent meta-analysis of temperament showed sex differences in temperament (Else-Quest, Hyde, Goldsmith, & Van Hulle, 2006). Girls showed higher levels of effortful control (e.g., attentional shifting, inhibitory control, ability to control inappropriate behavior), whereas boys demonstrated greater levels of surgency/extraversion (e.g., in ratings of activity, high-intensity pleasure, and impulsivity). However, no differences were seen in shyness, sociability, or broad negative affectivity, although girls had higher levels of fearfulness than boys.

Social Development

Starting early in life, boys' play tends to center on action, playing with objects, and achievement and power, whereas girls' play emphasizes relational and family themes (Maccoby, 2002). Boys tend to be more physically aggressive (e.g., hitting, punching, kicking) than girls (Coie & Dodge, 1998; Ruble & Martin, 1998), whereas girls aggression occurs more in indirect, social realms (i.e., relational aggression; Crick & Grotpeter, 1995; Crick, 1997; Underwood, 2003). Girls' focus on relationships, cooperation, and harmony persists from childhood into adolescence (Maccoby, 2002).

These sex differences are also observed in youths' interpersonal and social relationships (Rose & Rudolph, 2006). Generally, Western societies expect females to be more relationship-oriented than males, and males to be more assertive (Brody & Hall, 2000). For girls, as compared with boys, close interpersonal relationships are more important for their self-definition and identity (Gore, Aseltine, & Colten, 1993; Maccoby, 1990) and are used more as a source of emotional support (Buhrmester, 1996; Cross & Madson, 1997). Moreover, girls exhibit a stronger relational orientation and greater affiliative needs in adolescence as compared with boys (Cyranowski et al., 2000; Rudolph, 2002). Adolescent girls' relationships are characterized by greater levels of intimacy, emotional support, and self-disclosure than are boys' relationships (Buhrmester & Furman, 1987; Furman & Buhrmester, 1992; Rose & Rudolph, 2006), whereas such relationships among boys tend to be grounded in companionship and shared activities (Maccoby, 1990). Yet this general relational orientation for girls, although providing a source of support, also appears to carry a cost. Rose (2002) described the process of corumination, in which girls tend to disclose more emotional information as they seek support among peers, and which may contribute to internalizing problems. Girls' social orientation may contribute to their exposure to interpersonal stressors (Rose & Rudolph, 2006).

Parental Treatment and Socialization

The parental socialization literature suggests that parents accept greater levels of anger, assertiveness, and problematic behavior in boys, whereas they tend to encourage, reinforce, and respond more to girls' submissive emotions (e.g., sadness) and behaviors (Brody, 1999; Eisenberg, Cumberland, & Spinrad, 1998). Parents' differential treatment of sons and daughters appears to be subtle and outside their awareness, rather than overt, purposeful, or conscious (Eisenberg & Fabes, 1994; Fivush, 1989). Starting in their children's infancy, parents treat boys and girls differently in terms of modeling, instruction, training, and monitoring, although these interactions between child and parent are likely bidirectional (Leaper, 2002). Parents tend to enhance autonomy in sons, as compared with daughters, whereas daughters receive more physical affection in a manner that promotes relationships (Leaper, 2002). Parents also treat daughters and sons differently through their encouragement of sex-linked play. Fathers engage their sons via activity that is stimulating and physical in nature, whereas mothers more often interact with daughters in relational play involving shared activities (Leaper, 2002).

Parents also talk about affective experiences and use emotion words more often and in varied ways with daughters than with sons. Of particular importance to depression, parents discuss sadness more with girls and anger more with boys (Fivush, 1989); they accentuate the affective experience of emotions with girls, whereas the causes and consequences of emotions are highlighted for boys (Cervantes & Callanan, 1998); and they believe that girls are supposed to experience certain kinds of negative emotions (sadness, fear, and guilt), whereas boys are expected to display more anger (Brody & Hall, 1993). Mothers accept anger and physical retaliation more in toddler sons than daughters, but daughters are socialized more to resolve anger and to reestablish and to engage in damaged relationships (Fivush, 1989).

Sex Roles and Stereotypes

The real magnitude (i.e., effect size) in sex roles is relatively small (Hyde, 2005) and likely describe a subset of boys and girls who are at the tail end of a normally distributed sex role distribution. Still, it seems likely that these relatively atypical boys and girls at the ends of the sex role distribution may contribute to the formation and perpetuation of sex role stereotypes. In addition, those boys and girls who best represent the prototypic masculine and feminine traits, respectively, may be more likely to develop psychopathology.

Male sex role stereotypes include characteristics of competence and achievement denoted, for example, as "active," "aggressive," "athletic," "leader," and "assertive," whereas female sex role stereotypes include descriptions of their tendencies toward high levels of caring and involvement in relationships (e.g., "gentle," "sensitive," and "understanding"; Alfieri, Ruble, & Higgins, 1996; Bem, 1978). These sex role stereotypes begin early: Anger is viewed as a male characteristic, and sadness as a female feature, by the time of preschool (Karbon, Fabes, Carlo, & Martin, 1992). Moreover, traits that characterize the feminine stereotype (e.g., dependent, emotional, focused on relationships, helpless, passive) are most consistent with internalizing symptoms, whereas features of the male stereotype (active, assertive, independent, rational, self-motivated) are potentially more associated with externalizing problems (Hill & Lynch, 1983; Wichstrom, 1999).

DEVELOPMENTAL TIMELINE FOR THE EMERGENCE OF SEX DIFFERENCES IN DEPRESSION

Potential Sex Differences in Manifestation of Depression across Developmental Stages

Prior to delineating when the sex difference in depressive symptoms and disorders emerges, it is first important to evaluate and consider whether the construct or syndrome of depression is equivalent in boys and girls. This question can be broken down into subquestions:

1. Do clinically depressed boys and girls manifest the same depressive symptoms?
2. Is there a reporting bias in depression such that girls are more likely than boys to report or discuss depressive symptoms?
3. Do boys and girls respond to depression assessment measures equivalently?
4. Are the developmental pathways for depression similar for boys and girls?

Before reviewing the evidence available on these questions, we highlight the importance of these issues and call for more research to address them, because much of the research has been insufficiently rigorous and has produced inconclusive results. This means that the field has not been able to rule out rigorously the possibility that the sex difference in depression is not as real and as substantial as it is believed to be and portrayed. There is reason to suspect sex differences in symptom presentation at any particular developmental stage, as well as a potential reporting bias, because girls are socialized to express more sadness and to be more comfortable talking about sadness, whereas boys are socialized to inhibit expressions of sadness.

First, there is evidence showing that clinically depressed males and females exhibit a different pattern of depressive symptoms. Most of this evidence is based on adult samples (e.g., Angst & Dobler-Mikola, 1984; Frank, Carpenter, & Kupfer, 1988; Kornstein et al., 2000a; Silverstein, 2002). As compared with depressed men, depressed women tend to exhibit more anxiety, somatic complaints, hypersomnia, increased appetite and weight gain, fatigue, psychomotor retardation, and concerns about body image and physical appearance, although these exact symptom differences are not always found (Khan, Gardner, Prescott, & Kendler, 2002). There is little sex difference in functional impairment (Angst & Dobler-Mikola, 1984; Kornstein et al., 2000a). Fewer sex differences in symptoms are found among clinically depressed adolescents, although most studies have limited power, owing to small sample sizes (e.g., Kovacs, 2001; Mitchell, McCauley, Burke, & Moss, 1988; Roberts, Lewinsohn, & Seeley, 1995; Sorensen, Mors, & Thomsen, 2005). The largest study to date (Bennett, Ambrosini, Kudes, Metz, & Rabinovich, 2005) of clinically depressed adolescents found that adolescent girls reported more guilt, body image dissatisfaction, self-blame and disappointment, beliefs of failure, concentration difficulties, sadness/depressed mood, sleep problems, and fatigue, whereas boys reported more problems with anhedonia as well as diurnal variation (with greater levels of sadness and fatigue in the morning). Kovacs, Obrosky, and Sherrill (2003) followed their clinically referred sample of depressed children (49 girls and 38 boys) from age 10 to age 21 to examine this issue longitudinally. They found that girls were more likely to exhibit irritability during midadolescence, which then declined into adulthood, but most of the boys were consistently irritable throughout the follow-up; that girls were at greater risk for suicide in midadolescence, but boys during later adolescence; and that girls displayed more somatic symptoms than boys, and these complaints increased with age. Only negative body image and dysphoric mood displayed significant sex differences in manifestation equally across age (more typical among girls than boys).

Second, the issue of a possible reporting bias in willingness to discuss depressive symptoms has been examined indirectly. For example, the evidence that an equal proportion of adult men and women are likely to seek help or to be referred for treatment (Gater et al., 1998; Olfson, Zarin, Mittman, & McIntyre, 2001) has been inferred to mean that there is not a substantial sex difference in openness to report depression. We located no study that examined this issue among youth, so it remains an open question.

Third, males and females exhibit some differences in how they respond to assessments of depression (i.e., possibility of sex bias in measurement). The main issue is that the observed mean level sex difference found in certain symptoms or clusters of depression (e.g., anxious/somatic symptoms or concerns about body image) could be the result of a sex bias in reporting those symptoms rather than a true sex difference in depression manifestation. Data analytic methods, such as item response theory (IRT) and differential item functioning (DIF), can be used to differentiate the possible sex difference in manifestation of symptoms from the potential sex bias in measurement, yet few researchers have used them to examine this issue (Santor & Ramsay, 1998). In an examination of the Beck Depression Inventory (BDI) among depressed outpatient and nonpatient college samples, there was little evidence of a sex bias (Santor, Ramsay, & Zuroff, 1994), although some BDI items, especially the symptom concerning distorted body image, revealed a sex bias such that women were more likely to endorse it than men. A second study of a community sample of late adolescents (Hankin, Conrad, & Wang, 2006) examined this issue with the BDI and the Mood and Anxiety Symptoms Questionnaire (MASQ; Watson et al., 1995), which assesses both general distress and anhedonic symptoms of depression. This study found that boys were less likely to endorse some BDI items (sadness, episodes of crying, and change in body image), and other items were less likely to be endorsed by girls (insomnia, loss of appetite, and loss of weight). On the MASQ, boys were less likely to respond to the items indicating affective distress (e.g., felt sad, felt like crying, felt unattractive), whereas girls were less likely to respond to more behavioral/nonaffective items (e.g., felt really bored, felt as if it took extra effort to get started) and positively worded affective items (e.g., felt cheerful, felt as though I was having a lot of fun). It is important to note, however, that the sex difference in depression remained even after removing these potentially sex-biased items. Additional research examining the psychometric properties of depression assessments and possible sex-linked biases in responding is needed to evaluate this issue.

Fourth, there may be sex differences in depression manifestation over time in terms of developmental pathways (i.e., homotypic and heterotypic continuity). In their longitudinal research, Gjerde and colleagues (Gjerde, 1995; Block, Gjerde, & Block, 1991) showed that the manifestation and developmental antecedents of depressed mood may differ for boys and girls. Dysphoric boys expressed their unhappiness directly, whereas girls hid their unhappiness through introspection, greater self-preoccupation, and lack of direct hostility. Earlier in life, these dysphoric boys were described as undercontrolled and aggressive, whereas the girls tended to be oversocialized and overcontrolled. Rowe and colleagues (Rowe, Maughan, Pickles, Costello, & Angold, 2002) found that early oppositional behavior characterized a pathway that led to conduct disorder for boys, but depression for girls.

Finally, we highlight an additional methodological and conceptual difficulty in addressing whether depressive symptoms manifest themselves the same way in boys and girls. A significant complication is the fact that the symptoms and general syndrome of depression appear to change across development from preadolescence through adolescence (Weiss & Garber, 2003; Hankin & Abela, 2005). Thus, at present, the degree of continuity (either homotypic or heterotypic) in depression is uncertain, although the best available evidence is consistent with heterotypic continuity, such that depression is believed to be the same underlying construct across development despite some changes in manifest symptoms across development (e.g., anhedonia being less common in children but more prevalent starting in adolescence). As a result, the conundrum of establishing continuity in the syndrome of depression in general makes the investigation of potential sex differences in the manifestation of depression across development all the more difficult and complicated (e.g., presentation of depression in preadolescent girls versus boys and adolescent girls versus boys).

In sum, the available evidence suggests some small but replicable sex difference in the manifestation of depressive symptoms among youth and adults. However, the relatively small size of these differences in a few symptoms suggests that although the overall sex difference in depression is a real phenomenon, further research would help to determine the degree to which the sex difference in the manifestation and measurement of these particular symptoms affects the overall strength of the sex difference in depression across age.

Emergence of Sex Differences in Depression

We selectively focus our review on relatively large, community-based samples, in contrast to smaller convenience samples or psychiatric and clinically referred samples that are less representative and exhibit greater comorbidity (Newman et al., 1996). Overall, depressed mood is fairly common during adolescence, particularly among adolescent girls, with the likelihood of depressed mood ranging between 25 and 40% for girls and between 20 and 35% for boys (Petersen et al., 1993). Prospective longitudinal studies from preadolescence to young adulthood show that girls' depressive symptoms and depressed mood increase after age 13, whereas boys' symptoms and mood remain relatively constant or increase at a lower rate than girls' (Angold, Erkanli, Silberg, Eaves, & Costello, 2002; Petersen, Sarigiani, & Kennedy, 1991; Ge, Lorenz, Conger, Elder, & Simons, 1994; Cole, Martin, Peeke, Seroczynski, & Fier, 1999; Wade, Cairney, & Pevalin, 2002). Twenge and Nolen-Hoeksema (2002), in a meta-analytic review of self-reported symptoms, found this same pattern: Girls' depressive symptoms increased starting at age 13, whereas boys' levels of depressive symptoms remained relatively stable during adolescence.

Cross-sectional studies of children and adolescents provide evidence that more girls than boys are diagnosed with clinical depression after age 13 (Lewinsohn, Hops, Roberts, Seeley, & Andrews, 1993; Silberg et al., 1999; Angold, Costello, & Worthman, 1998). Prospective community studies indicate that more girls than boys show clinical depression beginning after age 13 (Cohen, Cohen, Kasen, & Velez, 1993; Costello, Mustillo, Erkanli, Keeler, & Angold, 2003; Hankin et al., 1998; Reinherz, Giaconia, Lefkowitz, Pakiz, & Frost, 1993; Weissman, Warner, Wickramaratne, Moreau, & Oflson, 1997). For example, one study (Hankin et al., 1998) showed that both boys and girls became increasingly more depressed between the ages of 15 and 18 (from 3 to 17%), and this increase was greater for girls (from 4 to 23%) than for boys (from 1 to 11%).

In addition to age as a developmental index, pubertal development and timing have also been studied as factors that may affect the time when more girls become depressed than boys (Angold, Worthman, & Costello, 2003; Hayward & Sanborn, 2002). Pubertal development (measured by Tanner stages) predicted the emergence of the sex difference in depression better than age: Girls reported increased rates of depressive disorders after Tanner Stage III (Angold et al., 1998). Regarding pubertal timing, most studies find that early puberty in girls, but not boys, is linked with elevated depression (e.g., Ge, Conger, & Elder, 1996; Graber, Lewinsohn, Seeley, & Brooks-Gunn, 1997; Paikoff, Brooks-Gunn, & Warren, 1991; but see Angold, et al.,1998, for contrary evidence). Stice, Presnell, and Bearman (2001) showed that body dissatisfaction, dieting, and high body mass partially explained why early puberty is linked with depression in girls. Still, it is worth noting that early pubertal timing is a complex phenomenon resulting from various biological, social, and contextual factors: Genetics and environmental influences (e.g., nutrition and exercise) affect pubertal timing (Hayward, 2003). However, Crick and Zahn-Waxler (2003) note that researchers must look beyond only a biological examination to understand the role of puberty in onset of depression. For example, maternal depression contributes to early puberty in daughters (Ellis & Garber, 2000).

Other research has examined whether ethnicity influences the unfolding of the sex difference in depression. One study (Kistner, David, & White, 2003) found that boys were more depressed than girls among African American youth (grades 3–5), whereas European American girls were more depressed than boys. Yet other studies (Schraedley, Gotlib, & Hayward, 1999; Siegel, Aneshensel, Taub, Cantwell, & Driscoll, 1998; Twenge & Nolen-Hoeksema, 2002) found that Hispanic adolescents reported the greatest level of depressed mood, as compared with European Americans or African Americans, but that there was no significant interaction between ethnicity and sex in predicting depressed mood. Hayward, Gotlib, Schraedley, and Litt (1999) found that menarche was associated with depressed mood only among European American girls, not among Hispanic or African American girls. Thus, these few studies highlight the need for further research on how ethnicity may influence the sex difference in depression.

Sex Differences and Comorbidity of Depression with Other Psychopathologies

It is well known that depression co-occurs with other common emotional and behavioral symptoms and problems. A comprehensive review of comorbidity is beyond the scope of this chapter (see Avenevoli, Knight, Kessler, & Merikangas, Chapter 2, this volume; Angold, Costello, & Erkanli, 1999); briefly, some of the most common comorbidities occur between depression, anxiety, externalizing behaviors such as attention-deficit/hyperactivity disorder (ADHD) and conduct disorder (CD), and eating disorders. In this section we review how sex influences the co-occurrence of depression with these psychopathologies and whether there are sex-linked developmental trajectories linking these comorbid conditions.

Overall, Rutter and colleagues (2003) have argued that the sex difference in psychopathology can be roughly categorized: Early-onset psychiatric disorders, such as ADHD, CD, autism, and language disorders, are more prevalent among boys, whereas adolescent-onset emotional disorders, such as depression, eating disorders, and anxiety, are more prevalent among girls. As a general rule describing the prototypic onset of these disorders and their association with sex, this dichotomy is accurate, yet it may obscure the investigation of issues important for advancing a more complete understanding of the development of the sex difference in depression. It is important to study the early onset of problems in girls and the later onset of symptoms in boys that may not fit into the prototypic pattern. Moreover, there may be important prodromal indicators and developmental precursors of problems in both boys and girls that are less likely to be noticed because they are subsyndromal and thus not diagnosed. As we discuss in greater detail later in the chapter, there has been increasing theoretical and empirical attention to the preadolescent precursors of the sex difference in depression (e.g., Keenan & Hipwell, 2005; Zahn-Waxler, 2000), and this line of research centers on subtle and early predictors of depression well before the substantial surge of depression among adolescent girls. A focus on only *when* the sex difference in modal patterns of marked, diagnosable syndromes occurs may obscure the study of early signs and predictors of problems.

Comorbidity of depression and anxiety is more common among girls than boys (Lewinsohn, Rohde, & Seeley, 1995). Prospective community studies (Cohen et al., 1993; Cole et al., 1999; Lewinsohn, Gotlib, Lewinsohn, Seeley, & Allen, 1998; Reinherz et al., 1993; Pine, Cohen, Gurley, Brook, & Ma, 1998) show that more girls than boys have an anxiety disorder, and the anxiety disorder often precedes the onset of a depressive disorder. In particular, certain anxiety disorders, including generalized anxiety disorder and panic disorder, tend to precede depression, especially in early adolescence and among girls (Parker & Hadzi-Pavlovic, 2004). Moreover, co-occurrence of depression with more than one anxiety disorders tends to occur primarily among girls (Parker & Hadzi-Pavlovic, 2004). Taken together, these results suggest that there may be a developmental pathway for girls from anxiety to depression.

In contrast, more boys than girls show overt, physically aggressive, externalizing behaviors (Loeber & Keenan, 1994; Keiley, Bates, Dodge, & Pettit, 2000; Moffitt, Caspi, Rutter, & Silva, 2001; Rutter et al., 2003). The co-occurrence of depression with disruptive behavioral problems (CD and oppositional defiant disorder) was found to be more likely among clinically depressed boys than girls (Rohde, Lewinsohn, & Seeley, 1991), and this likelihood holds longitudinally over time (Kovacs, Obrosky, & Sherrill, 2003). Yet the sex difference in aggression seems to diminish when both indirect/relational and direct/physical aggression are considered (Crick et al., 1999). Starting in preschool, girls show more indirect aggressive behaviors (e.g., threatening to end a friendship unless demands are met; retaliating by socially excluding others) than boys within interpersonal relationships (Crick & Grotpeter, 1995; Crick et al., 1999).

More adolescent girls than boys have been diagnosed with lifetime histories of eating disorders (Lewinsohn et al., 1993; Steiner & Lock, 1998). There is evidence that eating disorders co-occur among clinically depressed girls more than boys (Rohde et al., 1991) and that depressed girls, but not boys, are at elevated risk for developing eating disorders as they become young adults (Kovacs et al., 2003).

ETIOLOGICAL FACTORS AND CONCEPTUAL MODELS

Evaluating Proposed Causal Explanations for the Sex Difference in Depression

Prior to reviewing the various possible explanations for the emerging sex difference in depression, it is important to note that no comprehensive theory of depression has been offered that adequately accounts for the multiple facets of depression, including when and why sex differences in depression emerge. Multiple processes (i.e., equifinality and multifinality) likely contribute to the development of sex differences in depression. This review focuses on extant research examining those factors that may explain why the sex difference in depression emerges during early adolescence. Other factors may contribute to the sex difference in depression at different points during the lifespan. For example, gender role inequality in marital relationships may explain why more adult women are depressed than men (Strazdins, Galligan, & Scannell, 1997), but this association would not account for why more girls start becoming depressed around midpuberty. Similarly, factors associated with the emergence of the sex difference in depression may be developmentally specific to adolescence and may not apply to adults.

The potential range of studies to be reviewed is immense and beyond the scope of this chapter. In theory, any factor that has been shown to predict depression could be relevant for understanding why more girls are depressed than boys. We limited our focus to those major depression vulnerabilities and stressors that have received sufficient theoretical and empirical attention and for which there is a reasonable basis to expect a potential sex difference. We organized our review around mediational and moderational models when possible. We start by reviewing what *mediation* and *moderation* mean (Baron & Kenny, 1986), specifically in reference to understanding the sex difference in youth depression.

Mediation indicates that (1) there is a sex difference in levels of depression, (2) there is a sex difference in levels of a given etiological factor, (3) the factor leads to depression, and (4) the association between sex and depression is accounted for (i.e., reduced) by the mediating variable. Manipulating the mediating variable (e.g., by lowering levels of the etiological factor through intervention) would provide further support that this mediator explains the sex difference in depression, because reducing the etiological factor directly would result in lowered levels of depression. Most of the research conducted to date has examined only one mediating factor, even though it is most likely that multiple mediators may be involved as part of a developmental causal chain leading to the emerging sex difference in depression. Moreover, many studies that we reviewed did not conduct the appropriate mediational analyses, so it is unknown whether hypothesized factors account for the sex difference in depression. It is recommended that future studies conduct mediational analyses to evaluate whether a hypothesized factor or mechanism truly accounts for the sex difference in depression.

Moderation signifies that the association between depression and a causal factor varies as a function of sex (e.g., the strength of the relationship between depression and an etiological factor may be stronger in girls than in boys). Moderating variables, by themselves, cannot explain why the sex difference in depression occurs, because moderation indicates that the association between depression and an explanatory factor varies by level of sex (Baron & Kenny, 1986). Several of the studies we reviewed reported how sex moderated the association between a particular factor and depression and then suggested that this statistical interaction supported an *explanation* for why girls are more depressed than boys. However, obtaining a significant interaction between sex and a factor does not necessarily qualify as support for an explanation of the sex difference in depression, because moderation indicates several different possible patterns between sex and the factor (could hold for one sex but not the other, or the strength of the association is stronger for boys or girls). Additional research would still be required to elucidate why (i.e., the processes, mediation) a particular association is stronger among girls than boys (the moderation effect) in order to provide an explanation for the sex difference in depression.

Complicating any etiological explanation is the timing of a hypothesized mediating or moderating factor. A complete explanation of the sex difference in depression needs to account for the developmental unfolding of causal factors over time that leads to girls becoming more depressed than boys at about age 13. A comprehensive account of the *emergence* of the sex difference in depression around age 13 (or Tanner Stage III) would specify whether there is a developmental rise in the mediating variable occurring prior to or at about the same time that girls become depressed. Further, a mediating or moderating variable may vary along a temporal dimension from more distal to more proximal. A distal factor can mediate the sex difference in depression, but other more proximal factors need to be incorporated to explain why girls become more depressed at a particular developmental time point (age 13). For example, demonstrating that childhood abuse mediates the sex difference in depression constitutes an important finding, but this by itself may not provide a comprehensive explanation, because childhood abuse is likely a more distal factor (especially if the abuse occurred early in childhood). Further research would still need to explicate the other more proximal mediating factors in the developmental pathway occurring closer in time to when girls begin to become more depressed.

It is important to consider how different mediating and moderating variables may fit together in a larger etiological developmental pathway from childhood into young adulthood. A mediating factor may interact with a moderating factor so that the particular mediating factor predicts increases in depression more strongly for some individuals than others. For example, stressors may mediate the sex difference in depression, but early pubertal onset may moderate the association between sex and stressors. In this example, then, a subset of girls (those going through puberty early) is at especially high risk for experiencing stressors, and these early pubertal girls may account for a substantial portion of the sex difference in depression. Unfortunately, most of the research to date has, at best, examined only one mediating mechanism or one moderating variable in isolation to explain the sex difference in depression. Future research needs to expand beyond simple, one-factor explanations of the sex difference in depression to a more developmentally sensitive, transactional model with various mediating and moderating factors and pathways. Given the current state of knowledge, we next review the different, isolated explanatory constructs and mechanisms intended to account for the rise of depression in girls.

Stressors

Research suggests that stressors precede and predict depression (Grant, Compas, Thurm, McMahon, & Gipson, 2004). The association between stressors and depression can be broken down into four conceptually different models: stress exposure, reactivity, generation, and depression contagion.

Stress Exposure

The stress exposure hypothesis is a mediational model in, that girls experience more stressors than boys, and as a result, become more depressed. Data from multiple studies support this model and show that adolescent girls report more stressors overall than boys (e.g., Allgood-Merten, Lewinsohn, & Hops, 1990; Davies & Windle, 1997; Ge et al., 1994; Graber, Brooks-Gunn, & Warren, 1995; Hankin, Mermelstein, & Roesch, 2007). Girls also report more interpersonal stressors, including peers, romantic partners, and family members, whereas boys experience more achievement and self-relevant stressors (Gore et al., 1993; Hankin et al., 2007; Larson & Ham, 1993; Leadbeater, Blatt, & Quinlan, 1995; Rudolph, 2002; Rudolph & Hammen, 1999; Shih, Eberhart, Hammen, & Brennan, 2006; Towbes, Cohen, & Glyshaw, 1989; Wagner & Compas, 1990; Windle, 1992). The sex difference in adolescent depression is mediated, at least in part, by adolescent girls' greater exposure to interpersonal peer (Liu & Kaplan, 1999; Hankin et al., 2007; Rudolph, 2002; Rudolph & Hammen, 1999; Shih et al., 2006) and family (Davies & Windle, 1999) stressors.

Stress Reactivity

The stress reactivity hypothesis is a moderational model, in that girls are expected to exhibit greater levels of depression than boys in response to stressors. Evidence is somewhat consistent, but more mixed, with this model. Some studies find that adolescent girls respond to general stressors with greater depression than boys (Achenbach, Howell, & McConaughy, 1995; Ge et al., 1996; Hankin et al., 2007; Marcotte, Fortin, Potvin, & Papillon, 2002; Rudolph, 2002; Schraedley et al., 1999; Shih et al., 2006; see review by Grant et al., 2006), whereas others have not found a sex difference in stress reactivity (Burt, Cohen, & Bjorck, 1988; Cauce, Hannan, & Sargeant, 1992; Larson & Ham, 1993; Leadbeater, Kuperminc, Blatt, & Hertzog, 1999; Wagner & Compas, 1990). To interpersonal stressors, girls respond with higher levels of depressive symptoms, as compared with boys (Goodyer & Altham, 1991; Hankin et al., 2007; Moran & Eckenrode, 1991; Leadbeater et al., 1995; Shih et al., 2006), whereas boys react to school stressors with higher depression than girls (Sund, Larsson, & Wichstrom, 2003).

An important consideration is *why* girls may react to stressors with elevated depression, as compared with boys. It is likely that certain vulnerabilities, especially those risks (e.g., genetic, cognitive, etc.) that girls have more than boys, may help account for girls' greater stress reactivity. These vulnerabilities are reviewed later in the chapter.

Stress Generation

The stress generation hypothesis is a transactional model that suggests that characteristics of the individual youth (e.g., elevated depression, temperament/personality traits) precede and contribute to increases in the experience of stressors, called "dependent" stressors (Hammen, 1991). Stress generation theories suggest that interpersonal, dependent stressors are most typically experienced in adolescence, especially among girls (Hankin & Abramson, 2001; Rudolph, 2002). The few studies available show that girls experience more dependent stressors than boys (Hankin et al., 2007; Rudolph & Hammen, 1999; Rudolph, 2002), but less research has examined whether depressive symptoms are associated with future dependent stressors (see Shih et al., 2006, for evidence with young adults). Among youth, a three-wave prospective study examined the longitudinal direction of effects between depressive symptoms and contextually coded stressors in different developmentally salient domains over a 1-year follow-up (Hankin et al., 2007). Evidence for stress generation was observed: Initial depressive symptoms at baseline significantly predicted future increases in romantic stressors and overall dependent stressors. In contrast, evidence was also observed for the stress exposure model: Initial levels of independent, peer, and general interpersonal stressors predicted prospective increases in depressive symptoms over time. Taken together, these findings show that there are sex differences in different domains of stressors (e.g., peer and romantic) and stressor type (independent and dependent), but the longitudinal associations between depressive symptoms and stressors is not simple and straightforward. It is important to consider the particular stress model (e.g., generation and exposure) to understand more fully how stressors help to explain the sex difference in depression because the longitudinal direction of effects varies, depending on the stressor type and domain.

Depression Contagion

The depression contagion model pertains to the "contagion" of depression between adolescents and others in the context of an interpersonal relationship. Research shows a temporal synchrony between mothers' and daughters' depressive episodes (e.g., Hammen, Burge, & Adrian, 1991) and depressive symptoms between youth and parents longitudinally over time (e.g., Abela, Skitch, Adams, & Hankin, 2006). Other research has found that depressive symptoms among adolescents' best friends prospectively predict adolescents' own reported depressive symptoms (Hogue & Steinberg, 1995; Stevens & Prinstein, 2005), especially among girls (Prinstein, Borelli, Cheah, Simon, & Aikins, 2005). Depression in a parent (typically studied among mothers; see Goodman & Tully, Chapter 17, this volume) is a significant context for stressors. Girls, as compared with boys, of depressed mothers are more likely to develop anxiety and depression (Boyle & Pickles, 1997; Conger et al., 1993; Cummings, DeArth-Pendley, Du-Rocher-Schudlich, & Smith, 2001; Sheeber, Davis, & Hops, 2002). Furthermore, girls' greater reactivity to mothers' depression exhibits effects over time; maternal depression prospectively predicts later depression among girls but not boys (Davies & Windle, 1997; Duggal, Carlson, & Sroufe, & Egeland, 2001; Fergusson, Horwood, & Lynskey, 1995). Finally, girls react to family discord and conflict with greater depression as compared with boys (Crawford, Cohen, Midlarsky, & Brook, 2001; Essex, Klein, Cho, & Kraemer, 2003).

Child Abuse and Maltreatment as Severe Negative Events

The vast majority of studies examining abuse have utilized samples of adults who have retrospectively reported on these abusive events. There is little discernible retrospective bias in recalling abusive experiences or bias affecting reports of depression (Brewin, Andrews, & Gotlib, 1993; Maughan & Rutter, 1997). Depressed mood and depressive disorders are more likely to be reported among adults retrospectively reporting childhood abuse (see Harkness & Lumley, Chapter 19, this volume). Sex differences in child abuse also exist, especially in childhood sexual abuse (CSA) (Cutler & Nolen-Hoeksema, 1991; Levitan et al., 1998). A meta-analysis (Rind, Tromovitch, & Bauserman, 1998) of adults retrospectively recalling CSA concluded that 14% of men and 27% of women reported CSA. There is some evidence that CSA mediates the sex difference in depression (Whiffen & Clark, 1997). In this study, only childhood abuse, but not further adult victimization, was associated with depression. However, most of the studies of adults retrospectively recalling abusive experiences do not clearly consider *when* the abuse occurred as a potential factor. Given the importance of and interest in studying childhood maltreatment as a potential explanation of the sex difference in depression, especially its emergence in early adolescence, it will be important for future studies to indicate whether and how age influences any associations between abuse, sex, and depression, because abuse experienced early in childhood may serve as a more distal, rather than proximal, mediator.

Cognitive Vulnerabilities

There are various cognitive vulnerabilities (Abela & Hankin, Chapter 1, this volume), and some research has examined potential sex differences in these cognitive factors. The corpus of research has focused on a negative cognitive, or attributional, style (Abramson, Metalsky, & Alloy, 1989), dysfunctional attitudes (Beck, 1987), rumination (Nolen-Hoeksema, 1991), and interpersonal dependency/sociotropy (Blatt & Zuroff, 1992).

Among adult samples, women tend to score higher than men on measures of negative attributional/cognitive style (Angell et al., 1999; Nolen-Hoeksema, Larson, & Grayson, 1999), whereas men exhibit more dysfunctional attitudes than women (Angell et al., 1999; Gotlib, 1984; Haeffel et al., 2003). Women are more likely than men to ruminate in response to sad or anxious moods (Roberts, Gotlib, & Kassel, 1996; Mezulis, Abramson, & Hyde, 2002; Nolen-Hoeksema et al., 1999; Tamres, Janicki, & Helgeson, 2002). Women display higher scores than men on some measures of sociotropy (Leadbeater et al., 1995; McBride, Bacchiochi, & Bagby, 2005; Shih et al., 2006). Among adolescents, the evidence is consistent with the adult studies. Girls exhibit more cognitive vulnerability than boys on measures assessing a negative cognitive style (Hankin & Abramson, 2002; Hankin, 2006), rumination (Broderick, 1998; Hankin, 2006; Schwartz & Koenig, 1996; Ziegert & Kistner, 2002), whereas boys display more dysfunctional attitudes than girls (Hankin, 2006). Girls are more cognitively vulnerable in interpersonal domains than boys (Bandura, Pastorelli, Barbaranelli, & Caprara, 1999; Leadbeater et al., 1995, 1999). The research with children appears to be less consistent, such that sex differences in these cognitive vulnerabilities often are not observed (Abela, 2001; Abela, Brozina, & Haigh, 2002; Abela, Vanderbilt, & Rochon, 2004). This suggests the possibility that girls may become more cognitively vulnerable to depression than boys, starting in early adolescence, with such vulnerability lasting throughout adulthood. Indeed, a meta-analysis showed that girls exhibit a more negative attributional style than boys that starts in early adolescence and continues in adulthood (Mezulis, Abramson, Hyde, & Hankin, 2004).

Research examining mediational models shows that a negative cognitive style among adolescents (Hankin & Abramson, 2002), rumination among youth (Grant et al., 2004; Schwartz & Koenig, 1996) and adults (Nolen-Hoeksema et al., 1999), and interpersonal/social-evaluative concerns (Rudolph & Conley, 2005) partially explain why more girls are depressed than boys. Shih et al. (2006) found that female young adults with high interpersonal dependency experienced more dependent interpersonal stressors and that this stress generation effect partially mediated the association between sociotropy and depression among women. Among girls transitioning into high school, a greater interpersonal orientation was associated with increases in depressive symptoms after their experiencing interpersonal stressors (Little & Garber, 2004). Adolescent girls' negative interpretations of their peer experiences predicted future levels of depression (Prinstein & Aikins, 2004; Prinstein, Cheah, & Guyer, 2005; Quiggle, Garber, Panak, & Dodge, 1992).

Cognitive theories postulate different domains of vulnerability, and a particularly important domain for understanding the sex difference in depression is beliefs about physical attractiveness and body image (Hankin & Abramson, 2001). There is a marked sex difference in perceptions of physical appearance, and it occurs prior to the emergence of the sex difference in depression (Harter, 1999; Kostanski & Gullone, 1998). Cross-sectional (Kostanski & Gullone, 1998) and longitudinal (Cole, Martin, Peeke, Seroczynski, & Hoffman, 1998) research shows that beliefs about physical unattractiveness predicted depressed mood for girls more than boys, but mediation was not reported. Other research conducting mediational analyses demonstrates that girls' excessive body dissatisfaction partially explains the sex difference in depressive symptoms (Allgood-Merten et al., 1990; Wichstrom, 1999).

Adolescent girls have more cognitive vulnerability to depression than boys, but how do girls develop such cognitive risk factors? We note two possible mechanisms, although there are certainly others. First, adolescent girls are more likely to experience negative events, especially interpersonal stressors, than adolescent boys. Researchers have hypothesized that individuals confronted with repeated occurrences of negative life events in a wide variety of domains should develop a more stable, global attributional style for negative events over time, and hence increases in cognitive vulnerability to depression (e.g., Coyne & Whiffen, 1995; Just, Abramson, & Alloy, 2001; Rose & Abramson, 1991). Thus, girls' greater likelihood of experiencing negative events, especially during the transition from early to middle adolescence, may contribute to their greater cognitive vulnerability to depression, which may become more depressogenic around early adolescence (Mezulis et al., 2004). Second, females encode life events involving emotional memory, but not nonemotional memory, in more detail than males (Seidlitz & Diener, 1998; Davis, 1999). Parents discuss emotional material in more detail with their daughters than with their sons, and mothers discuss sadness in longer and more detailed conversations with daughters. Females having greater cognitive vulnerability than males may be the result, in part, of parents' sex-linked socialization practices and girls' encoding negative events in more emotional detail than boys. Girls' negative beliefs about themselves, their world and future may be more accessible and more tightly interconnected in associative cognitive networks linked with affective nodes.

Emotion and Temperament

An extensive literature grounded in temperament and personality research has identified three broad, innate temperamental traits that may be relevant to psychopathology: positive affectivity, negative affectivity, and disinhibition (Clark, 2005). Higher levels of negative affectivity and reduced levels of positive affectivity predict the development of depression (see, e.g., Caspi, Moffitt, Newman, & Silva, 1996; Krueger, 1999; Lonigan, Phillips, & Hooe, 2003); disinhibition has not been shown to have strong and reliable associations with depression. However, fewer studies have explicitly reported sex differences in these temperament dimensions. Some research shows age and sex differences in both negative and positive affectivity, such that adolescent girls exhibit less positive affectivity and greater negative affectivity than adolescent boys, with little sex difference during childhood (e.g., Jacques & Mash, 2004; Lonigan, Hooe, David, & Kistner, 1999), whereas other research shows sex differences in negative, but not positive, affectivity (Chorpita, Plummer, & Moffitt, 2000).

In addition to these temperament dimensions, other emotion constructs have been proposed as risks for depression, some of which may exhibit a sex difference (Keenan & Hipwell, 2005). First, theoretically, excessive empathy may predispose a person to the development of depression, so that individuals who experience high levels of empathy are more likely to take on others' problems as if they were their own, causing them to experience feelings of guilt and responsibility, placing them at risk for depression (Zahn-Waxler, 2000). Starting in early childhood, girls demonstrate higher levels of empathy and prosocial behavior than boys (Zahn-Waxler, Cole, & Barrett, 1991; Eisenberg & Fabes, 1998). Cross-sectional research shows that scores on an excessive empathy questionnaire uniquely predicted depressive symptoms (Robins & Hinkley, 1989), although no prospective longitudinal study has tested this association from childhood into adolescence. Second, girls demonstrate higher levels of compliance than boys as early as the toddler period and extending throughout childhood (see, e.g., Briggs-Gowan, Carter, Moye Skuban, & McCue Horwitz, 2001; Kochanska, Coy, & Murray, 2001; Mistry, Vanderwater, Huston, & McLoyd, 2002). Excessive compliance is associated with internalizing symptoms in children (e.g., Grant & Compas, 1995; Kochanska et al., 2001), although the evidence is predominantly indirect and there is a lack of prospective research in this area. Third, deficits in emotion regulation (i.e., over- or underregulation of emotion) may serve as distal risk factors for the development of internalizing disorders (John & Gross, 2004; Chaplin & Cole, 2005). Specifically, individuals who suppress negative emotions (e.g., sadness, anger) are at an increased risk of experiencing depressive symptoms (Zeman, Shipman, & Suveg, 2002; Penza-Clyve & Zeman, 2002), have low levels of well-being and life satisfaction, and are more pessimistic about their future (Gross & John, 2003). Research also indicates the presence of sex differences in emotion regulation. Girls demonstrate higher levels of regulation of negative emotions (e.g., anger) as compared with boys (e.g., Cole, Zahn-Waxler, & Smith, 1994; Underwood, Hurley, Johanson, & Mosley, 1999; Durbin & Shafir, Chapter 7, this volume; Chaplin & Cole, 2005).

Biological Factors

Genetics

The evidence is mixed with respect to sex differences in heritability estimates for depression. Some studies find no differences in adulthood (e.g., Lyons et al., 1998; Kendler & Prescott, 1999) or childhood/adolescence (Eaves et al., 1997; Rutter, Silberg, O'Connor, & Siminoff, 1999), whereas others have revealed mean level heritability differences (Bierut et al., 1999; Jacobson & Rowe, 1999; Kendler, Gardner, Neale, & Prescott, 2001; Tambs, Harris, & Magnus, 1995). Silberg and colleagues (Silberg et al., 1999; Silberg,

Rutter, & Eaves, 2001) found that genetic influences had a larger effect on the emergence of depression among postpubertal adolescent girls who had experienced stress and that the stability of depression was more genetically mediated for these girls than for boys. All of these studies employed behavioral genetic designs, and given the limitations that accompany behavioral genetics (i.e., investigation of abstract, nonspecific, latent genetic influence; see Rutter, Moffitt, & Caspi, 2006; Lau & Eley, 2006; Chapter 6, this volume), it will be important to investigate potential sex differences in measured genes using molecular genetics techniques.

Sex Hormones

The evidence for hormonal explanations is mixed, although mostly negative. Little evidence supports the hypothesis that rising hormonal levels (e.g., progesterone, estrogen) mediate the sex difference in depression (see Bebbington, 1998, for a review). Brooks-Gunn and Warren (1989) found that the effect of estradiol was minimal as compared with the influence of social factors (negative life events) in predicting depressed mood among girls (ages 10–14). Moreover, Susman's research (Susman, Inoff, Germain, Nottlemann, & Loriaux, 1987; Susman, Dorn, & Choursos, 1991) found that there was no sex difference in sex hormones or cortisol levels and that estradiol was not associated with depressive affect, so these sex hormones could not mediate the sex difference in depression. Despite little support for mediation, these hormones could affect boys and girls differently (i.e., moderation). Susman and colleagues (1991) found that boys reporting higher levels of negative affect had lower testosterone and higher androstenedione levels, whereas girls with higher levels of negative affect had higher levels of testosterone and lower levels of dehydroepiandrosterone sulfate (DHEAS). Angold, Costello, Erklani, and Worthman (1999) found that testosterone and estradiol were associated with depression in an all-girls sample, but moderation could not be tested because boys were not included. Taken together, these results suggest that different gonadal and adrenal hormones may provide some limited risk for later negative affect for boys and girls, separately (Brooks-Gunn, Graber, & Paikoff, 1994).

Cortisol

Results from adult studies examining the biological stress response of the HPA axis have shown increases in the stress hormone, cortisol, among depressed individuals as compared with controls (Thase, Jindal, & Howland, 2002), yet similar research with depressed adolescents has not found HPA axis dysfunction or elevations of cortisol, as compared with controls (Dahl, Kaufman, Ryan, & Perel, 1992; Dorn, Burgess, Susman, & von Eye, 1996). Although most studies (e.g., Birmaher, Rabin, Garcia, & Jain, 1994; Goodyer et al., 1996; Susman et al., 1987, 1991) have found comparable cortisol levels for boys and girls, and thus mediation seems unlikely, other research using uncertain and challenging conditions found evidence for increased cortisol levels and higher emotional distress in girls, as compared with boys (Susman, Dorn, Inoff-Germain, Nottlemann, & Chrousos, 1997). In a longitudinal study of children, girls exhibited higher cortisol levels than boys, and elevated cortisol predicted greater depressive and anxiety symptoms 18 months later in girls only (Smider et al., 2002). Other research showed that depressed girls exhibited a flattened diurnal rhythm, whereas normal controls and depressed youth with comorbid externalizing problems displayed the expected diurnal pattern of early morning cortisol elevations and a significant decline throughout the day (Klimes-Dougan,

Hastings, Granger, Usher, & Zahn-Waxler, 2001). Thus, the evidence for cortisol and biological stress reactivity as an explanation for sex differences in depression is intriguing but mixed.

In summary, existing studies of biological explanations have provided equivocal evidence that sex hormones or cortisol levels mediate the sex difference in depression (see Hayward & Sanborn, 2002; Seeman, 1997; Steiner et al., 2003, for other reviews). Hormonal changes, by themselves, are not likely to lead to significant alterations in mood or poor adjustment (Buchanan, Eccles, & Becker, 1992). The mixed evidence may be due to several factors. Many of the studies conducted to date have utilized small sample sizes, so the lack of statistically significant sex differences may result from a lack of statistical power. Moreover, most of the studies have considered only simple linear models in which hormonal changes directly influence depressive symptoms or negative affect (Brooks-Gunn et al., 1994), although it is unlikely that such a direct hormonal model would capture the complexity of the hormonal system. Brooks-Gunn and colleagues (1994) highlight the interdependencies among hormones and indicate that it may not be appropriate to consider independent effects of specific hormones. They recommend a transactional model involving bidirectional effects between hormonal changes, negative affect, pubertal timing, and social events to examine how hormones and other factors may influence negative affect.

Integrated Conceptual Models of the Sex Difference in Youth Depression

As noted earlier, there are few theoretical models that have been proposed to integrate coherently the various etiological influences contributing to the sex difference in depression in children and adolescents. In this section, we summarize the central conceptual models, review the available empirical research in support of them, and discuss each theory briefly.

Nolen-Hoeksema and Girgus (1994) were the first to review systematically the literature on etiological factors underlying the emergence of the sex difference in depression. Their seminal review stimulated the field and advanced knowledge by organizing previously disparate etiological factors into three coherent and distinct conceptual models. The first model proposes that although the same factors cause depression in both boys and girls, girls experience an increase in these factors in early adolescence, whereas boys do not. The second model suggests that the causes of depression are different for boys and girls, and that in early adolescence the causes of depression in females become more prevalent than the causes of depression in males. The third model follows a vulnerability–stress framework. Girls exhibit greater risk for depression than boys in childhood, but it is not until early adolescence, when girls experience additional stressors, that their greater levels of risks for depression interact with the increase in stressors to contribute to elevated levels of depression among girls.

After reviewing evidence from various literatures, Nolen-Hoeksema and Girgus (1994) concluded that the available evidence best supported the third model, but there was little direct evidence to support this assertion. Support for this model was based on the individual effects of different etiological constructs, what the authors framed as personality characteristics, biological challenges, and social challenges. Unfortunately, at the time their article was published, the interaction of personality and biological factors with the challenges of adolescence had not been studied directly. Since then, much of the research reviewed earlier in this chapter lends support to aspects of their third model (e.g., sex differences in rumination, social challenges, and stressors, including sexual abuse). However, few studies exist that have sought to test any of the three models in totality (but see Seiffge-Krenke & Stemmler, 2002, for a comprehensive test of their models); rather, the preponderance of the supporting evidence is based on individual aspects of their vulnerability–stress model. To adequately test the third model, longitudinal data using repeated measures of many vulnerabilities and stressors would be required, spanning childhood through the adolescent transition and into adulthood, when the sex difference grows.

Similar to Nolen-Hoeksema and Girgus's (1994) third model, *Cyranowski, Frank, Young, and Shear (2000)* propose that females possess an interpersonally oriented vulnerability that interacts with particular negative life events to contribute to higher levels of depression. Females' vulnerability consists of a high affiliative focus, low attachment security, high anxiety, and low instrumentality. When girls with this vulnerability encounter stressors, especially those that have interpersonal consequences, they are likely to become depressed. More distally, insecure parental attachments, anxious or inhibited temperaments, and low instrumental coping skills can lead to a more difficult transition into adolescence, especially for girls. Difficulty with this transition can produce increased anxiety, which, when combined with traditional female gender socialization and the hormonal changes of puberty (especially the increased release of oxytocin in females), can lead to an increase in affiliative need for girls (the basis of their vulnerability).

One study (Stemmler & Peterson, 2005) tested this model using growth curve modeling and found that the risk factors, such as insecure parental attachment, low instrumental coping skills, an anxious or inhibited temperament, and early physical maturation, differentiated the development of adolescents' emotional tone, or level of positive/negative affect. Results of other research, reviewed earlier, such as girls (as compared with boys) encountering more interpersonal stressors, exhibiting more fearful temperament, and displaying more anxiety, are all consistent with this theory.

Another related model is *Taylor et al. (2000)* bioevolutionary theory, although it is not specifically formulated to explain the sex difference in depression. Taylor and colleagues postulate that females possess a stress response different from the traditional male response of "fight or flight." The female stress response, as a result of biological and behavioral differences, is better characterized as "tend and befriend." Females are more apt to "tend" to relationships and act in ways that will protect themselves and their offspring, thus improving the likelihood that these traits will be passed on to future generations. Furthermore, females are more likely to "befriend" and to create social networks that provide resources, safety, and support under conditions of stress. Like Cyranowski et al.'s (2000) model, this framework highlights the role of oxytocin as a primary mechanism underlying these biobehavioral differences. Oxytocin is related to the attachment–caregiving system that underlies the theory (Taylor et al., 2000). This model holds promise for understanding why more girls become depressed than boys, especially from an interpersonal and biobehavioral perspective, but because it was not formulated to explain the ontogeny of depression, no research has yet examined whether the hypothesized processes are associated with depression or can explain the sex difference in depression.

Hankin and Abramson (2001) proposed an elaborated cognitive vulnerability–transactional stress model. They argued that a general depression model, based on existing and empirically supported depression theories, could be elaborated and expanded to include developmentally sensitive influences that improve the understanding of why more girls become depressed than boys. They emphasized the scientific goal of parsimony—

having a general theory capable of explaining disparate research findings (e.g., the sex difference in depression), rather than postulating sex-specific theories of depression (i.e., one model for boys, another for girls).

They stated that females encounter more negative life events than males and that this increase in stressors leads to elevations in depressed mood. Females exhibit more cognitive vulnerabilities to depression (e.g., negative cognitive style, rumination, negative cognitions about perceptions of physical attractiveness) than males. Females' greater cognitive vulnerability enhances the likelihood that they will experience depression when they encounter negative events, consistent with existing cognitive vulnerability–stress theories (Abela & Hankin, Chapter 1, this volume).

In addition, they elaborated on the traditional vulnerability–stress model to incorporate developmentally sensitive factors that may explain why girls encounter more stressors and exhibit more negative cognitive vulnerabilities. Girls are hypothesized to possess more distal preexisting vulnerabilities, such as genetic influences, temperament/personality factors, and environmental adversities like childhood maltreatment, and these contribute to girls' greater proximal vulnerabilities and exposure to stressors. Moreover, the traditional vulnerability–stress model was expanded to include initial negative affect and stress generation processes in the proximal etiological chain. Most individuals are expected to experience initial elevations in general negative affect (e.g., anger, anxiety, sad mood, frustration, etc.) after experiencing stressors, but depression is hypothesized to result more specifically when individuals possess cognitive vulnerabilities. The inclusion of initial negative affect may account for the observed comorbidity of depression; exposure to stressors is a general risk factor for the development of many psychopathologies, but cognitive vulnerabilities are hypothesized to be depression-specific risks, such that they moderate the likelihood that the initial negative affect after a stressor will progress to full-blown depression, specifically. Finally, the model incorporates a transactional stress generation mechanism, consistent with interpersonal models of depression (e.g., Hammen, 1991; Joiner & Coyne, 1999). As levels of depression rise, it is hypothesized that they will contribute to the generation of additional stressors, particularly in interpersonal contexts.

Evidence reviewed earlier in the chapter is consistent with many of the tenets of this theory. Girls exhibit greater cognitive vulnerabilities (e.g., negative cognitive style, rumination, negative beliefs and perceptions of physical attractiveness) than boys. Girls encounter more stressors (overall, interpersonal, and dependent) than boys. There may be a sex difference in genetic risk, so that girls may exhibit stronger heritability to depression than boys, particularly starting in adolescence. Finally, girls experience more of the hypothesized distal risk factors (e.g., maltreatment, such as sexual abuse, and perhaps negative emotionality) than boys. However, no published research has directly tested more than one component of the model at a time, so it is uncertain how well it explains the sex difference.

Keenan and Hipwell (2005) propose a framework to identify preadolescent precursors to individual differences in risk for depression in girls. In contrast to the other conceptual models that emphasize etiological influences primarily during adolescence, their model mostly focuses on sex differences in childhood. The authors extend previous theories on sex differences in depression, specifically building on the theoretical foundation provided by Zahn-Waxler and colleagues (Zahn-Waxler et al., 1991; Zahn-Waxler, 2000), and identify three constructs that may function, either singularly or in combination, as preadolescent precursors to depression: excessive empathy, compliance, and overregulation of emotions. The authors use a vulnerability–stress perspective in which these three factors act as the vulnerability and the psychological onset of puberty acts as a stressor in the development of depression. The results reviewed earlier in this chapter support these factors as putative vulnerabilities.

In addition to these preadolescent vulnerabilities, Keenan and Hipwell (2005) postulate two contexts, family conflict and maternal depression, that may trigger depression in girls. The evidence reviewed earlier is consistent with this aspect of their model as well. The presence of stressors may affect girls differently and at different times, and certain stressors may even be causally related to the precursors to depression.

This model is relatively new, so understandably there is no specific test of it. The theory is particularly innovative and has great potential for advancing knowledge about the preadolescent precursors that may contribute to more girls becoming depressed than boys.

TREATMENT AND PREVENTION

Most of the available literature on the effects of sex on interventions is based on research with adults, so we review this evidence briefly and highlight pertinent research with youth when available. Treatment studies have not found evidence for substantial sex differences in response to treatment (Garfield, 1994; Sinha & Rush, 2006; Zlotnick, Elkin, & Shea, 1998). For example, the National Institute of Mental Health's Treatment of Depression Collaborative Research Program (Zlotnick et al., 1998) shows that the depressed patient's sex did not affect the process or outcome of treatment (psychotherapy or pharmacotherapy). Still, most past studies were not designed to examine sex differences in treatment.

Among children and adolescents, the largest treatment outcome study to date is the Treatment for Adolescents with Depression Study (Treatment for Adolescents with Depression Study [TADS] Team, 2004), and the influence of sex was not reported. As this is the largest efficacy study of depression in youth, it has the greatest power to examine sex as a potential moderator of effects (psychotherapy or pharmacotherapy). Other investigators have suggested that group-based treatment of depression that includes only girls may be more effective than mixed-sex groups, and studies have been initiated to test the efficacy of psychosocial interventions in all-girls groups (Stark et al., 2006). For example, Stark and his colleagues have evaluated the effects of group-based cognitive-behavioral therapy (CBT) for clinically depressed girls only and reported remarkable success in their efficacy trial. To our knowledge, only one study has examined all-girl groups versus coed groups (Chaplin et al., 2006), and it was found that all-girl groups were better at reducing hopelessness and increasing girls' therapy attendance, although no differences were found between groups for reducing depressive symptoms (both types of group significantly reduced depression). Thus, the influence of sex on outcome in efficacy trials among youth and the sexual composition of group-based interventions are important areas for research.

With respect to antidepressant medication, the Institute of Medicine (2001) highlighted that little is known about potential sex differences in pharmacokinetics and pharmacodynamics, both of which are highly relevant to understanding possible sex differences in treatment with antidepressant medication. The available studies show that adult women are more likely than men to be diagnosed with atypical depression, and as a result, tend to be prescribed tricyclic antidepressants, whereas men more often receive selective serotonin reuptake inhibitors (SSRIs; Yonkers, Kando, & Cole, 1992). Women show a more potent response to sertraline than imipramine, whereas men respond better to imipramine (Kornstein, et al., 2000b). These results may be related to sex differences in the metabolism of sertraline (Ronfeld, Tremaine, & Wilner, 1997). A different study found that men and women had equal responses to fluoxetine and tricyclic antidepressants, but women responded better to monoamine oxidase (MAO) inhibitors (Quitkin, Stewart, & McGrath, 2002).

Results from two meta-analyses (Horowitz & Garber, 2006; Merry, McDowell, Hetrick, Bir, & Muller, 2004) of prevention studies of depression among youth reveal somewhat conflicting findings regarding possible sex differences. Merry and colleagues reported that boys had reduced depressive symptoms scores immediately after intervention, whereas girls did not; no sex data were reported for any follow-ups. In contrast to findings for depressive symptoms, prevention results for depressive disorder show that girls responded to intervention immediately after prevention but boys did not. Horowitz and Garber (2006) found that prevention studies with a greater percentage of girls in the samples showed larger effect sizes at immediate postintervention but no sex effect at follow-up. The reasons for this discrepancy in sex effects for depressive symptoms versus disorder are unclear. It is recommended that future research include individual difference characteristics, especially age and sex, as potential moderators of the effects of interventions, so as to improve our understanding of whether and how these affect interventions for individual youth.

SUMMARY, FUTURE DIRECTIONS, AND BROAD ISSUES CONFRONTING THE FIELD

In summary, it is clear that many robust results have been found and replicated in the field. It is now fairly well established that more girls than boys begin to become depressed starting in early adolescence (ages 12–13 or middle puberty). From an early age, there is a sex difference in social and emotional factors that is seen in both normal and abnormal development. On the average, girls tend to be more interpersonally oriented and emotionally focused than boys (see also Rose & Rudolph, 2006). This sex difference in girls' greater socioemotional orientation can be seen in many of the findings reviewed here. As compared with boys, girls experience more stressors, especially interpersonal peer events; girls ruminate and coruminate; girls exhibit more cognitive vulnerabilities to depression; girls exhibit more socially submissive emotions (e.g., fear and sadness) and are less likely to deny these affects; girls display stronger affiliative needs and have more intimate, emotional social relationships in which they are more invested; and girls exhibit higher levels of oxytocin, a hormone that enhances caregiving. Many of the etiological conceptual models highlight various aspects of this general sex difference, although each of the causal theories emphasizes different variations of girls' greater socioemotional vulnerability. Girls' relatively greater socioemotional orientation may contribute to some of the differences in manifestation of depressive symptoms (e.g., girls reporting more sadness and body image concerns).

Clearly, much has been learned in the past several decades about sex difference in normal and abnormal development, yet to advance understanding of why more girls than boys become depressed at a particular developmental point, more research is required. In this final section, we discuss some broad issues that could enhance research and present opportunities for future study.

First, in regard to methodology, we encourage all investigators to report findings (means and standard deviations) on all central variables separately by sex, even if there is no significant sex difference (see also the recommendation by the Institute of Medicine, 2001). Many published articles in the depression and normal child development literatures have statistically controlled for sex and removed any potential influence of sex on effects. This practice implies that sex is a nuisance variable to be controlled. However, we suggest that the practice is unwise for at least two reasons. First, meta-analyses of sex differences of different constructs often reveal small effect size differences that may not be statistically significant in individual studies with small to modest sample sizes (Hyde, 2005). By not reporting central findings separately by sex, the accrual of knowledge is impeded and makes a cumulative science, via meta-analysis, substantially more difficult. Second, conceptually, sex differences should not be viewed merely as a nuisance to be controlled statistically but, rather, as an opportunity for studying causal processes that can illuminate the complex etiological influences contributing to depression (Hankin & Abramson, 2001; Rutter et al., 2003). Understanding why more girls than boys become depressed can provide vital clues as to why individuals in general develop depression. Some of the sex differences in vulnerabilities and contextual developmental changes that may be relevant for explaining the sex difference in depression can provide windows that offer potentially important insights into the etiology of depression more broadly. By evaluating and reporting potential sex differences routinely in research, even when they are not the primary focus of a study, the field may unearth new and unexpected findings that can advance knowledge in this area.

Second, in regard to statistics, we recommend that investigators conduct appropriate mediational and moderational analyses to test properly and rigorously their hypotheses and theoretical models. Practically, this means conducting research with samples of both boys and girls, as opposed to a unisex sample, so that the appropriate statistical analyses can be conducted. Moreover, integrating multiple etiological factors, as opposed to single variable explanations, in combination with examination of more complex models that involve both mediation and moderation at different points along the developmental pathway, would be more informative and contribute more substantially to understanding the sex difference in depression. Testing these more complicated models can be accomplished with recent data analytic innovations (see, e.g., Collins & Sayer, 2001; Curran & Willoughby, 2003) as well as conceptual and statistical advancements in developmental pathways (Pickles & Hill, 2006).

Third, with respect to theory, we believe there are areas of research that to date have received less attention, but may provide important advances in understanding the developmental pathways leading to the sex difference in depression. First, developmental psychopathological research and theory suggest that the causes of depression may be different in children versus adolescents and adults irrespective of sex (e.g., Duggal et al., 2001; Jaffee, Moffitt, & Caspi, 2002; Hankin & Abela, 2005). Moreover, as reviewed earlier in this chapter, there is a switch in the sex difference in depression such that more boys are depressed than girls in childhood, and then more girls become depressed than boys starting in early adolescence. These findings suggest that the etiological influences in prepubertal-onset depression (predominantly more boys) versus postpubertal-onset depression (preponderance of girls) may be different. Existing theories do not address these potentially different pathways very well. The fact that the direction of the sex difference in depression switches at about the same time (i.e., early adolescence) that the some of the general causal factors contributing to depression are changing is suggestive and potentially informative. Second, the apparent sex-linked developmental unfolding of patterns of sequential comorbidity of depression, especially girls showing increased levels of anxiety in childhood and anxiety preceding and predicting later depression, is another area ripe for future research. What accounts for this sex-linked developmental pathway of comorbid patterns in depression? Is the likely heterotypic continuity from anxiety to depression stronger for girls than boys? Third, an emphasis on developmental pathways should include investigation of both the manifest symptomatic presentation of depression as well as the underlying causal processes contributing to depression over time. Taking the possible developmental pathway from anxiety to depression as an example, it is unknown whether the apparent pathway is the result of (1) an overlapping symptom manifestation (e.g., broad negative affect is common to both anxiety and depression; Clark & Watson, 1991), (2) similar etiological influences (e.g., shared genetic liability to experience broad negative affects of anxiety and depression [Thapar & McGuffin, 1997] or exposure to stressors contributing to emotional distress [Hankin & Abramson, 2001]), or (3) both manifest symptom and latent etiological influences. As noted earlier, there is some sex difference in the manifestation of depressive symptoms, and addressing this issue from a developmental pathways perspective could shed needed light on the reasons. Finally, it is important to integrate the many potential explanatory influences into a coherent developmental psychopathological model of the sex difference in youth depression. Some have postulated a sex-specific model (e.g., Keenan & Hipwell, 2005; Zahn-Waxler, 2000), whereas others have argued for a general depression model that posits factors that highlight sex differences (e.g., Hankin & Abramson, 2001). It will be interesting and informative for future research to evaluate these theories' hypotheses to ascertain whether sex-specific or general depression models more accurately explain why more girls become depressed in adolescence. It may be the case that both approaches are correct at different points along development trajectories. Perhaps the sex-specific preadolescent precursors to depression predominate in childhood and the general depression etiologic influences prevail in adolescence and beyond. We look forward to future conceptual and empirical advancements in the study of sex differences in depression that address the normal and abnormal development of such differences.

REFERENCES

Abela, J. R. Z. (2001). The hopelessness theory of depression: A test of the diathesis–stress and causal mediation components in third and seventh grade children. *Journal of Abnormal Child Psychology, 29*(3), 241–254.

Abela, J. R. Z., Brozina, K., & Haigh, E. P. (2002). An examination of the response styles theory of depression in third- and seventh-grade children: A short-term longitudinal study. *Journal of Abnormal Child Psychology, 30*(5), 515–527.

Abela, J. R. Z., Skitch, S. A., Adams, P., & Hankin, B. L. (2006). The timing of parent and child depression: A hopelessness theory perspective. *Journal of Clinical Child and Adolescent Psychology, 35*(2), 253–263.

Abela, J. R. Z., Vanderbilt, E., & Rochon, A. (2004). A test of the integration of the response styles and social support theories of depression in third and seventh grade children. *Journal of Social and Clinical Psychology, 23*(5), 653–674.

Abramson, L. Y., Metalsky, G. I., & Alloy, L. B. (1989). Hopelessness depression: A theory-based subtype of depression. *Psychological Review, 96*, 358–372.

Achenbach, T. M., Howell, C. T., & McConaughy, S. H. (1995). Six-year predictors of problems in a national sample of children and youth: II. Signs of disturbance. *Journal of the American Academy of Child and Adolescent Psychiatry, 34*(4), 488–498.

Alfieri, T., Ruble, D. N., & Higgins, E. T. (1996). Gender stereotypes during adolescence: Developmental changes and the transition to junior high school. *Developmental Psychology, 32*(6), 1129–1137.

Allgood-Merten, B., Lewinsohn, P. M., & Hops, H. (1990). Sex differences and adolescent depression. *Journal of Abnormal Psychology, 99*(1), 55–63.

Angell, K. E., Abramson, L. Y., Alloy, L. B., Hankin, B. L., Hogan, M. E., Whitehouse, W. G., et al. (1999, November). *Gender differences in dysphoria and etiological factors: Ethnic variations.* Paper presented at the 33rd Annual Meeting of the Association for Advancement of Behavior Therapy, Toronto, Canada.

Angold, A., Costello, E. J., & Erkanli, A. E. (1999). Comorbidity. *Journal of Child Psychology and Psychiatry, 40*(1), 57–87.

Angold, A., Costello, E., Erkanli, A., & Worthman, C. (1999). Pubertal changes in hormone levels and depression in girls. *Psychological Medicine, 29*(5), 1043–1053.

Angold, A., Costello, E. J., & Worthman, C. M. (1998). Puberty and depression: The roles of age, pubertal status and pubertal timing. *Psychological Medicine, 28*(1), 51–61.

Angold, A., Erkanli, A., Silberg, J., Eaves, L., & Costello, J. E. (2002). Depression scale scores in 8–17-year-olds: Effects of age and gender. *Journal of Child Psychology and Psychiatry, 43*(8), 1052–1063.

Angold, A., Worthman, C., & Costello, E. J. (2003). Puberty and depression. In C. Hayward (Ed.), *Gender differences at puberty* (pp. 137–164). New York: Cambridge University Press.

Angst, J., & Dobler-Mikola, A. (1984). Do the diagnostic criteria determine the sex ratio in depression? *Journal of Affective Disorders, 7,* 189–198.

Bandura, A., Pastorelli, C., Barbaranelli, C., & Caprara, G. V. (1999). Self-efficacy pathways to childhood depression. *Journal of Personality and Social Psychology, 76,* 258–269.

Baron, R. M., & Kenny, D. A. (1986). The moderator–mediator variable distinction in social psychological research: Conceptual, strategic, and statistical considerations. *Journal of Personality and Social Psychology, 51*(6), 1173–1182.

Bebbington, P. E. (1998). Sex and depression. *Psychological Medicine, 28,* 1–8.

Beck, A. T. (1987). Cognitive models of depression. *Journal of Cognitive Psychotherapy, 1,* 5–37.

Bem, A. (1978). *Social behavior: Fact and falsehoods about common sense, hypnotism, obedience, altruism, beauty, racism, and sexism.* Oxford, UK: Nelson-Hall.

Bennett, D. S., Ambrosini, P. J., Kudes, D., Metz, C., & Rabinovich, H. (2005). Gender differences in adolescent depression: Do symptoms differ for boys and girls? *Journal of Affective Disorders, 89,* 35–44.

Bierut, L. J., Heath, A. C., Bucholz, K. K., Dinwiddie, S. H., Madden, P. A. F., Statham, D. J., et al. (1999). Major depressive disorder in a community-based twin sample: Are there different genetic and environmental contributions for men and women? *Archives of General Psychiatry, 56*(6), 557–563.

Birmaher, B., Rabin, B., Garcia, M., & Jain, U. (1994). Cellular immunity in depressed, conduct disorder, and normal adolescents: Role of adverse life events. *Journal of the American Academy of Child and Adolescent Psychiatry, 33*(5), 671–678.

Blatt, S. J., & Zuroff, D. C. (1992). Interpersonal relatedness and self-definition: Two prototypes for depression. *Clinical Psychology Review, 12*(5), 527–562.

Block, J. H., Gjerde, P. H., & Block, J. H. (1991). Personality antecedents of depressive tendencies in 18-year-olds: A prospective study. *Journal of Personality and Social Psychology, 60*(5), 726–738.

Boyle, M. H., & Pickles, A. (1997). Maternal depressive symptoms and ratings of emotional disorder symptoms in children and adolescents. *Journal of Child Psychology and Psychiatry, 38*(8), 981–992.

Brewin, C. R., Andrews, B., & Gotlib, I. H. (1993). Psychopathology and early experience: A reappraisal of retrospective reports. *Psychological Bulletin, 113*(1), 82–98.

Briggs-Gowan, M. J., Carter, A. S., Moye Skuban, E., & McCue Horwitz, S. (2001). Prevalence of social-emotional and behavioral problems in a community sample of 1- and 2-year-old children. *Journal of the American Academy of Child and Adolescent Psychiatry, 40*, 811–819.

Broderick, P. C. (1998). Early adolescent gender differences in the use of ruminative and distracting coping strategies. *Journal of Early Adolescence, 18*, 173–191.

Brody, L. R. (1985). Conceptualizing gender in personality theory and research. *Journal of Personality, 53*(2), 102–149.

Brody, L. R. (1999). *Gender, emotion, and the family.* Cambridge, MA: Harvard University Press.

Brody, L. R., & Hall, J. A. (1993). Gender and emotion. In M. Lewis & J. M. Haviland (Eds.), *Handbook of emotions* (pp. 447–460). New York: Guilford Press.

Brody, L. R., & Hall, J. A. (2000). Gender, emotion, and expression. In M. Lewis & J. M. Haviland-Jones (Eds.), *Handbook of emotions* (2nd ed., pp. 325–414). New York: Guilford Press.

Brooks-Gunn, J., Graber, J., & Paikoff, R. (1994). Studying links between hormones and negative affect: Models and measures. *Journal of Research on Adolescence, 4*(4), 469–486.

Brooks-Gunn, J., & Warren, M. (1989). Biological and social contributions to negative affect in young adolescent girls. *Child Development, 60*(1), 40–55.

Buchanan, C. M., Eccles, J. S., & Becker, J. B. (1992). Are adolescents the victims of raging hormones? Evidence for activational effects of hormones on moods and behavior at adolescence. *Psychological Bulletin, 111*, 62–107.

Buhrmester, D. (1996). Need fulfillment, interpersonal competence, and the developmental contexts of early adolescent friendship. In W. M. Bukowski, A. F. Newcomb, & W. W. Hartup (Eds.), *The company they keep: Friendship in childhood and adolescence* (pp. 158–185). New York: Cambridge University Press.

Buhrmester, D., & Furman, W. (1987). The development of companionship and intimacy. *Child Development, 58*(4), 1101–1113.

Burt, C. E., Cohen, L. H., & Bjorck, J. P. (1988). Perceived family environment as a moderator of young adolescents' life stress adjustment. *American Journal of Community Psychology, 16*(1), 101–122.

Caspi, A., Moffitt, T. E., Newman, D. L., & Silva, P. A. (1996). Behavioral observations at age 3 years predict adult psychiatric disorders. *Archives of General Psychiatry, 53*, 1033–1039.

Cauce, A. M., Hannan, K., & Sargeant, M. (1992). Life stress, social support, and locus of control during early adolescence: Interactive effects. *American Journal of Community Psychology, 20*(6), 787–798.

Cervantes, C. A., & Callanan, M. A. (1998). Labels and explanations in mother–child emotion talk: Age and gender differentiation. *Developmental Psychology, 34*, 88–98.

Chaplin, T. M., & Cole, P. M. (2005). The role of emotion regulation in the development of psychopathology. In B. L. Hankin & J. R. Z. Abela (Eds.), *Development of psychopathology: A vulnerability–stress perspective* (pp. 49–74). Thousand Oaks, CA: Sage.

Chaplin, T. M., Gillham, J. E., Reivich, K., Elkon, A. G. L., Samuels, B., Freres, D. R., et al. (2006). Depression prevention for early adolescent girls: A pilot study of all girls versus co-ed groups. *Journal of Early Adolescence, 26*(1), 110–126.

Chorpita, B. F., Plummer, C. M., & Moffitt, C. E. (2000). Relations of tripartite dimensions of emotion to childhood anxiety and mood disorders. *Journal of Abnormal Child Psychology, 28*, 299–310.

Cicchetti, D. (2006). Development and psychopathology. In D. Cicchetti & D. J. Cohen (Eds.), *Developmental psychopathology: Vol. 1. Theory and method* (2nd ed., pp. 1–23). Hoboken, NJ: Wiley.

Cicchetti, D., & Rogosch, F. A. (2002). A developmental psychopathology perspective on adolescence. *Journal of Consulting and Clinical Psychology, 70*(1), 6–20.

Clark, L. A. (2005). Temperament as a unifying basis for personality and psychopathology. *Journal of Abnormal Psychology, 114*(4), 505–521.

Clark, L. A., & Watson, D. (1991). Tripartite model of anxiety and depression: Psychometric evidence and taxonomic implications. *Journal of Abnormal Psychology, 100,* 316–336.

Cohen, P., Cohen, J., Kasen, S., & Velez, C. N. (1993). An epidemiological study of disorders in late childhood and adolescence: I. Age and gender specific prevalence. *Journal of Child Psychology and Psychiatry and Allied Disciplines, 34,* 851–867.

Coie, J. D., & Dodge, K. A. (1998). Aggression and antisocial behavior. In W. Damon & N. Eisenberg (Eds.), *Handbook of child psychology: Vol. 3. Social, emotional, and personality development* (5th ed., pp. 779–862). Hoboken, NJ: Wiley.

Cole, D. A., Martin, J. M., Peeke, L. A., Seroczynski, A. D., & Fier, J. (1999). Children's over- and underestimation of academic competence: A longitudinal study of gender differences, depression, and anxiety. *Child Development, 70*(2), 459–473.

Cole, D. A., Martin, J. M., Peeke, L. G., Seroczynski, A. D., & Hoffman, K. (1998). Are cognitive errors of underestimation predictive or reflective of depressive symptoms in children?: A longitudinal study. *Journal of Abnormal Psychology, 107*(3), 481–496.

Cole, P. M., Zahn-Waxler, C., & Smith, K. D. (1994). Expressive control during disappointment: Variations related to preschoolers' behavior problems. *Developmental Psychology, 30,* 835–846.

Collins, L. M., & Sayer, A. G. (2001). *New methods for the analysis of change.* Washington, DC: American Psychological Association.

Conger, R. D., Conger, K. J., Elder, G. H., Lorenz, F. O., Simons, R. L., & Whitbeck, L. B. (1993). Family economic stress and adjustment of early adolescent girls. *Developmental Psychology, 29*(2), 206–219.

Costello, E. J., Mustillo, S., Erkanli, A., Keeler, G., & Angold, A. (2003). Prevalence and development of psychiatric disorders in childhood and adolescence. *Archives of General Psychiatry, 60*(8), 837–844.

Coyne, J. C., & Whiffen, V. E. (1995). Issues in personality as diathesis for depression: The case of sociotropy-dependency and autonomy-self-criticism. *Psychological Bulletin, 118,* 358–378.

Crawford T. N., Cohen, P., Midlarsky, E., & Brook, J. S. (2001). Internalizing symptoms in adolescents: Gender differences in vulnerability to parental distress and discord. *Journal of Research on Adolescence, 11*(1), 95–118.

Crick, N. R. (1997). Engagement in gender normative versus nonnormative forms of aggression: Links to social-psychological adjustment. *Developmental Psychology, 33*(4), 610–617.

Crick, N. R., & Grotpeter, J. K. (1995). Relational aggression, gender, and social-psychological adjustment. *Child Development, 66*(3), 710–722.

Crick, N. R., Werner, N. E., Casas, J. F., O'Brien, K. M., Nelson, D. A., Grotpeter, J. K., et al. (1999). Childhood aggression and gender: A new look at an old problem. In D. Bernstein (Ed.), *Gender and motivation: Nebraska Symposium on Motivation* (pp. 75–141). Lincoln: University of Nebraska Press.

Crick, N. R., & Zahn-Waxler, C. (2003). The development of psychopathology in females and males: Current progress and future challenges. *Development and Psychopathology, 15,* 719–742.

Cross, S. E., & Madson, L. (1997). Models of the self: Self-construals and gender. *Psychological Bulletin, 122,* 5–37.

Cummings, E. M., DeArth-Pendley, G., Du-Rocher-Schudlich, T., & Smith, D. A. (2001). Parental depression and family functioning: Toward a process-oriented model of children's adjustment. In S. R. H. Beach (Ed.), *Marital and family processes in depression: A scientific foundation for clinical practice* (pp. 89–110). Washington, DC: American Psychological Association.

Curran, P. J., & Willoughby, M. T. (2003). Implications of latent trajectory models for the study of developmental psychopathology. *Development and Psychopathology, 15*(3), 581–612.

Cutler, S. E., & Nolen-Hoeksema, S. (1991). Accounting for sex differences in depression through female victimization: Childhood sexual abuse. *Sex Roles, 24,* 425–438.

Cyranowski, J. M., Frank, E., Young, E., & Shear, K. (2000). Adolescent onset of the gender difference in lifetime rates of major depression. *Archives of General Psychiatry, 57,* 21–27.

Dahl, R., Kaufman, J., Ryan, N., & Perel, J. (1992). The dexamethasone suppression test in children and adolescents: A review and a controlled study. *Biological Psychiatry, 32*(2), 109–126.

Davies, P. T., & Windle, M. (1997). Gender-specific pathways between maternal depressive symptoms, family discord, and adolescent adjustment. *Developmental Psychology, 33*(4), 657–668.

Davis, P. J. (1999). Gender differences in autobiographical memory for childhood emotional experiences. *Journal of Personality and Social Psychology, 76,* 498–510.

Dorn, L., Burgess, E., Susman, E., & von Eye, A. (1996). Response to oCRH in depressed and nondepressed adolescents: Does gender make a difference? *Journal of the American Academy of Child and Adolescent Psychiatry, 35*(6), 764–773.

Duggal, S., Carlson, E. A., Sroufe, L. A., & Egeland, B. (2001). Depressive symptomatology in childhood and adolescence. *Development and Psychopathology, 13*(1), 143–164.

Eaves, L. J., Silberg, J. L., Maes, H. H., Simonoff, E., Pickles, A., Rutter, M., et al. (1997). Genetics and developmental psychopathology: II. The main effects of genes and environment on behavioral problems in the Virginia Twin Study of Adolescent Behavioral Development. *Journal of Child Psychology and Psychiatry, 38*(8), 965–980.

Eisenberg, N., Cumberland, A., & Spinrad, T. L. (1998). Parental socialization of emotion. *Psychological Inquiry, 9*(4), 241–273.

Eisenberg, N., & Fabes, R. A. (1994). Mothers' reactions to children's negative emotions: Relations to children's temperament and anger behavior. *Merrill Palmer Quarterly, 40,* 138–156.

Eisenberg, N., & Fabes, R. A. (1998). Prosocial development. In W. Damon & N. Eisenberg (Eds.), *Handbook of child psychology: Vol. 3. Social, emotional, and personality development* (pp. 701–778). Hoboken, NJ: Wiley.

Ellis, B. J., & Garber, J. (2000). Psychosocial antecedents of variation in girls' pubertal timing: Maternal depression, stepfather presence, and marital and family stress. *Child Development, 71*(2), 485–501.

Else-Quest, N. M., Hyde, J. S., Goldsmith, H. H., & Van Hulle, C. A. (2006). Gender differences in temperament: A meta-analysis. *Psychological Bulletin, 132,* 33–72.

Essex, M. J., Klein, M. H., Cho, E., & Kraemer, H. C. (2003). Exposure to maternal depression and marital conflict: Gender differences in children's later mental health symptoms. *Journal of the American Academy of Child and Adolescent Psychiatry, 42*(6), 728–737.

Fergusson, D. M., Horwood, J. L., & Lynskey, M. T. (1995). Maternal depressive symptoms and depressive symptoms in adolescents. *Journal of Child Psychology and Psychiatry, 36*(7), 1161–1178.

Fivush, R. (1989). Exploring sex differences in the emotional content of mother–child conversations about the past. *Sex Roles, 20,* 675–691.

Frank, E., Carpenter, L. L., & Kupfer, D. J. (1988). Sex differences in recurrent depression: Are there any that are significant? *American Journal of Psychiatry, 145,* 41–45.

Furman, W., & Buhrmester, D. (1992). Age and sex differences in perceptions of networks of personal relationships. *Child Development, 63,* 103–115.

Garfield, S. L. (1994). Research on client variables in psychotherapy. In A. E. Bergin & S. L. Garfield (Eds.), *Handbook of psychotherapy and behavior change* (4th ed., pp. 190–228). Oxford, UK: Wiley.

Gater, R., Tansella, M., Korten, A., Tiemens, B. G., Maureas, V. G., & Olatawura, M. O. (1998). Sex differences in the prevalence and detection of depressive and anxiety disorders in general health care settings: Report from the World Health Organization collaborative study on psychological problems in general health care. *Archives of General Psychiatry, 55*(5), 405–413.

Ge, X., Conger, R. D., & Elder, G. H. (1996). Coming of age too early: Pubertal influences on girls' vulnerability to psychological distress. *Child Development, 67,* 3386–3400.

Ge, X., Lorenz, F. O., Conger, R. D., Elder, G. H., & Simons, R. L. (1994). Trajectories of stressful life events and depressive symptoms during adolescence. *Developmental Psychology, 30*(4), 467–483.

Gjerde, P. F. (1995). Alternative pathways to chronic depressive symptoms in young adults: Gender differences in developmental trajectories. *Child Development, 66*(5), 1277–1300.

Goodyer, I. M., & Altham, P. M. (1991). Lifetime exit events and recent social and family adversities in anxious and depressed school-age children and adolescents: I. *Journal of Affective Disorders, 21*(4), 219–228.

Goodyer, I., Herbert, J., Altham, P., Pearson, J., Secher, S., & Shiers, H. (1996). Adrenal secretion during major depression in 8- to 16-year-olds: I. Altered diurnal rhythms in salivary cortisol and dehydroepiandrosterone (DHEA) at presentation. *PsychologicalMedicine, 26*(2), 245–256.

Gore, A., Aseltine, R. H., & Colten, M. E. (1993). Gender, social-relational involvement, and depression. *Journal of Research on Adolescence, 3*(2), 101–125.

Gotlib, I. H. (1984). Depression and general psychopathology in university students. *Journal of Abnormal Psychology, 93*(1), 19–30.

Graber, J. A., Brooks-Gunn, J., & Warren, M. P. (1995). The antecedents of menarcheal age: Heredity, family environment, and stressful life events. *Child Development, 66*, 346–359.

Graber, J. A., Lewinsohn, P. M., Seeley, J. R., & Brooks-Gunn, J. (1997). Is psychopathology associated with the timing of pubertal development? *Journal of the American Academy of Child and Adolescent Psychiatry, 36*, 1768–1776.

Grant, K. E., & Compas, B. E. (1995). Stress and anxious-depressed symptoms among adolescents: Searching for mechanisms of risk. *Journal of Consulting and Clinical Psychology, 63*, 1015–1021.

Grant, K. E., Compas, B. E., Thurm, A. E., McMahon, S. D., & Gipson, P. Y. (2004). Stressors and child and adolescent psychopathology: Measurement issues and prospective effects. *Journal of Clinical Child and Adolescent Psychology, 33*(2), 412–425.

Grant, K. E., Compas, B. E., Thurm, A. E., McMahon, S. D., Gipson, P. Y., Campbell, A. J., et al. (2006). Stressors and child and adolescent psychopathology: Evidence of moderating and mediating effects. *Clinical Psychology Review, 26*(3), 257–283.

Gross, J. J., & John, O. P. (2003). Individual differences in two emotion regulation processes: Implications for affect, relationships, and well-being. *Journal of Personality and Social Psychology, 85*, 348–362.

Haeffel, G. J., Abramson, L. Y., Voelz, Z. R., Metalsky, G. I., Halberstadt, L., Dykman, B. M., et al. (2003). Cognitive vulnerability to depression and lifetime history of Axis I psychopathology: A comparison of negative cognitive styles (CSQ) and dysfunctional attitudes (DAS). *Journal of Cognitive Psychotherapy, 17*(1), 3–22.

Hammen, C. (1991). The generation of stress in the course of unipolar depression. *Journal of Abnormal Psychology, 100*, 555–561.

Hammen, C., Burge, D., & Adrian, C. (1991). Timing of mother and child depression in a longitudinal study of children at risk. *Journal of Consulting and Clinical Psychology, 59*, 341–345.

Hankin, B. L. (2006). Adolescent depression: Description, causes, and interventions. *Epilepsy and Behavior, 8*(1), 102–114.

Hankin, B. L., & Abela, J. R. Z. (2005). Depression from childhood through adolescence and adulthood: A developmental vulnerability and stress perspective. In B. L. Hankin & J. R. Z. Abela (Eds.), *Development of psychopathology: A vulnerability–stress perspective* (pp. 245–288). Thousand Oaks, CA: Sage.

Hankin, B. L., & Abramson, L. Y. (1999). Development of gender differences in depression: Description and possible explanations. *Annals of Medicine, 31*, 372–379.

Hankin, B. L., & Abramson, L. Y. (2001). Development of gender differences in depression: An elaborated cognitive vulnerability–transactional stress theory. *Psychological Bulletin, 127*, 773–796.

Hankin, B. L., & Abramson, L. Y. (2002). Measuring cognitive vulnerability to depression in adolescence: Reliability, validity and gender differences. *Journal of Clinical Child and Adolescent Psychology, 31*(4), 491–504.

Hankin, B. L., Abramson, L. Y., Moffitt, T. E., McGee, R., Silva, P. A., & Angell, K. E. (1998).

Development of depression from preadolescence to young adulthood: Emerging gender differences in a 10-year longitudinal study. *Journal of Abnormal Psychology, 107*, 128–140.

Hankin, B. L., Conrad, K., & Wang, Z. (2006). *Sex differences in anhedonic and general domains
of depression: True differences or bias in measurement?* Unpublished manuscript.

Hankin, B. L., Mermelstein, R., & Roesch, L. (2007). Sex differences in adolescent depression:
Stress exposure and reactivity models in interpersonal and achievement contextual domains.
Child Development, 78, 279–295.

Harter, S. (1999). *The construction of the self: A developmental perspective.* New York: Guilford
Press.

Hayward, C. (2003). *Gender differences at puberty.* New York: Cambridge University Press.

Hayward, C., Gotlib, I. H., Schraedley, P. K., & Litt, I. F. (1999). Ethnic differences in the association between pubertal status and symptoms of depression in adolescent girls. *Journal of Adolescent Health, 25*(2), 143–149.

Hayward, C., & Sanborn, K. (2002). Puberty and the emergence of gender differences in psychopathology. *Journal of Adolescent Health, 30*(4), 49–58.

Hill, J. P., & Lynch, M. E. (1983). The intensification of gender-related role expectations during
adolescence. In J. Brooks-Gunn & A. Petersen (Eds.), *Girls at puberty: Biological and
psychosocial perspectives* (pp. 201–228). New York: Plenum Press.

Hogue, A., & Steinberg, L. (1995). Homophily of internalized distress in adolescent peer groups.
Developmental Psychology, 31(6), 897–906.

Horowitz, J. L., & Garber, J. (2006). The prevention of depressive symptoms in children and adolescents: A meta-analytic review. *Journal of Consulting and Clinical Psychology, 74*(3), 401–
415.

Hyde, J. S. (2005). The gender similarities hypothesis. *American Psychologist, 60*(6), 581–592.

Insel, T. R., & Fernald, R. D. (2004). How the brain processes social information: Searching for the
social brain. *Annual Review of Neuroscience, 27*, 697–722.

Institute of Medicine. (2001). *Exploring the biological contributions to human health: Does sex
matter?* Washington, DC: National Academy Press.

Jacobson, K., & Rowe, D. (1999). Genetic and environmental influences on the relationships
between family connectedness, school connectedness, and adolescent depressed mood: Sex differences. *Developmental Psychology, 35*(4), 926–939.

Jacques, H. A. K., & Mash, E. J. (2004). A test of the tripartite model of anxiety and depression in
elementary and high school boys and girls. *Journal of Abnormal Child Psychology, 32*(1), 13–
25.

Jaffee, S. R., Moffitt, T. E., & Caspi, A. (2002). Differences in early childhood risk factors for
juvenile-onset and adult-onset depression. *Archives of General Psychiatry, 59*(3), 215–222.

John, O. P., & Gross, J. J. (2004). Healthy and unhealthy emotion regulation: Personality processes, individual differences, and life span development. *Journal of Personality, 72*, 1301–
1333.

Joiner, T., & Coyne, J. C. (1999). *The interactional nature of depression: Advances in interpersonal
approaches.* Washington, DC: American Psychological Association.

Just, N., Abramson, L. Y., & Alloy, L. B. (2001). Remitted depression studies as tests of the cognitive vulnerability hypotheses of depression onset: A critique and conceptual analysis. *Clinical
Psychology Review, 21*, 63–83.

Karbon, M., Fabes, R. A., Carlo, G., & Martin, C. L. (1992). Preschoolers' beliefs about sex and
age differences in emotionality. *Sex Roles, 27*, 377–390.

Keenan, K., & Hipwell, A. E. (2005). Preadolescent clues to understanding depression in girls.
Clinical Child and Family Psychology Review, 8(2), 89–105.

Keiley, M. K., Bates, J. E., Dodge, K. A., & Pettit, G. S. (2000). A cross-domain growth analysis:
Externalizing and internalizing behaviors during 8 years of childhood. *Journal of Abnormal
Child Psychology, 28*(2), 161–179.

Kendler, K., Gardner, C., Neale, M., & Prescott, C. (2001). Genetic risk factors for major depression in men and women: Similar or different heritabilities and same or partly distinct genes? *Psychological Medicine, 31*(4), 605–616.

Kendler, K., & Prescott, C. (1999). A population-based twin study of lifetime major depression in men and women. *Archives of General Psychiatry, 56*(1), 39–44.

Keyes, C. L. M., & Goodman, S. H. (2006). *Women and depression: A handbook for the social, behavioral, and biomedical sciences.* New York: Cambridge University Press.

Khan, A. A., Gardner, C. O., Prescott, C. A., & Kendler, K. S. (2002). Gender differences in the symptoms of major depression in opposite-sex dizygotic twin pairs. *American Journal of Psychiatry, 159*(8), 1427–1429.

Kistner, C. F., David, C. F., & White, B. A. (2003). Ethnic and sex differences in children's depressive symptoms: Mediating effects of perceived and actual competence. *Journal of Clinical Child and Adolescent Psychology, 32*(3), 341–350.

Klimes-Dougan, B., Hastings, P., Granger, D., Usher, B., & Zahn-Waxler, C. (2001). Adrenocortical activity in at-risk and normally developing adolescents: Individual differences in salivary cortisol basal levels, diurnal variation, and responses to social challenges. *Development and Psychopathology, 13*(3), 695–719.

Kochanska, G., Coy, K. C., & Murray, K. (2001). The development of self-regulation in the first four years of life. *Child Development, 72,* 1091–1111.

Kornstein, S. G., Schatzberg, A. F., Thase, M. E., Yonkers, K. A., McCullough, J. P., Keitner, G. I., et al. (2000a). Gender differences in chronic major and double depression. *Journal of Affective Disorders, 60,* 1–11.

Kornstein, S. G., Schatzberg, A. F., Thase, M. E., Yonkers, K. A., McCulough, J. P., Keitner, G. I., et al. (2000b). Gender differences in treatment response to sertraline versus imipramine in chronic depression. *American Journal of Psychiatry, 157,* 1445–1452.

Kostanski, M., & Gullone, E. (1998). Adolescent body image dissatisfaction: Relationships with self-esteem, anxiety, and depression controlling for body mass. *Journal of ChildPsychology and Psychiatry, 39*(2), 255–262.

Kovacs, M. (2001). Gender and the course of major depressive disorder through adolescence inclinically referred youngsters. *Journal of the American Academy of Child and Adolescent Psychiatry, 40*(9), 1079–1085.

Kovacs, M., Obrosky, D. S., & Sherrill, J. (2003). Developmental changes in the phenomenology of depression in girls compared to boys from childhood onward. *Journal of Affective Disorders, 74,* 33–48.

Krueger, R. F. (1999). Personality traits in late adolescence predict mental disorders in early adulthood: A prospective-epidemiological study. *Journal of Personality, 67*(1), 39–65.

Kuehner, C. (2003). Gender differences in unipolar depression: An update of epidemiological findings and possible explanations. *Acta Psychiatrica Scandinavica, 108,* 163–174.

Larson, R., & Ham, M. (1993). Stress and "storm and stress" in early adolescence: The relationship of negative events with dysphoric affect. *Developmental Psychology, 29,* 130–140.

Lau, J., & Eley, T. (2006). A cognitive-behavioral genetic approach to emotional development in childhood and adolescence. In T. Canli (Ed.), *Biology of personality and individual differences* (pp. 335–352). New York: Guilford Press.

Leadbeater, B. J., Blatt, S. J., & Quinlan, D. M. (1995). Gender-linked vulnerabilities to depressive symptoms, stress, and problem behaviors in adolescents. *Journal of Research on Adolescence, 5,* 1–29.

Leadbeater, B. J., Kuperminc, G. P., Blatt, S. J., & Hertzog, C. (1999). A multivariate model of gender differences in adolescents' internalizing and externalizing disorders. *Developmental Psychology, 35,* 1268–1282.

Leaper, C. (2002). Parenting girls and boys. In M. H. Borstein (Ed.), *Handbook of parenting: Vol. 1. Children and parenting* (2nd ed., 189–225). Mahwah, NJ: Erlbaum.

Levitan, R. D., Parikh, S. V., Lesage, A. D., Hegadoren, K. M., Adams, M., Kennedy, S. H., et al. (1998). Major depression in individuals with a history of childhood physical or sexual abuse:

Relationship to neurovegetative features, mania, and gender. *American Journal of Psychiatry,* *155*(12), 1746–1752.

Lewinsohn, P. M., Gotlib, I. H., Lewinsohn, M., Seeley, J. R., & Allen, N. B. (1998). Gender differences in anxiety disorders and anxiety symptoms in adolescents. *Journal of Abnormal Psychology, 107*(1), 109–117.

Lewinsohn, P. M., Hops, H., Roberts, R. E., Seeley, J. R., & Andrews, J. A. (1993). Adolescent psychopathology: I. Prevalence and incidence of depression and other DSM-III-R disorders in high school students. *Journal of Abnormal Psychology, 102*(1), 133–144.

Lewinsohn, P. M., Rohde, P., & Seeley, J. R. (1995). Adolescent psychopathology: III. The clinical consequences of comorbidity. *Journal of the American Academy of Child and Adolescent Psychiatry, 34*(4), 510–519.

Little, S. A., & Garber, J. (2004). Interpersonal and achievement orientations and specific stressors predict depressive and aggressive symptoms. *Journal of Adolescent Research, 19*(1), 63–84.

Liu, X., & Kaplan, H. B. (1999). Explaining gender differences in symptoms of subjective distress in young adolescents. *Stress Medicine, 15,* 41–51.

Loeber, R., & Keenan, K. (1994). Interaction between conduct disorder and its comorbid conditions: Effects of age and gender. *Clinical Psychology Review, 14*(6), 497–523.

Lonigan, C. J., Hooe, E. S., David, C. F., & Kistner, J. A. (1999). Positive and negative affectivity in children: Confirmatory factor analysis of a two-factor model and its relation to symptoms of anxiety and depression. *Journal of Consulting and Clinical Psychology, 67,* 374–386.

Lonigan, C. J., Phillips, B. M., & Hooe, E. S. (2003). Relations of positive and negative affectivity to anxiety and depression in children: Evidence from a latent variable longitudinal study. *Journal of Consulting and Clinical Psychology, 71*(3), 465–481.

Lyons, M. J., Eisen, S. A., Goldberg, J., True, W., Lin, N., Meyer, J. M., et al. (1998). A registry-based twin study of depression in men. *Archives of General Psychiatry, 55*(5), 468–472.

Maccoby, E. E. (1990). Gender and relationships: A developmental account. *American Psychologist, 45,* 513–520.

Maccoby, E. E. (2002). Gender and group processes: A developmental perspective. *Current Directions in Psychological Science, 11,* 54–58.

Marcotte, D., Fortin, L., Potvin, P., & Papillon, M. (2002). Gender differences in depressive symptoms during adolescence: Role of gender-typed characteristics, self-esteem, body image, stressful life events, and pubertal status. *Journal of Emotional and Behavioral Disorders, 10*(1), 29–42.

Maughan, B., & Rutter, M. (1997). Retrospective reporting of childhood adversity: Assessing long-term recall. *Journal of Personality Disorders, 11*(1), 19–33.

Mazure, C. M., & Keita, G. P. (2006). *Understanding depression in women: Applying empirical research to practice and policy.* Washington, DC: American Psychological Association.

McBride, C., Bacchiochi, J. R., & Bagby, R. M. (2005). Gender differences in the manifestation of sociotropy and autonomy personality traits. *Personality and Individual Differences, 38*(1), 129–136.

McEwen, B. S. (1992). Steroid hormones: Effect on brain development and function. *Hormone Research, 37,* S1–S10.

McEwen, B. S. (2001). From molecules to mind: Stress, individual differences, and the social environment. *Annals of the New York Academy of Sciences, 935*(1), 42–49.

McEwen, B. S., & Alves, S. E. (1999). Estrogen actions in the central nervous system. *Endocrine Reviews, 20,* 279–307.

Merry, S., McDowell, H., Hetrick, S., Bir, J., & Muller, N. (2004). Psychological and/or educational interventions for the prevention of depression in children and adolescents. *The Cochrane Library,* 1–104.

Mezulis, A. H., Abramson, L. Y., & Hyde, J. S. (2002). Domain specificity of gender differences in rumination. *Journal of Cognitive Psychotherapy, 16*(4), 421–434.

Mezulis, A. H., Abramson, L. Y., Hyde, J. S., & Hankin, B. L. (2004). Is there a universal positivity bias in attributions? A meta-analytic review of individual, developmental, and cultural differences in the self-serving attributional bias. *Psychological Bulletin, 30*(5), 711–747.

Mistry, R. S., Vandewater, E. A., Huston, A. C., & McLoyd, V. (2002). Economic well-being and children's social adjustment: The role of family process in an ethnically diverse low-income sample. *Child Development, 73*, 935–951.

Mitchell, J. R., McCauley, E., Burke, P. M., & Moss, S. J. (1988). Phenomenology of depression in children and adolescents. *Journal of the American Academy of Child and Adolescent Psychiatry, 27*(1), 12–20.

Moffitt, T. E., Caspi, A., Rutter, M., & Silva, P. A. (Eds.). (2001). *Sex differences in antisocial behavior: Conduct disorder, delinquency, and violence in the Dunedin Longitudinal Study.* New York: Cambridge University Press.

Moran, P. B., & Eckenrode, J. (1991). Gender differences in the costs and benefits of peer relationships during adolescence. *Journal of Adolescent Research, 6*(4), 396–409.

Newman, D. L., Moffitt, T. E., Caspi, A., Magdol, L., Silva, P. A., & Stanton, W. R. (1996). Psychiatric disorder in a birth cohort of young adults: Prevalence, comorbidity, clinical significance, and new case incidence from ages 11 to 21. *Journal of Consulting and Clinical Psychology, 64*(3), 552–562.

Nolen-Hoeksema, S. (1990). *Sex differences in depression.* Stanford, CA: Stanford University Press.

Nolen-Hoeksema, S. (1991). Responses to depression and their effects on the duration of depressive episodes. *Journal of Abnormal Psychology, 100,* 569–582.

Nolen-Hoeksema, S. (2002). Gender differences in depression. In I. H. Gotlib & C. L. Hammen (Eds.), *Handbook of depression* (pp. 492–509). New York: Guilford Press.

Nolen-Hoeksema, S., & Girgus, J. S. (1994). The emergence of gender differences in depression during adolescence. *Psychological Bulletin, 115*(3), 424–443.

Nolen-Hoeksema, S., Larson, J., & Grayson, C. (1999). Explaining the gender difference in depressive symptoms. *Journal of Personality and Social Psychology, 77,* 1061–1072.

Olfson, M., Zarin, D. A., Mittman, B. S., & McIntyre, J. S. (2001). Is gender a factor in psychiatrists' evaluation and treatment of patients with major depression? *Journal of Affective Disorders, 63,* 149–157.

Paikoff, R. L., Brooks-Gunn, J., & Warren, M. P. (1991). Effects of girls' hormonal status on depressive and aggressive symptoms over the course of one year. *Journal of Youth and Adolescence, 20,* 191–215.

Parker, G., & Hadzi-Pavlovic, D. (2004). Is the female preponderance in major depression secondary to a gender difference in specific anxiety disorders? *Psychological Medicine, 34*(3), 461–470.

Penza-Clyve, S., & Zeman, J. (2002). Initial validation of the emotion expression scale for children (EESC). *Journal of Clinical Child and Adolescent Psychology, 31*(4), 540–547.

Petersen, A. C., Compas, B. E., Brooks-Gunn, J., Stemmler, M., Ey, S., & Grant, K. E. (1993). Depression in adolescence. *American Psychologist, 48*(2), 155–168.

Petersen, A. C., Sarigiani, P. A., & Kennedy, R. E. (1991). Adolescent depression: Why more girls? *Journal of Youth and Adolescence, 20*(2), 247–271.

Pickles, A., & Hill, J. (2006). Developmental pathways. In D. Cicchetti & D. J. Cohen (Eds.), *Developmental psychopathology: Vol. 1. Theory and method* (2nd ed., pp. 211–243). Hoboken, NJ: Wiley.

Pine, D. S., Cohen, P., Gurley, D., Brook, J., & Ma, Y. (1998). The risk for early-adulthood anxiety and depressive disorders in adolescents with anxiety and depressive disorders. *Archives of General Psychiatry, 55*(1), 56–64.

Prinstein, M. J., & Aikins, J. W. (2004). Cognitive moderators of the longitudinal association between peer rejection and adolescent depressive symptoms. *Journal of Abnormal Child Psychology, 32*(2), 147–158.

Prinstein, M. J., Borelli, J. L., Cheah, C. S. L., Simon, V. A., & Aikins, J. W. (2005). Adolescent girls' interpersonal vulnerability to depressive symptoms: A longitudinal examination of reassurance-seeking and peer relationships. *Journal of Abnormal Psychology, 114*(4), 676–688.

Prinstein, M. J., Cheah, C. S. L., & Guyer, A. E. (2005). Peer victimization, cue interpretation, and internalizing symptoms: Preliminary concurrent and longitudinal findings for children and adolescents. *Journal of Clinical Child and Adolescent Psychology, 34*(1), 11–24.

Quiggle, N. L., Garber, J., Panak, W. F., & Dodge, K. A. (1992). Social information processing in aggressive and depressed children. *Child Development, 63*(6), 1305–1320.

Quitkin, F. M., Stewart, J. W., & McGrath, P. J. (2002). Are there differences between women's and men's antidepressant responses? *American Journal of Psychiatry, 159*(11), 1848–1854.

Reinherz, H. Z., Giaconia, R. M., Lefkowitz, E. S., Pakiz, B., & Frost, A. K. (1993). Prevalence of psychiatric disorders in a community population of older adolescents. *Journal of the American Academy of Child and Adolescent Psychiatry, 32*, 369–377.

Rhodes, M. E., & Rubin, R. T. (1999). Functional sex differences ("sexual diergism") of CNS cholinergic systems, vasopressin, and hypothalamic–pituitary–adrenal axis activity in mammals: A selective review. *Brain Research Reviews, 30*, 135–152.

Rind, B., Tromovitch, P., & Bauserman, R. (1998). A meta-analytic examination of assumed properties of child sexual abuse using college samples. *Psychological Bulletin, 124*(1), 22–53.

Roberts, J. E., Gotlib, I. H., & Kassel, J. D. (1996). Adult attachment security and symptoms of depression: The mediating roles of dysfunctional attitudes and low self-esteem. *Journal of Personality and Social Psychology, 70*(2), 310–320.

Roberts, R. E., Lewinsohn, P. M., & Seeley, J. R. (1995). Symptoms of DSM-III-R major depression in adolescence: Evidence from an epidemiological survey. *Journal of the American Academy of Child and Adolescent Psychiatry, 34*(12), 1608–1617.

Robins, C. J., & Hinkley, K. (1989). Social-cognitive processing and depressive symptoms in children: A comparison of measures. *Journal of Abnormal Child Psychology, 17*, 29–36.

Rohde, P., Lewinsohn, P. M., & Seeley, J. R. (1991). Comorbidity of unipolar depression: II. Comorbidity with other mental disorders in adolescents and adults. *Journal of Abnormal Psychology, 100*(2), 214–222.

Ronfeld, R. A., Tremaine, L. M., & Wilner, K. D. (1997). Pharmacokinetics of sertraline and its N-demethyl metabolite in elderly and young male and female volunteers. *Clinical Pharmacokinetics, 32*, 22–30.

Rose, A. J. (2002). Co-rumination in the friendships of girls and boys. *Child Development, 33*(6), 1830–1843.

Rose, A. J., & Abramson, L. Y. 1991). Developmental predictors of depressive cognitive style: Research and theory. In D. Cicchetti & S. L. Toth (Eds.), *Developmental perspectives on depression* (pp. 323–349). Rochester, NY: University of Rochester Press.

Rose, A. J., & Rudolph, K. D. (2006). A review of sex differences in peer relationship processes: Potential trade-offs for the emotional and behavioral development of girls and boys. *Psychological Bulletin, 132*, 98–131.

Rowe, R., Maughan, B., Pickles, A., Costello, E. J., & Angold, A. (2002). The relationship between DSM-IV oppositional defiant disorder and conduct disorder: Findings from the Great Smoky Mountains Study. *Journal of Child Psychiatry and Psychology, 43*(3), 365–373.

Ruble, D. N., & Martin, C. L. (1998). Gender development. In W. Damon (Series Ed.) & N. Eisenberg (Vol. Ed.), *Handbook of child psychology: Vol. 3. Social, emotional, and personality development* (5th ed., pp. 933–1016). New York: Wiley.

Ruble, D. N., Martin, C. L., & Berebaum, S. A. (2006). Gender development. In W. Damon, R. M. Lerner, & N. Eisenberg (Eds.), *Handbook of child psychology: Vol. 3. Social, emotional, and personality development* (6th ed., pp. 858–932). New York: Wiley.

Rudolph, K. D. (2002). Gender differences in emotional responses to interpersonal stress during adolescence. *Journal of Adolescent Health, 30*(3), 3–13.

Rudolph, K. D., & Conley, C. S. (2005). The socioemotional costs and benefits of social-evaluative concerns: Do girls care too much? *Journal of Personality, 73*(1), 115–137.

Rudolph, K. D., & Hammen, C. (1999). Age and gender as determinants of stress exposure, generation, and reactions in youngsters: A transactional perspective. *Child Development, 70,* 660–677.

Rutter, M., Caspi, A., & Moffitt, T. E. (2003). Using sex differences in psychopathology to study causal mechanisms: Unifying issues and research. *Journal of Child Psychiatry and Psychology, 44*(8), 1092–1115.

Rutter, M., Moffitt, T., & Caspi, A. (2006). Gene–environment interplay and psychopathology: Multiple varieties but real effects. *Journal of Child Psychology and Psychiatry, 47*(3), 226–261.

Rutter, M., Silberg, J., O'Connor, T., & Siminoff, E. (1999). Genetics and child psychiatry: II. Empirical research findings. *Journal of Child Psychology and Psychiatry, 40*(1), 19–55.

Santor, D. A., & Ramsay, J. O. (1998). Progress in the technology of measurement: Applications of item response models. *Psychological Assessment, 10*(4), 345–359.

Santor, D. A., Ramsay, J. O., & Zuroff, D. C. (1994). Nonparametric item analyses of the Beck Depression Inventory: Evaluating gender item bias and response option weights. *Psychological Assessment, 6*(3), 255–270.

Schraedley, P. K., Gotlib, I. H., & Hayward, C. (1999). Gender differences in correlates of depressive symptoms in adolescents. *Journal of Adolescent Health, 25*(2), 98–108.

Schwartz, J. A. J., & Koenig, L. J. (1996). Response styles and negative affect among adolescents. *Cognitive Therapy and Research, 20,* 13–36.

Seeman, M. (1997). Psychopathology in women and men: Focus on female hormones. *American Journal of Psychiatry, 154*(12), 1641–1647.

Seidlitz, L., & Diener, E. (1998). Sex differences in the recall of affective experiences. *Journal of Personality and Social Psychology, 74,* 262–271.

Seiffge-Krenke, I., & Stemmler, M. (2002). Factors contributing to gender differences in depressive symptoms: A test of three developmental models. *Journal of Youth and Adolescence, 31*(6), 405–417.

Sheeber, L., Davis, B., & Hops, H. (2002). Gender-specific vulnerability to depression in children of depressed mothers. In S. H. Goodman & I. H. Gotlib (Eds.), *Children of depressed parents: Mechanisms of risk and implications for treatment* (pp. 253–274). Washington, DC: American Psychological Association.

Shih, J. H., Eberhart, N. K., Hammen, C. L., & Brennan, P. A. (2006). Differential exposure and reactivity to interpersonal stress predict sex differences in adolescent depression. *Journal of Clinical Child and Adolescent Psychology, 35*(1), 103–115.

Siegel, J. M., Aneshensel, C. S., Taub, B., Cantwell, D. P., & Driscoll, A. K. (1998). Adolescent depressed mood in a multiethnic sample. *Journal of Youth and Adolescence, 27*(4), 413–427.

Silberg, J. L., Pickles, A., Rutter, M., Hewitt, J., Simonoff, E., Maes, H., et al. (1999). The influence of genetic factors and life stress on depression among adolescent girls. *Archives of General Psychiatry, 56*(3), 225–232.

Silberg, J., Rutter, M., & Eaves, L. (2001). Genetic and environmental influences on the temporal association between earlier anxiety and later depression in girls. *Biological Psychiatry, 49*(12), 1040–1049.

Silverstein, B. (2002). Gender differences in the prevalence of somatic versus pure depression: A replication. *American Journal of Psychiatry, 159*(6), 1051–1052.

Sinha, R., & Rush, A. J. (2006). Treatment and prevention of depression in women. In C. M. Mazure & G. W. Keita (Eds.), *Understanding depression in women: Applying empirical research to practice and policy* (pp. 45–70). Washington, DC: American Psychological Association.

Smider, N. A., Essex, M. J., Kalin, N. H., Buss, K. A., Klein, M. H., Davidson, R. J., et al. (2002). Salivary cortisol as a predictor of socioemotional adjustment during kindergarten: A prospective study. *Child Development, 73*(1), 75–92.

Sorensen, M. J., Mors, O., & Thomsen, P. H. (2005). DSM-IV or ICD-10-DCR diagnoses in child and adolescent psychiatry: Does it matter? *European Child and Adolescent Psychiatry, 14*(6), 335–340.

Stark, K. D., Sander, J., Hauser, M., Simpson, J., Schnoebelen, S., Glenn, R., et al. (2006). Depressive disorders during childhood and adolescence. In E. J. Mash & R. A. Barkley (Eds.), *Treatment of childhood disorders* (3rd ed., pp. 336–407). New York: Guilford Press.

Steiner, H., & Lock, J. (1998). Anorexia nervosa and bulimia nervosa in children and adolescents: A review of the past 10 years. *Journal of the American Academy of Child and Adolescent Psychiatry, 37*(4), 352–359.

Steiner, M., Dunn, E., & Born, L. (2003). Hormones and mood: From menarche to menopause and beyond. *Journal of Affective Disorders, 74*, 67–82.

Stemmler, M., & Petersen, A. C. (2005). Gender differential influences of early adolescent risk factors for the development of depressive affect. *Journal of Youth and Adolescence, 34*(3), 175–183.

Stevens, E. A., & Prinstein, M. J. (2005). Peer contagion of depressogenic attributional styles among adolescents: A longitudinal study. *Journal of Abnormal Child Psychology, 33*(1), 25–37.

Stice, E., Presnell, K., & Bearman, S. K. (2001). Relation of early menarche to depression, eating disorders, substance abuse, and comorbid psychopathology among adolescent girls. *Developmental Psychology, 37*(5), 608–619.

Strazdins, L. M., Galligan, R. F., & Scannell, E. D. (1997). Gender and depressive symptoms: Parents' sharing of instrumental and expressive tasks when their children are young. *Journal of Family Psychology, 11*(2), 222–233.

Sund, A. M., Larsson, B., & Wichstrom, L. (2003). Psychosocial correlates of depressive symptoms among 12–14-year-old Norwegian adolescents. *Journal of Child Psychology and Psychiatry, 44*(4), 588–597.

Susman, E., Dorn, L., & Chrousos, G. (1991). Negative affect and hormone levels in young adolescents: Concurrent and predictive perspectives. *Journal of Youth and Adolescence, 20*(2), 167–190.

Susman, E., Dorn, L., Inoff-Germain, G., Nottelmann, E., & Chrousos, G. (1997). Cortisol reactivity, distress behavior, and behavioral and psychological problems in young adolescents: A longitudinal perspective. *Journal of Research on Adolescence, 7*(1), 81–105.

Susman, E., Inoff-Germain, G., Nottelmann, E., & Loriaux, D. (1987). Hormones, emotional dispositions, and aggressive attributes in young adolescents. *Child Development, 58*(4), 1114–1134.

Tambs, K., Harris, J., & Magnus, P. (1995). Sex-specific causal factors and effects of common environment for symptoms of anxiety and depression in twins. *Behavior Genetics, 25*(1), 33–44.

Tamres, L. K., Janicki, D., & Helgeson, V. S. (2002). Sex differences in coping behavior: A meta-analytic review and an examination of relative coping. *Personality and Social Psychology Review, 6*(1), 2–30.

Taylor, S. E., Dickerson, S. S., & Klein, L. C. (2002). Toward a biology of social support. In C. R. Snyder & S. J. Lopez (Eds.), *Handbook of positive psychology* (pp. 556–569). New York: Oxford University Press.

Taylor, S. E., Klein, L. C., Lewis, B. P., Gruenewald, T. L., Gurun, R. A. R., & Updegraff, J. A. (2000). Biobehavioral responses to stress in females: Tend-and-befriend, not fight-or-flight. *Psychological Review, 107*, 411–429.

Thapar, A., & McGuffin, P. (1997). Anxiety and depressive symptoms in childhood: A genetic study of comorbidity. *Journal of Child Psychology and Psychiatry, 38*(6), 651–656.

Thase, M. E., Jindal, R., & Howland, R. H. (2002). Biological aspects of depression. In I. H. Gotlib & C. L. Hammen (Eds.), *Handbook of depression* (pp. 192–218). New York: Guilford Press.

Towbes, L. C., Cohen, L. H., & Glyshaw, K. (1989). Coping strategies and psychological distress: Prospective analyses of early and middle adolescents. *American Journal of Community Psychology, 17*(5), 607–623.

Treatment for Adolescents with Depression Study (TADS) Team. (2004). Fluoxetine, cognitive-behavioral therapy, and their combination for adolescents with depression: Treatment for Adolescents with Depression Study (TADS) randomized controlled trial. *Journal of the American Medical Association, 292*(7), 807–820.

Twenge, J. M., & Nolen-Hoeksema, S. (2002). Age, gender, race, socioeconomic status, and birth cohort difference on the Children's Depression Inventory: A meta-analysis. *Journal of Abnormal Psychology, 111*(4), 578–588.

Udry, R. J. (2000). Biological limits of gender construction. *American Sociological Review, 65*(3), 443–457.

Underwood, M. K. (2003). *Social aggression among girls.* New York: Guilford Press.

Underwood, M. K., Hurley, J. C., Johanson, C. A., & Mosley, J. E. (1999). An experimental observation investigation of children's responses to peer provocation: Developmental and gender differences in middle childhood. *Child Development, 70,* 1428–1446.

Wade, T. J., Cairney, J., & Pevalin, D. J. (2002). Emergence of gender differences in depression during adolescence: National panel results from three countries. *Journal of the American Academy of Child and Adolescent Psychiatry, 41*(2), 190–198.

Wagner, B. M., & Compas, B. E. (1990). Gender, instrumentality, and expressivity: Moderators of the relation between stress and psychological symptoms during adolescence. *American Journal of Community Psychology, 18,* 383–406.

Watson, D., Weber, K., Assenheimer, J. S., Clark, L. A., Strauss, M. E., & McCormick, R. A. (1995). Testing a tripartite model: I. Evaluating the convergent and discriminant validity of anxiety and depression symptom scales. *Journal of Abnormal Psychology, 104,* 3–14.

Weiss, B., & Garber, J. (2003). Developmental differences in the phenomenology of depression. *Development and Psychopathology, 15*(12), 403–430.

Weissman, M. M., Warner, V., Wickramaratne, P., Moreau, D., & Olfson, M. (1997). Offspring of depressed parents: 10 years later. *Archives of General Psychiatry, 54,* 932–942.

Whiffen, V. E., & Clark, S. E. (1997). Does victimization account for sex differences in depressive symptoms? *British Journal of Clinical Psychology, 36*(2), 185–193.

Wichstrom, L. (1999). The emergence of gender difference in depressed mood during adolescence: The role of intensified gender socialization. *Developmental Psychology, 35,* 232–245.

Windle, M. (1992). A longitudinal study of stress buffering for adolescent problem behaviors. *Developmental Psychology, 28,* 522–530.

Yonkers, K. A., Kando, J. C., & Cole, J. O. (1992). Gender differences in pharmacokinetics and pharmacodynamics of psychotropic medication. *American Journal of Psychiatry, 149*(5), 587–595.

Zahn-Waxler, C. (2000). The development of empathy, guilt, and internalization of distress: Implications for gender differences in internalizing and externalizing problems. In R. Davidson (Ed.), *Anxiety, depression, and emotion* (pp. 222–265). New York: Oxford University Press.

Zahn-Waxler, C., Cole, P. M., & Barrett, K. C. (1991). Guilt and empathy: Sex differences and implications for the development of depression. In J. Garber & K. A. Dodge (Eds.), *Cambridge studies in social and emotional development* (pp. 243–272). New York: Cambridge University Press.

Zahn-Waxler, C., Crick, N. R., Shirtcliff, E. A., & Woods, K. E. (2006). The origins and development of psychopathology in females and males. In D. Cicchetti & D. J. Cohen (Eds.), *Developmental psychopathology: Vol. 1. Theory and method* (2nd ed., pp. 76–138). Hoboken, NJ: Wiley.

Zahn-Waxler, C., Robinson, J. L., & Emde, R. N. (1992). The development of empathy in twins. *Developmental Psychology, 28*(6), 1038–1047.

Zahn-Waxler, C., Schmitz, S., Fulker, D., Robinson, J. L., & Emde, R. N. (1996). Behavior problems in 5-year-old monozygotic and dizygotic twins: Genetic and environmental influences, patterns of regulation, and internalization of control. *Development andPsychopathology, 8,* 103–122.

Zeman, J., & Shipman, K. (1997). Social-contextual influences on expectancies for managing anger and sadness: The transition from middle childhood to adolescence. *Developmental Psychology, 33*(6), 917–924.

Zeman, J., Shipman, K., & Suveg, C. (2002). Anger and sadness regulation: Predictions to internalizing and externalizing symptoms in children. *Journal of Clinical Child and Adolescent Psychology, 31*, 393–398.

Ziegert, D. I., & Kistner, J. A. (2002). Response styles theory: Downward extension to children. *Journal of Clinical Child and Adolescent Psychology, 31*(3), 325–334.

Zlotnick, C., Elkin, I., & Shea, M. T. (1998). Does the gender of a patient or the gender of a therapist affect the treatment of patients with major depression? *Journal of Consulting and Clinical Psychology, 66*(4), 655–659.

17 Children of Depressed Mothers

Implications for the Etiology, Treatment, and Prevention of Depression in Children and Adolescents

Sherryl H. Goodman and Erin Tully

The high-risk paradigm (Mednick & Schulsinger, 1968) has provided the foundation for the current line of research on psychopathology. This method emphasizes the identification of both mechanisms and moderators of risk in the transmission of psychopathology from depressed parents to their offspring. The primary goal of this chapter is to examine the research on children of depressed parents for what it has revealed, or has promise to reveal in the future, about the etiology as well as the treatment and prevention of depression in children and adolescents.

NATURE AND EXTENT OF THE PROBLEM

Depression is one of the most common psychiatric disorders in adults. Between 6 and 17% of women experience an episode of major depression at some point in their lifetimes, a rate that is between one and a half to three times higher than in men (Kessler, 2006). Moreover, depression is the leading cause of both economic and social disability in early to middle adulthood (Wilhelm, 2006), the primary childbearing and child-rearing years. The aspect of disability that has particular implications for depression in children of depressed mothers is depression's interference with quality of parenting. This has been the subject of a large body of research that is reviewed later in this chapter, and it has also been the subject of a meta-analysis (Lovejoy, Graczyk, O'Hare, & Neuman, 2000).

The higher prevalence of depression in women than in men is only one of the reasons that most researchers have focused their attention on children of depressed mothers relative to depressed fathers. Another reason is concern about fetal exposure to depression in mothers, as reviewed later in this chapter. Furthermore, despite significant changes in recent years, mothers are still the primary caregivers of children and thus have more opportunities, relative to fathers, for potential influence in terms of inadequate parenting or modeling (Lamb, 2000). Finally, the data are consistent with these suggestions. That is, although depression in both mothers and fathers has been shown to affect children's psychological functioning, a meta-analysis of 134 samples, with a total of more than 60,000 parent–child dyads, showed that both internalizing and externalizing problems in children are more strongly associated with depression in mothers relative to depression in fathers (Connell & Goodman, 2002).

A review of the range of outcomes in children found to be associated with depression in mothers, and the strength of those associations, is beyond the scope of this chapter; the subject has been addressed in recent reviews (Goodman, Connell, Broth, & Hall, 2007; Goodman & Tully, 2006). Most relevant to this volume are two sets of findings. First, from the earliest ages when depression can reliably be measured in children, rates of depression are significantly higher in children with depressed mothers relative to a range of groups to which they have been compared (Beardslee et al., 1988; Billings & Moos, 1985; Brennan, Hammen, Katz, & Le Brocque, 2002; Goodman, Adamson, Riniti, & Cole, 1994; Hammen et al., 1987; Lee & Gotlib, 1989; Malcarne, Hamilton, Ingram, & Taylor, 2000; Orvaschel, Walsh-Allis, & Ye, 1988; Radke-Yarrow & Klimes-Dougan, 2002; Weissman et al., 1984; Welner, Welner, McCrary, & Leonard, 1977). Overall, rates of depression in the school-age and adolescent children of depressed mothers have been estimated at between 20 and 41%, with the variability within that range explained by the severity or impairment of the parent's depression, whether the father is also depressed, and a number of other sociodemographic variables.

Second, beginning in infancy and then throughout development, depression in mothers is associated with emotional and behavioral problems and wide-ranging problems in affective, cognitive, interpersonal, neuroendocrine, and brain functioning, as reviewed recently (Goodman & Tully, 2006). Any of these problems may represent either vulnerabilities to or early signs of (markers for) the later development of depression or other disorders. These problems identified in young children are of particular concern, because problems identified early in development are strongly predictive of psychopathology in later years (Campbell, 1995).

A discussion of the nature and extent of risk for the development of psychopathology in children of depressed mothers would be incomplete without consideration of comorbidity. First, depression, especially in women, is often comorbid with anxiety (Clark, 1989; Kessler, 2006). Second, prior anxiety strongly predicts depression in women (whereas prior substance use disorders or conduct disorders typify the pathway to depression for men) (Hettema, Prescott, & Kendler, 2003). Third, although the focus of this chapter is depression in child or adolescent offspring of depressed mothers, depression in the offspring, as in the mothers, is often comorbid both with other internalizing disorders such as anxiety, as well as with externalizing disorders. Thus, it is essential to take into account all of these aspects of comorbidity when thinking about the implications of depression in mothers for the etiology, treatment, and prevention of depression in children and adolescents. In the next section of this chapter, we examine the data on children of depressed mothers for its implications for the etiology of depression in children and adolescents. Later sections focus on implications for treatment and prevention.

IMPLICATIONS FOR THE ETIOLOGY OF DEPRESSION IN CHILDREN AND ADOLESCENTS

Although it is well accepted that any model of risk for the development of depression in children whose mothers have been depressed involves multiple interacting mechanisms, it is nonetheless essential to identify the primary mechanisms that are the key components of a model of risk. The empirically supported mechanisms then become components in a model that must account for multiple interacting influences, best described in terms of transactional processes (Sameroff, 1975, 1995). One such model is the integrative model for the transmission of risk to children of depressed mothers, shown in Figure 17.1 (Goodman & Gotlib, 1999). In this section, we first review the core etiological mechanisms proposed in the model, each of which has been gaining support in explaining the transmission of depression from mothers to their children. Then we review the ideas that take into account the interacting influences of the individual mechanisms and likely moderators of risk and examine the extent to which research has supported those influences. In a later section, we consider the role of vulnerabilities to depression in the possible developmental pathways from maternal depression to the emergence of depression in children and adolescents.

Core Mechanisms

Biological Mechanisms

Work on biological mechanisms that may explain the transmission of depression from mothers to their children has focused on two lines of research. First, much research has centered on genetic influences, not only in depression as a disorder, but also in vulnerabilities to depression. A second line of research has investigated the idea that fetal or postnatal exposures or experiences among children of depressed mothers may adversely influence brain development or hormonal functioning related to neuroregulatory mechanisms, thereby increasing risk for depression in the offspring. Support for both of those lines of research is reviewed in the following sections.

GENETIC INFLUENCES

Research based on family studies, quantitative genetic studies (twin and adoption designs), and molecular genetic studies all provide strong support for heritability of depression in adults, although some evidence suggests that the specific genes related to risk for depression may differ for men as compared with women (Caspi et al., 2003; Kendler, Gardner, Neale, & Prescott, 2001). Evidence for the heritability of depression in children and adolescents, however, is mixed. As based on family studies, strictly defined depression in children and adolescents is associated with increased rates of depression in relatives (Harrington, 1996; Harrington et al., 1997). According to twin studies, heritability is higher in those whose levels of symptoms were below rather than above clinical cutoffs (Rende, Plomin, Reiss, & Hetherington, 1993), for depression in adolescents rather than in children (Eley & Stevenson, 1999; Murray & Sines, 1996; Scourfield et al., 2003; Silberg et al., 2001; Thapar & McGuffin, 1994), for parent-reported rather than child-reported symptoms (Eaves et al., 1997), and for parent-reported symptoms in girls relative to boys (Murray & Sines, 1996; Scourfield et al., 2003). In addition, because heritability of depression is probably not specific to depression, heritability likely contrib-

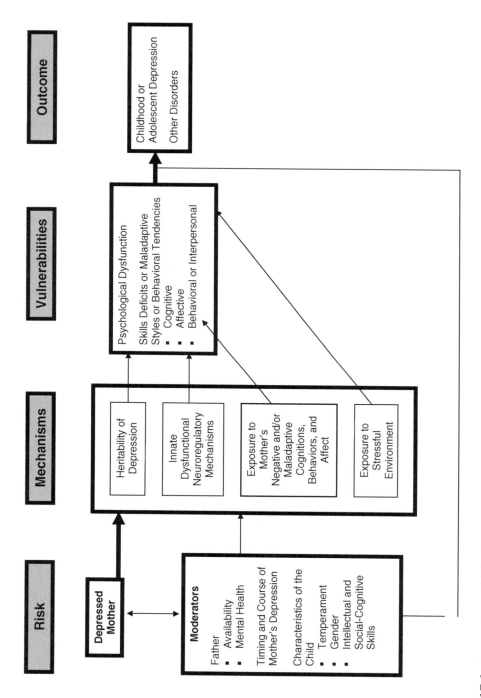

FIGURE 17.1. Integrative model for the transmission of risk to children of depressed mothers. From Goodman and Gotlib (1999). Copyright 1999 by the American Psychological Association. Reprinted by permission.

utes to risk for other disorders that are identified at higher rates in children of depressed mothers relative to controls (Moldin, 1999; Tsuang & Faraone, 1990). Thus, heritability likely contributes to the risk for depression in children and adolescents with depressed mothers, although more research is needed to clarify the nature and extent (or, conversely, the specificity) of the contribution.

An alternative to the notion that children with depressed mothers inherit a likelihood for depression per se is the idea that heritability contributes significantly to vulnerabilities to depression, such as those proposed in the Goodman and Gotlib (1999) model. In particular, high levels of heritability, based on behavior genetics studies, are found for behavioral inhibition and shyness (Cherny, Fulker, Corley, Plomin, & DeFries, 1994), low self-esteem (Loehlin & Nichols, 1976), neuroticism (Tellegen et al., 1988), sociability (Plomin et al., 1993), subjective well-being (Lykken & Tellegen, 1996), and expression of negative emotion (Plomin et al., 1993). This body of research suggests the possible genetic transmission of affective, cognitive, and interpersonal vulnerabilities for depression.

NEUROREGULATORY MECHANISMS

Biology may also play a role in the development of depression in offspring of depressed mothers, in that both prenatal and postnatal experiences may influence aspects of hormonal functioning and brain development, each of which may increase vulnerability to depression (Ashman & Dawson, 2002). Much of the evidence for this premise is based on research examining the role of early (neonatal) life stress in the development of psychopathology, emphasizing neuroregulatory processes and especially hypothalamic–pituitary–adrenal (HPA) axis functioning (Graham, Heim, Goodman, Miller, & Nemeroff, 1999). HPA functioning, typically measured in terms of abnormal cortisol responses to stress, but sometimes as a baseline cortisol measure, has been associated with depression in adults (Ressler & Nemeroff, 2000) and may suggest vulnerability mechanisms for the development of depression in children of depressed mothers.

Several lines of research point to a role of HPA functioning in the development of depression in children whose mothers were depressed during pregnancy. Studies from Field's lab show that depression during pregnancy increases a woman's level of cortisol (Field, 2002). Elevated stress hormones levels in pregnant women are of concern because they have been associated with impaired neurodevelopment in the fetus (Wadhwa et al., 2002). Furthermore, evidence implicating prenatal influences on fetal development of neuroregulatory mechanisms includes findings that pregnant women's levels of cortisol account for 50% of the variance in fetuses' levels of cortisol (Glover, 1999), that mothers' prenatal levels of cortisol predict newborns' cortisol levels (Lundy et al., 1999), and that number of months depressed during pregnancy predicts preschool-age children's baseline cortisol levels (Ashman & Dawson, 2002). Stress-related physiological dysregulation in children may index children's sensitivity to stress, suggesting a particular pathway through which maternal depression during pregnancy may increase children's later development of depression (Sanchez, Ladd, & Plotsky, 2001).

In addition to the possible disruption of HPA regulatory processes through fetal exposure to depression or stress, postnatal exposure to stressors associated with maternal depression may also disrupt HPA processes (Ashman & Dawson, 2002). In particular, depressed mothers' insensitive or unresponsive behavior, discussed in a later section of this chapter, may mediate the association between maternal depression and children's emotion regulation abilities, which in turn increases risk for the development of depression that may emerge in childhood or adolescence.

Along with disruptions in hormonal functioning, abnormal brain development (frontal lobe activity) is a second biological mechanism implicated in the development of depression in children of depressed mothers. Of particular interest is the abnormal electroencephalographic (EEG) pattern of relatively greater baseline right (as compared with left) frontal activation, which is a stable individual difference factor by adolescence (Tomarken, Davidson, Wheeler, & Kinney, 1992) and has been associated with the tendency in children to experience withdrawal emotions such as sadness or fear (Davidson & Fox, 1989) and with depression in adolescents and adults (Davidson, Ekman, Saron, Senulis, & Friesen, 1990). Particularly strong evidence for this mechanism in children of depressed mothers comes from Dawson and colleagues' findings showing associations between frontal lobe activity and affective expressions in infants of depressed mothers (Dawson, Grofer Klinger, Panagiotides, Hill, & Spieker, 1992) and, further, that 3-year-olds' frontal brain activation mediated the relation between maternal depression and children's level of behavior problems (Dawson et al., 2003). Further research is needed to reveal the extent to which genetics and fetal or early postnatal experiences contribute to the abnormal brain activation patterns. This work is especially needed, given that the frontal lobe develops rapidly during the first 2 years of life (Chugani & Phelps, 1986), suggesting sensitivity to early adverse experiences such as exposure to a mother whose depression interferes with her providing the sensitive and responsive parenting required by an infant. Also intriguing is emerging evidence linking these two behavioral mechanisms. Buss and colleagues found that in 6-month-old infants, higher basal and stressor reactive cortisol levels were associated with relatively greater right EEG asymmetry (Buss et al., 2003).

Parenting

MODELING OF COGNITIVE, AFFECTIVE, AND BEHAVIORAL ASPECTS OF DEPRESSION

Exposure to depressed mothers' negative affect, behavior, and cognitions is another potential mechanism for transmission of risk of depression from parents to offspring. Through social learning processes, including modeling, observational learning, and reinforcement, children of depressed mothers may acquire cognitions, behaviors, and affect that resemble those of the depressed parent. These acquired depressotypic cognitions, behaviors, and affect may place the children at elevated risk for developing depression.

Much evidence supports the different processes involved in this mechanism. First, children have ample opportunities to be exposed to negative cognitions, behaviors, and affect associated with depression in their mothers. In terms of affect and behavior, a meta-analysis of 46 observation studies revealed that maternal depression is strongly associated with negative (hostile/coercive) parenting behavior, moderately associated with parenting characterized as disengagement, and shows a small association with lower levels of positive behavior (Lovejoy et al., 2000). In terms of cognitions, the negatively biased cognitions associated with depression in adults (Gotlib, Gilboa, & Sommerfeld, 2000) emerge in parenting in depressed mothers' (1) more negative views of themselves as parents (Gelfand & Teti, 1990; Goodman, Sewell, Cooley, & Leavitt, 1993), (2) less confidence in being able to positively influence their children (Kochanska, Radke-Yarrow, Kuczynski, & Friedman, 1987), and (3) more negative, critical perceptions of their children (Goodman et al., 1994), relative to controls.

Second, these aspects of depression in mothers are associated with the development of both vulnerabilities to depression and depression per se in their children and adolescent offspring. In terms of vulnerabilities, depressed mothers' negative, critical perceptions of their children are associated with children's self-blaming attributions for negative events and with lowered perceived self-worth (Goodman et al., 1994; Jaenicke et al., 1987; Kochanska et al., 1987; Radke-Yarrow, Belmont, Nottelmann, & Bottomly, 1990). That is, children seem to be internalizing their depressed mother's negative views of them, thereby acquiring a cognitive vulnerability to depression (Beck, Rush, Shaw, & Emery, 1979). Depressed mothers' greater criticism and hostility (Frye & Garber, 2005; Webster-Stratton & Hammond, 1988) may also contribute to the emergence of coercive processes not dissimilar to those implicated in the development of not only externalizing behavior problems but also depression (Davis, Sheeber, & Hops, 2002; Hops, Sherman, & Biglan, 1990). However, family coercion was not found to mediate associations between maternal depression in the early school years and adolescent boys' or girls' depression (Compton, Snyder, Schrepferman, Bank, & Shortt, 2003).

INADEQUATE PARENTING

In addition to social learning processes linking depressed mothers' affect, behavior, and cognition to the development of depression in their offspring, other mechanisms may also explain how qualities of parenting contribute to the development of depression and how they interact with vulnerabilities in children to foster the development of depression. These other mechanisms include inadequate parenting (especially if early in child's life) as a stressor, which was touched on earlier in this chapter, and some alternative ways in which inadequate parenting may contribute to the development of cognitive vulnerabilities. The latter, although not incompatible with social learning processes, are addressed by a different tradition of research, emphasizing interpersonal processes such as the depressed mother's being an inadequate social partner for the child, and the mother being unable to meet the child's stage-salient social and emotional needs (Cicchetti & Toth, 1998). This inadequate parenting, in turn, negatively affects the child's development of social and cognitive skills.

In this model, inadequate parenting refers to the mother's being unable to meet the needs associated with healthy psychological development in any phase of child development, although with an emphasis on infancy, given infants' dependence on their caregivers to meet their basic needs (Sroufe, Egeland, Carlson, & Collins, 2005). This research is consistent with the idea that depression in mothers is a stressor for their infants, which is related to the literature on HPA activity and EEG asymmetries reviewed earlier. Mothers may be stressors as a function of being unresponsive or inconsistent (unpredictable in their responsiveness) in relating to their infants, thereby interfering with the infants' development of emotion regulation skills (Fox, 1994) and secure attachment relationships (Cicchetti, Rogosch, & Toth, 1998; Sroufe & Waters, 1977). Both of the latter may increase risk for the development of depression in childhood or adolescence.

STRESS

In addition to inadequate parenting of depressed mothers acting as a stressor, especially for infants, maternal depression increases children's exposure to stress in several other ways (Hammen, 2002). These include the stressfulness for children of the symptoms and episodic course of depression in their mothers (Compas, Langrock, Keller, Merchant, & Copeland, 2002), the chronic and episodic stressors that are often the context for depression (Monroe & Hadjiyannakis, 2002), and the stress-generating quality found to be associated with depression (Hammen, 1991). Furthermore, both episodic and chronic stressors are associated with depression symptoms and depressive disorders in children and adolescents (Grant et al., 2003). Finally, support is beginning to emerge for the role of stressors as a mediator of the association between maternal depression and children's depression (Brennan et al., 2002).

Interacting Etiological Mechanisms, Pathways to Depression, and Moderating Influences

Interacting Etiological Mechanisms

Complicating the model of risk for depression in offspring of depressed mothers, the individual mechanisms of risk interact in complex ways to create diverse pathways to disorder. Diverse pathways may lead to the same outcome, a concept termed *equifinality*; and similar developmental pathways may lead to diverse outcomes, a concept termed *multifinality* (Cicchetti & Rogosch, 1996; Harrington, Rutter, & Fombonne, 1996). Transactional models are particularly helpful for understanding these individual, complex pathways. Transactional models emphasize the interaction of genetic, neurobiological, biochemical, psychological, and sociological factors that, through mutual exchange between characteristics of the child and the environment, result in the development of psychopathology (Cicchetti & Toth, 1995).

As we reviewed previously, researchers have proposed several theoretical models involving the interface between two or more mechanisms, and empirical support for these models is beginning to appear (Goodman, 2003). These include passive, reactive, and active gene–environment correlation or covariation (Goldsmith, Gottesman, & Lemery, 1997; Rutter et al., 1997), gene–environment interactions such as stress–diathesis models (Monroe & Simons, 1991), genetic vulnerabilities interacting with other biological vulnerabilities or cognitive vulnerabilities (Coccaro, Silverman, Klar, Horvath, & Siever, 1994), genes interacting with other genes (Goldsmith, Gottesman, & Lemery, 1997), stress–diathesis models with diatheses other than genetics (such as temperament; Cicchetti & Toth, 1998; Goldsmith, Buss, & Lemery, 1997; Sameroff, 1995), and child qualities (e.g., negative affectivity) evoking environmental qualities (e.g., harsh parenting; Field, Healy, Goldstein, & Guthertz, 1990; Teti & Gelfand, 1991). A further example of interacting mechanisms that has gained recent interest is the finding that in a birth cohort of young adults, a functional polymorphism of the serotonin transporter gene (5-HTTLPR) moderated the prospective association between stressful life events and depression (Caspi et al., 2003).

Pathways to Depression: The Role of Children's Vulnerabilities

From a developmental psychopathology perspective, psychopathology should be conceptualized in terms of processes that extend through time and should be considered in the context of normal developmental processes (Cicchetti, 1984; Sroufe & Rutter, 1984). Moreover, understanding the mechanisms of risk in children of depressed parents requires understanding the processes underlying individual patterns of adaptation and the consequences of the individual patterns for the development of depression. Early in the developmental pathways, children of depressed mothers may develop *vulnerabilities* for depression, which, in turn, increase the likelihood of developing depression. For these reasons, vulnerabilities were a prominent component of the integrative model for the transmission of risk to children of depressed mothers (Goodman & Gotlib, 1999). In this section, we outline possible alternative pathways to depression in children of depressed mothers, tied to specific, known vulnerabilities to depression, specifically affective, interpersonal, and cognitive vulnerabilities.

First, children of depressed mothers may develop affective vulnerabilities for depression, particularly early in development. Physiological affect dysregulation is evident from the very first stages of development in offspring of depressed mothers. Fetuses of depressed women have higher baseline heart rates and delayed return to baseline after a vibroacoustic stimulus (Allister, Lester, Carr, & Liu, 2001). Infants of depressed mothers have delayed development of autonomic regulation, as evidenced by lower vagal tone, higher mean heart rates, particularly in stressful situations, and lower heart rate variability (Field, 1994; Field, Healy, & LeBlanc, 1989; Field et al., 1996; Field, Pickens, Fox, Nawrocki, & Gonzalez, 1995). Mothers' ratings and behavioral observations of affective arousal and dysregulation in infants also suggest difficulty with self-quieting, less social responsiveness, more irritability, lower activity levels, and more negative affect in infants of depressed mothers as compared with control infants (Cummings & Davies, 1994; Field, 1992; Sameroff, Seifer, & Zax, 1982). The few studies of affect regulation in developmental periods beyond infancy also support greater vulnerability in offspring of depressed mothers. For example, Zahn-Waxler and colleagues found that 5- to 9-year-old children of depressed mothers displayed greater emotional arousal to stimuli depicting hypothetical situations of distress and interpersonal conflict (Zahn-Waxler, Kochanska, Krupnick, & McKnew, 1990). Furthermore, children's ability to maintain low heart rate (a physiological indicator of emotion regulation) during stressful interactions with their parents at ages 4 and 5 has been found to be related to their emotion regulation skills at age 8 (Gottman & Katz, 2002). This finding may be particularly relevant for children of depressed mothers who are likely to have more stressful interactions with their mothers. Thus, these early affective vulnerabilities have implications for the development of later abilities to regulate affect and modulate behavior, increasing risk for the development of depression.

Second, children of depressed mothers may also develop interpersonal and behavioral vulnerabilities for depression. They may be more likely than other children to develop both a sense of responsibility and feelings of guilt for causing their mothers' distress, as well as patterns of behavioral responding to mothers' distress. Young children, even toddlers and preschoolers, of depressed mothers have been observed to intervene more and show higher levels of prosocial behavior toward their mothers in response to their mothers' sadness than children of well mothers (Radke-Yarrow, Zahn-Waxler, Richardson, Susman, & Martinez, 1994; Zahn-Waxler, Cole, Welsh, & Fox, 1995). Children of depressed mothers, relative to controls, also have elevated levels of interpersonal responsibility and guilt when interpreting hypothetical situations of interpersonal conflict and distress (Zahn-Waxler et al., 1990). This excessive empathy, guilt, and sense of interpersonal responsibility for the emotional well-being of others may place the children of depressed mothers at particular risk for developing depression.

Third, children of depressed mothers are at risk for developing cognitive vulnerabilities. According to cognitive models of depression, such as Beck's cognitive distortion model (Beck, 1967, 1976) and the learned helplessness and hopelessness models of depression (Abramson, Metalsky, & Alloy, 1989; Abramson, Seligman, & Teasdale, 1978), habitual patterns of thinking and processing information, most often habitual ways of explaining stressful life events, constitute a vulnerability for depression that is activated by the experience of negative life events. Children of depressed mothers tend to have more of these cognitive vulnerabilities, such as more negative views of the self, less positive self-schemas, and more stable and global attributional styles about negative events, than children of well parents (for a review, see Garber & Martin, 2002). Studies have also shown that, as compared with controls, children of depressed mothers have more maladaptive ways of processing information. For example, these children recall more negative self-descriptive words and fewer positive self-descriptive words than children of nondepressed mothers (Hammen & Zupan, 1984; Taylor & Ingram, 1999; Whitman & Leitenberg, 1990; Zupan, Hammen, & Jaenicke, 1987). Thus, depression in children of depressed mothers typically emerges over time through pathways, such as these affective, interpersonal, and cognitive vulnerability mechanisms, that likely begin early in development and unfold via transactional pathways over time.

Moderators

The processes underlying the developmental pathways that lead to depression are likely to be affected by multiple moderating variables, which not only create pathways unique to each child but also exacerbate or lessen the extent of risk associated with depression in the mother more generally (Kraemer, Stice, Kazdin, Offord, & Kupfer, 2001). A transactional perspective suggests that through a process of continuous reciprocation, characteristics and traits of the child influence the child's experiences in the environment, which, in turn, influence the child's characteristics and traits (Sameroff, 1975). Thus, from the perspective of transactional models, various factors may moderate the associations between mothers' depression and children's depression and account for differences in risk for depression among children of depressed mothers. These factors may include (1) qualities of the children, such as temperament, gender, and various cognitive variables, (2) the broader context of the children's environment, such as the presence and mental health of fathers and the quality of the marital relationship, and (3) characteristics of the mothers' depression, such as timing, course, and chronicity. For the most part, the moderating roles of these factors have been proposed but not empirically investigated in the literature. Nevertheless, each of these factors is reviewed here in turn.

QUALITIES OF CHILDREN

Temperament is one child characteristic hypothesized to influence risk for depression, although studies have not directly tested the moderating role of temperament in associations between depression in mothers and their offspring. Nonetheless, research suggests that children with difficult temperaments are more vulnerable to the effects of inadequate parenting such as that shown by depressed mothers (Goldsmith, Buss, & Lemery, 1997). Furthermore, mothers' depressive symptoms have been associated with their perceptions of infant temperament, particularly infant negativity (Pesonen, Raikkonen, Strandberg, Keltikangas-Jarvinen, & Jarvenpaa, 2004) and difficulty (Cutrona & Troutman, 1986; Edhborg, Seimyr, Lundh, & Widstrom, 2000), and with observational measures of infant difficulty (Cutrona & Troutman, 1986). Mothers of more difficult infants perceive their parenting to be less efficacious, which in turn is linked to depression in mothers (Cutrona & Troutman, 1986; Porter & Hsu, 2003). Although much of the focus in regard to temperament has been on infants' negativity, behavioral inhibition is also of concern. Inhibition has been associated with the development of anxiety and depression in children (Biederman et al., 1990; Kagan, Arcus, & Snidman, 1993). In samples of children of depressed mothers, behavioral inhibition may interact with problematic parenting, such as being harsh or critical, to increase the risk to infants of depressed mothers. Infants with greater behavioral inhibition are more difficult to soothe, perhaps particularly for depressed mothers, who may have limited capacity to be sensitive and responsive. Thus, although not tested as a moderator in associations between depression in mothers and depression in children, children's temperament has been associated with both depression in mothers and with the mechanisms for the transmission of risk, suggesting the potential for temperament to be a moderator.

Gender of the offspring is one characteristic that has been shown to moderate the association between mothers' and children's depression, albeit a recent review revealed that support for gender as a moderator is predominantly limited to depression that emerges in adolescent offspring of depressed mothers (Sheeber, Davis, & Hops, 2002). Adolescent daughters of depressed mothers have more dysphoric and less happy affect than adolescent daughters of nondepressed mothers, whereas no significant difference in affect was found for adolescent boys of depressed mothers as compared with non-depressed mothers (Hops et al., 1990). In the smaller body of support for gender differences among younger children, depressed mothers and their daughters, but not depressed mothers and their sons, have been shown to have synchronous bouts of depression (Radke-Yarrow, Nottelmann, Belmont, & Welsh, 1993). Moreover, in community samples, levels of depression in mothers and daughters are interrelated, but levels of depression in mothers and sons are not related (Davies & Windle, 1997; Fergusson, Horwood, & Lynskey, 1995). The mechanisms that explain increased risk for depression in daughters, as compared with sons, of depressed mothers are likely not independent from the mechanisms of risk for depression in adolescent girls, as compared with adolescent boys, in general populations (see the reviews by Goodman & Tully, 2006; Sheeber et al., 2002). Those mechanisms are likely to be gender-stereotyped socialization processes, especially early socialization of emotion expression, coping styles, and relationship orientation and possibly greater exposure of girls than boys to family discord.

A number of cognitive variables have also been studied as potential child qualities that may moderate the link between depression in parents and in children. These cognitive factors include both variables related to cognitive abilities, such as IQ, and cognitive vulnerabilities, such as depressogenic attributions. Children of depressed parents may be protected against adverse outcome concurrently and prospectively if they are more intelligent (Radke-Yarrow & Sherman, 1990) or have better social-cognitive skills (Beardslee, Schultz, & Selman, 1987). Other cognitive variables, such as those proposed by cognitive theories of depression, have also been proposed as moderating variables. For example, risk for depression may be affected by children's perceptions and beliefs about their parents' depression (e.g., (Beardslee, 1989; Beardslee & Podorefsky, 1989; Compas et al., 2002; Garber & Martin, 2002; Klimes-Dougan & Bolger, 1998). As children become aware of the signs and symptoms of their mothers' depression, they begin to develop their own conceptualizations to fit their observations and experiences. Children may have exaggerated recall of the frequency and severity of mothers' depression, self-blame for mothers' depression, inflated interpretations of threat related to their mothers' depression, and expectations that they will be unable to cope with their mothers' depression, which may contribute to maladjustment. These conceptualizations may guide children's emotional and coping responses and then influence the impact of the mothers' depression on the children's development of depression.

We are developing a measure of children's conceptualizations of the signs and symptoms of their parents' depression, the Children's Perceptions of Parental Sadness Scale

(ChiPPS). The measure yields scores on nine scales, including Impaired Parenting (the frequency with which the child sees the mother's depression as interfering with her being an available and responsive parent), Perceived Threat (the child's fears and worries about his or her own well-being in association with the mother's depression), and Self-Blame (the extent to which the child blames him- or herself for the mother's depression). Preliminary data support the internal consistency, reliability, and several aspects of validity of the ChiPPS: discriminant (relative to attributional style), convergent (relative to mothers' stressors and symptoms of depression), and criterion-related (in relation to child internalizing and externalizing problems) (Tully, Goodman, & Brooks-DeWeese, 2005). In ongoing work, we are testing the measure to determine whether these perceptions moderate the association between depression in mothers and in children, with the expectation that children who are more aware of their mothers' depressive symptomatology, blame themselves for their mothers' depression, and doubt their ability to cope will be more likely to develop depression.

Children's ability to cope with their mothers' depression and the stress associated with having a depressed parent may also be an important moderator. Compas and colleagues have found support for the mediating role of coping strategies in the relationship between parental stress and children's depression among children of depressed parents (Jaser et al., 2005). More specifically, they found that secondary control coping strategies, such as acceptance, distraction, positive thinking, and cognitive restructuring, were associated with lower levels of depression, whereas involuntary engagement responses, such as rumination and intrusive thoughts, were associated with higher levels of depression (Langrock, Compas, Keller, Merchant, & Copeland, 2002).

CONTEXT

Studies of depression are increasingly taking into account the broader context in which depression occurs (Keyes & Goodman, 2006). Particularly relevant to the risk for depression in children and adolescents whose mothers have been depressed are the roles of the father and of marital discord. With regard to fathers, both the quantity and quality of their involvement and their mental health have been the factors considered as potential moderators of risk associated with maternal depression (Goodman & Gotlib, 1999). In a study of families not selected for maternal depression, a greater quantity of involvement by fathers with high levels of antisocial behavior was associated with more conduct problems in the children (Jaffee, Moffitt, Caspi, & Taylor, 2003). In studies specific to the effects of maternal depression, although there is some evidence for the moderating effect of fathers' mental health (Thomas & Forehand, 1991), other studies suggest that a more complex model may be needed, such as one that takes into account transactional relationships over time (Hops et al., 1990). In addition to attention to transactional relationships, an adequate conceptualization of the role of fathers needs to take into account the quality and quantity of their involvement and their mental health.

Marital discord is also essential to consider, in that it is a common contextual factor with depression in women and by itself is related to increased risk for psychopathology in children. Davies and colleagues provided some intriguing findings on the role of marital discord in a model of risk for depression in children of depressed mothers. In one study, they found that marital discord significantly mediated the association between histories of maternal depression symptoms and symptoms of depression in children at middle adolescence, but only in girls (Davies & Windle, 1997). In a later study with a longitudinal design, they found that maternal depressive symptoms mediated the effects of marital distress on adolescents' depressive symptoms, implicating a pathway from marital distress through maternal depression (rather than vice versa) to adolescents' depression (Davies & Dumenci, 1999). Furthermore, parents' use of specific conflict strategies involving depressive behaviors such as physical distress, withdrawal, sadness, and fear mediate associations between maternal depression and children's depression, in contrast to destructive or constructive marital conflict strategies (Du Rocher Schudlich & Cummings, 2003). These findings strongly support the importance of context and the need to develop and test models that consider the potentially moderating and mediating roles of marital discord and how it is expressed.

CHARACTERISTICS OF MOTHERS' DEPRESSION

The timing and course of mothers' depression may also account for differences in risk among children of depressed mothers. In terms of timing, mothers' depression may have a stronger and more negative impact if children's first exposure occurs earlier in the developmental pathways. In other words, it is expected that younger children, who have fewer resources to cope with their mothers' depression, will be less able to cope with and recover from the impact of their mothers' depression. The exact role of timing may be complicated, with some research suggesting that the effect of timing varies with the type of psychopathology and by the child's gender (Essex, Klein, Miech, & Smider, 2001). In a meta-analysis, we found a negative correlation between children's age and effect size, such that maternal depression was more strongly associated with internalizing and externalizing problems in younger children (Connell & Goodman, 2002).

Timing is, naturally, related to course, given the episodic nature of depression disorders. Thus, children who are exposed earlier in their lives are also likely to be exposed more often. More chronic depression in mothers is related to children's more chronic exposure to their mothers' depressed affect, behavior, and cognitions and, likely, to greater, more chronic stress and other correlates of the mothers' depression, such as marital difficulty, all of which place the children at greater risk for depression. There may also be some critical periods when episodes of depression in mothers, perhaps particularly severe and chronic episodes, may have implications for the development of certain vulnerabilities in the children. Some examples were previously mentioned in terms of infant development. Another example is that mothers play an important role in young children's learning about emotions and how to regulate emotion (see, e.g., Denham & Kochanoff, 2002). Depression that impairs a mother's ability to facilitate emotional development in her young child may lead to the development of an affective vulnerability during this period. Also of concern and needing further study is the effect on children of the unpredictable course of their mothers' depression.

IMPLICATIONS FOR TREATMENT AND PREVENTION OF DEPRESSION

Taking into account cogent warnings that not all predictors are causal (Kraemer et al., 1997; Rutter, Pickles, Murray, & Eaves, 2001), empirically supported risk factors offer promising windows of opportunity for interventions to minimize the likelihood of depression developing in children or adolescents whose mothers have been depressed. Interventions designed to modify risk factors not only have a high likelihood of changing the outcome of concern, such as depression in children of depressed mothers, but also have the potential to further empirically support the causal role of the risk factor in the theoretical model of transmission of depression from mothers to children. A recent review summarized the limited work that has been conducted on prevention or treatment of depression in children of depressed parents (Gladstone & Beardslee, 2002). Next, we highlight some of the key ideas from that chapter and add some further suggestions, organizing these thoughts according to whether the immediate target of the intervention is the child, the depressed mother, or the family.

Child-Level Interventions: Targeting the Vulnerabilities

Given concerns about inherited or acquired vulnerabilities to depression in children with depressed mothers, and the role the vulnerabilities may play in pathways to disorder, those vulnerabilities are a promising target of intervention. Interventions to lessen affective vulnerabilities may include massage to help infants experience positive affect and develop homeostatic regulation (Field, 2002). With older children, interventions may focus on their learning skills for emotion regulation. Targets for these interventions come from knowledge that depressed mothers have difficulty in facilitating emotion regulation abilities and that the ability to maintain low heart rate during stressful interactions with parents is related to later emotion regulation abilities (Gottman & Katz, 2002). Thus, children of depressed mothers may benefit from interventions targeting emotion regulation abilities, including family-focused interventions that teach skills for family communication about emotions and coping during stressful interactions, and parent-focused interventions to help mothers learn to facilitate emotion regulation in their children. Using methods similar to those used by Gottman (1999) in his work with couples, heart rate monitoring during treatment may help families learn to recognize their children's physiological arousal as a cue for emotion dysregulation and an indicator of internal affect dysregulation to facilitate learning to express emotions externally in socially acceptable ways. For adolescents, treatment may target cognitive vulnerabilities through cognitive behavioral interventions, such as Clarke and Lewinsohn's interventions for children at risk for depression. For example, Clarke and colleagues found that a brief group cognitive-behavioral intervention was effective in reducing subsyndromal depression in offspring of depressed mothers to the normal range (Clarke et al., 2001). Seligman's learned optimism interventions, which focus on promoting more accurate cognitive styles, problem-solving skills, and supportive family relationships, has shown promise in preventing depression and anxiety and may also be an effective approach to prevention in children of depressed mothers (Chaplin et al., 2006; Jaycox, Reivich, Gillham, & Seligman, 1994; Seligman, Schulman, DeRubeis, & Hollon, 1999).

Interventions Targeting the Mothers

Treating Her Depression

To the extent that exposure to depression in mothers—to its symptoms, impairment, or correlated stressors—is implicated in the transmission of risk for depression, it is compelling to consider that quickly and effectively treating the depression in mothers decreases the children's exposure and, thereby, their risk for developing depression themselves. This topic was the basis of a recent symposium (Coiro, 2005), a recent *Journal of the American Medical Association* publication (Weissman et al., 2006) and a series of articles in a special issue of the *Infant Mental Health Journal* (Clark, in press), although these articles are specific to postpartum depression. Overall, the evidence is promising.

O'Hara and colleagues, with a controlled trial of interpersonal psychotherapy (IPT) in postpartum women with major depression, not only significantly reduced levels of depression in the mothers but also significantly enhanced the mothers' reports of their relationships with their children, even though the women did not achieve the levels of quality of parenting relationships typical of women with no history of depression (O'Hara, Stuart, Gorman, & Wenzel, 2000). Similarly, Cooper and Murray (1997) treated a community sample of depressed mothers (randomly assigned to nondirective counseling, cognitive-behavioral therapy, or dynamic psychotherapy) and found that despite significant improvement in mood, treated mothers were not observed to differ from untreated mothers or early-remission mothers on either sensitive–insensitive or intrusive–withdrawn dimensions in face-to-face interactions with their infants. Initial low levels of disturbances in parenting in these samples may have restricted their ability to find an impact of treatment on parenting. In a third study, Fleming, Klein, and Corter (1992) investigated a community sample of women with self-reported depression who were treated with group therapy. Despite limited changes in ratings of depression, the treated mothers made more noninstrumental approaches to their infants, and the infants decreased in amounts of crying and increased in non-cry vocalizations. Although all three of these studies relied on psychotherapy as the mode of treatment, antidepressant medications are also effective in the treatment of depression (Hollon, Thase, & Markowitz, 2002) and thus were the focus of interventions recently conducted in our lab. We found that regardless of initial levels of parenting quality and depression, mothers' reduced levels of depression, after 12 weeks of antidepressant treatment, were associated with improvements in the quality of their interactions with their infants and with improvements in their infants' quality of play (Goodman, Broth, Hall, & Stowe, in press). In a much larger-scale study of the effects of antidepressant medication treatment of mothers of 7- to 17-year-old children, remission of maternal depression symptoms was significantly correlated with children's decreases in both rates of depression and levels of depression symptoms (Weissman et al., 2006). Similarly, Garber and colleagues, in three independent samples of depressed parents treated with cognitive therapy or medication, showed that remission of parental depression predicted a significant decrease in children's depressive symptoms and was also associated with improvements in family environment (Garber, 2006; McCauley, Garber, Diamond, & Schloredt, 2005). In contrast, among a group of low-income minority mothers, successful treatment of their depression did not affect child behavior problems or social competence, parenting or family stress levels (Coiro, Riley, & Broitman, 2005). Given the mixed findings, further research is needed to determine whether the timing, type of therapy (IPT, cognitive-behavioral therapy [CBT], medication, or combinations), or sampling characteristics (e.g., poverty, severity, etc.) influence the likelihood of children's risk for depression decreasing in association with their mothers' receiving treatment for their depression.

Treating the Context of Her Depression

Also promising, although less often a topic of study, is the idea of treating the contextual factors that have been implicated as moderators or mediators of the association between maternal depression and children's development of depression. These treatments may include stress reduction techniques, interventions to minimize stress generation, and enhancing problem-solving skills in the women (Hammen, 2002). Also promising is the idea of treating the depressed mothers' parenting efficacy beliefs by, for example, training the women in cognitive coping skills (Sanders & McFarland, 2000). Improving the quality of the marital or couple relationship also has the potential benefits of increasing the depressed woman's perceived support from her husband/partner, decreasing her level of stress, and increasing the husband/partner's involvement with the children (Katz & Gottman, 1993). Another important consideration is that couple therapy designed to improve the quality of the marriage may be an effective treatment for depression in women (Epstein & Baucom, 2002). Any intervention designed to minimize the development of depression in offspring of depressed mothers may benefit from involving the husbands/partners (Dadds, Sanders, & James, 1987). Finally, the context of depression was the target of interventions involving the provision of home visitor services to mothers of infants or toddlers. Results have been mixed, with one study having found no effects on infants' cognitive development (Gelfand, Teti, Seiner, & Jameson, 1996), and another, among participants of low socioeconomic status (SES), having found prevention of cognitive-intellectual decline relative to no-intervention controls (Lyons-Ruth, Connell, Grunebaum, & Botein, 1990).

Enhancing the Quality of Parenting

To the extent that parenting practices can be considered causal of depression or depression vulnerabilities in children with depressed mothers (Davis et al., 2002), parenting interventions designed to change such practices should decrease risk for depression. In contrast to the strong support for the effectiveness of parent management training in reducing risk for conduct disorder, there is less support provided by the research on parenting interventions to reduce risk for depression. Ideally, such intervention studies would test specific theoretical models, such as the role of contingencies (which child behaviors do or do not get rewarded), rather than targeting broadly defined inadequate parenting.

A few studies have targeted parenting by depressed mothers. Among these, infants of depressed mothers have been found to benefit from their mothers having been instructed in recognizing their infants' abilities (Hart, Field, & Nearing, 1998), coached to enhance the sensitivity and responsiveness of their interactions with their infants (Malphurs et al., 1996), or taught to massage their infants (Field, Grizzle, et al., 1996). These interventions may have the further benefit of helping the infants to regulate their emotions, addressing one of our proposed vulnerabilities in the pathways from maternal to child depression. With toddlers of depressed mothers, an intervention designed to enhance the quality of the mother–child relationship, including responsivity and communication, toddler–parent psychotherapy (Lieberman, 1992), improved children's cognitive development (Cicchetti, Rogosch, & Toth, 2000) and attachment security (Cicchetti, Toth, & Rogosch, 2000).

Interventions Targeting the Families

Beardslee and colleagues have taken a family-based approach in interventions designed to minimize the risk of depression in adolescents of parents with depression (Beardslee et al., 1993). Building on their work identifying self-understanding and relationships as keys to resilience in adolescents of depressed parents, their intervention is designed to both decrease the effects associated with the contextual variables (family and marital risk factors) and encourage the promotion of resilience in the children (Beardslee et al., 1987). The latter includes providing psychoeducational material about depression and helping the children to feel less guilt and self-blame, while facilitating their development of relationships and activities independent of the family. The intervention is proving to be effective in increasing adolescents' understanding of depression, enhancing communication with their parents, increasing participation in adaptive activities, and lowering scores on depressive symptoms (Gladstone & Beardslee, 2002).

UNRESOLVED QUESTIONS/FUTURE DIRECTIONS

Although much has been learned about depression in children and adolescents from studies of children with depressed mothers, there are also many unanswered questions. In particular, although there is fairly extensive research on the mechanisms of risk, more work is needed on each of the core mechanisms and on their interactions. In particular, tests are needed of their actual mediating roles in associations between depression in mothers and children and on developmental pathways. Relative to work on mechanisms, there is considerably less research on potential moderators. Research on moderators, such as fathers' quality and quantity of involvement and mental health, and children's temperament, cognitive abilities and social-cognitive skills, is promising, but more research is needed to clarify the importance of these moderators and the role of development in these associations.

Also given little attention are the potential roles of race/ethnicity and poverty. Although a few studies targeted minority ethnicities or those in poverty (see the work by Karlen Lyons-Ruth [Lyons-Ruth et al., 1998] and Tiffany Field [Field, 1992] as examples), most sampled white, middle-SES families. The influence of the mechanisms of risk may vary among ethnic and SES groups. There may be differences in the severity of the risk mechanisms and moderators, and possibly additional mechanisms of risk, among these groups (Downey & Coyne, 1990). For example, there may be different or more extreme stressors associated with depression in mothers in low-income populations, greater deficits in the ability to provide for children's social-emotional needs, and more harsh and inconsistent parenting. The severity of the mechanisms may be influenced by more extreme versions of various moderators, such as lack of resources, child care, education, availability of fathers, and stable social supports. There may also be additional risks among some low-income families that compound the risks due to having a depressed mother, such as maltreatment or teen mothering.

The research on the mechanisms of risk provides ideas for interventions for children of depressed mothers. However, there are few studies of interventions in this population. Research on the development of interventions that address these mechanisms has promise not only to provide further empirical tests of our theoretical models, but also to minimize the risk for the development of depression in these children.

REFERENCES

Abramson, L. Y., Metalsky, G. I., & Alloy, L. B. (1989). Hopelessness depression: A theory-based subtype of depression. *Psychological Review, 96*, 358–372.

Abramson, L. Y., Seligman, M. E. P., & Teasdale, J. (1978). Learned helplessness in humans: Critique and reformulation. *Journal of Abnormal Psychology, 87*, 49–74.

Allister, L., Lester, B. M., Carr, S., & Liu, J. (2001). The effects of maternal depression on fetal heart rate responses to vibroacoustic stimulation. *Developmental Neuropsychology, 20*, 639–651.

Ashman, S. B., & Dawson, G. (2002). Maternal depression, infant psychobiological development, and risk for depression. In S. H. Goodman & I. H. Gotlib (Eds.), *Children of depressed parents: Mechanisms of risk and implications for treatment* (pp. 37–58). Washington, DC: American Psychological Association.

Beardslee, W. R. (1989). The role of self-understanding in resilient individuals: The development of a perspective. *American Journal of Orthopsychiatry, 59*(2), 266–278.

Beardslee, W. R., Keller, M. B., Lavori, P. W., Klerman, G. K., Dorer, D. J., & Samuelson, H. (1988). Psychiatric disorder in adolescent offspring of parents with affective disorder in a non-referred sample. *Journal of Affective Disorders, 15,* 313–322.

Beardslee, W. R., & Podorefsky, D. (1989). Resilient adolescents whose parents have serious affective and other psychiatric disorders: Importance of self-understanding and relationships. *American Journal of Psychiatry, 145,* 63–69.

Beardslee, W. R., Salt, P., Porterfield, K., Rothberg, P. C., van de Velde, P., Swatling, S., et al. (1993). Comparison of preventive interventions for families with parental affective disorder. *Journal of the American Academy of Child and Adolescent Psychiatry, 32,* 254–263.

Beardslee, W. R., Schultz, L. H., & Selman, R. L. (1987). Level of social-cognitive development, adaptive functioning, and DSM-III diagnoses in adolescent offspring of parents with affective disorders: Implications of the development of the capacity for mutuality. *Developmental Psychology, 23*(6), 807–815.

Beck, A. T. (1967). *Depression: Clinical, experimental, and theoretical aspects.* New York: Hoeber.

Beck, A. T. (1976). *Cognitive therapy and emotional disorders.* New York: International Universities Press.

Beck, A. T., Rush, A. J., Shaw, B. F., & Emery, G. (1979). *Cognitive therapy of depression.* New York: Guilford Press.

Biederman, J., Rosenbaum, J. F., Hirshfeld, D. R., Faraone, S. V., Bolduc, E. A., Gersten, M., et al. (1990). Psychiatric correlates of behavioral inhibition in young children of parents with and without psychiatric disorders. *Archives of General Psychiatry, 47*(1), 21–26.

Billings, A. G., & Moos, R. H. (1985). Children of parents with unipolar depression: A controlled 1-year follow-up. *Journal of Abnormal Child Psychology, 14*(1), 149–166.

Brennan, P. A., Hammen, C., Katz, A. R., & Le Brocque, R. M. (2002). Maternal depression, paternal psychopathology, and adolescent diagnostic outcomes. *Journal of Consulting and Clinical Psychology, 70*(5), 1075–1085.

Buss, K. A., Malmstadt Schumacher, J. R., Dolski, I., Kalin, N. H., Goldsmith, H. H., & Davidson, R. J. (2003). Right frontal brain activity, cortisol, and withdrawal behavior in 6-month-old infants. *Behavioral Neuroscience, 117,* 11–20.

Campbell, S. B. (1995). Behavior problems in preschool children: A review of recent research. *Journal of Child Psychology and Psychiatry, 36,* 113–149.

Caspi, A., Sugden, K., Moffitt, T. E., Taylor, A., Craig, I. W., Harrington, H., et al. (2003). Influence of life stress on depression: Moderation by a polymorphism in the 5-HTT gene. *Science, 301,* 386–389.

Chaplin, T. M., Gillham, J. E., Reivich, K., Elkon, A. G., Samuels, B., Freres, D. R., et al. (2006). Depression prevention for early adolescent girls: A pilot study of all girls versus co-ed groups. *Journal of Early Adolescence, 26*(1), 110–126.

Cherny, S. S., Fulker, D. W., Corley, R. P., Plomin, R., & DeFries, J. C. (1994). Continuity and change in infant shyness from 14 to 20 months. *Behavior Genetics, 24,* 365–379.

Chugani, H. T., & Phelps, M. E. (1986). Maturational changes in cerebral function in infants determined by 18FDG positron emission tomography. *Science, 231,* 840–843.

Cicchetti, D. (1984). The emergence of developmental psychology. *Child Development, 55*(1), 1–7.

Cicchetti, D., & Rogosch, F. A. (1996). Equifinality and multifinality in developmental psychopathology. *Development and Psychopathology, 8,* 597–600.

Cicchetti, D., Rogosch, F. A., & Toth, S. L. (1998). Maternal depressive disorder and contextual risk: Contributions to the development of attachment insecurity and behavior problems in toddlerhood. *Development and Psychopathology, 10,* 283–300.

Cicchetti, D., Rogosch, F. A., & Toth, S. L. (2000). The efficacy of toddler–parent psychotherapy for fostering cognitive development in offspring of depressed mothers. *Journal of Abnormal Child Psychology, 28,* 135–148.

Cicchetti, D., & Toth, S., L. (1995). Developmental psychopathology and disorders of affect. In D. Cicchetti & D. J. Cohen (Eds.), *Developmental psychopathology: Vol. 2. Risk, disorder, and adaptation* (pp. 369–420). Oxford, UK: Wiley.

Cicchetti, D., & Toth, S. (1998). The development of depression in children and adolescents. *American Psychologist, 53,* 221–241.

Cicchetti, D., Toth, S. L., & Rogosch, F. A. (2000). The effectiveness of toddler–parent psychotherapy to increase attachment security in offspring of depressed mothers. *Attachment and Human Development, 28,* 135–148.

Clark, L. A. (1989). The anxiety and depressive disorders: Descriptive psychopathology and differential diagnoses. In P. C. Kendall & D. Watson (Eds.), *Anxiety and depression: Distinctive and overlapping features* (pp. 83–129). San Diego: Academic Press.

Clark, R. (in press). *Infant Mental Health Journal* [Special Issue].

Clarke, G. N., Hornbrook, M., Lynch, F., Polen, M., Gale, J., Beardslee, W., et al. (2001). A randomized trial of a group cognitive intervention for preventing depression in adolescent offspring of depressed parents. *Archives of General Psychiatry, 58*(12), 1127–1134.

Coccaro, E. F., Silverman, J. M., Klar, H. M., Horvath, T. B., & Siever, L. J. (1994). Familial correlates of reduced central serotonergic system function in patients with personality disorders. *Archives of General Psychiatry, 51,* 318–324.

Coiro, M. J. (2005). *Treating parents' depression: How does it affect their children?* Paper presented at biennial meeting of the Society for Research in Child Development, Atlanta.

Coiro, M. J., Riley, A. W., & Broitman, M. (2005). *Treating maternal depression: Effects on children's behavior problems, social competence, and family environment.* Paper presented at the biennial meeting of the Society for Research in Child Development, Atlanta.

Compas, B. E., Langrock, A. M., Keller, G., Merchant, M. J., & Copeland, M. E. (2002). Children coping with parental depression: Processes of adaptation to family stress. In S. H. Goodman & I. H. Gotlib (Eds.), *Children of depressed parents: Mechanisms of risk and implications for treatment* (pp. 227–252). Washington, DC: American Psychological Association.

Compton, K., Snyder, J., Schrepferman, L., Bank, L., & Shortt, J. W. (2003). The contribution of parents and siblings to antisocial and depressive behavior in adolescents: A double jeopardy coercion model. *Development and Psychopathology, 15,* 163–182.

Connell, A. M., & Goodman, S. H. (2002). The association between psychopathology in fathers versus mothers and children's internalizing and externalizing behavior problems: A meta-analysis. *Psychological Bulletin, 128,* 746–773.

Cooper, P., & Murray, L. (1997). The impact of psychological treatments of post-partum depression on maternal mood and infant development. In L. Murray & P. Cooper (Eds.), *Postpartum depression and child development* (pp. 201–220). New York: Guilford Press.

Cummings, E. M., & Davies, P. T. (1994). Maternal depression and child development. *Journal of Child Psychology and Psychiatry, 35,* 73–112.

Cutrona, C. E., & Troutman, B. R. (1986). Social support, infant temperament, and parenting self-efficacy: A mediational model of postpartum depression. *Child Development, 57,* 1507–1518.

Dadds, M. R., Sanders, M. R., & James, J. E. (1987). The generalization of treatment effects in parent training with multidistressed parents. *Behavioural Psychotherapy, 15,* 289–313.

Davidson, R. J., Ekman, P., Saron, C., Senulis, R., & Friesen, W. V. (1990). Approach–withdrawal and cerebral asymmetry: Emotional expression and brain physiology: I. *Journal of Personality and Social Psychology, 58,* 330–341.

Davidson, R. J., & Fox, N. A. (1989). Frontal brain asymmetry predicts infants' response to maternal separation. *Journal of Abnormal Psychology, 98,* 127–131.

Davies, P. T., & Dumenci, L. (1999). The interplay between maternal depressive symptoms and marital distress in the prediction of adolescent adjustment. *Journal of Marriage and the Family, 61,* 238–254.

Davies, P. T., & Windle, M. (1997). Gender-specific pathways between maternal depressive symptoms, family discord, and adolescent adjustment. *Developmental Psychology, 33,* 657–668.

Davis, B., Sheeber, L., & Hops, H. (2002). Coercive family processes and adolescent depression. In J. B. Reid, G. R. Patterson, & J. J. Snyder (Eds.), *Antisocial behavior in children and adolescents: Developmental analysis and the Oregon model for intervention* (pp. 173–194). Washington, DC: American Psychological Association.

Dawson, G., Ashman, S. B., Panagiotides, H., Hessl, D., Self, J., Yamada, E., et al. (2003). Preschool outcomes of children of depressed mothers: Role of maternal behavior, contextual risk, and children's brain activity. *Child Development, 74,* 1158–1175.

Dawson, G., Grofer Klinger, L., Panagiotides, H., Hill, D., & Spieker, S. (1992). Frontal lobe activity and affective behavior of infants of mothers with depressive symptoms. *Child Development, 63,* 725–737.

Denham, S., & Kochanoff, A. T. (2002). Parental contributions to preschoolers' understanding of emotion. *Marriage and Family Review, 3/4,* 213–242.

Downey, G., & Coyne, J. C. (1990). Children of depressed parents: An integrative review. *Psychological Bulletin, 108,* 50–76.

Du Rocher Schudlich, T. D., & Cummings, E. M. (2003). Parental dysphoria and children's internalizing symptoms: Marital conflict styles as mediators of risk. *Child Development, 74,* 1663–1681.

Eaves, L. J., Silberg, J. L., Meyer, J. M., Maes, H. H., Simonoff, E., Pickles, A., et al. (1997). Genetics and developmental psychopathology: II. The main effects of genes and environment on behavioral problems in the Virginia Twin Study of Adolescent Behavioral Development. *Journal of Child Psychology and Psychiatry, 38,* 965–980.

Edhborg, M., Seimyr, L., Lundh, W., & Widstrom, A. M. (2000). Fussy child—difficult parenthood? Comparisons between families with a "depressed" mother and non-depressed mother 2 months postpartum. *Journal of Reproductive and Infant Psychology, 18*(3), 225–238.

Eley, T. C., & Stevenson, J. (1999). Exploring the covariation between anxiety and depression symptoms: A genetic analysis of the effect of age and sex. *Journal of Child Psychology and Psychiatry, 40,* 1273–1284.

Epstein, N. B., & Baucom, D. H. (2002). Addressing individual psychopathology, unresolved issues, and interpersonal traumas within couple therapy. In N. B. Epstein & D. H. Baucom (Eds.), *Enhanced cognitive-behavioral therapy for couples: A contextual approach* (pp. 441–473). Washington, DC: American Psychological Association.

Essex, M. J., Klein, M. H., Miech, R., & Smider, N. A. (2001). Timing of initial exposure to maternal major depression and children's mental health symptoms in kindergarten. *British Journal of Psychiatry, 179,* 151–156.

Fergusson, D. M., Horwood, L. J., & Lynskey, M. T. (1995). Maternal depressive symptoms and depressive symptoms in adolescents. *Journal of Child Psychology and Psychiatry, 36,* 1161–1178.

Field, T. (1992). Infants of depressed mothers. *Development and Psychopathology, 4,* 49–66.

Field, T. (1994). The effects of mother's physical and emotional unavailability on emotion regulation. *Monographs of the Society for Research in Child Development, 59,* 209–227.

Field, T. (2002). Prenatal effects of maternal depression. In S. H. Goodman & I. H. Gotlib (Eds.), *Children of depressed parents: Mechanisms of risk and implications for treatment* (pp. 59–88). Washington, DC: American Psychological Association.

Field, T., Grizzle, N., Scafidi, F., Abrams, S. M., Richardson, S., Kuhn, C., et al. (1996). Massage therapy for infants of depressed mothers. *Infant Behavior and Development, 19,* 107–112.

Field, T., Healy, B., Goldstein, S., & Guthertz, M. (1990). Behavior–state matching and synchrony in mother–infant interactions of nondepressed versus depressed dyads. *Developmental Psychology, 26,* 7–14.

Field, T., Healy, B. T., & LeBlanc, W. G. (1989). Sharing and synchrony of behavior states and heart rate in nondepressed versus depressed mother–infant interactions. *Infant Behavior and Development, 12,* 357–376.

Field, T., Lang, C., Martinez, A., Yando, R., Pickens, J., & Bendell, D. (1996). Preschool follow-up of infants of dysphoric mothers. *Journal of Clinical Child Psychology, 25,* 272–279.

Field, T., Pickens, J., Fox, N. A., Nawrocki, T., & Gonzalez, J. (1995). Vagal tone in infants of depressed mothers. *Development and Psychopathology, 7,* 227–231.

Fleming, A., Klein, E., & Corter, C. (1992). The effects of a social support group on depression, maternal attitudes and behavior in new mothers. *Journal of Child Psychology and Psychiatry, 33,* 685–698.

Fox, N. A. (1994). The development of emotion regulation: Biological and behavioral considerations. *Monographs of the Society for Research in Child Development (Vol. 59).* Chicago: University of Chicago Press.

Frye, A., & Garber, J. (2005). The relations among maternal depression, maternal criticism, and adolescents' externalizing and internalizing symptoms. *Journal of Abnormal Child Psychology, 33,* 1–11.

Garber, J. (2006). Depression in children and adolescents: Linking risk research and prevention. *American Journal of Preventive Medicine, 31*(6, Suppl.), 104–125.

Garber, J., & Martin, N. C. (2002). Negative cognitions in offspring of depressed parents: Mechanisms of risk. In S. H. Goodman & I. H. Gotlib (Eds.), *Children of depressed parents: Mechanisms of risk and implications for treatment* (pp. 121–154). Washington, DC: American Psychological Association.

Gelfand, D. M., & Teti, D. M. (1990). The effects of maternal depression on children. *Clinical Psychology Review, 10,* 329–353.

Gelfand, D. M., Teti, D. M., Seiner, S. A., & Jameson, P. B. (1996). Helping mother fight depression: Evaluation of a home-based intervention for depressed mothers and their infants. *Journal of Clinical Child Psychology, 24,* 406–422.

Gladstone, T. R. G., & Beardslee, W. R. (2002). Treatment, intervention, and prevention with children of depressed parents: A developmental perspective. In S. H. Goodman & I. H. Gotlib (Eds.), *Children of Depressed Parents: Mechanisms of Risk and Implications for Treatment* (pp. 277–305). Washington, DC: American Psychological Association.

Glover, V. (1999). Mechanisms by which maternal mood in pregnancy may affect the fetus. *Contemporary Reviews in Obstetrics and Gynecology, 11,* 155–160.

Goldsmith, H. H., Buss, K. A., & Lemery, K. S. (1997). Toddler and childhood temperament: Expanded content, stronger genetic evidence, new evidence for the importance of environment. *Developmental Psychology, 33,* 891–905.

Goldsmith, H. H., Gottesman, I. I., & Lemery, K. S. (1997). Epigenetic approaches to developmental psychopathology. *Development and Psychopathology, 9,* 365–387.

Goodman, S. H. (2003). Genesis and epigenisis of psychopathology in children with depressed mothers: Toward an integrative biopsychosocial perspective. In D. Cicchetti & E. Walker (Eds.), *Neurodevelopmental mechanisms in the genesis and epigenesis of psychopathology: Future research directions* (pp. 428–460). New York: Cambridge University Press.

Goodman, S. H., Adamson, L. B., Riniti, J., & Cole, S. (1994). Mothers' expressed attitudes: Associations with maternal depression and children's self-esteem and psychopathology. *Journal of the American Academy of Child and Adolescent Psychiatry, 33,* 1265–1274.

Goodman, S. H., Broth, M., Hall, C. M., & Stowe, Z. N. (in press). Treatment of postpartum depression in mothers: Secondary benefits to the infants. *Infant Mental Health Journal.*

Goodman, S. H., Connell, A. M., Broth, M. R., & Hall, C. M. (2007). *The association between psychopathology and competence in children and depression in mothers: A meta-analysis.* Manuscript in preparation.

Goodman, S. H., & Gotlib, I. H. (1999). Risk for psychopathology in the children of depressed mothers: A developmental model for understanding mechanisms of transmission. *Psychological Review, 106,* 458–490.

Goodman, S. H., Sewell, D. R., Cooley, E. L., & Leavitt, N. (1993). Assessing levels of adaptive functioning: The Role Functioning Scale. *Community Mental Health Journal, 29,* 119–131.

Goodman, S. H., & Tully, E. C. (2006). Depression in women who are mothers: An integrative model of risk for the development of psychopathology in their sons and daughters. In C. L. M. Keyes & S. H. Goodman (Eds.), *Women and depression: A handbook for the social, behavioral, and biomedical sciences* (pp. 241–282). Cambridge, UK: Cambridge University Press.

Gotlib, I. H., Gilboa, E., & Sommerfeld, B. K. (2000). Cognitive functioning in depression: Nature and origins. In R. J. Davidson (Ed.), *Wisconsin Symposium on Emotion* (Vol. 1, pp. 133–163). New York: Oxford University Press.

Gottman, J. M. (1999). *The marriage clinic: A scientifically based marital therapy.* New York: Norton.

Gottman, J. M., & Katz, L. F. (2002). Children's emotional reactions to stressful parent–child interactions: The link between emotion regulation and vagal tone. *Marriage and Family Review, 34*(3–4), 265–283.

Graham, Y. P., Heim, C., Goodman, S. H., Miller, A. H., & Nemeroff, C. B. (1999). The effects of neonatal stress on brain development: Implications for psychopathology. *Development and Psychopathology, 11,* 545–565.

Grant, K. E., Compas, B. E., Stuhlmacher, A. F., Thurm, A. E., McMahon, S. D., & Halpert, J. A. (2003). Stressors and child and adolescent psychopathology: Moving from markers to mechanisms of risk. *Psychological Bulletin, 129,* 447–466.

Hammen, C. L. (1991). Generation of stress in the course of unipolar depression. *Journal of Abnormal Psychology, 100,* 555–561.

Hammen, C. (2002). Context of stress in families of children with depressed parents. In S. H. Goodman & I. H. Gotlib (Eds.), *Children of depressed parents: Mechanisms of risk and implications for treatment* (pp. 175–202). Washington, DC: American Psychological Association.

Hammen, C., Gordon, D., Burge, D., Adrian, C., Jaenicke, C., & Hiroto, D. (1987). Maternal affective disorders, illness, and stress: Risk for children's psychopathology. *American Journal of Psychiatry, 144*(6), 736–741.

Hammen, C., & Zupan, B. A. (1984). Self-schemas, depression, and the processing of personal information in children. *Jouranl of Experimental Child Psychology, 37,* 598–608.

Harrington, R. (1996). Family-genetic findings in child and adolescent depressive disorders. *International Review of Psychiatry, 8,* 355–368.

Harrington, R., Rutter, M., & Fombonne, E. (1996). Developmental pathways in depression: Multiple meanings, antecedents, and endpoints. *Development and Psychopathology, 8,* 601–616.

Harrington, R., Rutter, M., Weissman, M. M., Fudge, H., Groothues, C., Bredenkamp, D., et al. (1997). Psychiatric disorders in the relatives of depressed probands: I. Comparison of prepubertal, adolescent and early adult onset cases. *Journal of Affective Disorders, 42,* 9–22.

Hart, S., Field, T., & Nearing, G. (1998). Depressed mothers' neonates improve following the MABI and a Brazelton demonstration. *Journal of Pediatric Psychology, 23,* 351–356.

Hettema, J. M., Prescott, C. A., & Kendler, K. S. (2003). The effects of anxiety, substance use and conduct disorders on risk of major depressive disorder. *Psychological Medicine, 33,* 1423–1432.

Hollon, S. D., Thase, M. E., & Markowitz, J. C. (2002). Treatment and prevention of depression. *Psychological Science in the Public Interest, 3,* 39–77.

Hops, H., Sherman, L., & Biglan, A. (1990). Maternal depression, marital discord, and children's behavior: A developmental perspective. In G. R. Patterson (Ed.), *Depression and aggression in family interaction* (pp. 185–208). Hillsdale, NJ: Erlbaum.

Jaenicke, C., Hammen, C. L., Zupan, B., Hiroto, D., Gordon, D., Adrian, C., et al. (1987). Cognitive vulnerability in children at risk for depression. *Journal of Abnormal Child Psychology, 15,* 559–572.

Jaffee, S. R., Moffitt, T. E., Caspi, A., & Taylor, A. (2003). Life with (or without) father: The benefits of living with two biological parents depend on the father's antisocial behavior. *Child Development, 74,* 109–126.

Jaser, S. S., Langrock, A. M., Keller, G., Merchant, M. J., Benson, M. A., Reeslund, K., et al. (2005). Coping with the stress of parental depression: II. Adolescent and parent reports of coping and adjustment. *Journal of Clinical Child and Adolescent Psychology, 34*(1), 193–205.

Jaycox, L. H., Reivich, K. J., Gillham, J., & Seligman, M. E. (1994). Prevention of depressive symptoms in school children. *Behaviour Research and Therapy, 32*(8), 801–816.

Kagan, J., Arcus, D., & Snidman, N. (1993). The idea of temperament: Where do we go from here? In R. Plomin & G. E. McClearn (Eds.), *Nature, nurture, and psychology* (pp. 197–210). Washington, DC: American Psychological Association.

Katz, L. F., & Gottman, J. M. (1993). Patterns of marital conflict predict children's internalizing and externalizing behaviors. *Developmental Psychology, 29*, 940–950.

Kendler, K. S., Gardner, C. O., Neale, M. C., & Prescott, C. A. (2001). Genetic risk factors for major depression in men and women: Similar or different heritabilities and same or partly distinct genes? *Psychological Medicine, 31*, 605–616.

Kessler, R. C. (2006). The epidemiology of depression among women. In C. L. M. Keyes & S. H. Goodman (Eds.), *Women and depression: A handbook for the social, behavior, and biomedical sciences* (pp. 22–40). New York: Cambridge University Press.

Keyes, C. L. M., & Goodman, S. H. (2006). *Women and depression: A handbook for the social, behavioral, and biomedical sciences.* New York: Cambridge University Press.

Klimes-Dougan, B., & Bolger, A. K. (1998). Coping with maternal depressed affect and depression: Adolescent children of depressed and well mothers. *Journal of Youth and Adolescence, 27*, 1–15.

Kochanska, G., Radke-Yarrow, M., Kuczynski, L., & Friedman, S. (1987). Normal and affectively ill mothers' beliefs about their children. *American Journal of Orthopsychiatry, 57*, 345–350.

Kraemer, H. C., Kazdin, A. E., Offord, D. R., Kessler, R. C., Jensen, P. S., & Kupfer, D. J. (1997). Coming to terms with the terms of risk. *Archives of General Psychiatry, 54*, 337–343.

Kraemer, H. C., Stice, E., Kazdin, A., Offord, D., & Kupfer, D. J. (2001). How do risk factors work together? Mediators, moderators, and independent, overlapping, and proxy risk factors. *American Journal of Psychiatry, 158*, 848–856.

Lamb, M. E. (2000). The history of research on father involvement: An overview. *Marriage and Family Review, 29*, 23–42.

Langrock, A. M., Compas, B. E., Keller, G., Merchant, M. J., & Copeland, M. E. (2002). Coping with the stress of parental depression: Parents' reports of children's coping, emotional, and behavioral problems. *Journal of Clinical Child and Adolescent Psychology, 31*(3), 312–324.

Lee, C. M., & Gotlib, I. H. (1989). Clinical status and emotional adjustment of children of depressed mothers. *American Journal of Psychiatry, 146*, 478–483.

Lieberman, A. F. (1992). Infant–parent psychotherapy with toddlers. *Development and Psychopathology, 4*, 559–574.

Loehlin, J. C., & Nichols, R. C. (1976). *Heredity, environment, and personality.* Austin: University of Texas Press.

Lovejoy, M. C., Graczyk, P. A., O'Hare, E., & Neuman, G. (2000). Maternal depression and parenting behavior: A meta-analytic review. *Clinical Psychology Review, 20*, 561–592.

Lundy, B., Jones, N., Field, T., Pietro, P., Nearing, G., Davalos, M., et al. (1999). Prenatal depression effects on neonates. *Infant Behavior and Development, 22*, 119–129.

Lykken, D. T., & Tellegen, A. (1996). Happiness is a stochatic phenomenon. *Psychological Science, 7*, 186–189.

Lyons-Ruth, K., Connell, D. B., Grunebaum, H. U., & Botein, S. (1990). Infants at social risk: Maternal depression and family support as mediators of infant development and security of attachment. *Child Development, 61*, 85–98.

Malcarne, V. L., Hamilton, N. A., Ingram, R. E., & Taylor, L. (2000). Correlates of distress in children at risk for affective disorder: Exploring predictors in the offspring of depressed and nondepressed mothers. *Journal of Affective Disorders, 59*(3), 243–251.

Malphurs, J. E., Field, T. M., Larraine, C., Pickens, J., Pelaez-Nogueras, M., Yando, R., et al. (1996). Altering withdrawn and intrusive interaction behavior of depressed mothers. *Infant Mental Health Journal, 17*, 152–160.

McCauley, E., Garber, J., Diamond, G., & Schloredt, K. (2005). *Changes in family environment and child functioning in relation to changes in parental depression.* Paper presented at the biennial meeting of the Society for Research in Child Development, Atlanta.

Mednick, S. A., & Schulsinger, F. (1968). Some premorbid characteristics related to breakdown in children with schizophrenic mothers. In R. Rosenthal & S. S. Kety (Eds.), *The transmission of schizophrenia* (pp. 267–291). Oxford, UK: Pergamon Press.

Moldin, S. O. (1999). Report of the NIMH's genetic workgroups: Summary of research. *Biological Psychiatry, 45,* 559–602.

Monroe, S. M., & Hadjiyannakis, K. (2002). The social environment and depression: Focusing on severe life stress. In I. H. Gotlib & C. L. Hammen (Eds.), *Handbook of depression* (pp. 314–340). New York: Guilford Press.

Monroe, S. M., & Simons, A. D. (1991). Diathesis–stress theories in the context of life-stress research: Implications for depressive disorders. *Psychological Bulletin, 110,* 406–425.

Murray, K. T., & Sines, J. O. (1996). Parsing the genetic and nongenetic variance in children's depressive behavior. *Journal of Affective Disorders, 38,* 23–34.

O'Hara, M. W., Stuart, S., Gorman, L., & Wenzel, A. (2000). Efficacy of interpersonal psychotherapy for postpartum depression. *Archives of General Psychiatry, 57,* 1039–1045.

Orvaschel, H., Walsh-Allis, G., & Ye, W. (1988). Psychopathology in children of parents with recurrent depression. *Journal of Abnormal Child Psychology, 16*(1), 17–28.

Pesonen, A. K., Raikkonen, K., Strandberg, T., Keltikangas-Jarvinen, L., & Jarvenpaa, A. L. (2004). Insecure adult attachment style and depressive symptoms: Implications for parental perceptions of infant temperament. *Infant Mental Health Journal, 25*(2), 99–116.

Plomin, R., Emde, R. N., Braungart, J. M., Campos, J., Corley, R. P., Fulker, D. W., et al. (1993). Genetic change and continuity from fourteen to twenty months: The MacArthur Longitudinal Twin Study. *Child Development, 64,* 1354–1376.

Porter, C. L., & Hsu, H. C. (2003). First-time mothers' perceptions of efficacy during the transition to motherhood: Links to infant temperament. *Journal of Family Psychology, 17*(1), 54–64.

Radke-Yarrow, M., Belmont, B., Nottelmann, E., & Bottomly, L. (1990). Young children's self-conceptions: Origins in the natural discourse of depressed and normal mothers and their children. In D. Cicchetti & M. Beeghly (Eds.), *The self in transition: Infancy to childhood* (pp. 345–361). Chicago: University of Chicago Press.

Radke-Yarrow, M., & Klimes-Dougan, B. (2002). Parental depression and offspring disorders: A developmental perspective. In S. H. Goodman & I. H. Gotlib (Eds.), *Children of depressed parents: Mechanisms of risk and implications for treatment* (pp. 155–174). Washington, DC: American Psychological Association.

Radke-Yarrow, M., Nottelmann, E., Belmont, B., & Welsh, J. D. (1993). Affective interactions of depressed and nondepressed mothers and their children. *Journal of Abnormal Child Psychology, 21,* 683–695.

Radke-Yarrow, M., & Sherman, T. (1990). Hard growing: Children who survive. In J. Rolf, A. S. Masten, D. Cicchetti, K. H. Nuechterlein, & S. Weintraub (Eds.), *Risk and protective factors in the development of psychopathology* (pp. 97–119). Cambridge, UK: Cambridge University Press.

Radke-Yarrow, M., Zahn-Waxler, C., Richardson, D. T., Susman, A., & Martinez, P. (1994). Caring behavior in children of clinically depressed and well mothers. *Child Development, 65,* 1405–1414.

Rende, R. D., Plomin, R., Reiss, D., & Hetherington, E. M. (1993). Genetic and environmental influences on depressive symptomatology in adolescence: Individual differences and extreme scores. *Journal of Child Psychology and Psychiatry, 34,* 1387–1398.

Ressler, K. J., & Nemeroff, C. B. (2000). Role of serotonergic and noradrenergic systems in the pathophysiology of depression and anxiety disorders. *Depression and Anxiety, 12*(Suppl. 1), 2–19.

Rutter, M., Dunn, J., Plomin, R., Simonoff, E., Pickles, A., Maughan, B., et al. (1997). Integrating nature and nurture: Implications of person–environment correlations and interactions for developmental psychopathology. *Development and Psychopathology, 9,* 335–364.

Rutter, M., Pickles, A., Murray, R., & Eaves, L. (2001). Testing hypotheses on specific environmental causal effects on behavior. *Psychological Bulletin, 127,* 291–324.

Sameroff, A. J. (1975). Transactional models in early social relations. *Human Development, 18,* 65–79.

Sameroff, A. J. (1995). General systems theories and developmental psychopathology. In D. Cicchetti & D. J. Cohen (Eds.), *Developmental psychopathology: Vol. 1. Theory and methods* (pp. 659–695). New York: Wiley.

Sameroff, A. J., Seifer, R., & Zax, M. (1982). Early development of children at risk for emotional disorder. *Monographs of the Society for Research in Child Development, 47*(Serial No. 199).

Sanchez, M. M., Ladd, C. O., & Plotsky, P. M. (2001). Early adverse experience as a developmental risk factor for later psychopathology: Evidence from rodent and primate models. *Development and Psychopathology, 13,* 419–449.

Sanders, M. R., & McFarland, M. (2000). Treatment of depressed mothers with disruptive children: A controlled evaluation of cognitive behavioral family intervention. *Behavior Therapy, 31,* 89–112.

Scourfield, J., Rice, F., Thapar, A., Harold, G. T., Martin, N. C., & McGuffin, P. (2003). Depressive symptoms in children and adolescents: Changing aetiological influences with development. *Journal of Child Psychology and Psychiatry and Allied Disciplines, 44,* 968–976.

Seligman, M. E., Schulman, P., DeRubeis, R. J., & Hollon, S. D. (1999). The prevention of depression and anxiety. *Prevention and Treatment, 2.*

Sheeber, L., Davis, B., & Hops, H. (2002). Gender-specific vulnerability to depression in children of depressed mothers. In S. H. Goodman & I. H. Gotlib (Eds.), *Children of depressed parents: Mechanisms of risk and implications for treatment* (pp. 253–274). Washington, DC: American Psychological Association.

Silberg, J., Pickles, A., Rutter, M., Hewitt, J., Simonoff, E., Maes, H., et al. (2001). The influence of genetic factors and life stress on depression among adolescent girls. *Archives of General Psychiatry, 56,* 225–232.

Sroufe, L. A., Egeland, B., Carlson, E. A., & Collins, W. A. (2005). *The development of the person: The Minnesota study of risk and adaptation from birth to adulthood.* New York: Guilford Press.

Sroufe, L. A., & Rutter, M. (1984). The domain of developmental psychopathology. *Child Development, 55,* 17–29.

Sroufe, L. A., & Waters, E. (1977). Attachment as an organizational construct. *Child Development, 48,* 1184–1199.

Taylor, L., & Ingram, R. E. (1999). Cognitive reactivity and depressotypic information processing in children of depressed mothers. *Journal of Abnormal Psychology, 108*(2), 202–210.

Tellegen, A., Lykken, D. T., Bouchard, T. J., Wilcox, K. J., Segal, N. L., & Rich, S. (1988). Personality similarity in twins reared apart and together. *Journal of Personality and Social Psychology, 54,* 1031–1039.

Teti, D. M., & Gelfand, D. M. (1991). Behavioral competence among mothers of infants in the first year: The mediational role of maternal self-efficacy. *Child Development, 62,* 918–929.

Thapar, A., & McGuffin, P. (1994). A twin study of depressive symptoms in childhood. *British Journal of Psychiatry, 165,* 259–265.

Thomas, A. M., & Forehand, R. (1991). The relationship between paternal depressive mood and early adolescent functioning. *Journal of Family Psychology, 4,* 43–52.

Tomarken, A. J., Davidson, R. J., Wheeler, R. E., & Kinney, L. (1992). Psychometric properties of resting anterior EEG asymmetry: Temporal stability and internal consistency. *Psychophysiology, 29,* 576–592.

Tsuang, M. T., & Faraone, S. V. (1990). *The genetics of mood disorders.* Baltimore: Johns Hopkins University Press.

Tully, E. C., Goodman, S. H., & Brooks-DeWeese, A. (2005). *Measuring children's perceptions of mothers' depression: The CHiPPS measure.* Paper presented at the biennial meeting of the International Society for Research in Child and Adolescent Psychopathology, New York.

Wadhwa, P. D., Glynn, L., Hobel, C. J., Garite, T. J., Porto, M., Chicz-DeMet, A., et al. (2002). Behavioral perinatology: Biobehavioral processes in human fetal development. *Regulatory Peptides, 108,* 149–157.

Webster-Stratton, C., & Hammond, M. (1988). Maternal depression and its relationship to life stress, perceptions of child behavior problems, parenting behaviors, and child conduct problems. *Journal of Abnormal Child Psychology, 16,* 299–315.

Weissman, M. M., Prusoff, B., Gammon, G. D., Merikangas, K. R., Leckman, J. F., & Kidd, K. K. (1984). Psychopathology in the children (ages 6–18) of depressed and normal parents. *Journal of the American Academy of Child and Adolescent Psychiatry, 23*(1), 78–84.

Weissman, M. W., Pilowsky, D. J., Wickramaratne, P. J., Talati, A., Wisniewski, S. R., Fava, M., et al. (2006). Remissions in maternal depression and child psychopathology: A STAR*D-Child report. *Journal of the American Medical Association, 295,* 1389–1398.

Welner, Z., Welner, A., McCrary, M., & Leonard, M. A. (1977). Psychopathology in children of inpatients with depression: A controlled study. *Journal of Nervous and Mental Disease, 164,* 408–413.

Whitman, P. B., & Leitenberg, H. (1990). Negatively biased recall in children with self-reported symptoms of depression. *Journal of Abnormal Psychology, 18,* 15–27.

Wilhelm, K. (2006). Depression: From nosology to global burden. In C. L. M. Keyes & S. H. Goodman (Eds.), *Women and depression: A handbook for the social, behavior, and biomedical sciences* (pp. 3–21). New York: Cambridge University Press.

Zahn-Waxler, C., Cole, P., M., Welsh, J. D., & Fox, N. A. (1995). Psychophysiological correlates of empathy and prosocial behaviors in preschool children with behavior problems. *Development and Psychopathology, 7,* 27–48.

Zahn-Waxler, C., Kochanska, G., Krupnick, J., & McKnew, D. (1990). Patterns of guilt in children of depressed and well mothers. *Developmental Psychology, 26*(1), 51–59.

Zupan, B. A., Hammen, C., & Jaenicke, C. (1987). The effects of current mood and prior depressive history on self-schematic processing in children. *Journal of Experimental Child Psychology, 43,* 149–158.

18 Suicidal Behavior in Youth

Kimberly A. Van Orden, Tracy K. Witte,
Edward A. Selby, Theodore W. Bender,
and Thomas E. Joiner, Jr.

Every 2 hours and 4 minutes, a person under the age of 25 dies by suicide (as based on data from 2003; McIntosh, 2006). One of the strongest risk factors for suicide in youth is the presence of a psychiatric disorder, especially depression (Shaffer & Pfeffer, 2001). One of the symptoms of major depressive disorder, according to the American Psychiatric Association (2000) is suicidal thoughts or behaviors. According to the practice parameters for the assessment and treatment of children and adolescents with depressive disorders (American Academy of Child and Adolescent Psychiatry [AACAP], 1998), youth suffering from major depressive disorder are at increased risk for suicidal thoughts and behaviors, thus necessitating the assessment of suicide risk with depressed youth (see, e.g., Wagner, 2003). Depression in youth continues to increase risk for suicide attempts (lethal and nonlethal) into adulthood (Weissman et al., 1999), suggesting that the relationship between depression and suicide in youth is robust and persistent. Therefore, a comprehensive account of depression in youth must consider the assessment, treatment, and prevention of suicidal behavior. In 2002, deaths by suicide accounted for 6.3% of deaths in children (ages 10–14) and 11% of deaths in adolescents (ages 15–19; Arias, Anderson, Kung, Murphy, & Kochanek, 2003). In 2002, suicide was the third leading cause of death in children and the fourth leading cause in adolescents. Acknowledging the gravity of this health problem, the U.S. Department of Heath and Human Services (2001) set forth specific methods aimed at reducing suicide rates. Methods specifically targeting suicide rates in youth were included, such as increasing the proportion of school districts with empirically supported programs designed to prevent suicide. In this chapter, we seek to provide an overview of what constitutes an empirically supported program for the treatment and prevention of suicidal behavior in youth. To accomplish this goal, we first provide a brief introduction to the epidemiology of suicidal behavior in youth. Next, we provide an overview of theoretical models of suicidal behavior that can contribute to our understanding of suicidal behavior in youth and discuss the empirical support for these models. We focus on one theory in particular, *the interpersonal–psychological theory of suicidal behavior* (Joiner, 2005). We then provide empirically informed recommendations the risk assessment, crisis intervention, and long-term psychotherapy with suicidal youth. Finally, we conclude with future directions and an overview of the status of programs for the prevention of suicide in youth.

EPIDEMIOLOGY OF YOUTH SUICIDAL BEHAVIOR

In this section, we briefly review *prevalence* (the number of lethal and nonlethal suicide attempts), *rates* (the number of cases of suicide in a group divided by the number of individuals in the group, standardized to a base of 100,000), *patterns* of suicidal behavior (e.g., comparisons by age, gender, ethnicity), and documented *risk factors* for suicidal behaviors in children and adolescents. Readers interested in greater depth of coverage of this topic are encouraged to consult the following resources: Gould, Shaffer, and Greenberg (2003), Berman, Jobes, and Silverman (2006), and the American Academy of Child and Adolescent Psychiatry (AACAP) practice parameters for the treatment of suicidal behavior in children and adolescents (Shaffer & Pfeffer, 2001).

The prevalence of suicidal behavior can be estimated from official mortality statistics compiled by government agencies, published reports of psychological autopsies, and epidemiological studies of suicidal ideation and attempts (Gould et al., 2003). The Centers for Disease Control and Prevention (CDC) compile official mortality statistics for the U.S. population each year. The number of deaths due to suicide is provided for all individuals, grouped by age, gender, and ethnicity. These data are available online (*wonder.cdc.gov/welcome.html*) and are updated when new information is available. The following statistics on prevalence and rates are compiled from the CDC data base for 2002 (U.S Department of Health and Human Services, 2004). In 2002, no lethal suicide attempts were reported for children 4 years old or younger. For children ages 5–9, 4 lethal suicide attempts were reported (1 female). For children ages 10–14, 260 lethal suicide attempts were reported (33% female), accounting for 6.3% of all deaths occurring in this age group. The age-specific rate of mortality due to suicide was 1.2 per 100,000. For adolescents 15 through 19 years of age, 1,513 lethal suicide attempts were reported (18% female), accounting for 11% of all deaths occurring in this age group. The age-specific rate of mortality due to suicide was 7.4 per 100,000.

Although uncommon, suicidal behavior can occur in very young children; for example, Rosenthal and Rosenthal (1984) describe the characteristics of 16 preschoolers (ages 2.5–5 years) who engaged in nonlethal attempts. However, suicidal behavior is more common in older youth: Within the group of 10- to 14 year-olds, most deaths by suicide occur in children ages 12–14 and the rate of suicide deaths increases sharply in the late teen years and continues to increase until the early twenties (Gould et al., 2003). The rate plateaus in the early twenties until it rises again in later life (Gould et al., 2003). More boys than girls die by suicide; however, estimates suggest that in childhood and adolescence, as in adulthood, more females engage in nonlethal attempts (CDC, 2004; Gould et al., 2003). Thus, the landscape of suicide in youth varies, depending on both age and gender.

The CDC conducts a nationwide survey of high school students in the United States—the Youth Risk Behavior Surveillance System (YRBSS)—that reports on the prevalence of those seriously considering suicide, making a suicide plan, attempting suicide, and attempting suicide with a need for medical attention. These statistics allow for a consideration of patterns in the prevalence of nonlethal attempts. In 2003 estimates from the YRBSS (Centers for Disease Control and Prevention, 2004) suggested that 16.5% of U.S. high school students seriously considered attempting suicide (21.3% of females and 12.8% of males). The number of those considering a suicide attempt also varied by ethnicity: Prevalence was higher in white (16.5%) and Hispanic youth (18.1%) than in black youth (12.5%). In 2003, 8.5% of U.S. high school students attempted suicide one or more times (11.5% of females and 5.4% of males). The prevalence of suicide attempts was higher among Hispanic youth (10.6%) than among white (6.9%) or black youth (8.4%). Suicide attempts requiring medical attention occurred in 2.9% of youth. For attempts requiring medical attention, prevalence was higher in Hispanic females (5.7%) than in white females (2.4%) or black females (2.2%). Prevalence was also higher in black males (5.2%) and Hispanic males (4.2%) than in white males (1.1%).

A striking finding from the YRBSS is the elevated prevalence of suicidal behavior in Hispanic youth. Zayas, Lester, Cabassa, and Fortuna (2005) suggest that suicidal behavior in these youth may be explained by an examination of interpersonal variables: A conflict may exist between a cultural emphasis on family unity and an individual desire for autonomy.

RISK FACTORS FOR SUICIDAL BEHAVIOR

Variables that explain or predict suicidal behavior can be grouped into two broad categories: long-standing *risk factors* that may predispose individuals to suicidal behavior and *warning signs*, which are more dynamic and proximal factors that indicate the presence of a current suicidal crisis (Rudd, Berman, et al., 2006). Numerous risk factors for suicidal behavior in youth have been identified. One of the most reliable and robust risk factors is the presence of psychopathology: Findings from psychological autopsy studies estimate that at least 90% of youth who die by suicide experienced at least one mental disorder (Gould et al., 2003). Data from a psychological autopsy study, the Utah Youth Suicide Study (Moskos, Olson, Halbern, Keller, & Gray, 2005), indicate that mood disorders and substance use disorders are the most common diagnoses in youth who have died by suicide. In a psychological autopsy of adolescents who died by suicide, significant psychiatric risk factors were major depression, bipolar mixed state, substance abuse, and conduct disorder (Brent et al., 1993). A psychological autopsy conducted by Shaffer and colleagues (Shaffer et al., 1996) found that mood disorders—alone or comorbid with substance use disorders or conduct disorder—were the most common diagnoses among adolescents who died by suicide. Mood disorders with childhood onset (i.e., prepubertal onset) have been found to relate to a 3.5 increased risk for a nonlethal suicide attempt (as compared with an absence of mood disorder; Pfeffer et al., 1993). Both mood disorders and anxiety disorders with childhood onset (prior to age 13) have been found to elevate risk for multiple nonlethal attempts in young adulthood (Rudd, Joiner, & Rumzek, 2004). Personality disorders have been found to confer risk for lethal attempts in adolescents, particularly Cluster B (impulsive-dramatic) and Cluster C (avoidant-dependent) disorders (Brent et al., 1994). Reith, Whyte, Carter, and McPherson (2003) investigated factors predictive of death by suicide in young adulthood in a sample of individuals with a history of a nonlethal suicide attempt in adolescence. Disorders classified as "usually first diagnosed in infancy, childhood, or adolescence" increased risk for lethal attempts in adolescence. Research also suggests that disorders in this category may confer risk for nonlethal suicide attempts: Oppositional and conduct disorders were found to increase risk for nonlethal attempts in adolescence (Apter, Bleich, Plutchik, Mendelsohn, & Tyano, 1988).

Research on adult samples has demonstrated that the relationship between past and future suicidal behavior is robust and that previous suicidal behavior elevates risk for future suicidal behavior (Joiner et al., 2005). This relationship has also been found in youth samples. Borowsky, Ireland, and Resnick (2001) found that the presence of a prior attempt significantly elevated risk for future suicide attempts in adolescence.

A working group convened by the American Association of Suicidology (AAS) reviewed the empirical literature and reached consensus on a set of warning signs for suicide (see Rudd, Berman, et al., 2006). These warning signs, designed to educate the public about suicidal crises, and are presented in Figure 18.1. These warning signs were not developed specifically for youth, thus future research is needed to determine if signs of acute suicide risk differ for youth and adults.

A host of cognitive and interpersonal variables have also been found to confer risk for suicidal behavior in youth. We discuss these factors below, in relation to theories of suicidal behavior. Kurt Lewin (1951) wrote: "There is nothing so practical as a good theory" (p. 169). The rest of the chapter uses theory to organize empirical evidence on risk factors and allow us to present empirically informed recommendations on risk assessment, crisis intervention, and psychotherapy with suicidal youth.

Are you or someone you love at risk for suicide? Get the facts and take action.

Call 911 or seek immediate help from a mental health provider when you hear, say, or see any one of these behaviors:
- Someone threatening to hurt or kill him- or herself
- Someone looking for ways to kill him- or herself: seeking access to pills, weapons, or other means
- Someone talking or writing about death, dying, or suicide

Seek help by contacting a mental health professional or calling 1-800-273-TALK for a referral should you witness, hear, say, or see anyone exhibiting any one or more of these behaviors:
- Hopelessness
- Rage, anger, seeking revenge
- Acting reckless or engaging in risky activities, seemingly without thinking
- Feeling trapped—as if there's no way out
- Increasing alcohol or drug use
- Withdrawing from friends, family, or society
- Anxiety, agitation, unable to sleep or sleeping all the time
- Dramatic changes in mood
- No reason for living; no sense of purpose in life

FIGURE 18.1. Consensus warning signs for suicide. Developed by the American Association of Suicidology. See Rudd, Berman, et al. (2006).

THEORIES OF YOUTH SUICIDAL BEHAVIOR

Many theories of suicidal behavior in general, and suicidal behavior in youth in particular, have been put forth. The five theories we review below have received empirical support and/or present falsifiable and coherent predictions suitable for empirical testing. Readers interested in a more comprehensive overview of the status of theory in youth suicidal behavior are referred to Berman et al. (2006).

Hopelessness—a belief that circumstances will not improve in the future—involves expectations of negative outcomes combined with expectations that those negative outcomes are out of one's control (Abramson, Alloy, & Metalsky, 1989). According to the *hopelessness theory of suicide* (e.g., Cornette, Abramson, & Bardone, 2000), a negative cognitive style functions as a vulnerability for the development of hopelessness. Hopelessness, in turn, is a proximal cause of the symptoms of depression, including suicidal thoughts and behavior. In support of this hypothesis, improvements in attributional style (a type of cognitive style) in children and adolescents have been found to reduce suicidal ideation over the course of inpatient stays (Wagner, Rouleau, & Joiner, 2000). The relation between hopelessness and suicidality is one of the most consistent and robust findings in the suicidality literature (e.g., Joiner & Rudd, 1996). Empirical evidence from a number of studies using both adult and youth samples suggests that hopelessness is indeed a risk factor for lethal attempts. For example, in a large-scale prospective study of adult psychiatric outpatients, patients who scored high on the Beck Hopelessness Scale were 4 times more likely to die of suicide in a given year than those who scored lower (Brown, Beck, Steer, & Grisham, 2000). Similarly, a large community study of adults found that individuals who expressed hopelessness were 11.2 times more likely to die by suicide over a 13-year follow-up period (Kuo, Gallo, & Eaton, 2004). In a sample of youth psychiatric inpatients (ages 8–13), hopelessness predicted level of suicidal intent, while controlling for symptoms of depression (Kazdin, French, Unis, Esveldt-Dawson, & Sherick, 1983).However, hopelessness has been found to have low predictive power for suicidal behaviors (Brown et al., 2000). In terms of risk assessment, this suggests that most youth engaging in suicidal behaviors are hopeless, but that most hopeless youth do not engage in suicidal behaviors.

Shneidman's (1985) *psychache theory* suggests that individuals engage in suicidal behavior because of intolerable psychological and emotion pain (i.e., psychache), which results from unmet psychological needs. Shneidman (1998) proposes an extensive list of basic needs, seven of which, he argues, are most commonly thwarted in suicidal individuals, ranging from "affiliation" to "shame avoidance" to "order and understanding." Shneidman (1985) proposes that all individuals who die by suicide experience psychache just prior to their deaths, but that only a small proportion of all individuals who experience psychache will die by suicide. Thus, psychache is not sufficient to cause death by suicide. Shneidman's theory posits that another factor, lethality, contributes to risk for suicide and must also be present for someone to die by suicide. Shneidman (1996) describes lethality as the idea that "I can stop this pain; I can kill myself" (p. 8). However, Shneidman's theory does not specify the components of lethality nor what contributes to higher levels of lethality.

Empirical findings provide support for the role of psychache in both youth and adults. Orbach, Mikulincer, Gilboa-Schechtman, and Sirota (2003) found that adult psychiatric inpatients who attempted suicide prior to hospital admission scored higher on a measure of mental pain than nonsuicidal psychiatric inpatients and community controls.

Kienhorst, De Wilde, Diekstra, and Wolters (1995) reported that adolescents most frequently name mental pain as the cause for their suicidal behavior. Boergers, Spirito, and Donaldson (1998) surveyed a sample of adolescents who had recently attempted suicide about their reasons for the attempt: In addition to a desire for death, "relief from a terrible state of mind" and "escape for a while from an impossible situation" were the most cited reasons for the attempts. Data thus support the psychache component of Shneidman's theory and suggest that mental pain is a necessary, but not sufficient cause of suicide. Additional research is needed to determine under what conditions psychache is most likely to result in death by suicide.

Baumeister's (1990) *escape theory of suicidal behavior* also posits that mental pain is a key factor in such behavior. For Baumeister, mental pain takes the form of "aversive self-awareness." In contrast to Shneidman's theory, Baumeister's theory describes in detail a sequence of steps leading up to serious suicidal behavior. The sequence begins with an individual's experiencing a negative and severe discrepancy between expected and actual outcomes (e.g., failures, unmet goals, disappointments). In the next step, the individual attributes this disappointment internally and blames him- or herself—not only are recent outcomes not meeting expectations, but the *self* is perceived as not meeting self-standards and is thus inadequate. In the third step, an aversive state of high self-awareness develops, which leads to step four, the experience of negative affect. The experience of negative affect due to aversive self-awareness is conceptually similar to Shneidman's construct of psychache.

In Baumeister's next step, the individual attempts to escape from this negative affect, as well as from the aversive self-awareness, by retreating into a numb state of "cognitive deconstruction." In this state, meaningful thought about the self, including painful self-awareness and failed standards, is replaced by a lower-level awareness of concrete sensations and movements and of immediate, proximal goals and tasks. Finally, the important consequence of this state of cognitive deconstruction is reduced inhibitions, and especially a lack of impulse control, for suicidal behavior. According to Baumeister, when people are in the lower-level state of focusing on concrete behaviors, their ability to identify other options is impaired and suicide may be viewed as the only means available to escape mental pain. According to both Shneidman and Baumeister, suicide is an attempt to escape mental pain. Insofar as mental pain is a key component in the escape theory, the studies described above that are consistent with Shneidman's theory are consistent with the escape theory as well. However, we are not aware of any direct tests of the other components of Baumeister's theory. Regarding its utility in understanding suicide in youth, we suggest that tests of the theory utilizing a developmental framework are needed. For example, many children may not possess the level of cognitive sophistication required to experience discrepancies between desired and actual outcomes. It may be that the content of mental pain depends on developmental considerations, such as the development of information-processing abilities, emotion regulation skills, and awareness of self. The escape theory proposes a set of coherent and falsifiable predictions, making it a potentially useful theory in terms of generating suicide research applicable to treatment and prevention efforts (see Higgins, 2004, for a discussion of properties of useful theories). However, empirical tests of the escape theory utilizing a developmental framework are needed.

The desire to escape negative affect is similar to the primary risk factor in Linehan's (1993) theory of suicidal behavior, *emotional dysregulation*, which involves an inability to adaptively modulate one's emotions. Self-injury, according to Linehan, is an attempt to regulate emotions—an attempt that becomes necessary because the usual emotion regulation mechanisms have broken down or have never developed adequately. Linehan theorizes that emotion dysregulation—the proximal cause of suicidal behavior—results from the joint influences of biological predispositions and invalidating environments. Biological predispositions to emotional dysregulation result in abnormal responses to negative emotional stimuli: high emotional sensitivity, an intense emotional experience, and a slow return to emotional baseline. Emotion dysregulation resulting from biological predispositions is amplified by invalidating environments. Invalidating environments are those in which the communication of private experiences is met by erratic, inappropriate, and extreme responses. An example of an invalidating environment is childhood abuse. Consistent with Linehan's theory, childhood abuse has been found to be a risk factor for suicidal behavior (Brown, Cohen, Johnson, & Smailes, 1999; Joiner, Sachs-Ericsson, Wingate, & Brown, 2007; Rosenthal & Rosenthal, 1984).

Linehan has also applied this theory to affective and behavioral problems seen in borderline personality disorder (Linehan, 1993). Borderline personality disorder is one of two disorders in the *Diagnostic and Statistical Manual* (along with major depressive disorder; American Psychiatric Association, 2000) to include suicidal behavior as a diagnostic criterion. Although the criteria for borderline personality disorder are polythetic—thus suicidal behavior is not a necessary symptom for the diagnosis—suicidal behavior is common among individuals with borderline personality disorder and is a key feature of the disorder (see, e.g., Linehan et al., 2006). Dialectical behavior therapy (DBT; Linehan, 1993) was developed from Linehan's theory of emotion dysregulation and has been applied to the treatment of suicidal adolescents (Miller, Rathus, Linehan, Wetzler, & Leigh, 1997) and suicidal adults (Linehan et al., 2006). More detail on the application to adolescents is provided later in the section "Psychotherapy." DBT has been shown to be effective in six randomized controlled trials with adults (Koons et al., 2001; Linehan, Armstrong, Suarez, Allmon, & Heard, 1991; Linehan et al., 1999; Linehan et al., 2002; Linehan et al., 2006; Verheul et al., 2003). The efficacy of DBT provides indirect support for Linehan's theory. Direct empirical evidence testing the etiological role of emotional dysregulation, biological dispositions, and invalidating environments is needed. Research on mechanisms of change in DBT is a potential means of providing a more precise test of the theory.

Joiner's (2005) *interpersonal–psychological theory of suicidal behavior* (hereafter referred to as the interpersonal–psychological theory) proposes that an individual will not die from suicide unless he or she has both the desire to die by suicide and the ability to do so (see Figure 18.2).

The theory further proposes that suicidal desire results from the presence of two interpersonal constructs, thwarted belongingness and perceived burdensomeness. These result from an unmet need to belong (Baumeister & Leary, 1995) and an unmet need to contribute to the welfare of close others (Joiner et al., 2002). The theory also proposes that suicidal desire is not sufficient to result in death by suicide: Individuals must also have the ability to enact lethal self-injury. This ability can be acquired over time through exposure to painful and provocative experiences, including the physical and mental pain involved in self-injury. Through repeated practice and exposure, an individual can habituate to the painful and fearful aspects of self-harm, making it possible for him or her to engage in increasingly painful, damaging, and lethal forms of self-harm. Such a process is consistent with opponent process theory (Solomon & Corbit, 1974), which states that with repetition, the negative and provocative aspects of a behavior may diminish while the opposite effects (i.e., the opponent processes) are amplified and strengthened. Thus, what was originally a fear-inducing and painful experience (e.g., self-injury) can become a

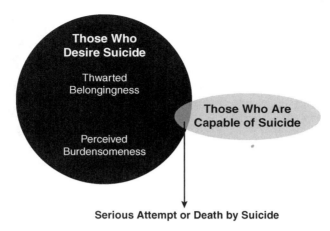

FIGURE 18.2. Joiner's (2005) Interpersonal–psychological theory of suicidal behavior.

source of calming emotions and emotional relief. The interpersonal–psychological theory posits that the most direct pathway to an acquired capability is through previous suicidal behavior: As one becomes more practiced via suicide attempts, the punishing aspects of self-injury may diminish (i.e., fear and the experience of physical pain), while the reinforcing aspects may increase (i.e., emotional relief). In line with this hypothesis, a past suicide attempt is one of the strongest and most reliable predictors of future attempts (Borowsky et al., 2001; Joiner, Walker, Rudd, & Jobes, 1999).

The theory also proposes that other less direct pathways may also exist through the experience of other fear-inducing, risky behaviors, such as self-injecting drug use, nonsuicidal self-injury, or exposure to physical violence. Data suggest that these pathways are operative in youth suicidal behavior. For example, three studies conducted by Nock and colleagues (Nock, Joiner, Gordon, Lloyd-Richardson, & Prinstein, 2006; Nock & Prinstein, 2004, 2005) suggest that the experience of nonsuicidal self-injury (NSSI) may also be relevant for youth suicidal behavior. Estimates of adolescent NSSI (i.e., self-injurious behavior without suicidal intent) have been shown to be as high as 39% in community samples (see, e.g., Lloyd, Kelley, & Hope, 1997) and as high as 61% in psychiatric samples (see, e.g., DiClemente, Ponton, & Hartley, 1991). Nock and Prinstein (2004) investigated functions of NSSI by asking participants (adolescent psychiatric inpatients) how often they had engaged in NSSI for a series of 22 reasons. These reasons were collapsed into four subscales (supported by confirmatory factor analysis): automatic negative reinforcement, automatic positive reinforcement, social negative reinforcement, and social positive reinforcement. *Automatic* refers to internal, psychologically reinforcing effects of NSSI, and *social* refers to interpersonally reinforcing effects of self-injury. Automatic negative reinforcement was the most common reason adolescents reported for engaging in NSSI. Nock and Prinstein (2005), also in a sample of adolescent psychiatric inpatients, found that NSSI done for the purpose of automatic negative reinforcement was related to a history of suicide attempts; none of the other functions were related to a history of suicide attempts. They also found that most adolescents reported experiencing little or no pain during the NSSI. Regarding the implications of these results, Nock and Prinstein (2005) propose that the most common form of NSSI among adolescents—NSSI performed in order to experience automatic negative reinforcement—is a predictor of suicidal behavior and may serve the same function as suicidal behavior. They suggest that automatic negative reinforcement is a motive similar to that of escaping mental pain—a link also theorized by Shneidman and Baumeister, as discussed above.

The potential functional equivalence of NSSI and suicidal behavior suggests that data on NSSI may be relevant to models of suicidal behavior. In a test of this hypothesis, Nock et al. (2006) investigated the relationship between NSSI and nonlethal attempts in a sample of inpatient adolescents. They found that a longer history of NSSI and the use of more methods of NSSI were both associated with higher rates of lifetime suicide attempts. In addition, the absence of physical pain during NSSI was also associated with a higher rate of lifetime suicide attempts: Adolescents who reported experiencing no pain during NSSI reported nearly twice as many lifetime suicide attempts, as compared with adolescents who reporting experiencing pain during NSSI. Although this study was cross-sectional, thus necessitating that conclusions be interpreted with caution, these results are consistent with the hypothesis that NSSI may represent an indirect pathway to an acquired capability for lethal self-injury.

How may NSSI function as an indirect pathway to an acquired capability? The finding by Nock and colleagues (2006) that the absence of pain during NSSI was a predictor of a greater number of lifetime nonlethal attempts is consistent with the hypothesis that through repeated exposure to the pain of self-injury, individuals may habituate to the pain involved and thus be capable of increasingly painful acts of self-injury. For example, adolescents may begin with less painful, damaging, and fear-inducing forms of NSSI, and after habituating to these behaviors, may escalate to more painful, damaging, and fear-inducing behaviors such as suicide attempts. Nock and Prinstein (2005) report that the majority of individuals in their sample of adolescent psychiatric inpatients reported engaging in NSSI impulsively (i.e., contemplating the behavior for a few minutes or less) and without the influence of drugs or alcohol. This finding is consistent with the hypothesis of the interpersonal–psychological theory that the relationship between impulsivity and suicide attempts may be indirect. Longitudinal studies are needed to directly address these hypotheses.

Research also suggests that there may be other less direct pathways to the acquired capability in youth. For example, a diagnosis of conduct disorder has been found to increase risk for lethal suicide attempts in adolescents (Shaffer et al., 1996; Brent et al., 1993), and risk is especially elevated for youth with a diagnosis of conduct disorder as well as a prior attempt and comorbid substance use (Renaud, Brent, Birmaher, Chiapetta, & Bridge, 1999). Conduct disorder is characterized by violence, cruelty, impulsivity, and overall disruptive behavior, according to the *Diagnostic and Statistical Manual of Mental Disorders* (4th ed., text rev. [DSM-IV-TR]; American Psychiatric Association, 2000). The impulsive and disruptive behaviors involved in conduct disorder may expose youth to physical pain and cause them to witness the physical pain of others. These provocative experiences, coupled with substance use disorders—another form of impulsive and potentially painful behavior—may place youth on a trajectory toward an acquired capability for lethal self-injury by engaging processes of habituation to physical pain and accompanying fear.

Research also suggests that even young children may begin to habituate to painful experiences through the experience of physical and sexual abuse, thereby acquiring the capability for suicidal behavior. Rosenthal and Rosenthal (1984) compared a group of preschool children who had engaged in suicidal behavior with a group of preschool children with behavioral problems (who had not engaged in suicidal behavior). The suicidal children had more often been abused by parents. Joiner et al. (2007) found that both childhood physical abuse and childhood sexual abuse predicted greater number of lifetime suicide attempts, while controlling for such factors as age, gender, psychiatric history, and family psychiatric history. Brown et al. (1999) found that the risk for multiple suicide attempts was found to be eight times higher for individuals with a history of childhood sexual abuse. Rosenthal and Rosenthal (1984) found that a majority of the suicidal children in their sample did not cry after being physically injured. This suggests that these children may have acquired increased pain tolerance through such experiences as abuse, thus making them more vulnerable to suicidal behavior.

Research indicates that feelings of thwarted belongingness may play a role in the etiology of youth suicide, as hypothesized by the interpersonal–psychological theory. The definition of the construct of thwarted belongingness used in the interpersonal–psychological theory was put forth by Baumeister and Leary (1995): To fully satisfy the need to belong, an individual must frequently have positive interactions with others and feel cared about by others. Individuals whose social interactions are predominantly unpleasant, unstable, infrequent, or lacking face-to-face contact, as well as individuals who do not feel connected to others or cared about by others, are likely to experience thwarted belongingness.

One source of thwarted belongingness in youth may be the experience of peer rejection, which has been indicated in the development of loneliness (Cassidy & Asher, 1992; Crick & Ladd, 1993; Parkhurst & Asher, 1992). In a test of the interpersonal-psychological theory, Van Orden and Joiner (2005) found that loneliness and thwarted belongingness are highly related, but distinct constructs, and suggest that loneliness may be one component of thwarted belongingness. In this study, both loneliness and a measure of thwarted belongingness predicted suicidal ideation. The association between loneliness and suicide has been reported by numerous research groups (Bonner & Rich, 1987; Dieserud, Roysamb, Ekeberg, & Kraft, 2001; Koivumaa-Honkanen et al., 2001; Roberts, Roberts, & Chen, 1988; Stravynski & Boyer, 2001; Waern, Rubenowitz, & Wilhelmson, 2003). These data suggest that peer rejection in youth that leads to loneliness may be a risk factor for thwarted belongingness and suicidal desire. For example, loss of friends after disclosing one's sexual orientation is a strong predictor of suicide among gay, lesbian, and bisexual youth (Hershberger, Pilkington, & D'Augelli, 1997). A loss of friends through rejection may meet both criteria for a thwarted need to belong—a lack of positive interactions and not feeling cared about—making this form of rejection especially pernicious in regard to suicide. Finally, an increased level of parental involvement with children—which is likely to foster belongingness—has been found to serve as a protective factor against adolescent suicide attempts (Flouri & Buchanan, 2001). The studies presented above are consistent with the hypothesis of the interpersonal–psychological theory that the absence of belongingness may function as a risk factor for suicide in youth, and the presence of belongingness may function as a protective factor against suicide in youth.

Research also suggests that perceived burdensomeness may play a role in the etiology of youth suicide. For example, research has shown that members of families of suicidal children have often expressed to a child (directly or indirectly) that they feel he or she is a burden on the family and is unwanted. Sabbath (1969) described the "expendable child" construct as a "parental wish, conscious or unconscious, spoken or unspoken, that the child interprets as their [the parents'] desire to be rid of him, for him to die" (pp. 272–273). Woznica and Shapiro (1990) examined 20 adolescent outpatients who had a history of suicide attempts and/or were rated by psychotherapists as having a high degree of suicidal ideation, and 20 controls who had been treated with psychotherapy but had never attempted suicide and had no suicidal ideation, and found that the adolescents with a history of suicide attempts scored higher on a measure of perceived expendability. Further evidence for perceived burdensomeness in children and adolescents can be seen in higher rates of depression among children who exhibit deficits in social and academic competence (Cole, 1990, 1991).

RISK ASSESSMENT

The assessment of suicide risk in children in particular (and in adolescents to some degree) presents the clinician with some uniquely challenging issues. Younger children (i.e., those under age 12) may have difficulty in being able to verbalize their suicide intent (Pfeffer, 2003). Thus, it is critical that the clinician conduct a multi-informant (e.g., parents, teachers, friends, siblings) assessment in order to ascertain the severity of the child's suicidal intent. In addition, the use of a clinician-administered interview rather than a self-report measure enables the clinician to be more flexible in explaining suicide-related constructs to younger children (Allan, Kashani, Dahlmeier, Taghizadeh, & Reid, 1997). The use of one such interview, the Scale for Suicide Ideation (Beck, Kovacs, & Weissman, 1979), has been validated in both adolescent and child inpatients (Allan et al., 1997; Steer, Kumar, & Beck, 1993).

Several self-report measures have recently been validated as well. For a more detailed review of validated measures of suicide risk in children and adolescents, see Pfeffer, Jiang, and Kakuma (2000) as well as Shaffer and Pfeffer (2001). An example is the Child–Adolescent Suicide Potential Index (CASPI), which has been validated for use in children and adolescents between the ages of 8 and 17 (Pfeffer et al., 2000). A CASPI cutoff score of 11 showed adequate (although certainly not optimal) sensitivity (70%) and specificity (65%) in the identification of children or adolescents who had experienced either suicidal ideation or a suicide attempt within the past 6 months. The authors note that the CASPI can be utilized as a screening measure in community samples, but owing to the likely high number of false positives, further screening methods (e.g., interview) should be conducted once those at high risk are identified.

Although some children may not understand that death is final, Pfeffer (2003) emphasizes the importance of taking suicide threats in children seriously. For example, some children do not understand that certain suicidal acts are very likely to be lethal (e.g., jumping from the sixth floor of a building), and they make statements indicating that they expect to be taken to the doctor's office afterward to be healed (Pfeffer, 2003; Rosenthal & Rosenthal, 1984). If a child endorses a plan for suicide that is objectively lethal, clinicians should respond accordingly, regardless of the child's understanding of the finality of the act. Conversely, some acts that would not be objectively lethal (e.g., taking two aspirins) may be believed to be so by younger children. Pfeffer (2003) encourages clinicians to take such plans seriously so that intervention efforts can prevent future, more pernicious suicide attempts.

Joiner et al. (1999) developed the *Suicide Assessment Decision Tree*, a suicide risk assessment framework that illustrates one way to incorporate the components of the interpersonal–psychological theory into a standardized procedure for managing suicidal clients (for a detailed account of the procedures, see Cukrowicz, Wingate, Driscoll, & Joiner, 2004). Levels of risk vary from nonexistent, which is categorized by a lack of suicidal symptoms, to extreme, which indicates imminent risk for suicidal behavior. This framework considers previous suicidal behavior, current suicidal symptoms, and related domains with empirically demonstrated relationships with suicidal behavior (e.g., precipitant stressors, Axis I and II symptomatology, presence of hopelessness). In the framework, past suicidal behavior is used to "weight" information about current suicidal symptoms. Individuals with multiple attempts are designated at higher risk than other individuals because research has demonstrated empirical differences between single and multiple attempters on key suicide-related variables, including likelihood of future suicide completions. Because of the increased likelihood that multiple attempters have acquired the ability to accomplish lethal self-injury, for individuals who have attempted suicide multiple times, any other significant finding in the assessment constitutes at least moderate risk.

In addition to ascertaining the number of previous attempts, acquired capability is assessed in the Decision Tree by measuring levels of resolved plans and preparation for suicide, current level of impulsivity, history of drug abuse, and history of physical or sexual abuse (Stellrecht et al., 2006). The "resolved plans and preparations" factor is a group of suicidal symptoms that involves preparatory behaviors for suicide (e.g., specificity of a plan for attempt and having made preparations for an attempt), as well as courage and intention for suicidal behaviors (e.g., availability of means and perceived competence for an attempt). These symptoms have been found to be empirically distinct from symptoms such as a wish to die and frequency of ideation, which involve the "suicidal desire and ideation" factor (Joiner, Rudd, & Rajab, 1997). Youth who endorse symptoms of resolved plans and preparations may be farther along the trajectory for an acquired capability and thus may be more likely to engage in suicidal behavior, as compared with youth who exhibit only symptoms of suicidal desire and ideation. However, this factor structure of suicidal symptoms has not been replicated in youth samples. For example, Allan et al. (1997) found an "active" and a "passive" factor on the Scale for Suicide Ideation (Beck et al., 1979) in a sample of children and adolescents, rather than the "resolved plans and preparations" and "suicidal desire and ideation" factors. Thus, further research is needed on the factor space of suicidal symptoms in youth (i.e., how symptoms "hang together") in order to best inform risk assessment of suicidal youth.

Stellrecht et al. (2006) emphasize the importance of assessing the constructs of thwarted belongingness and perceived burdensomeness in adults in order to determine suicide risk with adults. We propose that the same considerations should apply in the risk assessment of children. According to the interpersonal–psychological theory, the presence of thwarted belongingness, perceived burdensomeness, and acquired capability for suicide dramatically increase a child's risk for suicide, as compared with any of these risk factors alone. How might thwarted belongingness and perceived burdensomeness be expressed in children? In the preceding discussion we described research on peer rejection in youth and how that experience may contribute to thwarted belongingness. In addition, there is a wide body of research that demonstrates a relationship between lack of family cohesion and suicide risk in children (e.g., Asarnow, Carlson, & Guthrie, 1987; Gould, Fisher, Parides, Flory, & Shaffer, 1996; Morano, Cisler, & Lemerond, 1993). Indeed, among children, lack of family support has been shown to be a more important predictor of suicide risk than lack of other types of social support (Morano et al., 1993). It may very well be that one reason for the lower prevalence of suicide in children is their greater sense of belonging, owing to their higher likelihood of living in a group of people (i.e., a family). When this sense of belonging is thwarted, such as in the case of children placed in out-of-home treatment programs, suicide attempt rates are dramatically higher (Ringle & Larzelere, 2001). Clinicians should therefore evaluate the state of the child/adolescent's social network, placing particular emphasis on the family. In order to assess for perceptions of burdensomeness, a clinician should inquire about a child's feeling of expendability in the context of his or her family. The Expendable Child Measure (Woznica & Shapiro, 1990) has been validated for use in outpatient adolescents and can be utilized to assess the construct of burdensomeness.

An additional correlate of suicidal behavior among children/adolescents is the experience of child abuse or neglect (Deykin, Alpert, & McNamarra, 1985; Brent & Mann, 2003). Child abuse and neglect may be an especially pernicious risk factor for suicide in youth because it may place youth at risk for all three components of the interpersonal–psychological theory—thwarted belongingness, perceived burdensomeness, and an acquired capability for lethal self-injury.

CRISIS INTERVENTION

Youth presenting with signs of acute risk for suicide are said to be experiencing *suicidal crises*. Crisis intervention strategies can be used to prevent youth from utilizing their capabilities for suicide and can be used to treat symptomatic manifestations of an acquired capability, such as severe symptoms of resolved plans and preparation. In this section, we briefly discuss the following strategies: hospitalization, removal of means for suicide, utilizing parents as monitors of the young person's behavior, and education about emergency mental health services.

Clinicians utilizing the Joiner et al. (1999) risk assessment procedure should consider hospitalization for youth in the midst of suicidal crises with risks that are categorized as *severe* or *extreme*. The imminence of risk must be considered, as well as the availability and willingness of parents or guardians to watch the youth and keep him or her safe at home. Shaffer and Pfeffer (2001) suggest that the following diagnostic features indicate the need for hospitalization in youth: major depressive disorder with psychotic features, rapid cycling with irritability and impulsivity, psychosis with command hallucinations, and alcohol or substance abuse. Youth with risk categorizations of *severe* or *extreme* must never be left alone: Parents must accompany and monitor these youth at all times. Parents should be given a rationale for the necessity of this precaution and helped to problem solve obstacles that could interfere. Clinicians should also meet with parents to ensure that firearms, lethal medications, or any means for suicide are removed from the home, or at the very least, inaccessible to the youth (Shaffer & Pfeffer, 2001). Research suggests that an explicit discussion of this precaution with parents is necessary to ensure that it is implemented (McManus et al., 1997). Shaffer and Pfeffer (2001) provide four steps that must be taken before a young person who has attempted suicide can be discharged from a hospital: (1) The patient and family must be given information about the dangerousness of the use of drugs and alcohol, because those substances can have disinhibiting effects on behavior; (2) firearms and lethal medications must be removed or effectively secured; (3) a supportive person must be present at home; and (4) a follow-up appointment must be scheduled.

Rudd, Mandrusiak, and Joiner (2006) reviewed the literature on the use of *no-suicide contracts* and suggest that empirical support for the efficacy of this intervention is lacking. They propose the use of *commitment to treatment statements* as an alternative. This involves an agreement between a clinician and patient on what the patient *should do*, versus what he or she should not do. Contracts can specify the roles, obligations, and expectations of both the patient and the clinician, including the expectation of open and honest communication about treatment (including the presence and nature of suicidal symptoms), as well as the expectation that emergency services will be accessed during periods of crisis. Rotheram-Borus et al. (1996) present findings that suggest that commitment to treatment statements may be effective in increasing compliance with treatment for suicidal youth. They describe an intervention for adolescents presenting at an emergency room after an attempt: The youth and his or her family were shown a video to increase understanding of adolescent suicidal behavior and how it is treated. A family therapy session was also held with a crisis therapist, who created a safety plan for the adolescent and provided case management services for the family and the follow-up treatment provider. This intervention increased compliance with attendance at the first outpatient therapy session. For suicidal youth, parents must be included in the creation and implementation of a commitment to treatment statement. When creating the statement, clinicians should work with the parents and the youth to devise a specific crisis plan, including guidance on when to utilize emergency mental health treatment. The parents and the youth should also be made aware of national and local crisis hotlines (e.g., 1-800-273-TALK).

For youth not requiring immediate hospitalization (or once a youth is hospitalized and partially stabilized), crisis intervention efforts should focus on alleviating feelings of thwarted belongingness and perceived burdensomeness (as opposed to the acquired capability for suicide), as these are likely to be the most malleable (Joiner, 2005). Although it will most likely not be possible to completely eliminate the experience of thwarted belongingness and perceived burdensomeness, there are techniques that can be used to "take the edge off" for the patient in crisis. The interpersonal–psychological theory proposes that if an individual experiences feelings of connection with others or effectiveness, he or she will *not* attempt suicide. Using basic principles of cognitive-behavioral therapy (CBT), the therapist can challenge the child's or adolescents' beliefs that he or she is disconnected from others, unwanted, and/or ineffective. It is important to concentrate not only on the child's current state of belonging/competence, but also on his or her past experiences. If possible, the family of the child/adolescent should be engaged in this process and encouraged to openly express the importance of their relationship with the individual in crisis.

The creation of a crisis card, the goal of which is to list helpful activities to be used when an individual is faced with a suicidal crisis, can be helpful as well (Joiner, 2005; Stellrecht et al., 2006). This should be done in a collaborative fashion, with the child/adolescent taking an active role in determining what should be included on the card. It is useful to include activities that will actively combat feelings of thwarted belongingness and perceived burdensomeness (e.g., playing a game with a sibling; recalling times when he or she was helpful to his or her family). For children younger than 7, it may be preferable to use drawings and pictures to represent activities on the crisis card. Chronically suicidal children and adolescents should also be encouraged to engage in enjoyable activities that have a high potential of fostering feelings of connection and effectiveness, such as participation in school activities.

PSYCHOTHERAPY

The AACAP's practice parameters for the assessment and treatment of children and adolescents with suicidal behavior indicate the following treatment modalities as "options": CBT, interpersonal psychotherapy for adolescents (IPT-A), DBT, psychodynamic therapy, and family therapy (Shaffer & Pfeffer, 2001). The parameters do not recommend a particular treatment, because of insufficient empirical evidence. Macgowan (2004) reviewed the literature on psychosocial treatments for youth suicidal behavior (i.e., all non-pharmacological treatments targeted at individuals 18 years old and younger) and concluded that, of 10 treatments, no current treatments for youth suicidal behavior meet the American Psychological Association's Division 12 Task Force's criteria for "well-established treatments." These criteria are outlined by Chambless and Hollon (1998). Two treatments met the criteria for "probably efficacious": developmental group psychotherapy (Wood, Trainor, Rothwell, Moore, & Harrington, 2001) and family communication and problem solving (Harrington et al., 1998).

Developmental group psychotherapy involves group sessions with youth who had engaged in self-harm in the past year. The treatment includes elements of many therapies, including CBT, DBT, problem solving, and psychodynamic group psychotherapy. Youth randomly assigned to developmental group psychotherapy were found to have significantly lower risk for a future episode of deliberate self-harm, as compared with those assigned to "routine care" (e.g., family sessions, nonspecific counseling, and psychotropic mediation). Family communication and problem solving involves family sessions with the youth (in the study, these youth had deliberately poisoned themselves) in the youth's home. This treatment significantly reduced suicidal ideation as compared with routine care (e.g., psychiatric consultations), but only in youth *without* major depression. We identified an additional study published after 2004 (Donaldson, Spirito, & Esposito-Smythers, 2005); however, this treatment (a skills-based treatment) did not produce greater decreases in suicidal ideation and depression in adolescent suicide attempters than a supportive relationship treatment group.

Other studies in Macgowan's (2004) review, although not meeting the stringent Chambless and Hollon (1998) criteria, are nonetheless suggestive of treatment effectiveness and point to future directions for treatment development and testing. Significant decreases in suicide attempts and deliberate self-harm were found in two studies (Gutstein & Rudd, 1990; Wood et al., 2001), and nonsignificant decreases were found in four others (Cotgrove, Zirinsky, Black, & Weston, 1995; Deykin & Buka, 1994; Rathus & Miller, 2002; Rotheram-Borus, Piacentini, Cantwell, Berlin, & Song, 2000). Reduction in suicidal ideation or threats were found in five studies (Brent et al., 1997; Greenfield, Larson, Hechtman, Rousseau, & Platt, 2002; Gutstein & Rudd, 1990; Rathus & Miller, 2002; Rotheram-Borus et al., 2000). Most treatments with positive effects involved a form of CBT and many included family involvement, which suggests that these components should be the focus of future research on youth suicidal behavior and that current treatments with these components are the current treatments of choice. Thus, we next briefly discuss CBT with suicidal youth and an example of treatment with family involvement (DBT with adolescents).

The efficacy of CBT in the treatment of major depressive disorder is well established (e.g., Butler & Beck, 2000). Rudd, Joiner, and Rajab (2004) have documented that cognitive therapy is the leading treatment for suicidal behavior. CBT has also been found to be efficacious in the treatment of depression in youth (see, e.g., TADS Team, 2004). Brent et al. (1997) revised Beck's approach (Beck, Rush, Shaw, & Emery, 1979) for use with depressed adolescents. The treatment involves 12–16 weekly sessions (plus booster sessions) in which the adolescent and therapist work collaboratively to identify and restructure negative automatic thoughts, maladaptive assumptions, and core beliefs relevant to depression. Both the adolescent and his or her parents are given psychoeducation on mood disorders and treatment. This modification of CBT was as effective as systemic family therapy and nondirective supportive therapy in the reduction of suicidal ideation. Rudd et al. (2004) provide a detailed guide to the treatment of suicidal behavior using

CBT techniques. Clients are taught problem-solving and distress tolerance skills in addition to cognitive restructuring skills. The cognitive restructuring skills are denoted by the acronym ICARE: Clients are taught to *identity* suicidal ideation (and other relevant thoughts), *connect* thoughts to cognitive distortion, *assess* the validity of the thoughts, *restructure* the thoughts, and *enact* the new, more accurate and helpful thoughts.

Stellrecht et al. (2006) suggest that an integrative form of cognitive therapy, the cognitive-behavioral analysis system of psychotherapy (CBASP; McCullough, 2003), may be well suited for treating suicidal ideation because it challenges clients to be goal oriented and planful in their approaches to problem solving and managing emotional distress. Clients are taught to identify discrete situations that are emotionally distressing and then to identify their "desired outcome" (i.e., goal) for a situation. Thoughts and behaviors are evaluated by the client (with help from the therapist) as either "helpful" or "hurtful" in terms of achieving the desired outcome. A goal in treatment is for clients to spontaneously utilize this goal-oriented approach "in the moment." In doing so, clients approach problems with a goal in mind and plan their actions to maximize chances of achieving this goal. This form of CBT may allow clinicians to address all components of the interpersonal–psychological theory: the impulsivity and lack of planfulness that places individuals along a trajectory toward the acquired capability for lethal self-injury can be addressed indirectly by encouraging a goal-oriented and problem-solving approach to emotional distress. In addition, cognitions related to themes of perceived burdensomeness and thwarted belongingness can be directly targeted in treatment (as helpful or hurtful thoughts).

Other treatments that utilize methods of CBT and target components of the interpersonal–psychological theory may be effective as well. For example, although treatment may not be able to directly alter the acquired capability component, skill deficits and maladaptive behaviors that can serve to promote or maintain an acquired capability, such as emotion regulation deficits, problem-solving deficits, and impulsive response styles, are amenable to psychotherapy. Cognitive-behavioral treatments with an emphasis on problem solving have been found to be effective in the treatment of suicidal behavior in young adults (Rudd et al., 1996). Data suggest that this treatment worked by compensating for skill deficits, specifically deficits in problem-solving skills (Wingate, Van Orden, Joiner, Williams, & Rudd, 2005). A brief problem-solving intervention consisting of a video focused on problem solving and coping styles was found to lead to more pronounced initial drops in suicidal ideation in young adults, as compared with a control condition consisting of a video on health-related issues (e.g., diet, exercise, and sleep habits; Fitzpatrick, Witte, & Schmidt, 2005). This suggests that even a brief, nonspecific problem-solving intervention may lead to reductions in suicidal symptoms.

DBT (Linehan, 1993) has shown potential in the treatment of suicidal adolescents, especially those with borderline personality disorder, perhaps owing to its focus on reducing life-threatening behaviors and therapy-interfering behaviors. It may also provide suicidal adolescents with beneficial skills, such as emotion regulation, mindfulness, interpersonal effectiveness, and distress tolerance, which can be used to increase their quality of life. Miller and colleagues (1997) have developed a model of DBT specifically aimed at treating suicidal adolescents. In this adaptation of DBT for suicidal adolescents, parents attend a skills training group to facilitate family involvement in treatment and promote generalization of skill usage. The treatment length was also shortened to facilitate treatment compliance in adolescents. The treatment adaptation was tested in a quasi-experimental study that compared DBT with treatment as usual for treating suicidal adolescents with borderline features (Rathus & Miller, 2002). The results of this study showed that DBT significantly reduced suicidal ideation, general psychiatric problems, and symptoms of borderline personality disorder, as compared with treatment as usual. In a similar study, Miller and colleagues (2000) found that the behavioral skills taught in DBT were effective in reducing borderline symptomatology, including impulsivity, in suicidal adolescents.

Antidepressant medications have been found to be efficacious in the treatment of depression in youth. For example, the TADS Team (2004) found that fluoxetine combined with CBT was more efficacious in the reduction of depressive symptoms than either CBT alone or fluoxetine alone, suggesting a role for pharmacotherapy in the treatment of depression in youth. However, the public health advisory issued by the Food and Drug Administration (FDA) in October 2004 on the potential danger of worsening depressive symptoms and suicidality in patients treated with antidepressants (U.S. Food and Drug Administration, 2004) alerted the field to potential safety issues related to the prescription of antidepressants in youth. Numerous studies have since been conducted on the safety profile of antidepressants in youth. Some studies have not found statistically significant higher levels of suicidal symptoms in youth prescribed antidepressants (e.g., Valuck, Libby, Sills, Giese, & Allen, 2004), suggesting that antidepressants do not increase risk for suicidal behaviors, whereas others did find such differences (e.g., Wohlfarth et al., 2005). Bostwick (2006) explored potential mechanisms for increases in suicidal behavior in children treated with antidepressants, including the presence of psychomotor agitation (a side effect of akathisia). He suggests that if vulnerability exists, it is most likely to occur in the first few weeks after beginning medication and that the longer youth take antidepressants, the lower their risk for suicide. Thus, he calls for increased monitoring of youth, especially in the initial weeks after beginning a prescription, as well as clear communication with youth and parents that they must contact the physician at the first signs of any troublesome changes in mood or behavior (also see Brent, 2004).

PREVENTION

The AACAP's practice parameters (Shaffer & Pfeffer, 2001) outlines approaches to suicide prevention. First, crisis hotlines should be available to individuals experiencing a suicidal crisis. Second, reducing the availability or accessibility of means for suicide may decrease the number of suicide attempts. Research on crisis hotlines is limited and has not demonstrated that they reduce suicidal behavior. Research on the effectiveness of method restriction has been mixed, with some researchers suggesting a preventative effect, such as with barriers on bridges (Beautrais, 2001), and others suggesting no effect, such as with gun security laws that restrict access to firearms (Cummings, Grossman, Rivara, & Koepsell, 1997). Both prevention methods merit further research. The interpersonal–psychological theory allows us to predict that crisis hotlines may be effective by decreasing perceptions of thwarted belongingness and that method restriction may be effective by preventing individuals from acting on acquired capabilities for suicide.

Third, the AACAP practice parameters suggest that gatekeeper training through education about warning signs may also be an avenue for prevention. Gatekeeper training involves educating laypersons in direct contact with youth (e.g., teachers, parents, clergy, and peers) about warning signs for suicide so that the gatekeepers can refer these youth to mental health professionals. Classes for high school students about suicide have not been found to increase help-seeking behavior (see, e.g., Shaffer, Garland, Vieland, Underwood, & Busner, 1991) and may increase distress in adolescents with a history of suicidal behavior (Shaffer, Vieland, Garland, Rojas, Underwood, & Busner, 1990). However, it is unclear from these studies as to what specific content caused distress. Two experimental studies involving the presentation of the AAS set of warning signs (listed in Figure 18.1) failed to find an effect of negative mood resulting from exposure to the warning signs (Rudd, Mandrusiak, et al., 2006; Van Orden et al., 2006). We suggest that the impact of straightforward presentations of warning signs for suicide, in combination with information on how to seek help, is an important area for future research on suicide prevention in youth.

Finally, the AACAP practice parameters suggest that screening 15- to 19-year-olds (the age group at greatest risk for attempts) for suicidal symptoms is a potentially effective method of suicide prevention. Obtaining information about past suicide attempts, current suicidal symptoms, depression, and alcohol and substance use is recommended. Preliminary research has demonstrated that school-wide screening for suicide risk can be efficacious in the prevention of suicide (Reynolds, 1991; Shaffer & Craft, 1999). However, school officials are often hesitant to do such screening because they believe that asking about suicide will encourage youth to engage in suicidal behavior (Miller, Eckert, DuPaul, & White, 1999). A randomized controlled trial of the effect of youth screening for suicide on suicidal behavior did not find iatrogenic effects of screening (Gould et al., 2005). The researchers concluded that screening for suicide in youth is a safe component of prevention programs.

FUTURE DIRECTIONS

Our review of empirical literature on suicidal behavior in youth indicates that psychopathology, past suicide attempts, hopelessness, mental pain, lack of family support, and feelings of expendability are robust predictors of suicidal behavior in youth. Given the association between depression and suicide in youth (American Academy of Child and Adolescent Psychiatry, 1998; Wagner, 2003), these data can inform our understanding of the causes, treatment, and prevention of depression in youth.

Our review suggests several future directions for research on suicidal behavior in youth. The factor space of suicidal symptoms in children and adolescents has not been adequately described. Work in this area could provide insights into suicidal symptoms that may indicate relatively more severe or imminent risk. Research on warning signs for suicidal crises has not yet been conducted specifically with youth. Work in this area could also aid risk assessment, as well as prevention efforts. Additional research is also needed to determine safe and efficacious methods of teaching youth, parents, and teachers about warning signs for suicide. Most research on suicidal behavior has focused on either youth or adults. We suggest that a developmental psychopathology framework in which developmental considerations are an explicit component of a theory may yield more generalizable data as well as provide greater insights into the etiology of suicidal behavior. This research could explore developmental factors relevant to suicidal symptoms and how these symptoms are experienced and expressed over the lifespan. Finally, the most common components of the effective treatments for suicidal behavior reviewed above were CBT techniques and family involvement. Additional research is needed on the treatment of suicidal symptoms in youth, as well as on mechanisms that explain treatment gains. Miller and colleagues' (1997) adaptation of DBT for adolescents includes both CBT techniques and family involvement and thus represents a promising avenue for future research. We suggest that theory-driven research on the causes and treatment of suicidal behavior is an approach likely to provide useful information for the treatment and prevention of suicidal behavior in youth.

REFERENCES

Abramson, L. Y., Alloy, L. B., & Metalsky, G. I. (1989). Hopelessness depression: A theory-based subtype of depression. *Psychological Review, 96,* 358–372.

Allan, W. D., Kashani, J. H., Dahlmeier, J., Taghizadeh, P., & Reid, J. C. (1997). Psychometric properties and clinical utility of the Scale for Suicide Ideation with inpatient children. *Journal of Abnormal Child Psychology, 25,* 465–473.

American Academy of Child and Adolescent Psychiatry. (1998). Practice parameters for the assessment and treatment of children and adolescents with depressive disorders. *Journal of the American Academy of Child and Adolescent Psychiatry, 37,* 63S–83S.

American Psychiatric Association. (2000). *Diagnostic and statistical manual of mental disorders* (4th ed., text rev.). Washington, DC: Author.

Apter, A., Bleich, A., Plutchik, R., Mendelsohn, S., & Tyano, S. (1988). Suicidal behavior, depression, and conduct disorder in hospitalized adolescents. *Journal of the America Academy of Child and Adolescent Psychiatry, 27,* 696–699.

Arias, E., Anderson, R. N., Kung, H. C., Murphy, S. L., & Kochanek, K. D. (2003). Deaths: Final data for 2001. *National Vital Statistics Reports, 52.* Hyattsville, MD: National Center for Health Statistics.

Asarnow, J. R., Carlson, G. A., & Guthrie, D. (1987). Coping strategies, self-perceptions, hopelessness, and perceived family environments in depressed and suicidal children. *Journal of Consulting and Clinical Psychology, 55,* 361–366.

Baumeister, R. F. (1990). Suicide as escape from self. *Psychological Review, 97,* 90–113.

Baumeister, R. F., & Leary, M. R. (1995). The need to belong: Desire for interpersonal attachments as a fundamental human motivation. *Psychological Bulletin, 117,* 497–529.

Beautrais, A. L. (2001). Effectiveness of barriers at suicide jumping sites: A case study. *Australian and New Zealand Journal of Psychiatry, 35,* 557–562.

Beck, A. T., Kovacs, M., & Weissman, A. (1979). Assessment of suicidal intention: The Scale for Suicide Ideation. *Journal of Consulting and Clinical Psychology, 47,* 343–352.

Beck, A. T., Rush, A. J., Shaw, B. F., & Emery, G. (1979). *Cognitive therapy of depression: A treatment manual.* New York: Guilford Press.

Berman, A. L., Jobes, D. A., & Silverman, M. M. (2006). *Adolescent suicide: Assessment and intervention* (2nd ed.). Washington, DC: American Psychological Association.

Boergers, J., Spirito, A., & Donaldson, D. (1998). Reasons for adolescent suicide attempts: Associations with psychological functioning. *Journal of the American Academy of Child and Adolescent Psychiatry, 37,* 1287–1293.

Bonner, R. L., & Rich, A. L. (1987). Toward a predictive model of suicidal ideation and behavior: Some preliminary data in college students. *Suicide and Life-Threatening Behavior, 17,* 50–63.

Borowsky, I. W., Ireland, M., & Resnick, M. D. (2001). Adolescent suicide attempts: Risks and protectors. *Pediatrics, 107,* 485–493.

Bostwick, J. M. (2006). Do SSRIs cause suicide in children?: The evidence is underwhelming. *Journal of Clinical Psychology, 62,* 235–241.

Brent, D. (2004). Antidepressants and pediatric depression—the risk of doing nothing. *New England Journal of Medicine, 351,* 1598–1601.

Brent, D. A., Holder, D., Kolko, D., Birmaher, B., Baugher, M., Roth, C., et al. (1997). A clinical psychotherapy trial for adolescent depression comparing cognitive, family, and supportive therapy. *Archives of General Psychiatry, 54,* 877–885.

Brent, D. A., Johnson, B. A., Perper, J., Connolly, J., Bridge, J., Bartle, S., et al. (1994). Personality disorder, personality traits, impulsive violence, and completed suicide in adolescents. *Journal of the American Academy of Child and Adolescent Psychiatry, 33,* 1080–1086.

Brent, D. A., & Mann, J. J. (2003). Familial factors in adolescent suicidal behavior. In R. A. King & A. Apter (Eds.), *Suicide in children and adolescents* (pp. 86–117). Cambridge, UK: Cambridge University Press.

Brent, D. A., Perper, A. J., Moritz, G., Allman, C., Friend, A., Roth, C., et al. (1993). Psychiatric risk factors for adolescent suicide: A case-control study. *Journal of the American Academy of Child and Adolescent Psychiatry, 32,* 521–529.

Brown, G. K., Beck, A. T., Steer, R. A., & Grisham, J. R. (2000). Risk factors for suicide in psychiatric outpatients: A 20-year prospective study. *Journal of Consulting and Clinical Psychology, 68,* 371–377.

Brown, J., Cohen, P., Johnson, J., & Smailes, M. (1999). Childhood abuse and neglect: Specificity of effects on adolescent and young adult depression and suicidality. *Journal of the American Academy of Child and Adolescent Psychiatry, 38,* 1490–1496.

Butler, A. C., & Beck, J. S. (2000). Cognitive therapy outcomes: A review of meta-analyses. *Journal of the Norwegian Psychological Association, 37,* 1–9.

Cassidy, J., & Asher, S. R. (1992). Loneliness and peer relations in young children. *Child Development, 63,* 350–365.

Centers for Disease Control and Prevention (CDC). (2004). Youth risk behavior surveillance—United States, 2003. *Morbidity and Mortality Weekly Report, 53*(SS02), 1–29).

Chambless, D. L., & Hollon, S. D. (1998). Defining empirically supported therapies. *Journal of Consulting and Clinical Psychology, 66,* 7–18.

Cole, D. A. (1990). Relation of social and academic competence to depressive symptoms in childhood. *Journal of Abnormal Psychology, 99,* 422–429.

Cole, D. A. (1991). Preliminary support for a competency-based model of depression in children. *Journal of Abnormal Psychology, 100,* 181–190.

Cornette, M., Abramson, L. Y., & Bardone, A. (2000). Toward an integrated theory of suicidal behaviors: Merging the hopelessness, self-discrepancy, and escape theories. In T. Joiner & M. D. Rudd (Eds.), *Suicide science: Expanding the boundaries* (pp. 43–66). Boston: Kluwer.

Cotgrove, A. J., Zirinsky, L., Black, D., & Weston, D. (1995). Secondary prevention of attempted suicide in adolescence. *Journal of Adolescence, 18,* 569–577.

Crick, N. R., & Ladd, G. W. (1993). Children's perceptions of their peer experiences: Attributions, loneliness, social anxiety, and social avoidance. *Developmental Psychology, 29,* 244–254.

Cukrowicz, K. C., Wingate, L. R., Driscoll, K. A., & Joiner, T. E. (2004). A standard of care for the assessment of suicide risk and associated treatment: The Florida State University psychology clinic as an example. *Journal of Contemporary Psychotherapy, 34,* 87–100.

Cummings, P., Grossman, D. C., Rivara, F. P., & Koepsell, T. D. (1997). State gun safe storage laws and child mortality due to firearms. *Journal of the American Medical Association, 278,* 1084–1086.

Deykin, E. Y., Alpert, J. J., & McNamarra, J. J. (1985). A pilot study of the effect of exposure to child abuse or neglect on adolescent suicidal behavior. *American Journal of Psychiatry, 142,* 1299–1303.

Deykin, E. Y., & Buka, S. L. (1994). Suicidal ideation and attempts among chemically dependent adolescents. *American Journal of Public Health, 84,* 634–639.

DiClemente, R. J., Ponton, L. E., & Hartley, D. (1991). Prevalence and correlates of cutting behavior: Risk for HIV transmission. *Journal of the American Academy of Child and Adolescent Psychiatry, 30,* 735–739.

Dieserud, G., Roysamb, E., Ekeberg, O., & Kraft, P. (2001). Toward an integrative model of suicide attempt: A cognitive psychological approach. *Suicide and Life-Threatening Behavior, 31,* 153–168.

Donaldson, D., Spirito, A., & Esposito-Smythers, C. (2005). Treatment for adolescents following a suicide attempt: Results of a pilot trial. *Journal of the American Academy of Child and Adolescent Psychiatry, 44,* 113–120.

Fitzpatrick, K. K., Witte, T. K., & Schmidt, N. B. (2005). Randomized controlled trial of a brief problem-orientation intervention for suicidal ideation. *Behavior Therapy, 36,* 323–333.

Flouri, E., & Buchanan, A. (2001). The protective role of parental involvement in adolescent suicide. *Crisis: The Journal of Crisis Intervention and Suicide Prevention, 23,* 17–22.

Gould, M. S., Fisher, P., Parides, M., Flory, M., & Shaffer, D. (1996). Psychosocial risk factors for child and adolescent completed suicide. *Archives of General Psychiatry, 53,* 1155–1162.

Gould, M. S., Marrocco, F. A., Kleinman, M., Thomas, J. G., Mostkoff, K., Cote, J., et al. (2005). Evaluating iatrogenic risk of youth suicide screening programs: A randomized controlled trial. *Journal of the American Medical Association, 293,* 1635–1643.

Gould, M. S., Shaffer, D., & Greenberg, T. (2003). The epidemiology of youth suicide. In R. A. King & A. Apter (Eds.), *Suicide in children and adolescents* (pp. 1–40). Cambridge, UK: Cambridge University Press.

Greenfield, B., Larson, C., Hechtman, L., Rousseau, C., & Platt, R. (2002). A rapid-response outpatient model for reducing hospitalization rates among suicidal adolescents. *Psychiatric Services, 53,* 1574–1579.

Gutstein, S. E., & Rudd, M. D. (1990). An outpatient treatment alternative for suicidal youth. *Journal of Adolescence, 13,* 265–277.

Harrington, R., Kerfoot, M., Dyer, E., McNiven, F., Gill, J., Harrington, V., et al. (1998). Randomized trial of a home-based family intervention for children who have deliberately poisoned themselves. *Journal of the American Academy of Child and Adolescent Psychiatry, 37,* 512–518.

Hershberger, S. L., Pilkington, N. W., & D'Augelli, A. R. (1997). Predictors of suicide attempts among gay, lesbian, and bisexual youth. *Journal of Adolescent Research, 12,* 477–497.

Higgins, E. T. (2004). Making a theory useful: Lessons handed down. *Personality and Social Psychology Review, 8,* 138–145.

Joiner, T. E. (2005). *Why people die by suicide.* Cambridge, MA: Harvard University Press.

Joiner, T. E., Jr., Conwell, Y., Fitzpatrick, K. K., Witte, T. K., Schmidt, N. B., Berlim, M. T., et al. (2005). Four studies on how past and current suicidality relate even when "everything but the kitchen sink" is covaried. *Journal of Abnormal Psychology, 114,* 291–303.

Joiner, T. E., Pettit, J. W., Walker, R. L., Voelz, Z. R., Cruz, J., Rudd, M. D., et al. (2002). Perceived burdensomeness and suicidality: Two studies on the suicide notes of those attempting and those completing suicide. *Journal of Social and Clinical Psychology, 21,* 531–545.

Joiner, T. E., Jr., & Rudd M. D. R. (1996). Disentangling the interrelations between hopelessness, loneliness, and suicidal ideation. *Suicide and Life-Threatening Behavior, 26,* 19–26.

Joiner, T. E., Rudd, M. D., & Rajab, M. H. (1997). The modified scale for suicidal ideation: Factors of suicidality and their relationship to clinical and diagnostic variables. *Journal of Abnormal Psychology, 106,* 260–265.

Joiner, T. E., Sachs-Ericsson, N. J., Wingate, L. R., & Brown, J. S. (2007). Childhood physical and sexual abuse and lifetime number of suicide attempts: A resilient and theoretically important relationship. *Behaviour Research and Therapy, 45,* 539–547.

Joiner, T. E., Walker, R. L., Rudd, M. D., & Jobes, D. A. (1999). Scientizing and routinizing the assessment of suicidality in outpatient practice. *Professional Psychology: Research and Practice, 30,* 447–453.

Kazdin, A. E., French, N. H., Unis, A. S., Esveldt-Dawson, K., & Sherick, R. B. (1983). Hopelessness, depression, and suicidal intent among psychiatrically disturbed inpatient children. *Journal of Consulting and Clinical Psychology, 51,* 504–510.

Kienhorst, I. C., De Wilde, E. J., Diekstra, R. F., & Wolters, W. H. (1995). Adolescents' image of their suicide attempt. *Journal of the American Academy of Child and Adolescent Psychiatry, 34,* 623–628.

Koivumaa-Honkanen, H., Honkanen, R., Viinamaki, H., Heikkila, K., Kaprio, J., & Koskenvuo, M. (2001). Life satisfaction and suicide: A 20-year follow-up study. *American Journal of Psychiatry, 158,* 433–439.

Koons, C. R., Robins, C. J., Tweed, J. L., Lynch, C. R., Gonzalez, A. M., Morse, J. Q., et al. (2001). Efficacy of dialectical behavior therapy in women veterans with borderline personality disorder. *Behavior Therapy, 32,* 371–390.

Kuo, W., Gallo, J. J., & Eaton, W. W. (2004). Hopelessness, depression, substance disorder, and suicidality. *Social Psychiatry and Psychiatric Epidemiology, 39*, 497–501.

Lewin, L. (1951). *Field theory in social science*. New York: Harper & Brothers.

Linehan, M. M. (1993). *Cognitive-behavioral treatment of borderline personality disorder*. New York: Guilford Press.

Linehan, M. M., Armstrong, H. E., Suarez, A., Allmon, D., & Heard, H. L. (1991). Cognitive-behavioral treatment of chronically parasuicidal borderline patients. *Archives of General Psychiatry, 48*, 1060–1064.

Linehan, M. M., Comtois, K. A., Murray, A. M., Brown, M. Z., Gallop, R. J., Heard, H. L., et al. (2006). Two-year randomized controlled trial and follow-up of dialectical behavior therapy vs therapy by experts for suicidal behaviors and borderline personality disorder. *Archives of General Psychiatry, 63*, 757–766.

Linehan, M. M., Dimeff, L. A., Reynolds, S. K., Comtois, K., Shaw-Welch, S., Heagerty, P., et al. (2002). Dialectical behavior therapy versus comprehensive validation plus 12-step for the treatment of opioid dependent women meeting criteria for borderline personality disorder. *Drug and Alcohol Dependence, 67*, 13–26.

Linehan, M. M., Schmidt, H., III, Dimeff, L. A, Craft, J. C., Kanter, J., & Comtois, K. A. (1999). Dialectical behavior therapy for patients with borderline personality disorder and drug-dependence. *American Journal on Addictions, 8*, 279–292.

Lloyd, E., Kelley, M. L., & Hope, T. (1997, April). *Self-mutilation in a community sample of adolescents: Descriptive characteristics and provisional prevalence rates*. Paper presented at the annual meeting of the Society for Behavioral Medicine, New Orleans.

Macgowan, M. J. (2004). Psychosocial treatment of youth suicide: A systematic review of the research. *Research on Social Work Practice, 14*, 147–162.

McCullough, J. P. (2003). *Treatment for chronic depression: Cognitive-behavioral analysis system of psychotherapy (CBASP)*. New York: Guilford Press.

McIntosh, J. L. (2006). *U.S.A. suicide statistics for the year 2003*. Washington, DC: American Association of Suicidology.

McManus, B. L., Kruesi, M. J., Dontes, A. E., Defazio, C. R., Piotrowski, J. T., & Woodward, P. J. (1997). Child and adolescent suicide attempts: An opportunity for emergency departments to provide injury prevention education. *American Journal of Emergency Medicine, 15*, 357–360.

Miller, A. L., Rathus, J. H., Linehan, M. M., Wetzler, S., & Leigh, E. (1997). Dialectical behavior therapy adapted for suicidal adolescents. *Journal of Practical Psychiatry and Behavioral Health, 3*, 78–86.

Miller, A. L., Wyman, S. E., Huppert, J. D., Glassman, S. L., & Rathus, J. H. (2000). Analysis of behavioral skills utilized by suicidal adolescents receiving dialectical behavior therapy. *Cognitive and Behavioral Practice, 7*, 183–187.

Miller, D. N., Eckert, T. L., DuPaul, G. J., & White, G. P. (1999). Adolescent suicide prevention: Acceptability of school-based programs among secondary school principles. *Suicide and Life-Threatening Behavior, 29*, 72–83.

Morano, C. D., Cisler, R. A., & Lemerond, J. (1993). Risk factors for adolescent suicidal behavior: Loss, insufficient familiar support, and hopelessness. *Adolescence, 28*, 851–865.

Moskos, M., Olson, L., Halbern, S., Keller, T., & Gray, D. (2005). Utah Youth Suicide Study: Psychological autopsy. *Suicide and Life-Threatening Behavior, 35*, 536–546.

Nock, M. K., Joiner, T. E., Gordon, K. H., Lloyd-Richardson, E., & Prinstein, M. J. (2006). Non-suicidal self-injury among adolescents: Diagnostic correlates and relation to suicide attempts. *Psychiatry Research, 144*, 65–72.

Nock, M. K., & Prinstein, M. J. (2004). A functional approach to the assessment of self-mutilative behavior. *Journal of Consulting and Clinical Psychology, 72*, 885–890.

Nock, M. K., & Prinstein, M. J. (2005). Contextual features and behavioral functions of self-mutilation among adolescents. *Journal of Abnormal Psychology, 114*, 140–146.

Orbach, I., Mikulincer, M., Gilboa-Schechtman, E., & Sirota, P. (2003). Mental pain and its relationship to suicidality and life meaning. *Suicide and Life-Threatening Behavior, 33*, 231–241.

Parkhurst, J. T., & Asher, S. R. (1992). Peer rejection in middle school: Subgroup differences in behavior, loneliness, and interpersonal concerns. *Developmental Psychology, 28,* 231–241.

Pfeffer, C. R. (2003). Assessing suicidal behavior in children and adolescents. In R. A. King & A. Apter (Eds.), *Suicide in children and adolescents* (pp. 211–226). Cambridge, UK: Cambridge University Press.

Pfeffer, C. R., Jiang, H., & Kakuma, T. (2000). Child–Adolescent Suicidal Potential Index (CASPI): A screen for risk for early onset suicidal behavior. *Psychological Assessment, 12,* 304–318.

Pfeffer, C. R., Klerman, G. L., Hurt, S. W., Kakuma, T., Peskin, J. R., & Siefker, C. A. (1993). Suicidal children grow up: Rates and psychosocial risk factors for suicide attempts during follow-up. *Journal of the American Academy of Child and Adolescent Psychiatry, 32,* 106–113.

Rathus, J. H., & Miller, A. L. (2002). Dialectical behavior therapy adapted for suicidal adolescents. *Suicide and Life-Threatening Behavior, 32,* 146–157.

Reith, D. M., Whyte, I., Carter, G., & McPherson, M. (2003). Adolescent self-poisoning: A cohort study of subsequent suicide and premature deaths. *Crisis, 24,* 79–84.

Renaud, J., Brent, D. A., Birmaher, B., Chiapetta, L., & Bridge, J. (1999). Suicide in adolescents with disruptive disorders. *Journal of the American Academy of Child and Adolescent Psychiatry, 38,* 846–851.

Reynolds, W. M. (1991). A school-based procedure for the identification of adolescents at risk for suicidal behaviors. *Family and Community Health, 14,* 64–75.

Ringle, J. L., & Larzelere, R. E. (2001). *Validity comparison of the Child Suicide Risk Assessment (CSRA) and Suicide Probability Scale (SPS) with pre-adolescents* (Tech. Rep. No. 01-05). Boys Town, NE: Girls and Boys Town National Research Institute for Child and Family Studies.

Roberts, R. E., Roberts, C. R., & Chen, Y. R. (1988). Suicidal thinking among adolescents with a history of attempted suicide. *Journal of the American Academy of Child and Adolescent Psychiatry, 37,* 1294–1300.

Rosenthal, P. A., & Rosenthal, S. (1984). Suicidal behavior by preschool children. *American Journal of Psychiatry, 141,* 520–525.

Rotheram-Borus, M. J., Piacentini, J., Cantwell, C., Belin, T. R., & Song, J. (2000). The 18-month impact of an emergency room intervention for adolescent female suicide attempters. *Journal of Consulting and Clinical Psychology, 68,* 1081–1093.

Rotheram-Borus, M. J., Piacentini, J., Van Rossem, R., Graae, F., Cantwell, C., Castro-Blanco, D., et al. (1996). Enhancing treatment adherence with a specialized emergency room program for adolescent suicide attempters. *Journal of the American Academy of Child and Adolescent Psychiatry, 35,* 654–663.

Rudd, M. D., Berman, L., Joiner, T. E., Nock, M., Mandrusiak, M., Van Orden, K., et al. (2006). Warning signs for suicide: Theory, research, and clinical application. *Suicide and Life-Threatening Behavior, 36,* 255–262.

Rudd, M. D., Joiner, T., & Rajab, M. H. (2004). *Treating suicidal behavior: An effective, time-limited approach.* New York: Guilford Press.

Rudd, M. D., Joiner, T. E., & Rumzek, H. (2004). Childhood diagnoses and later risk for multiple suicide attempts. *Suicide and Life-Threatening Behavior, 34,* 113–125.

Rudd, M. D., Mandrusiak, M., & Joiner, T. E. (2006). The case against no-suicide contracts: The commitment to treatment statement as a practice alternative. *Journal of Clinical Psychology, 62,* 243–251.

Rudd, M. D., Mandrusiak, M., Joiner, T. E., Berman, L., Van Orden, K., & Hollar, D. (2006). The emotional impact and ease of recall of warning signs for suicide: A controlled study. *Suicide and Life-Threatening Behavior, 36,* 288–295.

Rudd, M. D., Rajab, M. H., Orman, D. T., Stulman, D. A., Joiner, T., & Dixon, W. (1996). Effectiveness of an outpatient intervention targeting suicidal young adults: Preliminary results. *Journal of Consulting and Clinical Psychology, 64,* 179–190.

Sabbath, J. C. (1969). The suicidal adolescent—The expendable child. *Journal of the American Academy of Child and Adolescent Psychiatry, 8,* 272–285.

Shaffer, D., & Craft, L. (1999). Methods of adolescent suicide prevention. *Journal of Clinical Psychiatry, 60,* 70–74.

Shaffer, D., Garland, A., Vieland, V., Underwood, M., & Busner, C. (1991). The impact of curriculum-based suicide prevention programs for teenagers. *Journal of the American Academy of Child and Adolescent Psychiatry, 30,* 588–596.

Shaffer, D., Gould, M., Fisher, P., Trautman, P., Moreau, D., Kleinman, M., et al. (1996). Psychiatric diagnosis in child and adolescent suicide. *Archives of General Psychiatry, 53,* 339–348.

Shaffer, D., & Pfeffer, C. R. (2001). Practice parameter for the assessment and treatment of children and adolescents with suicidal behavior. *Journal of the American Academy of Child and Adolescent Psychiatry, 40*(Suppl.), 4S–23S.

Shaffer, D., Vieland, V., Garland, A., Rojas, M., Underwood, M., & Busner, C. (1990). Adolescent suicide attempters: Response to suicide prevention programs. *Journal of the American Medical Association, 264,* 3151–3155.

Shneidman, E. (1985). *Definition of suicide.* New York: Wiley.

Shneidman, E. S. (1996).*The suicidal mind.* New York: Oxford University Press.

Shneidman, E. S. (1998). Further reflections on suicide and psychache. *Suicide and Life-Threatening Behavior, 28,* 245–250.

Solomon, R. L., & Corbit, J. D. (1974). An opponent-process theory of motivation. *Psychological Review, 81,* 119–145.

Steer, R. A., Kumar, G., & Beck, A. T. (1993). Self-reported suicidal ideation in adolescent psychiatric inpatients. *Journal of Consulting and Clinical Psychology, 61,* 1096–1099.

Stellrecht, N. E., Gordon, K. H., Van Orden, K., Witte, T. K., Wingate, L., Cukrowicz, K. C., et al. (2006). Clinical applications of the interpersonal–psychological theory of attempted and completed suicide. *Journal of Clinical Psychology, 62,* 211–222.

Stravynski, A., & Boyer, R. (2001). Loneliness in relation to suicide ideation and parasuicide: A population-wide study. *Suicide and Life-Threatening Behavior, 31,* 32–40.

Treatment for Adolescents with Depression (TADS) Team. (2004). Fluoxetine, cognitive-behavioral therapy, and their combination for adolescents with depression: Treatment for Adolescents with Depression Study (TADS) randomized controlled trial. *Journal of the American Medical Association, 292,* 807–820.

U.S. Department of Heath and Human Services. (2001). *National strategy for suicide prevention: Goals and objectives for action.* Washington, DC: Author.

U.S. Department of Health and Human Services. (2004). Compressed mortality file (CMF) compiled from CMF 2002. *CDC WONDER on-line database.* Retrieved March 18, 2006. Washington, DC: Author.

U.S. Food and Drug Administration Public Health Advisory. (2004). Worsening depression and suicidality in patients being treated with antidepressant medications. Available at *www.fda.gov/cder/drug/antidepressants/AntidepressanstPHA.htm.* Retrieved November 15, 2004.

Valuck, R. J., Libby, A. M., Sills, M. R., Giese, A. A., & Allen, R. R. (2004). Antidepressant treatment and risk of suicide attempt by adolescents with major depressive disorder: A propensity-adjusted retrospective cohort study. *CNS Drugs, 18,* 1119–1132.

Van Orden, K. A., & Joiner, T. E., Jr. (2005). *Interpersonal beliefs and suicidality: The relationship between suicidal desire, a thwarted need to belong, and perceived burdensomeness.* Poster session presented at the meeting of the Association of Cognitive and Behavioral Therapists, Washington, DC.

Van Orden, K. A., Joiner, T. E., Jr., Hollar, D., Rudd, M. D., Mandrusiak, M., & Silverman, M. M. (2006). A test of the effectiveness of a list of suicide warning signs for the public. *Suicide and Life-Threatening Behavior, 36,* 272–287.

Verheul, R., van den Bosch, L. M. C., Koeter, M. W. J., de Ridder, M. A. J., Stijnen, T., & van den Brink, W. (2003). Dialectical behaviour therapy for women with borderline personality disorder: 12-month, randomised clinical trial in the Netherlands. *British Journal of Psychiatry, 182,* 135–140.

Waern, M., Rubenowitz, E., & Wilhelmson, K. (2003). Predictors of suicide in the old elderly. *Gerontology, 49,* 328–334.

Wagner, K. D. (2003). Major depression in children and adolescents. *Psychiatric Annals, 33,* 266–270.

Wagner, K. D., Rouleau, M., & Joiner, T. (2000). Cognitive factors related to suicidal ideation and resolution in psychiatrically hospitalized children and adolescents. *American Journal of Psychiatry, 157,* 2017–2021.

Weissman, M. M., Wolk, S., Wickramaratne, P., Goldstein, R. B., Adams, P., Greenwald, S., et al. (1999). Children with prepubertal-onset major depressive disorder and anxiety grown up. *Archives of General Psychiatry, 56,* 794–801.

Wingate, L. R., Van Orden, K. A., Joiner, T. E., Williams, F. M., & Rudd, M. D. (2005). Comparison of compensation and capitalization models when treating suicidality in young adults. *Journal of Consulting and Clinical Psychology, 73,* 756–762.

Wohlfarth, T. D., van Zwieten, B. J., Lekkerkerker, F. J., Gispen-de Wied, C. C., Ruis, J. R., Elferink, A. J. A., et al. (2005). Antidepressants use in children and adolescents and the risk of suicide. *European Neuropsychopharmacology, 16,* 79–83.

Wood, A., Trainor, G., Rothwell, J., Moore, A., & Harrington, R. (2001). Randomized trial of group therapy for repeated deliberate self-harm in adolescents. *Journal of the American Academy of Child and Adolescent Psychiatry, 40,* 1246–1263.

Woznica, J. G., & Shapiro, J. R. (1990). An analysis of adolescent suicide attempts: The expendable child. *Journal of Pediatric Psychology, 15,* 789–796.

Zayas, L. H., Lester, R. J., Cabassa, L. J., & Fortuna, L. R. (2005). Why do so many Latina teens attempt suicide? A conceptual model for research. *American Journal of Orthopsychiatry, 75,* 275–287.

19 Child Abuse and Neglect and the Development of Depression in Children and Adolescents

Kate L. Harkness and Margaret N. Lumley

According to the United States Department of Health and Human Services, 50,000 reports of suspected child abuse or neglect are made to child protective services agencies throughout the United States each week (U.S. Department of Health and Human Services, 2005). In 2003, 2.9 million reports concerning the welfare of approximately 5.5 million children were made. Investigations resulted from approximately two-thirds of these cases, and, from these investigations, 1.9 million cases were substantiated. That is, an average of more than 5,200 children per day were found to be the victims of abuse and neglect. Approximately 1,500 children died as a result of abuse or neglect in 2003, an average of nearly 4 children per day, with children under age 3 making up more than 75% of these fatalities. The numbers cited are likely underestimates of the true prevalence of child abuse and neglect, as epidemiological studies suggest that close to two-thirds of cases go unreported (London, Bruck, Ceci, & Shuman, 2005).

The experience of abuse is traumatic in and of itself. Even further, it places children at risk for a number of negative outcomes in later life, including increased rates of substance abuse and dependence, delinquency, early pregnancy, school dropout, and unemployment, as well as significant impairments in interpersonal relationships and physical health that persist into adulthood (e.g., Cicchetti & Toth, 2005; Simpson & Miller, 2002). Despite the pervasiveness of child maltreatment and the clear link to a lifelong pattern of dysfunction, researchers are still at a very early stage in understanding the *mechanisms* that translate maltreatment into later psychopathology. Elucidating such mechanisms is very important clinically: Understanding *how* a risk factor causes a particular disorder provides a clear target for intervention.

The purpose of this chapter is to review the literature regarding the association between child abuse and neglect and major depression in childhood and adolescence, and to examine three theorized causal mechanisms underlying this association. Specifically, we suggest that childhood adversity leads to major depression through its effects on (1) the development of negative cognitive schemas, (2) the disruption of neural pathways subserving the stress response, particularly the hypothalamic–pituitary–adrenal (HPA) axis, and (3) the sensitization to stressful life events that trigger depression onset. We argue further that these three mediating mechanisms are part of an integrated developmental model of major depression etiology.

Before proceeding, a few caveats are in order. First, we acknowledge that child abuse and neglect are associated with many pathological outcomes, such as substance dependence (Simpson & Miller, 2002) and personality disorders (Battle et al., 2004). Indeed, the breadth of their impact lends further urgency to research on their causes and consequences. Our research focuses specifically on major depression in an attempt to reduce the prevalence, and improve the treatment, of this devastating disorder. We believe that the knowledge gained from this targeted analysis can be used along with that bearing on other disorders to develop a broad-ranging model of risk associated with child maltreatment. Second, child maltreatment is associated with a number of other mediators, such as stress generation and disruptions in personality, emotion regulation, attachment, and coping (see, e.g., Whiffen & MacIntosh, 2005). We see these processes as complementary to those that we address in this chapter, and all could likely be integrated into a larger patho-developmental model of major depression. However, for the sake of parsimony we focus specifically on the mediating roles of cognitive schema development, HPA axis dysregulation, and stress sensitivity. We hope that researchers will take the ideas put forth here and apply them to the study of additional variables.

THE ASSESSMENT OF CHILD ABUSE AND NEGLECT

The validity of research examining the relation of child abuse and neglect to depression must be assessed within the context of the reliability and validity of the instruments employed to measure maltreatment. Studies in this area typically rely on retrospective self-reports and/or documented case records, such as Child Protective Services (CPS) or police records. The primary advantage of public documents is that they circumvent memory inaccuracies and biases that exist with retrospective self-reports. Furthermore, they are easily incorporated into prospective designs. That is, samples can be selected from documented reports at, or near to, the time of occurrence and can then be followed to assess longitudinal outcomes. The primary disadvantage of documented reports is that many incidents of adversity are not identified by CPS and may not be noticed by, or reported to, other sources. According to a recent review, the modal disclosure rate of child sexual abuse is 33% (London et al., 2005). That is, two-thirds of adults who retrospectively report having been sexually abused as children did not disclose their abuse at the time it occurred. Therefore, relying solely on documented reports may result in samples that are biased by other factors known to be associated with an increased likelihood of reporting (e.g., low socioeconomic status and non-white ethnicity) and may miss many cases of maltreatment.

Self-reports of adversity are assessed through either questionnaire or interview. Questionnaires can be administered to large groups and are not labor-intensive, nor do they require any expertise to administer. Questionnaires are also relatively anonymous, and thus individuals may be more willing to divulge details about societal taboos such as incest (e.g., Dill, Chu, Grob, & Eisen, 1991). Yet the questions posed on questionnaires are free to be (mis)interpreted in different ways by different people with no chance for clarification. Moreover, the rating scales used on most questionnaires may be interpreted differently by different people (e.g., "sometimes" may mean "twice" to one individual and "20 times" to another).

Most researchers agree that interviews have important advantages over questionnaires, including the ability to stress the importance of honesty, the ability of the interviewer to clarify questions and answers, and the possibility of collecting contextual information about the adversity (e.g., Bifulco, Brown, & Harris, 1994). However, interviews also demand a considerably greater investment of time and more expertise than questionnaires. Following an extensive review of the literature, Hardt and Rutter (2004) concluded that far more important than method of administration (e.g., interview vs. questionnaire) is having a clearly defined construct of adversity, asking multiple questions about the adversity, and avoiding vague language. For example, in a study reviewed below, youths were asked to self-report adversity based on two yes/no questions, "Have you ever been physically abused?" and "Have you ever been sexually abused?" (Schraedly, Gotlib, & Hayward, 1999). These questions are very broad and easily open to misinterpretation based on idiosyncratic notions of what constitutes "abuse." Questions with specific behavioral content are preferable (e.g., "Did an adult ever hit you with a belt?").

An important disadvantage of retrospective self-reports is that they are subject to memory degradation and biases. For example, evidence suggests that adults free of psychopathology may underreport documented abuse (see, e.g., Williams, 1994). Furthermore, mood-congruent recall biases are of particular concern when assessing for a history of childhood adversity in depressed participants (Brewin, Andrews, & Gotlib, 1993). To improve the validity of retrospective self-reports, researchers can compare self-reports with official records or sibling reports (see, e.g., Bifulco, Brown, Lillie, & Jarvis, 1997; Kendall-Tackett & Becker-Blease, 2004). In addition, researchers can structure their questions so that they focus on specific behavioral indicators (e.g., "Prior to age 18, were you spanked so forcefully that you sustained bruises or welts?") as opposed to general questions (e.g., "Prior to age 18, were you physically abused?").

The latter issue is particularly important when assessing childhood experiences that may not have clear-cut behavioral indicators (e.g., emotional neglect). The question, "Were your emotional needs met as a child?", for example, may provide information regarding the respondent's *perception* of the nurturance received from parents, but does little to clarify what actually happened, whether what happened meets the investigator's operationalization of emotional neglect, and thus whether responses can be compared across participants. An example of an interview that addresses this concern is the Childhood Experience of Care and Abuse (CECA) interview (Bifulco et al., 1994), which is based on the Bedford College contextual method of rating life experience. First, in this interview, respondents are given an opportunity to elaborate on their experience, thus priming autobiographical memory. Second, the interview probes for behavioral evidence to support respondents' impressions (e.g., "What did he do or say that makes you say that he was a 'bad' father?"). Third, these behavioral indicators, and not the respondent's perceptions, are used by raters blind to the respondent's mental health status to rate childhood experience based on a standardized rating system with clear guidelines. In this way, "the distinction can be made between parental neglectful [or abusive] behavior and the child's interpretation of such behavior (whether seen as neglectful or not) and report of the feelings evoked" (Bifulco et al., 1994, p. 1420), thereby enhancing validity.

In summary, documented reports and self-reports of adversity have unique advantages and disadvantages, and the choice of either type of report largely depends on the research design. For example, documented records may be more appropriate with young children, given the ethical issues related to mandatory reporting. In addition, self-reports in young children may be very susceptible to suggestion, manipulation, and confabulation, given the immaturity of children's memory systems. In contrast, retrospective self-reports may be more appropriate for late adolescent clients when youths are past the age at which mandatory reporting is an issue. Furthermore, in very large national surveys, gaining access to records, especially for abuse that may have occurred several years prior, would be very laborious. The more important issue in these studies is that the questions contained in the interviews be specific and behaviorally anchored.

CHILDHOOD ABUSE AND NEGLECT PREDICT MAJOR DEPRESSION

Substantial evidence from both cross-sectional and prospective studies suggests that child abuse and neglect are strongly associated with depression in both childhood and adolescence. The majority of these studies have been conducted with adolescent samples, but a handful of reports from studies with children have emerged. Studies with children have focused mainly on the relation of child maltreatment to depression *symptoms*, as assessed by self- or parent report, whereas studies with adolescents have generally investigated the prediction of the major depressive *syndrome*.

The Relation of Maltreatment to Depression in Children

In an early cross-sectional study of 81 children ages 7–12 with documented physical or sexual abuse or neglect, Toth, Manly, and Cicchetti (1992) found that the maltreated group scored significantly higher than a matched control group on measures of depression and significantly lower on self-esteem. Similarly, Lipovsky, Saunders, and Murphy (1989) reported that a sample of 88 children (mean age = 11.2 years) with documented sexual abuse reported higher parent- and self-rated depression symptoms, as assessed by the Child Behavior Checklist (CBCL; Achenbach & Edelbrock, 1983) and the Children's Depression Inventory (CDI; Kovacs, 1985), than their nonabused siblings.

Prospective studies confirm the aforementioned relations. Tebbutt, Swanston, Oates, and O'Toole (1997) followed a group of 84 children and early adolescents, ages 5–15, with documented sexual abuse for 5 years. Relative to a matched control group, the abused group had significantly higher depressive symptoms, as measured by the CBCL and the Youth Self-Report (YSR; Achenbach, 1991) 5 years later, even after controlling for other factors shown to predict depression, including family socioeconomic status, number of parent changes, mother's psychiatric history, and number of intervening life events. Similarly, Éthier, Lemelin, and Lacharité (2004) followed 49 children (mean age = 4.5 years), recruited through CPS, for 6 years. These children were all victims of severe emotional and/or material neglect. Children with chronic neglect over the longitudinal period had significantly higher levels of depression and anxiety, as assessed by mothers' reports on the CBCL, than those with transitory neglect.

The results of the latter study by Éthier and colleagues are consistent with a number of studies suggesting that chronic maltreatment has a stronger effect on depression than transitory abuse. For example, Thornberry, Ireland, and Smith (2001) assessed a sample of 738 12-year-olds every 6 months for 5 years. Abuse and neglect were documented through CPS records. They found that maltreatment that persisted from childhood through adolescence was a stronger predictor of internalizing and externalizing problems, as assessed by the CBCL, than was maltreatment experienced during childhood only. It is interesting to note that maltreatment that was experienced in *adolescence only* was an equally strong predictor of symptoms as chronic maltreatment, and was the *only* significant predictor of depressive symptoms (odds ratio = 2.62; Thornberry et al., 2001). Additional studies have confirmed this result, finding that child abuse and neglect have a significantly stronger relation to depression when experienced in adolescence than when experienced only in childhood (Feiring, Taska, & Lewis, 1999; Tebbutt et al., 1997).

The Relation of Maltreatment to Depression in Adolescents

The research cited above suggests that adolescence is a key developmental period during which maltreatment exerts its pathological effects. Adolescence is also a crucial period in the development of major depression. Point prevalence rates of major depression are approximately four times higher in adolescence than in childhood, and by adolescence, lifetime prevalence rates of major depression are comparable to those seen in adults (Birmaher et al., 1996). The profound developmental changes occurring in adolescence may account for these epidemiological trends, including, among others, changes in brain maturation and hormonal development, disruptions in socioemotional regulation and attachment patterns, and consolidation of cognitive schemas. Given the amount of "normal dysfunction" associated with the adolescent transition, it is not surprising that trauma occurring during this period is associated with severe and long-lasting effects.

There have now been several large-scale studies of the relation between child abuse and neglect and depression in adolescence, and the results of these are summarized in Table 19.1. All of these studies employed very large, and sometimes nationally representative, samples. All consistently document a strong relation between a history of child abuse and neglect and depression in adolescence. For example, Schraedley, Gotlib, and Hayward (1999), in a very large sample of 6,943 adolescents, found that those with a history of physical abuse were more than three times as likely to score high on the CDI, and those with sexual abuse were more than four times as likely to be in the high-depression range than those without this history. Of some interest is that boys with sexual abuse scored significantly higher on the CDI than girls, whereas no sex difference emerged among those with a history of physical abuse. However, this study suffered from very vague definitions of abuse, which may have led to an inflated association of abuse with depression if depressed individuals were biased to retrospectively label their experiences as "abuse."

A similarly strong relation of physical and sexual abuse to depression emerged in a study by Silverman, Reinherz, and Giaconia (1996): Girls who reported physical or sexual abuse prior to age 16 scored significantly higher on the CDI and YSR at age 15 than those without this history and were more than five times more likely to report a major depressive episode in the past year at age 21. Boys with a history of physical abuse were also more than five times more likely to report a major depressive episode at age 21, whereas no significant differences emerged between boys with, versus without, a history of physical abuse in CDI or YSQ depression scores at age 15. (There were too few boys who reported a history of sexual abuse in this study to examine the relation of sexual abuse to outcome separately for boys). However, again, physical and sexual abuse were

TABLE 19.1. Methodological Details of Studies Examining the Relation of Child Abuse and Neglect to Depression in Adolescence

Authors	Sample	Maltreatment and depression assessment	Results
Schraedley et al. (1999)	Nationally representative sample of 6,954 youths, grades 5–12, from the Commonwealth Fund Adolescent Survey	*Physical abuse (PA) and sexual abuse (SA):* lifetime retrospective self-report *Depression:* CDI scores	21% with PA vs. 6% without PA were in high depressive symptoms group; 27% with SA vs. 6% without SA were in high depressive symptoms group
Silverman et al. (1996)	Subsample of 375 youths from a Northeastern U.S. school system assessed five times over 17 years, from age 5 to age 21	*PA and SA:* lifetime retrospective self-report of abuse prior to age 18 based on interview at age 21 *Depression:* YSR and CDI administered at age 15; 1-year prevalence major depression diagnosis assessed at age 21	*Age 15:* Girls with PA or SA had significantly higher CDI and YSR depression scores than those without. No significant differences for boys. *Age 21:* 20% boys and 25% girls with PA vs. 3.9% boys and 5.1% girls without PA had 1-year depression diagnosis. 21.7% girls with SA vs. 4.3% girls with no SA had 1-year depression diagnosis.
Brown et al. (1999)	Subsample of 776 youths from Northeastern U.S. counties assessed four times over 17-year period, starting when youths were between 1 and 10 years	*PA, SA, and neglect:* CPS records and lifetime retrospective self-report based on interview during early adulthood *Depression:* DSM-III (American Psychiatric Association, 1980) diagnosis of major depression in adolescence or young adulthood	PA (OR = 2.37), SA (OR = 3.17), and neglect (OR = 2.49) significantly predicted depression, controlling for relevant covariates
Kilpatrick et al. (2003)	Nationally representative sample of 4,023 youths, ages 12–17, from the National Survey of Adolescents	*PA and SA:* lifetime retrospective self-report *Depression:* DSM-IV (American Psychiatric Association, 1994) Diagnosis of major depression in past year	PA (OR = 2.15) significantly associated with depression, controlling for relevant covariates; SA (OR = 2.76) significantly associated with comorbid depression and PTSD, controlling for relevant covariates
Fergusson et al. (1996)	Subsample of 1,019 youths from Christchurch Health and Development Study, assessed annually from birth to age 18.	*SA:* lifetime self-report of SA prior to age 16 based on interview at age 18 *Depression:* DSM-IV diagnosis of major depression from ages 16–18	Noncontact SA (OR = 3.6), contact SA (OR = 3.6), and intercourse SA (OR = 5.4) significantly predicted depression, controlling for relevant covariates
Boney-McCoy & Finkelhor (1996)	Nationally representative sample of 1,433 youths, ages 10–16, from the National Youth Victimization Prevention Study, assessed twice, 15 months apart	*PA and SA:* retrospective self-report *Depression:* diagnosis of DSM-III-R (American Psychiatric Association, 1987) major depression in past month	PA (OR = 2.82) and SA (OR = 4.21) assessed during time 1–time 2 period significantly predicted time 2 depression, controlling for time 1 victimization levels
Thornberry et al. (2001)	738 12-year-olds from the Rochester Youth Development Study followed longitudinally for 5 years	*PA, SA, and neglect:* retrospective self-report interview *Depression:* depressive symptoms checklist	Adolescent PA (OR = 2.07) and neglect (OR = 2.80), but *not* SA (OR = 1.34) significantly predicted early adolescent depressive symptoms, controlling for relevant covariates.

defined on the basis of only two questions: "At any time in your life were you physically abused (sexually abused)?" These questions leave room for misinterpretation and, in particular, may be interpreted differently among those with, versus without, depression.

Despite the limitations in the assessment of child abuse, the results of the two studies cited above were replicated in a number of subsequent studies that employed more rigorous assessment methods. Brown, Cohen, Johnson, and Smailes (1999) reported odds ratios ranging from 2.37 to 3.17 relating a lifetime history of physical abuse, sexual abuse, and neglect to a diagnosis of major depression in adolescence or young adulthood in a sample of 776 young adults. Child maltreatment was officially documented and then supplemented with self-reports. Furthermore, these results held even after controlling for age, sex, and a host of other "contextual factors" previously associated with both maltreatment and depression (e.g., sex, ethnicity, socioeconomic status, difficult childhood temperament, low maternal education, single parenthood).

Moreover, Kilpatrick et al. (2003), in a very large sample of 4,023 adolescents, found that youths with a history of physical or sexual abuse were more than two to three times as likely as those without such a history to have received a diagnosis of major depression in the past year. A finding of maltreatment in this study was based on a rigorous interview that included clear questions focused on particular abuse behaviors. These relations held even after controlling for gender, age, race, and family substance abuse. It is interesting to note that in a subsequent report, using a subsample of 548 youths from the aforementioned sample who met the criteria for major depression, Danielson, de Arellano, Kilpatrick, Saunders, and Resnick (2005) found that a history of both physical and sexual abuse, or sexual abuse alone, was associated with a more *severe* depression. Specific symptoms most strongly associated with abuse included guilt, thoughts of death or hurting oneself, appetite change, and sleep disturbance.

Even higher odds ratios were reported by Fergusson, Horwood, and Lynskey (1996) in their investigation of the relation of specific forms of child sexual abuse, as assessed by a detailed 2-hour interview, to major depression. Sexual abuse involving no contact, contact (but no intercourse), or intercourse was related to a 3.6- to 5.4-fold increase in the risk of major depression in late adolescence, even after controlling for a large number of prospectively measured "childhood and family factors" (e.g., socioeconomic status, changes of parents, parental conflict, parental attachment, family functioning, parental mental health). The larger odds ratios found in this study may be due to the increased specificity of the sexual abuse assessment, as well as the focus on a relatively circumscribed period of time for depression onset in late adolescence, when incidences of major depression are higher than in earlier adolescence. Finally, the results of these studies were confirmed in a further prospective report that included a detailed and lengthy abuse interview (Boney-McCoy & Finkelhor, 1996). Specifically, physical and sexual abuse assessed during a 15-month period in adolescence prospectively predicted the diagnosis of past-month major depression assessed at the end of the 15-month study period, even after controlling for Time 1 quality of the parent–child relationship, age, single parenthood, parental education status, community size, and race.

As reviewed above, Thornberry et al. (2001) found evidence that maltreatment experienced in adolescence had a stronger effect on later depression than maltreatment experienced in childhood only. This study also found relatively specific effects for maltreatment. In particular, physical abuse and neglect experienced in adolescence significantly predicted early adolescent depression outcomes, whereas sexual abuse did not.

In summary, the studies cited above provide compelling evidence for a strong association between a history of physical abuse, sexual abuse, or neglect and the development of depression symptoms, as well as the major depression syndrome, in adolescence. These studies employed samples of youths spanning the entire adolescent age range, drawn from diverse geographical regions, and relied on diverse assessments of child maltreatment and depression. A history of abuse and/or neglect was associated with a two- to five-fold increase in the risk of depression, even after controlling for a host of demographic and family contextual factors known to be associated with depression onset in this age group. As stated previously, the majority of adults with major depression have their first onset as adolescents, suggesting that maltreatment may be a risk factor for a lifelong course of dysfunction that has its onset in adolescence.

Specificity of Adversity

The evidence reviewed above suggests that childhood adversity places children and adolescents at risk for depression. However, it is unclear whether different forms of adversity (e.g., physical abuse vs. sexual abuse vs. emotional abuse/neglect) confer differential risk. The results reported in Table 19.1 suggest that physical abuse, neglect, and, in all but one case, sexual abuse are all associated with strong and significant effects in the prediction of depression in adolescence. However, these different forms of maltreatment often co-occur, and thus multivariate analyses are required to more conclusively determine the unique risk conferred by each form of adversity, controlling for all other forms.

A few research groups have taken such a multivariate approach in investigating the relation of child maltreatment to depression in adults. Two of these groups have found evidence in undergraduate samples that *emotional* abuse is more specifically associated with depression symptoms and the diagnosis of depression than physical or sexual abuse (Gibb et al., 2001; Hankin, 2005). In a sample of adult women with major depression, we reported that sexual abuse was specifically associated with comorbid anxiety (posttraumatic stress disorder [PTSD] or panic disorder), whereas, interestingly, both emotional *and* physical abuse were specifically associated with a pure and chronic depression presentation (Harkness & Wildes, 2002). The issue of specificity is an important question for future research in the area of child and adolescent depression. Demonstrating such fine-grained relationships between types of adversity and the development of symptoms may provide important clues to the etiological and pathological mechanisms in major depression, as well as aid in the development of more well-informed and specifically geared intervention strategies.

Contextual Factors

Individual differences in the nature of maltreatment, and in the characteristics of the victims, moderate the effect of child abuse and neglect on depression. Features of such abuse that have been consistently found to predict more severe outcomes include (1) higher severity, involving a greater use of force and higher likelihood of injury, or, in the case of sexual abuse, use of penetration (see, e.g., Fergusson et al., 1996), (2) a closer relationship of the perpetrator to the victim (see, e.g., Kendall-Tackett, Williams, & Finkelhor, 1993; Ruggiero, McLeer, & Dixon, 2000), and (3) a greater comorbidity of abuse. That is, individuals with multiple forms of maltreatment have significantly worse outcomes (and higher psychiatric comorbidity) than those who experience only one form of abuse (e.g., Danielson et al., 2005).

Victim characteristics that moderate the relation of child maltreatment to depression have also been examined. As discussed earlier, maltreatment occurring in adolescence or persisting throughout childhood and adolescence, is significantly more strongly predictive of depression than is maltreatment that occurs only in childhood (see, e.g., Éthier et al., 2004; Thornberry et al., 2001). This is an important finding as, currently, most public spending on prevention and intervention related to maltreatment is focused on younger children (Thornberry et al., 2001).

Furthermore, several studies have provided evidence that among children with a history of sexual abuse, boys report significantly more depression (Schraedley et al., 1999), suicidal ideation and attempts (see, e.g., Garnefski & Diekstra, 1997; Martin, Bergen, Richardson, Roeger, & Allison, 2004), and behavioral problems (see, e.g., Garnefski & Arends, 1998) than girls. This differential relation to outcome emerges despite epidemiological data from the National Incidence and Prevalence Study of Child Abuse and Neglect suggesting that girls are more than twice as likely to *report* sexual abuse than are boys (Cappelleri, Eckenrode, & Powers, 1993). Some research suggests that sexual abuse experienced by boys may be more severe than that experienced by girls, relying on force and occurring in the context of physical abuse (e.g., Watkins & Bentovim, 1992). In addition, most perpetrators of sexual abuse are men, and thus sexual identity conflict resulting from this experience may help to explain the stronger effects of sexual abuse in boys (Duncan & Williams, 1998). Indeed, Dhaliwal, Gauzas, Antonowicz, and Ross (1996) suggest that shame may be a particularly important factor for boys, given the same-sex nature of the assault and the fact that society has been slow to acknowledge the presence of male sexual abuse survivors. Regardless of the reason for this sex difference, it is clear that greater attention needs to be paid to male victims in both research and intervention programs.

Finally, epidemiological data suggest that the prevalence of abuse varies by race (Cappelleri et al., 1993). Although white children are most likely to have experienced sexual abuse, black children are most likely to be identified as physical abuse victims. Very few studies have examined race as a moderator of the relation of child abuse and neglect to mental health outcomes, and all have focused exclusively on sexual abuse. Two of these studies suggest a stronger relation of sexual abuse to negative outcomes, including depression, in Hispanic children relative to black children (Sanders-Phillips, Moisan, Wadlington, Morgan, & English, 1995; Shaw, Lewis, Loeb, Rosado, & Rodriguez, 2001). These reports attribute this differential relation to greater severity of the abuse and higher levels of family conflict in Hispanic children. Differences between white and non-white groups are less clear. Although Feiring, Coates, and Taska (2001) reported that a history of child sexual abuse was related to higher levels of shame and internal attributions of the abuse in white children than in Hispanic or black children, Mennen (1995) reported no differences between these three groups in depression or anxiety. All of these studies focused on documented sexual abuse in samples of a similar age range (~8–16) and employed similar measures of depression. Therefore, inconsistencies in the results are difficult to interpret. These studies were also small in scale, and thus ethnic differences in the outcomes associated with abuse should be investigated in large nationally representative data bases.

COGNITIVE MEDIATION OF THE RELATION OF CHILD ABUSE AND NEGLECT TO DEPRESSION

The studies reviewed in the previous section provide strong evidence that child abuse and neglect are potent vulnerability factors for future episodes of depression. However, not all young people who experience these adversities will become depressed, which leads to a search for mediating mechanisms. Several theories, including attachment theory (Bowlby, 1969), schema theory (Young, 1994), and the cognitive theory of depression (Beck, 1976), suggest that it is the cognitive representation of the early adversity that implicates it in negative long-term outcomes. For example, Beck's (1976) cognitive theory of depression posits that child maltreatment leads to the development of depressogenic cognitive schemas, or negative core beliefs about the self, world, and future that are enduring and resistant to change (e.g., "I'm worthless," "The world is a dangerous place"). Similarly, the revised hopelessness theory of depression (Rose & Abramson, 1992) predicts that chronically maltreated children learn to view the causes of their maltreatment as internal, stable, and global (e.g., "This happened because I am a flawed person and will always be flawed"), thus developing hopelessness-inducing inferences about the world in general. These negative cognitive processes subsequently set the stage for depression.

Results of several studies suggest that child abuse and neglect are associated with negative cognitions. Cross-sectional studies of children have found that those with documented abuse and/or neglect evidence a more negative attributional style than matched controls (Cerezo-Jimenez & Frias, 1994; Mannarino & Cohen, 1996). The relation of child maltreatment to negative cognitions has been documented even in very young children. For example, two examinations of preschooler narratives found that maltreated preschoolers evidenced more negative self and parent representations than did non-maltreated preschoolers (Toth, Cicchetti, Macfie, Maughan, & Vanmeenen, 2000; Toth, Cicchetti, Macfie, & Emde, 1997).

Interesting individual differences in the relation of maltreatment to negative cognition have also been reported. Using a sample of children ages 7–18, Kolko, Brown, and Berliner (2002) reported that sexual abuse was associated with significantly higher scores on a measure of negative abuse-specific attributions than was physical abuse. This is consistent with Gibb's (2002) review of the relation between child maltreatment and negative attributional style in the adult literature. In particular, he found the largest effect sizes for the relation of *emotional* abuse to negative attributional style. Small, but still significant effect sizes emerged for the relation of sexual abuse to attributional style, whereas no significant effect of physical abuse on attributional style was detected. Gibb and colleagues' prospective longitudinal work with undergraduate samples in the Temple–Wisconsin project also suggests that *emotional* abuse, but not physical or sexual abuse, is significantly associated with the development of a negative attributional style that prospectively mediates the development of depression (Gibb, Alloy, Abramson, & Marx, 2003; Gibb et al., 2001). Using two independent samples of undergraduates, Hankin (2005) also recently found that emotional abuse, but not physical or sexual abuse, was significantly associated with a negative cognitive style and an insecure attachment style, and these intervening variables mediated the prospective development of depressive symptoms. Finally, these findings were recently replicated in a sample of fourth and fifth graders, such that a negative attributional style significantly mediated the relation between verbal abuse, specifically, and the 6-month longitudinal change in depressive symptoms (Gibb & Alloy, 2006).

We recently investigated individual differences in the outcomes associated with particular cognitive schema themes resulting from maltreatment. Our sample included 76 adolescents with major depression, of whom 37% had a history of severe physical abuse and/or neglect, as assessed by the CECA interview (Lumley & Harkness, in press). In contrast to the findings pertaining to attributional style, we found that physical abuse, sexual abuse, and neglect were significantly associated with several negative cognitive schemas, as assessed by the Young Schema Questionnaire (YSQ; Young, 1994). Furthermore, negative cognitive schemas with themes of vulnerability (e.g., "I can't seem to escape the feeling that something bad is about to happen") preferentially mediated the relation of mal-treatment to the severity of *anxious* symptoms, and schemas with themes of emotional deprivation (e.g., "People have not been there to give me warmth, holding, and affec-tion"), social isolation (e.g., "I don't fit in"), and failure (e.g., "I'm incompetent when it comes to achievement") preferentially mediated the relation of maltreatment to the sever-ity of *depression* symptoms.

Several additional studies have tested the mechanistic prediction that a negative cognitive style mediates the relation between child abuse and neglect and depression. In a sample of 240 sixth graders, Garber, Robinson, and Valentiner (1997) reported that children's perceptions of self-worth partially mediated the relation between maternal parenting style, as assessed by child and mother reports on the Children's Report of Parental Behavior Inventory (CRPBI; Schaefer, 1965), and depression, defined as a composite of self-report, mother report, and clinician interview. Similarly, in a sample of 70 maltreated children (ages 6–13), Brown and Kolko (1999) found that abuse-specific attributions, as well as a general negative attributional style, significantly medi-ated the relation between the severity of maltreatment and children's internalizing and externalizing symptoms. Overall, physical abuse, attributions of self-blame and guilt, and general negative cognitive errors accounted for 28% of the variance in depressive symptomatology, as assessed by the CDI. This result was replicated subsequently in a sample of 160 adolescents with documented abuse or neglect (McGee, Wolfe, & Olson, 2001). Results of these cross-sectional studies are limited, however, as causal mediation cannot be determined.

Prospective studies supported the results of the cross-sectional reports. For example, Garber and Flynn (2001) followed their sample of sixth graders annually over 3 years, and found that maternal parenting style significantly prospectively predicted adolescents' self-worth, attributional style, and level of hopelessness, even after controlling for the effect of maternal depression. Although this study did not specifically address the ques-tion of mediation, it is important for establishing a prospective relation between maltreat-ment and negative cognition.

In two studies, both using the same sample of 147 child and adolescent victims of sexual abuse, Feiring and colleagues found that negative attributional style at abuse dis-covery significantly mediated the relation between sexual abuse severity and depressive symptoms, both cross-sectionally (Feiring, Taska, & Lewis, 1998) and prospectively, 1 year later (Feiring, Taska, & Lewis, 2002). The longitudinal pattern of results remained significant after controlling for level of psychopathology at abuse discovery. Similarly, in an 8-year longitudinal study of 363 mother–child dyads, Stuewig and McCloskey (2005) found that harsh parenting in childhood predicted the development of cognitions related to shame and guilt in early adolescence, indirectly through ongoing parental rejection. Shame and guilt subsequently mediated the relation of parental maltreatment to depres-sion symptoms in late adolescence.

The studies reviewed above suggest that children and adolescents with a history of maltreatment are more likely to endorse negative cognitions and are more likely to dis-play a negative abuse-specific and general attributional style, than those without this his-tory. Prospective studies suggest that these negative cognitive processes in turn mediate the development of depressive symptoms. As such, these findings implicate cognitive style as an important causal mechanism that translates early abuse and neglect into the symp-toms and syndrome of depression, thus providing a clear target for intervention. Spe-cifically, cognitive strategies that focus on changing negative attributions may be particu-larly helpful for youths with a history of maltreatment. Indeed, recent studies suggest that cognitive-behavioral interventions for sexually abused youths result in significant reductions in depression, anxiety, and posttraumatic symptomatology, as compared with nondirective supportive treatments (e.g., Cohen, Mannarino, & Knudsen, 2005; King et al., 2000) and child-centered treatment that is typically delivered in community agencies (Cohen, Deblinger, Mannarino, & Steer, 2004).

THE NEUROBIOLOGY OF CHILD ABUSE AND NEGLECT: HPA AXIS DYSREGULATION

In addition to significant changes in cognition associated with early abuse, there is now an impressive amount of evidence suggesting that child maltreatment is associated with critical changes in neural function and structure. The effects of child maltreatment on the developing brain are broad-ranging and likely affect the structure and function of a number of neural pathways (see De Bellis et al., 1999). In this section we focus specifically on the effect of child abuse and neglect on the HPA axis. The reason for this focused approach is that child abuse and neglect are potent, and often chronic, stressors. Therefore, the neural consequences of these experiences are likely strongly mediated by dysregulation of these critical brain areas subserving the stress response. Indeed, most of the research on the neurobiological effects of child maltreatment focuses on dysregulation of the structure and function of the HPA axis. First, we describe the normal function of the HPA axis, and then the changes that occur at a structural and functional level when this system goes awry in the face of chronic, severe stress.

The purpose of the HPA axis is to facilitate survival in response to acute stress (e.g., predator attack). In this normal system, acute stress results in an immediate release of corticotropin-releasing hormone (CRH) in the cortex, hypothalamus, and pituitary (Weiss & Kilts, 1998). This process then causes release of adrenocorticotropic hormone (ACTH) from the pituitary and, subsequently, release of the glucocorticoid hormone cortisol from the adrenal cortex. This acute stress response ensures survival by inducing critical physiologic changes (e.g., increased heart rate) that facilitate adaptive behavioral patterns (i.e., fighting, "flighting," or freezing; Sapolsky & Plotsky, 1990). This evolutionarily adaptive response system is time-limited and counterbalanced by various processes that inhibit arousal via negative feedback.

However, when stress is chronic, sustained elevation of glucocorticoids can result, which reduces negative feedback inhibition of the HPA axis (Sapolsky, Krey, & McEwen, 1984). As a result, glucocorticoid levels can remain chronically elevated and responses to further stressors exaggerated. Prolonged periods of glucocorticoid hypersecretion can cause cell death and permanent damage to the hippocampus (see, e.g., Sapolsky, Uno, Rebert, & Finch, 1990). Stressors early in development may have particularly marked neuropathological consequences. For example, maternal deprivation of young rodents results in long-lasting changes in the HPA axis response to stress (see, e.g., Ladd, Owens, & Nemeroff, 1996). Therefore, the presence of chronic stress, particularly early in development, can have profound consequences for the HPA axis response to stress. These may be indexed structurally in terms of hippocampal atrophy and functionally in terms of hypersecretion of cortisol in response to stress (i.e., an exaggerated HPA axis stress response). Evidence for the effect of child maltreatment on the dysregulation of the HPA axis, in terms of both its structure and function, is presented next.

A large amount of evidence has now accumulated documenting a relation between child maltreatment and hippocampal atrophy. Indeed, this series of structural magnetic resonance imaging (MRI) studies is perhaps the most compelling evidence for the effect of childhood trauma on the brain in humans. In the seminal study in this series, Bremner and colleagues (1997) reported that adult women with posttraumatic stress disorder (PTSD) and a history of childhood physical or sexual abuse had a 12% lower left hippocampal volume than women with PTSD and no history of abuse. The degree of hippocampal atrophy was significantly correlated with the duration of the abuse. This is important, as it supports the interpretation that the atrophy was *caused* by the abuse, as opposed to the alternative interpretation that small hippocampal volumes serve as a vulnerability to childhood abuse and PTSD. Bremner et al. (2003) also reported that the hippocampal volume of women with PTSD and a history of childhood physical or sexual abuse was 19% lower than that of controls and 16% lower than that of women with childhood trauma but no PTSD. This latter result suggests that the trauma in and of itself is not toxic, and that it exerts its neurotoxic effect only in the context of psychopathology. This is an important finding as it suggests that individuals who are psychologically resilient to trauma (i.e., they do not exhibit psychopathology) also show neurobiological resilience. An important question for future research is whether neurobiological resilience and symptomatic resilience are causally related. Finally, Vythilingam et al. (2002) extended the aforementioned results to depression, reporting that the hippocampal volumes of women with major depression and a history of abuse were 18% lower than those of women with major depression and no abuse, and 15% lower than those of controls. Researchers suggest, given these findings, that the observed hippocampal atrophy is caused by glucocorticoid neurotoxicity resulting from chronic traumatic stress (e.g., Sapolsky, 2000).

The evidence of hippocampal atrophy in *children* with abuse is less clear, however. In general, significant neurostructural changes have been observed in maltreated children. For example, De Bellis et al. (1999, 2002), in two independent samples, reported that children (ages 6–17) with PTSD and documented maltreatment had significantly lower intracranial volumes, significantly higher cortical and prefrontal cortical cerebrospinal fluid volumes, and significant lateral ventrical enlargement, as compared with non-maltreated controls. These structural differences were significantly correlated with the duration of abuse and PTSD. However, in neither of these two studies was there evidence for differences in *hippocampal* volume between groups. Hippocampal volume differences were also not observed in a longitudinal study of nine maltreated 10-year-olds with PTSD versus nine controls followed to age 13 (De Bellis, Hall, Boring, Frustaci, & Moritz, 2001).

The results of the studies cited are of great interest, as they suggest that the strong relation between child abuse and hippocampal volume loss reported consistently in studies with adults is *not* replicated in studies with children, despite the experience of similar adversity and psychopathology, and despite the presence of diffuse cortical neuron loss in children. On one hand, this result is helpful, as it provides evidence that the lower hippocampal volumes observed in adults with childhood trauma are not a vulnerability marker for trauma (otherwise they would be seen in the children as well), but instead are caused by the trauma itself. On the other hand, however, this result presents a paradox that has yet to be explained. This paradox is further evident in studies of the effect of childhood trauma on HPA axis *function*.

As reviewed above, chronic stress results in chronically elevated release of glucocorticoids and exaggerated cortisol response to acute stress (Sapolsky et al., 1984). In samples of adults with a history of child maltreatment, increased cortisol release has been documented in response to CRF challenge (Heim et al., 2002; Heim et al., 2000) and a psychosocial stress challenge (Heim, Newport, Bonsall, Miller, & Nemeroff, 2001). Again, it is the increased and sustained release of cortisol during chronic stress that is believed to be responsible for hippocampal cell death.

In samples of children, the results are again less clear. De Bellis and colleagues (1994) reported a significantly lower ACTH response to ovine CRH challenge in sexually abused girls (ages 7–15) versus matched controls. However, the two groups did not differ in cortisol levels either pre- or postchallenge. Kaufman et al. (1997) also reported differences in ACTH secretion following CRH challenge in a sample of maltreated children with major depression versus depressed children with no adversity and controls, but did not report cortisol differences. Therefore, the null results of De Bellis and his group regarding both hippocampal volume and hypercortisolemia require independent replication before any firm conclusions can be drawn.

Nevertheless, it is compelling that the profound effects of child abuse on hippocampal structure and cortisol function in adults with PTSD and major depression are not seen in children. The reason for this discrepancy is unclear and thus provides a very important avenue for further study. Indeed, this question cuts to the heart of our understanding of the pathological developmental effects of early adversity. The children with abuse studied by De Bellis and colleagues *become* the adults with a history of abuse in the samples studied by Bremner, Heim, and colleagues. Therefore, something must happen in the intervening transition.

Developmental changes in the rate of neurogenesis in the hippocampus may help to account for the inconsistencies. In particular, hippocampal neurogenesis is very dramatic through childhood, but then slows across adolescence and adulthood (Paus, 2005). Therefore, the high rate of neuron growth in this critical area in childhood may mask any neurotoxic effects of trauma. This may also help to explain why individuals who experience trauma only in childhood have lower rates of psychopathology than individuals who experience trauma in adolescence or chronically throughout the child–adolescent transition (Thornberry et al., 2001). That is, the early developing limbic system may be particularly plastic to the effects of trauma. Therefore, if the trauma resolves while limbic structures are still in the midst of massive neuronal growth, the effects on later cognitive-emotional development may not be as severe as if the trauma persists into a period of increasing neuronal stability (Harkness & Tucker, 2000). A crucial study needed to test this hypothesis is to examine the longitudinal changes in hippocampal volume and cortisol function in maltreated and nonmaltreated children as they make the transition from adolescence to young adulthood. In this way, researchers can chart the developmental time course of brain changes associated with adversity both within and between groups.

CHILD ABUSE AND NEGLECT INCREASE STRESS SENSITIVITY

Child abuse and neglect are associated with significant disruptions in cognitive schema development and in the neurological stress response. One consequence of these disruptions is that they render individuals more vulnerable to the effects of later stress. For example, animals with hypercortisolemia show an enhanced behavioral response to stress (Kalynchuk, Gregus, Boudreau, & Perrot-Sinal, 2004). Furthermore, there is ample evidence that negative cognitive schemas are easily primed by negative life events (see Segal, Williams, Teasdale, & Gemar, 1996). The strongest proximal trigger of major depression onset is the presence of stressful life events (Kendler, Gardner, & Prescott, 2002; Mazure,

1998). A logical question to ask next, then, is whether child maltreatment is associated with a heightened sensitivity to later stressors.

One of the most intriguing developments in the area of stress research is the finding that certain individuals are particularly sensitive to the effects of stress, so that (1) they are significantly more likely to develop depression in the face of stress and (2) they require a lower severity level of stress to precipitate an episode. That is, their threshold for a pathological response to stress is reduced, such that lower levels of stress are required to trigger onset. This stress sensitization, or "kindling," hypothesis was proposed by Post (1992) to explain the phenomenon of increased stress sensitivity over the recurrent course of major depression (see Monroe & Harkness, 2005). Subsequent investigators have proposed that childhood adversity may be a risk factor for stress sensitization. That is, the presence of early adversity may significantly increase individuals' response to stress, so that they (1) are more likely to develop depression in the face of stress and (2) require a lower severity level of stress to precipitate depression than those without this risk factor *even prior to the first onset of the syndrome.*

In support of this prediction, Kendler, Kuhn, and Prescott (2004) reported that adult women with a history of childhood physical or sexual abuse were significantly more likely to develop depression in the face of proximal stress than women without this history. Similarly, in studies of late adolescent girls (Hammen, Henry, & Daley, 2000) and younger children (Rudolph & Flynn, 2007), researchers found that those with a wide range of adversities (e.g., parental death, parental psychopathology, witnessing violence) required a lower level of stress to precipitate depression onset than those without this history. We have subsequently replicated this effect in a sample of adolescents with a history of childhood physical abuse, sexual abuse, or neglect, as assessed with the CECA interview (Harkness, Bruce, & Lumley, 2006). We further demonstrated that the effect of child abuse and neglect in sensitizing adolescents to proximal stress was specific to those with their *very first onset* of depression.

It is important to note that individuals with a history of childhood maltreatment are also at increased risk for the *generation* of stressful life events (see Hankin & Abramson, 2001). In particular, across two independent samples of undergraduates, Hankin (2005) recently found that a history of emotional abuse, as assessed by a self-report questionnaire, and a history of parental discord, as assessed by the CECA, were significantly associated with elevated rates of stressful life events experienced over a 10-week (sample 1) and a 2-year (sample 2) prospective period. The generation of stress mediated the change in depressive symptoms in both samples over the respective prospective periods. We recently replicated the relation of childhood adversity to stress generation in a sample of adolescents with major depression. We found that depressed adolescents with a history of physical abuse, sexual abuse, and/or neglect, as assessed by the CECA, were significantly more likely than depressed adolescents with no such history to report recent stressors, particularly in the interpersonal domain, as assessed by the Life Events and Difficulties Schedule (LEDS; Bifulco et al., 1989), a rigorous contextual interview and rating system (Harkness, Lumley, & Bruce, 2007). Several other studies have also documented a significant relation between child maltreatment and increased rates of interpersonal stressors, including peer rejection and social withdrawal (Finzi, Ram, Har-Even, Shnit, & Weizman, 2001; Salzinger, Feldman, Ng-Mak, Mojica, & Stockhammer, 2001), bullying victimization (Shields & Cicchetti, 2001), and conflict in peer and romantic relationships (Egeland, Yates, Appleyard, & van Dulmen, 2002). These associations held even when controlling for psychopathology. Therefore, childhood adversity may represent a "double threat" in promoting vulnerability to depression. That is, childhood adversity may be a potent risk factor for depression, possibly because it increases *sensitization* to the stressors that precede the onset of the syndrome, *and* may increase the *generation* of stressors that increase risk for recurrence.

The results of the studies reviewed above suggest that childhood adversity heightens sensitivity to future stress, so that depression is more likely to occur following stress, and is more likely to occur in the face of lower levels of stress in individuals with a history of adversity than in those without. We suggest that this process may be mediated by (1) an increase in cognitive schema consolidation and (2) an increase in the HPA axis stress response, both of which may stabilize during adolescence. Adolescence is a crucial period in cognitive-emotional development, when schemas related to the self and the self in the world are hypothesized to consolidate (see Gibb & Coles, 2005; Hankin & Abela, 2005). Furthermore, adolescence is a crucial period in brain development and a time when neurogenesis in critical limbic structures begins to stabilize. Therefore, we suggest that adolescence is a period of extreme vulnerability for the development of depression in the face of child maltreatment because it is during this important stage of development that the neural and cognitive-emotional consequences of adversity are most profound.

An Integrated Psychobiological Developmental Model of Child Adversity and Depression

Our model is depicted graphically in Figure 19.1. We predict that severe physical abuse, sexual abuse, emotional abuse, and/or neglect result in the development of core negative beliefs about the self and world and dysregulation of the HPA axis response to stress. These two processes interact throughout adolescence, especially in the face of chronic adversity, and stabilize through the general process of neurobiological and cognitive-emotional maturity. The resulting rigid depressogenic schema structure and hyper-responsive limbic system are kindled, or primed, to respond to future stressors in the environment with a heightened depressogenic response. That is, we predict that child abuse and neglect lead to depression, at least in part, because they are associated with (1) the consolidation of rigid depressogenic schema structures that become more easily primed by proximal life events and (2) the dysregulation of limbic brain structures that become hyperreactive in the face of proximal life events. As a result, these proximal

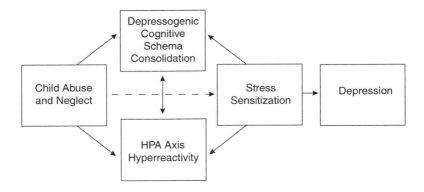

FIGURE 19.1. Integrated psychobiological developmental model of child adversity and depression.

stressors are more likely to trigger depression onset in adolescents with abuse than in those without.

Although the research reviewed here bears on various aspects of this theoretical framework, there are currently no studies, to our knowledge, that have tested the full developmental model. We hope that presenting it in this context will help stimulate multidisciplinary research into the psychobiological developmental *mechanisms* that translate early adversity into depression in vulnerable adolescents. What is particularly needed is longitudinal research that charts the within- and between-subject time course of these pathological processes that mediate depression in those with maltreatment. This work is crucial to explaining individual differences in the response to child abuse and neglect and to determining when and how best to focus intervention.

SUMMARY AND CONCLUSIONS

There is now a substantial body of literature demonstrating a strong prospective relation of physical abuse, sexual abuse, emotional abuse, and neglect to depression in children and adolescents. However, we are still at a very early stage in understanding (1) individual differences in the relation of maltreatment to depression and (2) the mechanisms that translate maltreatment into depression. In terms of individual differences, a limited number of studies suggest that the effect of abuse and neglect on depression is moderated by victim gender, age, and ethnicity, as well as by characteristics of the abuse itself (e.g., chronicity, severity, and relationship to perpetrator). Most of this research has been conducted with victims of sexual abuse. The pattern of moderators may differ in important ways for victims of physical abuse or neglect, and thus research into individual difference predictors of outcome for these adversities requires similar attention. Understanding the pattern of individual heterogeneity in the effects of child abuse and neglect will help to more effectively target vulnerable groups. For example, research suggesting that maltreatment may have a more pathological effect for adolescent than for child victims will, we hope, encourage more services targeted to this group.

In terms of mechanism, compelling evidence suggests that child abuse and neglect are associated with profound effects on cognition and neurobiology that may mediate the later development of depression. In particular, children and adolescents with a history of adversity endorse more negative views of themselves and a more negative attributional style than those without adversity, and these negative cognitions prospectively mediate the relation between adversity and depression symptoms and the major depression syndrome. Child abuse and neglect are also associated with general neuron loss across broad cortical areas in childhood, as well as dysregulation of the HPA axis response to stress. However, key indicators of neurotoxicity seen in adults (i.e., hypercortisolemia and hippocampal atrophy) are not seen in children. We have argued here that this paradox may be explained through greater attention to the adolescent transition. In particular, we suggest that the neurotoxic effects of child maltreatment may emerge gradually over this period as neurogenesis stabilizes in the hippocampus.

Finally, we suggest that the effects of trauma on neurobiological and cognitive development may increase victims' sensitivity to proximal stressful life event triggers. That is, individuals with a history of abuse and neglect may be cognitively and neurobiologically primed to react to future environmental stress with a stronger pathological response than those without this trauma history. We predict that stress sensitivity may be a crucial mechanism that results in higher rates of depression onset in adolescents who have been abused and neglected.

   Adolescence is a period of strong vulnerability to the pathological effects of trauma. However, for the same reason it is also a period of opportunity. Interventions during this period have the potential to produce change in the system, stabilizing it in a positive direction. In particular, interventions focused on (1) changing attributions of the trauma and general attributions of the world so as to prevent the consolidation of negative core schemas and (2) teaching self-efficacy skills to dampen sensitivity to proximal stressors hold promise for preventing the often lifelong pattern of devastation in young victims of abuse.

ACKNOWLEDGMENTS

This work was supported by a New Investigator Award from the Hospital for Sick Children Foundation (to Kate L. Harkness). We thank Mark A. Sabbagh for his very helpful comments on earlier drafts of this chapter.

REFERENCES

Achenbach, T. M. (1991). *Manual for the Youth Self-Report and 1991 profile.* Burlington: University of Vermont, Department of Psychiatry.

Achenbach, T. M., & Edelbrock, C. (1983). *Manual for the Child Behavior Checklist and revised child behavior profile.* Burlington, VT: Queen City.

American Psychiatric Association. (1980). *Diagnostic and statistical manual of mental disorders* (3rd ed.). Washington, DC: Author.

American Psychiatric Association. (1987). *Diagnostic and statistical manual of mental disorders* (3rd ed., rev.). Washington, DC: Author.

American Psychiatric Association. (1994). *Diagnostic and statistical manual of mental disorders* (4th ed.). Washington, DC: Author.

Battle, C. L., Shea, M. T., Johnson, D. M., Yen, S., Zlotnick, C., Zanarini, M. C., et al. (2004). Childhood maltreatment associated with adult personality disorders: Findings from the collaborative longitudinal personality disorders study. *Journal of Personality Disorders, 18,* 193–211.

Beck, A. T. (1976). *Cognitive therapy and the emotional disorders.* New York: International Universities Press.

Bifulco, A., Brown, G., Edwards, A., Harris, T., Neilson, E., Richards, C., et al. (1989). *Life Events and Difficulties Schedule (LEDS-2): Volume 1. Life events manual.* London: Royal Halloway and Bedford New College, University of London.

Bifulco, A., Brown, G. W., & Harris, T. O. (1994). Childhood Experience of Care and Abuse (CECA): A retrospective measure. *Journal of Child Psychology and Psychiatry, 35,* 1419–1435.

Bifulco, A., Brown, G. W., Lillie, A., & Jarvis, J. (1997). Memories of childhood neglect and abuse: Corroboration in a series of sisters. *Journal of Child Psychology and Psychiatry, 38,* 365–374.

Birmaher, B., Ryan, N. D., Williamson, D. E., Brent, D. A., Kaufman, J., Dahl, R. E., et al. (1996). Childhood and adolescent depression: A review of the past 10 years: I. *Journal of the American Academy of Child and Adolescent Psychiatry, 35,* 1427–1439.

Boney-McCoy, S., & Finkelhor, D. (1996). Is youth victimization related to trauma symptoms and depression after controlling for prior symptoms and family relationships? A longitudinal, prospective study. *Journal of Consulting and Clinical Psychology, 64,* 1406–1416.

Bowlby, J. (1969). *Attachment and loss: Vol. I. Attachment.* New York: Basic Books.

Bremner, J. D., Randall, P., Vermetten, E., Staib, L., Bronen R. A., Mazure C., et al. (1997). Magnetic resonance imaging-based measurement of hippocampal volume in posttraumatic stress disorder related to childhood physical and sexual abuse: A preliminary report. *Biological Psychiatry, 41,* 23–32.

Bremner, J. D., Vythilingam, M., Vermetten, E., Southwick, S. M., McGlashan, T., Nazeer, A., et al. (2003). MRI and PET study of deficits in hippocampal structure and function in women with childhood sexual abuse and posttraumatic stress disorder. *American Journal of Psychiatry, 160,* 924–932.

Brewin, C. R., Andrews, B., & Gotlib, I. H. (1993). Psychopathology and early experience: A reappraisal of retrospective reports. *Psychological Bulletin, 113,* 82–98.

Brown, E. J., & Kolko, D. J. (1999). Child victims' attributions about being physically abused: An examination of factors associated with symptom severity. *Journal of Abnormal Child Psychology, 27,* 311–322.

Brown, J., Cohen, P., Johnson, J. G., & Smailes, E. M. (1999). Childhood abuse and neglect: Specificity of effects on adolescent and young adult depression and suicidality. *Journal of the American Academy of Child and Adolescent Psychiatry, 38,* 1490–1496.

Cappelleri, J. C., Eckenrode, J., & Powers, J. L. (1993). The epidemiology of child abuse: Findings from the Second National Incidence and Prevalence Study of Child Abuse and Neglect. *American Journal of Public Health, 83,* 1622–1624.

Cerezo-Jimenez, M. A., & Frias, D. (1994). Emotional and cognitive adjustment in abused children. *Child Abuse and Neglect, 18,* 923–932.

Cicchetti, D., & Toth, S. L. (2005). Child maltreatment. *Annual Review of Clinical Psychology, 1,* 409–438.

Cohen, J. A., Deblinger, E., Mannarino, A. P., & Steer, R. A. (2004). A multisite, randomized controlled trial for children with sexual abuse-related PTSD symptoms. *Journal of the American Academy of Child and Adolescent Psychiatry, 43,* 393–402.

Cohen, J. A., Mannarino, A. P., & Knudsen, K. (2005). Treating sexually abused children: 1 year follow-up of a randomized controlled trial. *Child Abuse and Neglect, 29,* 135–145.

Danielson, C. K., de Arellano, M. A., Kilpatrick, D. G., Saunders, B. E., & Resnick, H. S. (2005). Child maltreatment in depressed adolescents: Differences in symptomatology based on history of abuse. *Child Maltreatment, 10,* 37–48.

De Bellis, M. D., Chrousos, G. P., Dorn, L. D., Burke, L., Helmers, K., Kling, M. A., et al. (1994). Hypothalamic–pituitary–adrenal axis dysregulation in sexually abused girls. *Journal of Clinical Endocrinology and Metabolism, 78,* 249–255.

De Bellis, M. D., Hall, J., Boring, A. M., Frustaci, K., & Moritz, G. (2001). A pilot longitudinal study of hippocampal volumes in pediatric maltreatment-related posttraumatic stress disorder. *Biological Psychiatry, 50,* 305–309.

De Bellis, M. D., Keshavan, M. S., Clark, D. B., Casey, B. J., Giedd, J. N., Boring, A. M., et al. (1999). Bennett Research Award. Developmental traumatology: Part II. Brain development. *Biological Psychiatry, 45,* 1271–1284.

De Bellis, M. D., Keshavan, M. S., Shifflett, H., Iyengar, S., Beers, S. R., Hall, J., et al. (2002). Brain structures in pediatric maltreatment-related posttraumatic stress disorder: A sociodemographically matched study. *Biological Psychiatry, 52,* 1066–1078.

Dhaliwal, G. K., Gauzas, L., Antonowicz, D. H., & Ross, R. R. (1996). Adult male survivors of childhood sexual abuse: Prevalence, sexual abuse characteristics, and long-term effects. *Child Abuse and Neglect, 16,* 765–785.

Dill, D. L., Chu, J. A., Grob, M. C., & Eisen, S. V. (1991). The reliability of abuse history reports: A comparison of two inquiry formats. *Comprehensive Psychiatry, 32,* 166–169.

Duncan, L. E., & Williams, L. M. (1998). Gender role socialization and male-on-male vs. female-on-male child sexual abuse. *Sex Roles, 39,* 765–785.

Egeland, B., Yates, T., Appleyard, K., & van Dulmen, M. (2002). The long-term consequences of maltreatment in the early years: A developmental pathway model to antisocial behavior. *Children's Services: Social Policy, Research, and Practice, 5,* 249–260.

Éthier, L. S., Lemelin, J., & Lacharité, C. (2004). A longitudinal study of the effects of chronic maltreatment on children's behavioral and emotional problems. *Child Abuse and Neglect, 28,* 1265–1278.

Feiring, C., Coates, D. L., & Taska, L. S. (2001). Ethnic status, stigmatization, support, and symptoms development following sexual abuse. *Journal of Interpersonal Violence, 16,* 1307–1329.

Feiring, C., Taska, L., & Lewis, M. (1998). The role of shame and attributional style in children's and adolescents' adaptation to sexual abuse. *Child Maltreatment, 3,* 129–142.

Feiring, C., Taska, L., & Lewis, M. (1999). Age and gender differences in children's and adolescents' adaptation to sexual abuse. *Child Abuse and Neglect, 23,* 115–128.

Feiring, C., Taska, L., & Lewis, M. (2002). Adjustment following sexual abuse discovery: The role of shame and attributional style. *Developmental Psychology, 38,* 79–92.

Fergusson, D. M., Horwood, L. J., & Lynskey, M. T. (1996). Childhood sexual abuse and psychiatric disorder in young adulthood: II. Psychiatric outcomes of childhood sexual abuse. *Journal of the American Academy of Child and Adolescent Psychiatry, 35,* 1365–1374.

Finzi, R., Ram, A., Har-Even, D., Shnit, D., & Weizman, A. (2001). Attachment styles and aggression in physically abused and neglected children. *Journal of Youth and Adolescence, 30,* 769–786.

Garber, J., & Flynn, C. (2001). Predictors of depressive cognitions in young adolescents. *Cognitive Therapy and Research, 25,* 353–376.

Garber, J., Robinson, N. S., & Valentiner, D. (1997). The relation between parenting and adolescent depression: Self-worth as a mediator. *Journal of Adolescent Research, 12,* 12–33.

Garnefski, N., & Arends, E. (1998). Sexual abuse, adolescent sexual behaviors, and sexual revictimization. *Child Abuse and Neglect, 21,* 789–803.

Garnefski, N., & Diekstra, R. F. W. (1997). Child sexual abuse and emotional and behavioral problems in adolescence: Gender differences. *Journal of the American Academy of Child and Adolescent Psychiatry, 36,* 323–329.

Gibb, B. E. (2002). Childhood maltreatment and negative cognitive styles: A quantitative and qualitative review. *Clinical Psychology Review, 22,* 223–246.

Gibb, B. E., & Alloy, L. B. (2006). A prospective test of the hopelessness theory of depression in children. *Journal of Clinical Child and Adolescent Psychology, 35,* 264–274.

Gibb, B. E., Alloy, L. B., Abramson, L. Y., & Marx, B. P. (2003). Childhood maltreatment and maltreatment-specific inferences: A test of Rose and Abramson's (1992) extension of the hopelessness theory. *Cognition and Emotion, 17,* 917–931.

Gibb, B. E., Alloy, L. B., Abramson, L. Y., Rose, D. T., Whitehouse, W. G., Donovan, P., et al. (2001). History of childhood maltreatment, negative cognitive styles, and episodes of depression in adulthood. *Cognitive Therapy and Research, 25,* 425–446.

Gibb, B. E., & Coles, M. E. (2005). Cognitive vulnerability–stress models of psychopathology: A developmental perspective. In B. L. Hankin & J. R. Z. Abela (Eds.), *Development of psychopathology: A vulnerability–stress perspective* (pp. 104–135). Thousand Oaks, CA: Sage.

Hammen, C., Henry, R., & Daley, S. E. (2000). Depression and sensitization to stressors among young women as a function of childhood adversity. *Journal of Consulting and Clinical Psychology, 68,* 782–787.

Hankin, B. L. (2005). Childhood maltreatment and psychopathology: Prospective tests of attachment, cognitive vulnerability, and stress as mediating processes. *Cognitive Therapy and Research, 29,* 645–671.

Hankin, B. L., & Abela, J. R. Z. (2005). *Development of psychopathology: A vulnerability–stress perspective.* Thousand Oaks, CA: Sage.

Hankin, B. L., & Abramson, L. Y. (2001). Development of gender differences in depression: An elaborated cognitive vulnerability–transactional stress theory. *Psychological Bulletin, 127,* 773–796.

Hardt, J., & Rutter, M. (2004). Validity of adult retrospective reports of adverse childhood experiences: Review of the evidence. *Journal of Child Psychology and Psychiatry, 45,* 260–273.

Harkness, K. L., Bruce, A. E., & Lumley, M. N. (2006). Childhood adversity and the sensitization to stressful life events in adolescent depression. *Journal of Abnormal Psychology, 115,* 730–741.

Harkness, K. L., Lumley, M. N., & Bruce, A. E. (2007). *Stress generation in adolescent depression: The moderating role of childhood adversity.* Manuscript under review.

Harkness, K. L., & Tucker, D. M. (2000). Adaptive organization of corticolimbic networks. In M. Lewis & I. Granic (Eds.), *Emotion, development, and self-organization* (pp. 186–208). New York: Cambridge University Press.

Harkness, K. L., & Wildes, J. (2002). Childhood adversity and anxiety versus dysthymia comorbidity in major depression. *Psychological Medicine, 32,* 1239–1249.

Heim, C., Newport, D. J., Bonsall, R., Miller, A. H., & Nemeroff, C. B. (2001). Altered pituitary-adrenal axis responses to provocative challenge tests in adult survivors of childhood abuse. *American Journal of Psychiatry, 158,* 575–581.

Heim, C., Newport, D. J., Heit, S., Graham, Y. P., Wilcox, M., Bonsall, R., et al. (2000). Pituitary-adrenal and autonomic responses to stress in women after sexual and physical abuse in childhood. *Journal of the American Medical Association, 284,* 592–597.

Heim, C., Newport, D., Wagner, D., Wilcox, M., Miller, A., & Nemeroff, C. B. (2002). The role of early adverse experience and adulthood stress in the prediction of neuroendocrine stressreactivity in women: A multiple regression analysis. *Depression and Anxiety, 15,* 117–125.

Kalynchuk, L. E., Gregus, A., Boudreau, D., & Perrot-Sinal, T. S. (2004). Corticosterone increases depression-like behavior, with some effects on predator odor-induced defensive behavior, in male and female rats. *Behavioral Neuroscience, 118,* 1365–1377.

Kaufman, J., Birmaher, B., Perel, J., Dahl, R. E., Moreci, P., Nelson, B., et al. (1997). The corticotropin-releasing hormone challenge in depressed abused, depressed nonabused, and normal control children. *Biological Psychiatry, 42,* 669–679.

Kendall-Tackett, K., & Becker-Blease, K. (2004). The importance of retrospective findings in child maltreatment research. *Child Abuse and Neglect, 28,* 723–727.

Kendall-Tackett, K. A., Williams, L. M., & Finkelhor, D. (1993). Impact of sexual abuse on children: A review and synthesis of recent empirical studies. *Psychological Bulletin, 113,* 164–180.

Kendler, K. S., Gardner, C. O., & Prescott, C. A. (2002). Toward a comprehensive developmental model for major depression in women. *American Journal of Psychiatry, 159,* 1133–1145.

Kendler, K. S., Kuhn, J. W., & Prescott, C. A. (2004). Childhood sexual abuse, stressful life events and risk for major depression in women. *Psychological Medicine, 34,* 1475–1482.

Kilpatrick, D. G., Ruggiero, K. J., Acierno, R., Saunders, B. E., Resnick, H. S., & Best, C. L. (2003). Violence and risk of PTSD, major depression, substance abuse/dependence, and comorbidity: Results from the National Survey of Adolescents. *Journal of Consulting and Clinical Psychology, 71,* 692–700.

King, N. J., Tonge, B. J., Mullen, P., Myerson, N., Heyne, D., Rollings, S., et al. (2000). Treating sexually abused children with posttraumatic stress symptoms: A randomized clinical trial. *Journal of the American Academy of Child and Adolescent Psychiatry, 39,* 1347–1355.

Kolko, D. J., Brown, E. J., & Berliner, L. (2002). Children's perceptions of their abusive experience: Measurement and preliminary findings. *Child Maltreatment, 7,* 42–55.

Kovacs, M. (1985). The Children's Depression Inventory. *Psychopharmacology Bulletin, 21,* 995–998.

Ladd, C. O., Owens, M. J., & Nemeroff, C. B. (1996). Persistent changes in corticotropin-releasing factor neuronal systems induced by maternal deprivation. *Endocrinology, 137,* 1212–1218.

Lipovsky, J. A., Saunders, B. E., & Murphy, S. M. (1989). Depression, anxiety, and behavior problems among victims of father–child sexual assault and nonabused siblings. *Journal of Interpersonal Violence, 4,* 452–468.

London, K., Bruck, M., Ceci, S. J., & Shuman, D. W. (2005). Disclosure of child sexual abuse: What does the research tell us? *Psychology, Public Policy, and Law, 11*, 194–226.

Lumley, M. N., & Harkness, K. L. (in press). Specificity in the relations among childhood adversity, early maladaptive schemas, and symptom profiles in adolescent depression. *Cognitive Therapy and Research*.

Mannarino, A. P., & Cohen, J. A. (1996). Abuse-related attributions and perceptions, general attributions, and locus of control in sexually abused girls. *Journal of Interpersonal Violence, 11*, 162–180.

Martin, G., Bergen, H. A., Richardson, A. S., Roeger, L., & Allison, S. (2004). Sexual abuse and suicidality: Gender differences in a large community sample of adolescents. *Child Abuse and Neglect, 28*, 491–503.

Mazure, C. M. (1998). Life stressors as risk factors in depression. *Clinical Psychology: Science and Practice, 5*, 291–313.

McGee, R., Wolfe, D., & Olson, J. (2001). Multiple maltreatment, attribution of blame, and adjustment among adolescents. *Development and Psychopathology, 13*, 827–846.

Mennen, F. E. (1995). The relationship of race/ethnicity to symptoms in childhood sexual abuse. *Child Abuse and Neglect, 19*, 115–124.

Monroe, S. M., & Harkness, K. L. (2005). Life stress, the "kindling" hypothesis, and the recurrence of depression: Considerations from a life stress perspective. *Psychological Review, 112*, 417–445.

Paus, T. (2005). Mapping brain maturation and cognitive development during adolescence. *Trends in Cognitive Sciences, 9*, 60–68.

Post, R. M. (1992). Transduction of psychosocial stress into the neurobiology of recurrent affective disorder. *American Journal of Psychiatry, 149*, 999–1010.

Rose, D. T., & Abramson, L. Y. (1992). Developmental predictors of depressive cognitive style: Research and theory. In D. Cicchetti & S. L. Toth (Eds.), *Developmental perspectives on depression* (pp. 323–349). Rochester, NY: University of Rochester Press.

Rudolph, K. D., & Flynn, M. (2007). Childhood adversity and youth depression: Influence of gender and pubertal status. *Development and Psychopathology, 19*, 497–521.

Ruggiero, K. J., McLeer, S. V., & Dixon, J. F. (2000). Sexual abuse characteristics associated with survivor psychopathology. *Child Abuse and Neglect, 24*, 951–964.

Salzinger, S., Feldman, R. S., Ng-Mak, D. S., Mojica, E., & Stockhammer, T. F. (2001). The effect of physical abuse on children's social and affective status: A model of cognitive and behavioral processes explaining the association. *Development and Psychopathology, 13*, 805–825.

Sanders-Phillips, K., Moisan, P. A., Wadlington, S., Morgan, S., & English, K. (1995). Ethnic differences in psychological functioning among black and Latino abused girls. *Child Abuse and Neglect, 19*, 691–706.

Sapolsky, R. M. (2000). Glucocorticoids and hippocampal atrophy in neuropsychiatric disorders. *Archives of General Psychiatry, 57*, 925–935.

Sapolsky, R. M., Krey, L., & McEwen, B. (1984). Glucocorticoid-sensitive hippocampal neurons are involved in terminating the adrenocortical stress response. *Proceedings of the National Academy of Science, 81*, 6174–6178.

Sapolsky, R. M., & Plotsky, P. M. (1990). Hypercortisolism and its possible neural basis. *Biological Psychiatry, 27*, 937–952.

Sapolsky, R. M., Uno, H., Rebert, C., & Finch, C. (1990). Hippocampal damage associated with prolonged glucocorticoid exposure in primates. *Journal of Neuroscience, 10*, 2897–2902.

Schaefer, E. S. (1965). Children's reports of parental behavior: An inventory. *Child Development, 36*, 413–424.

Schraedley, P. K., Gotlib, I. H., & Hayward, C. (1999). Gender differences in correlates of anhedonic symptoms in adolescents. *Journal of Adolescent Health, 25*, 98–108.

Segal, Z. V., Williams, J. M., Teasdale, J. D., & Gemar, M. (1996). A cognitive science perspective on kindling and episode sensitization in recurrent affective disorder. *Psychological Medicine, 26*, 371–380.

Shaw, J. A., Lewis, J. E., Loeb, A., Rosado, J., & Rodriguez, R. A. (2001). A comparison of His-panic and African-American sexually abused girls and their families. *Child Abuse and Neglect, 25,* 1363–1379.

Shields, A., & Cicchetti, D. (2001). Parental maltreatment and emotion dysregulation as risk fac-tors for bullying and victimization in middle childhood. *Journal of Clinical Child Psychology, 30,* 349–363.

Silverman, A. B., Reinherz, H. Z., & Giaconia, R. M. (1996). The long-term sequelae of child and adolescent abuse: A longitudinal community study. *Child Abuse and Neglect, 20,* 709–723.

Simpson, T. L., & Miller, W. R. (2002). Concomitance between childhood sexual and physical abuse and substance use problems: A review. *Clinical Psychology Review, 22,* 27–77.

Stuewig, J., & McCloskey, L. A. (2005). The relation of child maltreatment to shame and guilt among adolescents: Psychological routes to depression and delinquency. *Child Maltreatment, 10,* 324–336.

Tebbutt, J., Swanston, H., Oates, R. K., & O'Toole, B. I. (1997). Five years after child sexual abuse: Persisting dysfunction and problems of prediction. *Journal of the American Academy of Child and Adolescent Psychiatry, 36,* 330–339.

Thornberry, T. P., Ireland, T. O., & Smith, C. A. (2001). The importance of timing: The varying impact of childhood and adolescent maltreatment on multiple problem outcomes. *Develop-ment and Psychopathology, 13,* 957–979.

Toth, S. L., Cicchetti, D., Macfie, J., & Emde, R. N. (1997). Representations of self and other in the narratives of neglected, physically abused, and sexually abused preschoolers. *Development and Psychopathology, 9,* 781–796.

Toth, S. L., Cicchetti, D., Macfie, J., Maughan, A., & Vanmeenen, K. (2000). Narrative representa-tions of caregivers and self in maltreated pre-schoolers. *Attachment and Human Develop-ment, 2,* 271–305.

Toth, S. L., Manly, J. T., & Cicchetti, D. (1992). Child maltreatment and vulnerability to depres-sion. *Development and Psychopathology, 4,* 97–112.

U.S. Department of Health and Human Services, Administration on Children, Youth and Families. (2005). *Child maltreatment 2003.* Washington, DC: U.S. Government Printing Office.

Vythilingam, M., Heim, C., Newport, J., Miller, A. H., Anderson, E., Bronen, R. A., et al. (2002). Childhood trauma associated with smaller hippocampal volume in women with major depres-sion. *American Journal of Psychiatry, 159,* 2072–2080.

Watkins, W. G., & Bentovim, A. (1992). The sexual abuse of male children and adolescents: A review of current research. *Journal of Child Psychology and Psychiatry, 33,* 197–248.

Weiss, J. M., & Kilts, C. D. (1998). Animal models of depression and schizophrenia. In A. F. Schatzberg & C. B. Nemeroff (Eds.), *Textbook of psychopharmacology* (2nd ed., pp. 89–131). Washington, DC: American Psychiatric Press.

Whiffen, V. E., & MacIntosh, H. B. (2005). Mediators of the link between childhood sexual abuse and emotional distress: A critical review. *Trauma, Violence, and Abuse, 6,* 24–39.

Williams, L. M. (1994). Recall of childhood trauma: A prospective study of women's memories of child sexual abuse. *Journal of Consulting and Clinical Psychology, 62,* 1167–1176.

Young, J. E. (1994). *Cognitive therapy for personality disorders: A schema-focused approach* (rev. ed.). Sarasota, FL: Professional Resource Press.

Author Index

Abaied, J., 89
Abe, J. A., 158
Abela, J. R. Z., 20, 37, 38, 39, 40, 41, 42, 43, 44, 45, 47, 48, 49, 50, 51, 52, 53, 55, 56, 58, 59, 60, 61, 63–64, 65, 67, 68, 89, 90, 94, 157, 310, 311, 389, 390, 399, 481
Abramowicz, M., 210
Abramson, L. Y., 35, 36, 37, 38, 40, 47, 49, 51, 52, 56, 57, 58, 61, 63, 64, 65–66, 67, 68, 85, 86, 90, 142, 184, 274, 310, 311, 314, 333, 340, 377, 389, 390, 391, 395, 431, 445, 475, 480
Achenbach, T. M., 3, 8, 388, 469
Ackerman, S, 268
Adam, E. K., 166
Adam, T., 243
Adams, J., 340
Adams, M., 340
Adams, P., 39, 44, 45, 50, 55, 56, 61, 389
Adamson, L. B., 52, 84, 416
Adan, A. M., 365
Addy, C., 299
Adler, C. M., 108
Adrian, C., 19, 37, 389
Affleck, G., 273
Ahrens, A. H., 38, 40
Aikins, J. W., 38, 41, 82, 84, 90, 91, 389, 391
Ainsworth, M. D. S, 58, 88
Aitchison, K. J., 134
Alfieri, T., 381
Alford, B. A., 333
Allan, W. D., 451, 452
Allen, N. B., 20, 67, 385

Allen, R. R., 457
Allgood-Merten, B., 388, 391
Allison, S., 338, 474
Allister, L., 423
Allman, C., 229
Allmon, D., 447
Alloy, L. B., 35, 36, 37, 38, 49, 51, 58, 59, 68, 142, 156–157, 184, 274, 311, 390, 391, 423, 445, 475
Allport, G., 256, 259, 260
Alpert, A., 85–86, 230, 289
Alpert, J. J., 453
Altemus, M., 19
Altham, P., 83, 180, 184
Altmann, E., 82, 183
Altshuler, J. L., 228, 229
Alves, S. E., 379
Ambrosini, P., 8, 213, 382
Amir, N., 8
Andersen, S. L., 112, 113
Anderson, J., 9, 12, 14
Anderson, K. J., 92
Anderson, R. N., 441
Andreasen, N. C., 106
Andrews, B., 390, 468
Andrews, G., 7
Andrews, J., 3, 9, 83, 85–86, 179, 195, 230, 289, 333, 384
Aneshensel, C. S., 384
Angell, K. E., 390
Angold, A., 6, 7, 8, 9, 10, 14, 15, 16, 18, 21, 67–68, 114, 216, 229, 383, 384, 385, 393

Angst, J., 7, 15, 153, 382
Anjum, A., 270
Antonowicz, D. H, 474
Appleyard, K, 480
Apter, A., 444
Arcus, D., 424
Arends, E., 474
Arias, E., 441
Arieti, S., 229
Armistead, L., 82
Armitage, R., 19
Armstrong, H. E., 447
Armstrong, T. D., 15
Arthur, M. W., 365
Asarnow, J. R., 84, 230, 452
Aseltine, R. H., 92, 380, 388
Asher, S. R., 450
Ashman, S. B., 419
Assaad, J. M., 107
Audette, D. P., 227
Auerbach, R. P., 42, 43, 44, 45, 61
Avenevoli, S., 6, 7, 15, 16
Aydin, C., 49, 61

B

Bacchiochi, J. R., 390
Bagby, R. M., 390
Bailey, S. M., 326
Baker, M., 83
Baldus, C., 335
Bandura, A., 259, 390
Bank, L., 421
Barbaranelli, C., 390
Barber, B., 182
Bardone, A. J., 445
Bardone, A. M., 16, 17
Barlow, D. H., 153
Barnett, D., 229
Baron, R. M., 386, 387
Barrett, K. C., 392
Barrett, P. M., 252
Bartels, M., 133
Basturk, M., 111
Bates, J., 38, 39, 55, 152, 386
Battle, C. L., 467
Baucom, D. H., 430
Bauer, J., 275
Baumeister, R. F., 157, 251, 446, 447,
    450

Baumgart, E. P., 64
Bauserman, R., 390
Beach, S. R. H., 8, 82
Beardslee, W. , 18, 182–183, 326, 338, 358,
    416, 425, 428, 430, 431
Bearman, S. K., 384
Beautrais, A. L., 17, 447, 450
Bebbington, P., 20, 393
Bechner, A. M. P., 169
Beck, A. T., 35, 36, 37, 38, 44, 51, 58, 63,
    90, 180, 182, 185, 187, 191, 196, 213,
    225, 263, 270, 311, 333, 340, 390, 421,
    423, 445, 451, 452, 455, 457, 475
Beck, J., 240, 455
Becker, J. B., 394
Becker-Blease, K., 468
Beevers, C. J., 320
Beidel, D. C., 17
Belin, T. R., 455
Bell-Dolan, D. J., 82
Belmont, B., 421, 425
Belmonte, P. L., 19
Belsky, J., 88
Bem, A., 381
Bemporad, J. R., 229
Benkelfat, C., 112
Bennett, D., 8, 38, 39, 382
Benson, P. L., 355, 370
Bentovim, A., 474
Berebaum, S. A., 379
Bergeman, C. S., 127, 137
Bergen, H. A, 474
Berglund, M. L., 354, 356, 357, 358, 361,
    364, 365, 368, 370
Berglund, P., 14, 21
Bergmann, P. E., 21
Berkman, L. F., 268
Berlin, L., 167
Berliner, L., 475
Berman, A. L., 442, 445
Berman, L., 443, 444, 456
Bernal, G., 196, 298, 299, 303
Bettes, B. A., 229
Beyer, J. L., 109
Biederman, J., 210, 424
Bierut, L. J., 392
Bifulco, A., 468, 469, 480
Biglan, A., 421
Billings, A., 183, 416
Bir, J., 312, 354, 360, 384, 398
Bird, H. R., 10, 18

Birmaher, B., 16, 114, 131, 213, 215, 216, 393, 449, 470

Birmaher, D., 20

Bishop, B., 320

Bittner, A., 18

Bjorck, J. P., 388

Black, D., 191, 445, 455

Black, S. A., 254

Blackwell, J., 51–52

Blade, J., 12

Blalock, J., 81, 289

Blaney, P. H., 57

Blatt, S. J., 36, 37, 44, 56, 58, 63, 90, 388, 390

Blazer, D., 7, 9, 14

Blechman, E. A., 227

Blehar, M., 88

Bleich, A., 444

Block, J., 153, 155, 158, 165, 167, 383

Blyth, D., 92, 369, 370

Boergers, J., 446

Bohlin, G., 167

Boivin, M., 85

Bolger, A. K., 425

Bolhofner, K., 16

Bolognini, M., 157

Bolte, A., 263

Bolte, K., 213

Bonari, L., 113

Bond, L., 338, 343

Boney-McCoy, S, 471, 472

Bonner, R. L., 450

Bonsall, R, 479

Bonte, F. J., 111

Booji, L., 112

Boomsma, D. I., 131,132, 133

Boomsma, P., 157

Bor, W., 20

Borden, L., 369

Borelli, J. L., 82, 83, 85, 87, 389

Boring, A. M, 478

Borowsky, I. W., 444, 448

Bostwick, J. M., 457

Boswell, J., 225

Botein, S., 430

Botteron, K. N., 109

Bottomly, L., 421

Boudreau, D, 479

Boulos, C., 213

Bourjolly, J., 326

Bower, G. H., 57, 317

Bower, S. A., 317

Bowlby, J., 58, 88, 185, 475

Boyd, R. C., 326

Boyer, R., 450

Boyle, M. H., 3, 12, 14, 389

Braafladt, N., 85, 157, 168, 228–229

Brabeck, M., 183

Braet, C., 63

Branigan, C., 263

Braswell, L., 237

Bratslavsky, E., 251

Bremner, J. D., 478

Brendgen, M., 82, 83, 87, 91, 343

Brennan, P. A., 20, 82, 388, 416, 422

Brent, D., 131, 179, 184, 196, 200, 229, 443, 444, 449, 453, 455, 457

Brewin, C. R., 390, 468

Breznitz, Z., 229

Brickman, P., 276–277

Bridge, J., 449

Bridges, M., 290

Briggs-Gowan, M. J., 392

Broderick, P. C., 42, 43, 390

Brody, L. R., 379, 380, 381

Broitman, M., 429

Bronfenbrenner, U., 338

Brook, J., 9, 17, 18, 299, 385, 389

Brooks-DeWeese, A., 426

Brooks-Gunn, J., 354, 356, 384, 388, 393, 394

Brotchie, L., 114

Broth, M., 416, 429

Brown, B. B., 92

Brown, E. J, 475, 476

Brown, G. K., 445

Brown, G. W, 468

Brown, J., 228, 447, 450, 471, 472

Brown, T. A., 153

Brozina, K., 38, 40, 42, 43, 63, 64, 157, 390

Bruce, A. E., 58, 480

Bruck, M, 466

Bruder, G. E., 165

Bry, B., 59

Buchanan, A., 450

Buchanan, C. M., 394

Bucholz, K. K., 133

Buckley, M. E., 153

Buhrmester, D., 380

Buka, L., 18

Buka, S. L., 455

Bukowski, W. M., 85

Bumbarger, B., 359
Burge, D., 19, 82, 183, 389
Burgeson, R., 92
Burgess, E., 393
Burke, E. C., 9
Burke, J. D., 9
Burke, P., 7, 311, 382
Burney, E., 19
Burnham, B. L., 64
Burns, B., 7, 18, 21
Burns, J., 339
Burns, M. O., 53
Burt, C. E., 388
Burton, C. M., 265, 275
Burwell, R. A., 88
Busner, C., 457, 458
Buss, D. M., 251
Buss, K. A., 115, 152, 161, 420, 422, 424
Butler, A. C., 311, 455
Butler, E. A., 158
Butler, H., 343
Butler, L., 157, 195
Buttenweiser, P., 255
Byrd, D., 105
Byrum, C. E., 109

C

Cacioppo, J. T., 252
Cahill, H., 338
Cain, K. M., 59
Cairney, J., 384
Caldwell, M. S., 85, 90
Calhoun, L. G., 273
Calkins, S. D., 154, 163, 166
Callanan, M. A., 381
Campbell, F., 195
Campbell, S. B., 164, 229, 416
Campos, J. J., 150, 151, 152, 154, 162, 163
Campos, R. G., 150
Camras, L., 150, 154, 169
Canals, J., 12, 16, 17
Cane, D. B., 64
Canino, G., 10, 21
Canli, T., 66, 117
Cantwell, C., 455
Cantwell, D. P., 84, 384
Capaldi, D. M., 358
Cappelleri, J. C, 474
Caprara, G. V., 390

Carbajo, G., 12
Carbonell, D. M., 299
Cardamone, A. L., 56
Cardemil, E. V., 320, 321, 324, 337, 360
Cardno, A. G., 126
Carella, E. T., 227
Carey, G., 153
Carey, M. P., 153
Carlo, G., 381
Carlson, E. A., 164, 389, 421
Carlson, G. A., 229, 452
Carlson, N. R., 107–108
Carlton-Ford, S., 92
Carmola-Hauf, A. M., 11
Carpenter, L. L., 382
Carr, A., 179, 195
Carr, S., 423
Carson, S., 338
Carter, A. S., 392
Carter, G., 444
Carter, I., 50, 55
Casey, B. J., 105, 106
Casey, J., 167
Caspi, A., 9, 16, 17, 19, 20, 53, 55, 66, 116, 137, 139, 153, 162, 214, 378, 386, 392, 393, 399, 417, 422, 426
Cassidy, J., 84, 88, 450
Cassidy, K. W., 319
Catalano, R. F., 354, 356, 357, 358, 361, 364, 365, 368, 370
Catron, T., 68
Cauce, A. M., 388
Ceci, S. J, 466
Cerezo-Jimenez, M. A, 475
Cervantes, C. A., 381
Chalmers, D. T., 135
Chamber, D. B., 263
Chambers, W. J., 8
Chambless, D. L., 455
Champion, K., 169
Chang, E., 274
Chang, H. L., 13
Chaplin, T. M., 169, 311, 321, 323, 324, 327, 392, 397, 428
Chapman, D. A., 334
Chapman, J. E., 311
Charney, D., 17, 95, 135, 141, 160
Cheah, C. S. L., 82, 389, 391
Cheavens, J., 257
Chen, A. T., 13
Chen, T. H., 13

Chen, W. J., 13
Chen, Y. R., 450
Chernoff, J. J., 84
Cherny, S. S., 419
Chesney, M. A., 263
Cheung, A. H., 212, 213, 215, 220
Chiapetta, L., 449
Chicz-DeMet, A., 419
Cho, E., 389
Chong, M. Y., 13
Chorpita, B. F., 153, 392
Christiana, J. M., 21
Chrousos, G., 393
Chu, J. A, 468
Chugani, H. T., 420
Cicchetti, D., 7, 81, 86, 163, 164, 168, 169,
    229, 311, 377, 421, 422, 430, 466, 469,
    475, 480
Cisler, R. A., 452
Clark, A. G., 82, 83
Clark, D., 35, 63, 90, 180, 317, 333
Clark, E., 195
Clark, L. A., 149, 152, 153, 160, 260, 391,
    400, 416, 428
Clark, S. E., 390
Clarke, G., 180, 186, 190, 195, 196, 197,
    288, 289, 333, 360, 368, 428
Clayton, P. J., 153
Cleland, C. M., 8
Clements, C. M., 68
Clum, G., 195
Coates, D., 276–277, 474
Coats, K., 195
Coatsworth, J. D., 355
Cobb, R., 92
Coccaro, E. F., 422
Cohen, E., 17, 299
Cohen, J., 46, 322, 384
Cohen, J. A., 475, 477
Cohen, J. D., 107
Cohen, L. H., 157, 388
Cohen, P., 9, 14, 17, 18, 299, 384, 385, 389,
    447, 472
Cohn, J., 163
Cohn, J. F., 164, 229
Coie, J. D., 318, 380
Coiro, M. J., 428, 429
Colbus, D., 86, 227
Cole, D., 182
Cole, D. A., 47, 51, 52, 55, 65, 83, 85, 86,
    87, 92, 225, 229, 384, 385, 391, 451

Cole, E., 195
Cole, J. O, 397
Cole, P., 150, 228, 423
Cole, P. M., 164, 165, 169, 311, 327, 392
Cole, S., 84, 416
Coles, M., 47, 51
Coles, M. E., 481
Collins, L. M., 399
Collins, M. H., 52
Collins, P., 252
Collins, W. A., 421
Colten, M. E., 380, 388
Colton, M. E., 92
Compas, B., 184
Compas, B. E., 6, 82, 155, 388, 392, 421,
    425, 426
Compton, K., 421
Compton, W., 20
Conger, R. D., 91, 116, 153, 384, 389
Conley, C. S., 38, 40, 48, 52–53, 57, 82, 90,
    92, 391
Connell, A. M., 416, 427
Connell, D. B., 430
Connolly, J., 83, 86
Connor-Smith, J., 82, 155, 184
Conrad, K., 383
Conway, K. P., 20
Cooney, R. E., 66
Cooper, P., 13, 429
Cooper, T. B., 213
Cooper, V., 207
Copeland, M. E., 421, 426
Coppen, A., 135
Copping, W., 214
Corbit, J. D., 447
Corley, R. P., 419
Cornell, J., 253
Cornes, C., 289
Cornette, M., 445
Corrigan, R., 52
Corte, C., 35
Corter, C., 429
Costello, E., 6, 7, 9, 10, 14, 15, 16, 17, 18,
    20, 21, 67–68, 114, 229, 383, 384, 385,
    393
Cotgrove, A. J., 455
Cottrell, C. A., 251–252
Coy, K. C., 392
Coyne, J., 81, 82, 86, 168, 227, 289, 326,
    391, 396, 431
Craft, L., 458

Craig, I. W., 128
Craney, J., 16
Crawford T. N., 389
Crick, N. R., 83, 318, 327, 378, 380, 384, 386, 389, 450
Cris-Houran, M., 269
Crook, K., 227
Cross, S. E., 380
Crouse-Novak, M. A., 14
Csikszentmihalyi, M., 255, 259, 262, 266, 267
Cukrowicz, K. C., 451
Cumberland, A., 380
Cummings, E. M., 389, 423, 427
Cummings, P., 457
Cunliffe, R., 335, 360
Curran, P. J., 399
Curry, J., 179, 180, 181, 184, 185, 194, 199, 200
Curtin, J. J., 169
Cutler, S. E., 390
Cutrona, C. E., 424
Cutuli, J. J., 321, 323, 324
Cyranowski, J. M., 378, 380, 395

D

Dadds, M. R., 84, 325, 335, 337, 430
Dadds, V., 338
Dahl, R., 393
Dahl, R. E., 20, 166
Dahlmeier, J., 451
D'Alessandro, D. U., 41, 42
Daley, S. E., 82, 83, 84, 86, 87, 480
Damon, W., 311, 355
Danielson, C. K., 472, 473
Danner, D., 263
Darbes, L. A., 263
D'Augelli, A. R., 450
Davalos, M., 115
David, C. F., 384, 392
Davidson, R., 66, 107, 108, 109, 110, 111, 113, 149, 160, 165, 166, 172, 263, 420
Davidson, W., 59
Davies, M., 3, 11, 303
Davies, P. T., 85, 388, 389, 423, 425, 426, 427
Davila, J., 92
Davis, B., 85–86, 230, 289, 389, 421, 425, 430

Davis, C. G., 19, 20
Dawson, G., 89, 115, 116, 165, 419, 420
Dean, P., 112
de Arellano, M. A, 472
DeArth-Pendley, G., 389
Deater-Deckard, K., 131, 132, 133
Debats, D. L., 268
DeBellis, M. D., 113, 477, 478, 479
Debener, S., 165
Deblinger, E., 477
Dechef, M. L. E., 90
Deci, E. L., 256
Decker, D, 277
Dedmon, S. A., 166
DeFries, J. C., 125, 128, 137, 419
DelBello, M. P., 108
Delle Fave, A., 266
DelVecchio, W. F., 153, 162
Demler, O., 14
Denham, S., 427
Dennis, T., 150
DeRubeis, R. J., 428
de St. Aubin, E., 266, 268
Dewey, J., 255
De Wilde, E. J., 446
Deykin, E. Y., 10, 453, 455
Dhaliwal, G. K, 474
Diamond, A., 266, 268
Diamond, G., 326, 429
Dichter, G. S., 116
Dickerson, S. S., 379
Dickey, M., 326
Dickson, N., 16, 17
DiClemente, R. J., 448
Diego, M. A., 115
Diekstra, R. F., 446, 474
Diener, E., 260, 268, 270, 272, 277, 391, 253260
Diener, M. L., 88
Dierker, L., 15
Dieserud, G., 450
Dill, D. L., 468
Dinella, L., 91
Dinicola, V. F., 214
Dixon, J. F., 38, 40, 473
Dobler-Mikola, A., 382
Dobson, K., 179, 200, 312
Dodge, K. A., 68, 82, 229, 318, 380, 386, 391
Dolcini, M. N., 92
Doll, B., 328

Domenech, E., 12
Domenech-Llaberia, E., 12, 16, 17
Domitrovich, C., 359
Donaldson, D., 446, 455
Donelan-McCall, N., 164
Donenberg, G. R., 325
Donovan, C., 38, 41, 358
Dorn, L., 393
Dorta, K. P., 288, 290, 296, 298, 299, 300, 303
Downey, G., 168, 326, 431
Doyle, A., 88, 142
Dozois, D. J. A., 312
Drake, D. R., 370
Drevrets, W., 109, 110, 111, 135, 141
Driscoll, A. K., 384
Driscoll, K., 42, 43, 451
DuBois, D., 179, 182
Duckworth, A. L., 252, 253, 262
Duggal, S., 389, 399
Dulcan, M. K., 11
Dumenci, L., 427
Dumont, M., 343
Duncan, E. M., 9
Duncan, L. E., 474
Dunn, J., 228
DuPaul, G. J., 328, 458
Durbin, C. E., 153, 162
During, S., 169
Durlak, C., 254
Durlak, J. A., 359
Du Rocher Schudlich, T., 389, 427
Dweck, C. S., 59
Dyck, M., 180
Dziurawiec, S., 320, 337, 360

E

Earls, F., 6
Easterbrook, G., 269
Eaton, W. W., 445
Eaves, L., 18, 20, 126, 132, 137, 139, 153, 392, 417, 427
Eberhart, N. K., 388
Ebsworthy, G., 320, 337, 360
Eccles, J. S., 310, 394
Eccleston, E. G., 135
Eckenrode, J., 388, 474
Eckert, T. L., 458
Edelbrock, C., 469

Edhborg, M., 424
Egan, S. K., 85
Egeland, B., 389, 421, 480
Egger, H. L., 7, 15
Eisen, S. V., 468
Eisenberg, N., 165, 167, 380
Ekeberg, O., 450
Ekman, P., 420
Elder, G. G., 91
Elder, G. H., 153, 384
Eley, T., 19, 66, 95, 116, 128, 131, 132, 133, 137, 138, 140, 143, 393, 417
Elkin, I., 289, 397
Ellenbogen, M. A., 112
Ellis, A., 311, 312, 315, 326
Ellis, B. J., 384
Ellman, S. W., 360
Else-Quest, N. M., 379
Elster, A., 21
Emde, R. N., 379, 475
Emery, G., 184, 225, 263, 340, 421, 455
Emmons, R. A., 260, 265
Emslie, G., 198, 212, 216, 227
English, K., 474
Enna, B., 59
Epstein, N. B., 430
Erbaugh, J., 196, 213
Erickson, M., 132
Erikson, E., 364
Erkanli, A., 7, 9, 15, 16, 18, 67–68, 114, 137, 229, 384, 385, 393
Ernst, C., 153
Ernst, D., 180
Ervin, F., 104
Esposito-Smythers, C., 455
Essau, C., 179
Essex, M. J., 389, 427
Esveldt-Dawson, K., 52, 86, 227, 445
Éthier, L. S., 469, 474
Evans, D., 187, 361
Ey, S., 6, 184

F

Faber, R. J., 277
Fabes, R. A., 380, 381
Faraone, S. V., 142, 419
Farchione, T. R., 113
Farmer, E., 7, 18, 21
Fava, G. A., 252, 256, 257

Feehan, M., 9, 12, 14
Feeney, B. C., 88
Feeny, N., 185
Feiguine, R. J., 213
Feinberg, T. L., 14
Feiring, C, 58, 470, 474, 476
Feldman, D. B., 257
Feldman, R. S, 480
Felner, R. D., 227, 361, 365, 367, 368
Fendrich, M., 19, 229
Ferdinand, R. F., 9
Ferenz-Gillies, R., 82
Ferguson, H.B., 214
Fergusson, D. M., 12, 16, 17, 18, 21, 389,
    425, 471
Fernald, R. D., 379
Fernandez-Ballart, J., 12, 16, 17
Fichman, L., 56, 90
Field, T., 115, 165, 419, 422, 423, 428, 430,
    431
Fier, J., 384
Finch, A. J., 153
Finch, C., 477
Fincham, F., 59, 92
Finkelhor, D., 471, 472, 473
Finkelstein, R., 14
Finkenauer, C., 251
Finzi, R., 480
Fischer, S., 36
Fisher, C. B., 356
Fisher, P., 11, 452
Fitzmaurice, G., 9, 18
Fitzpatrick, K. K., 456
Fivush, R., 380, 381
Fleming, A., 429
Fleming, J. E., 3, 12, 14
Fleming, M., 21
Flora, J., 86
Flory, M., 452
Flouri, E., 450
Flynn, C., 56, 57, 58, 59, 83, 95, 476
Flynn, M., 480
Foa, C., 61
Foley, D. L., 6
Folkman, S., 273
Fombonne, E., 131, 207, 208, 214, 422
Fonagy, P., 195
Forbes, E. E., 116, 166
Fordyce, M. W., 256
Forehand, R., 82, 229, 426
Forman, E. M., 311

Fortin, L., 388
Fox, M., 364
Fox, N. A., 115, 154, 163, 165, 173, 420,
    421, 423
Fraley, C., 53
Fraley, R. C., 7, 37, 53
Frank, E., 289, 378, 380, 382, 395
Frankel, C. B., 150, 154
Frankl, V. E., 268
Franklin, J., 57
Franko, D. L., 20
Fraser, J., 196
Frauenknecht, M., 191
Fredrickson, B. L., 160, 263, 275
Freeman, A., 184
Freeman, J., 269
French, N. H., 52, 445
Freres, D. R., 310, 321, 325
Freud, S., 251
Frey, K., 165
Frias, D., 475
Friedberg, R., 188
Friedman, R., 195
Friedman, S., 420
Friend, A., 229
Friesen, W. V., 420
Frisch, M. B., 253, 257
Frombonne, E., 3
Frosch, C. A., 88
Frost, A., 11, 14, 384
Frustaci, K, 478
Frye, A., 83, 421
Fudge, H., 17, 214
Fujita, F., 277
Fulker, D., 128, 131, 379, 419
Furman, W., 380

G

Gable, S. L., 254, 265, 273, 278
Gallagher, T., 299, 300
Galligan, R. F., 386
Gallo, J. J., 445
Gallop, R., 321, 325
Gamble, W., 84, 343
Ganiban, J., 229
Garber, J., 7, 36, 38, 40, 41, 44, 45, 46, 51,
    56, 57, 58, 59, 64, 65, 67, 68, 82, 83,
    85, 87, 90, 116, 157, 168, 183, 228–229,
    300, 310, 312, 318, 321, 322, 323, 354,

359, 360, 368, 370, 383, 384, 391, 398, 421, 424, 425, 429, 476
Garcia, M., 393
Gardner, C., 392, 417, 479
Garfield, S. L., 397
Garfinkel, R., 298
Garite, T. J., 419
Garland, A., 457, 458
Garmezy, N., 339, 355
Garnefski, N., 168, 474
Garrison, C. Z., 9, 10, 17, 299
Gater, R., 382
Gates, L. L., 113
Gatsonis, C., 7, 179
Gau, J. M., 9
Gau, S. S., 13
Gauzas, L, 474
Gaynor, S., 179
Gazelle, H., 90
Ge, X., 91, 153, 384, 388
Geleijnse, J. M., 254
Gelfand, D. M., 420, 422, 430
Geller, B., 16, 210, 213
Geller, S., 83
Gemar, M., 479
Ghaziuddin, N., 112
Giaconia, R. M., 9, 11, 14, 18, 20, 299, 384, 470
Gibb, B. E., 38, 40, 47, 51, 57, 58, 59, 473, 475, 481
Giedd, J. N., 106, 107
Giese, A. A., 457
Gilbert, P., 88
Gilboa, E., 420
Gilboa-Schechtman, E., 445
Gill, K. L., 163
Gillham, J., 254, 309, 310, 312, 318, 319, 321, 323, 324, 325, 340, 361, 368, 428
Gilman, S. E., 18
Giltay, E. J., 254
Ginter, M., 365
Gipson, P. Y., 388
Girgus, J. S., 14, 38, 82, 311, 340, 394, 395
Gjerde, P. F., 153, 383
Gjerde, P. H., 383
Gjone, H., 133, 134
Gladstone, T., 36, 68, 182–183, 358, 428, 431
Glass, G. V., 322
Glover, S., 343
Glover, V., 419

Glowinski, A. L., 133
Glynn, L., 419
Glyshaw, K., 157, 388
Goldberg, C., 279
Goldsmith, H. H., 152, 161, 379, 422, 424
Goldstein, M. J., 230
Goldstein, S., 422
Golinis, G., 362
Gomez, C., 115
Gönül, A. S., 111
Gonzalez, A. M., 447
Gonzalez, J., 423
Gonzalez-Tejera, G., 7, 9, 10, 14, 15
Goodman, S. H., 19, 84, 89, 163, 164, 168, 340, 378, 416, 417, 419, 420, 421, 422, 423, 425, 426, 427, 429
Goodman-Brown, T., 45, 64, 182
Goodwin, J. S., 254
Goodyer, I., 13, 83, 180, 184, 393
Gordis, E., 184
Gordon, K. H., 448
Gordon, R. S., 299
Gore, A., 380, 388
Gore, S., 92
Gorman, L., 429
Goschke, T., 263
Gotlib, I. H., 15, 16, 19, 20, 47, 63, 64, 66, 67, 81, 82, 87, 89, 164, 168, 182, 183, 184, 185, 299, 310, 384, 385, 390, 416, 417, 419, 420, 423, 426, 468, 470
Gottesman, H., 66
Gottesman, I. I., 141, 422
Gottman, J. M., 164, 423, 428, 430
Gould, M. S., 442, 443, 452, 458
Gould, T. D., 66, 141
Gowers, S., 196
Graber, J., 384, 388, 393
Grace, D., 41, 42, 43
Graczyk, P. A., 89, 164
Graham, D., 213
Graham, S., 85
Graham, Y. P., 419
Granger, D., 393–394
Grant, B. F., 20
Grant, G., 257
Grant, K., 6, 184, 388, 391, 392, 422
Graves, D. J., 227
Gravitt, G. W., 340
Gray, D., 443
Grayson, C., 157, 390
Graziano, W. G., 155

Greenberg, M. T., 359
Greenberg, T., 442
Greenfield, B., 455
Gregory, A. G., 143
Gregus, A, 479
Griffin, S., 260
Grisham, J. R., 445
Grizzle, N., 430
Grob, M. C, 468
Groen, G., 334, 335
Grofer Klinger, L., 420
Groot, A., 94
Gross, A. M., 82, 84
Gross, J. J., 150, 154, 158, 164, 392
Grossman, D. C., 457
Grossman, J. B., 365
Grotpeter, J. K., 83, 327, 380, 386
Grunebaum, H. U., 430
Gudmundsen, G. R., 88
Gullone, E., 391
Gum, A., 257
Gunnar, M. R., 107, 108, 113
Gurley, D., 9, 385
Guthertz, M., 422
Guthrie, D., 230, 452
Gutkin, T. B., 328
Gutstein, S. E., 455
Guyer, A. E., 391

H

Haaga, D., 180
Haber, D., 269
Hadjiyannakis, K., 183, 421
Hadzi-Pavlovic, D., 385
Haeffel, G., 49, 390
Hagerty, B. M., 343
Haggerty, R. J., 299, 333, 355
Haidt, J., 254, 273, 277, 278
Haigh, E. P., 42, 43, 157, 390
Haines, B. A., 38, 56
Hains, A. A., 360
Halbern, S., 443
Halberstadt, L., 58, 64
Hall, C. M., 416, 429
Hall, J., 379, 380, 381, 478
Ham, D., 334
Ham, M., 388
Hamilton, J., 321, 325
Hamilton, M., 213, 217, 270

Hamilton, N. A., 416
Hammad, T. A., 219
Hammen, C. L., 3, 15, 19, 20, 36, 37, 38, 40,
    45, 47, 51, 57, 59, 64, 66, 67, 81, 82,
    83, 84, 86, 87, 89, 90, 91, 182, 183,
    184, 185, 289, 388, 389, 396, 416, 421,
    422, 424, 429, 480
Hammond, M., 421
Han, S. S., 325
Hankin, B. L., 7, 14, 20, 36, 37, 38, 39, 40,
    41, 42, 43, 44, 47, 49, 50, 51, 52, 53,
    55, 56, 57, 58, 59, 60, 61, 66, 67, 68,
    86, 87, 89, 90, 91, 92, 142, 310, 311,
    377, 383, 384, 388, 389, 391, 395, 399,
    473, 475, 480, 481
Hannan, K., 388
Hans, T. A., 362
Happonen, M., 133
Hardan, A., 112
Hardt, J, 468
Har-Evan, D., 480
Hargrave, J. L., 227
Hariri, A. R., 139
Harkness, K. L., 473, 475, 479, 480
Harlan, E. T., 155
Harnett, P. H., 325, 335, 337
Harold, G., 18, 131, 132, 133, 134, 137
Harrington, M., 184
Harrington, R., 3, 17, 195, 196, 207, 214,
    333, 417, 422, 455
Harris, J., 392
Harris, T. O., 468
Harrison, H. M., 83, 91
Hart, B., 320
Hart, D., 311
Hart, S., 430
Harter, S., 52, 391
Hartlage, S., 35, 37, 142
Hartley, D., 448
Haslam, N., 8
Hasler, G., 141
Hastings, P., 393–394
Hattie, J. A., 362, 363, 364
Hautzinger, M., 9, 334, 335
Hawkins, J. D., 354, 365
Hayden, E. P., 153, 162
Hays, R. D., 268
Hayward, C., 92, 379, 384, 385, 394, 468,
    470
Hazell, P., 214
Healy, B., 422, 423

Heard, H. L., 447
Heath, A., 20, 109, 126, 133, 153
Heathcote, D., 214
Hechtman, L., 455
Heffelfinger, A., 7
Heim, C., 116, 117, 419, 478, 479
Helgeson, V. S., 390
Helsel, W. J., 271
Heninger, G. R., 135
Henry, D., 214
Henry, R., 480
Hensley, R., 227
Herbert, J., 180
Herman-Stahl, M., 83, 340
Hernandez-Reif, M., 115
Hersen, M., 15
Hershberger, S. L., 450
Hessl, D., 165
Hetherington, E. M., 132, 133, 137, 290, 417
Hetrick, S., 312, 354, 359, 360, 361, 368, 370, 384, 398
Hettema, J. M., 416
Hewitt, J., 132, 133, 392–393
Higgins, E. T., 381, 446
Hilbert, S. M., 364
Hill, D., 420
Hill, J., 17, 214, 310, 381, 399
Hilsman, R., 38, 40, 41
Hilt, L. M., 38
Hinkley, K., 392
Hipwell, A. E., 378, 385, 392, 396, 397, 400
Hiroto, D., 37
Hirschfeld, R. M., 135, 153
Ho, M., 61
Ho, R., 56, 61
Hoagwood, K., 288, 325
Hobel, C. J., 419
Hoberman, H. M., 21
Hodulik, C. J., 58
Hoekstra, T., 254
Hoerster, K., 263
Hoffman, K., 86, 391
Hoffmann, R., 19
Hofstra, M. B., 17
Hogan, M. E., 49
Hogue, A., 84, 389
Hokanson, J., 289
Holahan, C. J., 86
Holdsworth, R., 338
Hollon, S., 180, 312, 428, 429, 455
Holmbeck, G. N., 229, 310

Holmes, C. J., 163
Homann, E., 56, 58, 90
Hooe, E. S., 392
Hoorens, V., 252
Hope, T., 448
Hopkins, J., 164
Hops, H., 3, 9, 16, 83, 85–86, 179, 195, 196, 230, 289, 333, 384, 388, 389, 421, 425, 426
Horn, A. B., 334, 335
Horowitz, J. L., 300, 303, 310, 312, 321, 322, 323, 354, 359, 360, 368, 370, 398
Horvath, T. B., 422
Horwath, E., 299
Horwood, J. L., 389
Horwood, L. J., 9, 17, 21, 425
Howard, M. S., 88
Howe, G. W., 137
Howell, C. T., 3, 8, 388
Howland, R. H., 393
Hoyle, K., 343
Hsu, H. C., 424
Hudson, J., 188
Hudziak, J. J., 132
Huebner, E. S., 271
Huezo-Diaz, P., 134, 135
Hughes, C. W., 213
Humphrey, L. L., 227
Hurley, J. C., 392
Huston, A. C., 392
Hyde, J. S., 379, 381, 390, 399
Hymel, S., 85
Hynan, L., 257

I

Iacono, W. G., 229
Ialongo, N., 361
Inghilleri, P., 266
Ingram, R. E., 36, 47, 56, 63, 181, 182, 185, 416, 424
Inhelder, B., 311
Inoff-Germain, G., 393
Insabella, G. M., 290
Insel, T. R., 379
Iosifescu, D. V., 109
Ireland, M., 444
Ireland, T. O, 470
Irons, C., 88
Isakson, K., 20

Ito, T. A., 252
Izard, C. E., 158

J

Jackson, D. C., 172
Jackson, K. L., 299
Jacobsen, R. H., 227
Jacobson, K., 133, 137, 392
Jacobson, N., 200, 325
Jacques, H. A. K., 392
Jaenicke, C., 58, 421, 424
Jaffee, S. R., 214, 399, 426
Jahoda, M., 256
Jain, U., 393
James, J., 320, 430
Jameson, P. B., 430
Jamieson, E., 230
Janicki, D., 390
Janoff-Bulman, R., 57, 276–277
Jarosik, J., 21
Jarvenpaa, A. L. t., 424
Jarvis, J., 468
Jarvis, P., 20
Jaser, S. S., 82, 155, 426
Jaycox, L., 309, 318, 319, 340, 361, 368, 428
Jayson, D., 196
Jensen, A. L., 325
Jensen, P. S., 15, 333, 424
Jenson, W., 195
Jernigan, T. L., 163
Jin, R., 14
Jindal, R., 393
Jobes, D. A., 442, 448
Johanson, C. A., 392
John, O. P., 152, 154, 158, 164, 392
Johnson, J., 299, 447, 472
Johnson, M. C., 163
Johnson, M. H., 162
Johnson, S., 63
Johnson, W., 255
Joiner, T., 56, 190, 289, 396, 445, 455
Joiner, T. E., 7, 38, 40, 41, 42, 50, 53, 55,
       81, 82, 83, 84, 85, 86, 225, 442, 443,
       444, 445, 447, 448, 449, 450, 451, 452,
       453, 454, 456
Jones, N., 115
Jones, P., 153
Joormann, J., 63, 66, 154
Jordan, C., 51–52

Jorgensen, J., 197
Judd, L. L., 299
Jung, C. G., 255
Jung. J. H., 109
Just, N., 156–157, 391
Juvonen, J., 85

K

Kabat-Zin, J., 262
Kachdourian, L., 92
Kagan, J., 16, 424
Kahn, J., 195
Kahneman, D., 251
Kalin, N. H., 172
Kalodner, C. R., 361
Kalynchuk, L. E, 479
Kandel, D. B., 3
Kando, J. C., 397
Kane, P., 229
Kane, R., 320, 337, 360
Kaplan, H. B., 388
Karbon, M., 381
Kasen, S., 384
Kashani, J. H., 7, 9, 10, 12, 14, 213, 229, 451
Kasius, M. C., 9
Kaslow, N., 36, 52, 58, 68, 195, 228, 340
Kassel, J. D., 390
Kasser, T., 256
Katz, A. R., 416
Katz, J., 82, 84
Katz, L. F., 164, 423, 428, 430
Katz, R., 20
Kaufman, J., 17, 95, 114, 131, 393, 479
Kawachi, I., 18, 268
Kazdin, A., 15, 52, 86, 200, 227, 252, 325,
       333, 424, 445
Keeler, G., 229, 384
Keenan, K., 378, 385, 386, 392, 396, 397,
       400
Keeves, J., 338
Kehle, T., 195
Keiley, M. K., 386
Keita, G. P., 377, 378
Kellam, S. G., 361
Keller, G., 9, 16, 421, 426
Keller, M., 18, 199, 215, 216
Keller, T., 443
Kelley, M. L., 448
Kelly, K. A., 68

Keltikangas-Jarvinen, L., 424
Kendall, P., 166, 188, 237, 243
Kendall-Tackett, K., 468, 473
Kendler, K., 18, 19, 20, 116, 126, 153, 392, 416, 417, 479, 480
Kenealy, P., 157
Kennard, B., 198
Kennedy, E., 227, 228
Kennedy, R. E., 14, 327, 384
Kenny, D. A., 53, 386, 387
Kenny, M., 183
Kermoian, R., 150
Kessler, R. C., 6, 7, 9, 10, 14, 18, 19, 20, 21, 126, 153, 288, 415, 416, 424
Keyes, C. L. M., 253, 378, 426
Khan, A. A., 382
Khan, S. C., 113
Kibar, M., 111
Kienhorst, I. C., 446
Kieras, J. E., 155
Killgore, W. D., 110
Kilpatrick, D., 11, 471, 472
Kilts, C. D., 477
Kim, D., 85
Kim-Cohen, J., 9, 12, 14, 16, 17, 18, 310
King, L., 265, 268, 273, 275
King, N. J., 477
King, R. A., 17, 95
Kinney, L., 420
Kistner, C. F., 384
Kistner, J., 42, 43, 49, 157, 164, 390, 392
Kitayama, S., 149
Klar, H. M., 422
Klausner, E., 257
Klein, D., 9, 16, 153, 162, 288
Klein, E., 429
Klein, L. C., 379
Klein, M. H., 159, 389, 427
Klein, R., 213, 215, 216
Klerman, G. L., 289, 299
Kliewer, W., 227
Klimes-Dougan, B., 393–394, 416, 425
Knauper, 64
Knudsen, K., 477
Kobak, R. R., 82, 84, 88, 343
Kochanek, K. D., 441
Kochanoff, A. T., 427
Kochanska, G., 88, 153, 155, 229, 392, 420, 421, 423
Koenig, L. J., 42, 43, 157, 390
Koepsell, T. D., 457

Koestner, R., 56, 58, 90
Koivumaa-Honkanen, H., 450
Kolb, B., 226
Kolko, D. J., 475, 476
Koons, C. R., 447
Koplewicz, H., 213
Kopp, C. B., 228
Kornstein, S. G., 382, 398
Korteland, C., 42, 43
Kostanski, M., 391
Kotsoni, E., 105
Kovacs, M., 7, 14, 16, 168, 179, 213, 215, 217, 322, 382, 386, 457, 469
Kowalenko, N., 336
Kowatch, R. A., 111
Kraaij, V., 168
Kraemer, H. C., 8, 333, 389, 424, 427
Kraft, P., 450
Kramer, A. D., 213
Krasnoperova, E., 63, 182
Kratochvil, C., 198
Krey, L., 47
Krishnan, K. R., 109
Kroll, L., 196
Krueger, R. F., 117, 392
Krupnick, J., 423
Kuczynski, L., 229, 420
Kudes, D., 382
Kuehner, C., 378
Kuhl, J., 263
Kuhn, J. W., 20, 116, 480
Kuiper, N. A., 64
Kumar, G., 451
Kung, H. C., 441
Kuo, P. H., 13
Kuo, W., 445
Kuperminc, G., 44
Kupfer, D. J., 289, 382, 424
Kurlakowsky, K. D., 57, 82
Kusumakar, V., 110, 113
Kutcher, S., 83, 113, 213, 215, 216
Kye, C. H., 213

L

Lacharité, C., 469
Lachner, G., 9
Ladd, C. O., 419, 477
Ladd, G., 9, 450
Ladouceur, C. D., 167

La Greca, A. M., 83, 91
Lahey, B. B., 7, 8, 37, 227
Lai, T.-J., 109
Lakdawalla, Z., 41, 42, 43, 47, 50, 68
Lamb, M. E., 416
Lambert, M. J., 252, 270
Lambrichs, R., 340
Langrock, A. M., 421, 426
Larsen, J. T., 252
Larsen, R. J., 162, 260
Larson, C., 455
Larson, D. W., 57
Larson, J., 157, 259, 390
Larson, R., 268, 388
Larsson, B., 386
Larzelere, R. E., 452
Last, C. G., 15
Lau, J., 66, 133, 137, 142, 393
Laurent, J., 225
Laursen, B., 92
Lavori, P. W., 18
Law, W., 213
Leadbeater, B. J., 44, 388, 390
Leahy, R., 180
Leaper, C., 92, 380
Leary, M. R., 447, 450
Lease, A. M., 227
LeBlanc, W. G., 423
Le Brocque, R. M., 416
Lee, A., 41, 42, 43
Lee, C. M., 416
Lee, H. K., 109
Leff, G., 58
Leffert, N., 370
Lefkowitz, E. S., 11, 14, 384
LeGagnoux, G., 197
Leibenluft, E., 66, 160
Leigh, E., 447
Leitenberg, H., 424
Lemelin, J, 469
Lemerond, J., 452
Lemery, K. S., 422, 424
Lennox, C., 270
Lent, R. W., 279
Leonard, M. A., 416
Lepper, H. S., 260
Lerner, M., 195
Lerner, R. M., 338, 356
Lesch, K. P., 139
Lester, B. M., 423
Levenson, R. W., 158

Leventhal, A., 92
Levinson, D. F., 19, 134, 135
Levitan, R. D., 390
Levy, J. C., 10
Lew, A. S., 84
Lewin, K., 444
Lewinsohn, M., 15, 68, 385
Lewinsohn, P., 3, 7, 8, 9, 11, 14, 15–16, 20,
    21, 36, 38, 40, 41, 42, 57, 60, 67, 68,
    83, 85, 86, 87, 153, 179, 180, 183, 195,
    196, 227, 288, 289, 299, 310, 333, 358,
    382, 384, 385, 386, 388
Lewis, G., 153
Lewis, H., 227
Lewis, J. E, 474
Lewis, K., 227
Lewis, M., 58, 81, 470, 476
Leyton, M., 112
Li, J., 15
Liang, H., 138
Libby, A. M., 457
Lieberman, A. F., 430
Lieberman, M., 88
Lillie, A, 468
Lin, E., 21
Linehan, M. M., 446, 447, 456
Liotti, M., 110
Litt, I. F., 385
Little, K. Y., 135
Little, S. A., 44, 45, 46, 64, 65, 67, 87, 90,
    391
Liu, J., 423
Liu, X., 388
Liu, Y., 58
Livingston, R., 225, 333
Lloyd, E., 448
Lloyd-Richardson, E., 448
Lochman, J. E., 318
Lock, J., 386
Loeb, A., 474
Loeber, R., 386
Loehlin, J. C., 419
Lomax, R., 183
Lombardo, E., 180
Lonczak, H. S., 354
London, K., 466, 467
Lonigan, C. J., 153, 392
Lopez, A. D., 21
Lopez, J. F., 135
Lopez, S., 253, 257, 260
Lorenz, F. O., 91, 384

Loriaux, D., 393
Losada, M., 263, 275
LoSciuto, L., 364, 365
Loughren, T., 219
Lovejoy, C. M., 89
Lovejoy, M. C., 164, 420
Low, N. C., 19
Luborsky, L., 261
Luby, J., 7
Luby, J. L., 114
Lumley, M. N., 475, 480
Lundh, W., 424
Lundy, B., 419
Lutz, J. G., 328
Luu, P., 252
Luxton, D. D., 36
Lykken, D. T., 419
Lynch, C. R., 447
Lynch, M. E., 381
Lynch-Sauer, J., 343
Lynd-Stevenson, R. M., 320, 337
Lynskey, M. T., 9, 133, 389, 425
Lyons, M. J., 392
Lyons-Ruth, K., 430, 431
Lyoo, I. K., 109
Lyubomirsky, S., 260, 265, 268

M

Ma, Y., 9, 385
Maccoby, E. E., 380
Mace, D., 197
Macfie, J, 475
Macgowan, M. J., 448
MacIntosh, H. B., 467
MacMaster, F. P., 110, 113
MacMillan, S., 110
Madden, P. A., 133
Maddux, J. E., 255
Madson, L, 380
Maes, H., 127, 392–393
Magdol, L., 9
Magnus, P., 392
Magnusson, D., 267
Mahoney, A., 268
Malcarne, V. L., 416
Malphurs, J. E., 430
Mancuso, R. A., 263
Mandoki, M., 212
Mandrusiak, M., 453, 458

Mangelsdorf, S. C., 88, 161, 162
Manji, H. K., 135, 141
Manly, J. T., 169, 469
Mann, J. J., 453
Mannarino, A. P., 475, 477
Manolis, M., 83
Mansfield, E., 266, 268
March, J., 198, 216, 219, 227
Marcotte, D., 388
Marczak, M., 369
Markides, K. S., 254
Markiewicz, D., 88
Markowitz, J., 180, 289, 429
Markus, H. R., 149
Marmorstein, N. R., 229
Marsh, H. W., 362
Marsteller, F., 213, 299
Marti-Henneberg, C., 12, 16, 17
Martin, A., 17, 95
Martin, C. L., 379, 380, 381
Martin, G., 338, 474
Martin, J., 85, 86, 214, 384, 391
Martin, N. C., 424, 425
Martin, S., 150
Martinez, P, 423
Marton, P., 83, 213
Marx, B. P., 475
Marx, E. M., 290
Marzolf, D., 161, 162
Mash, E. J., 392
Maslow, A. H., 255
Mason, C. A., 334
Massimini, F., 266
Masten, A. S., 355
Masters, J. C., 228
Mathews, C. A., 127, 135
Matias, R., 164
Matson, J. L., 271
Matt, G. E., 252
Matthews, H., 320
Maughan, A., 163, 475
Maughan, B., 16, 383, 390
Mayberg, H. S., 110
Mayer, L. S., 361
Mayes, T. L., 212
Mazure, C. M., 377, 378, 479
McAdams, D. P., 268, 275
McBride, C., 390
McCabe, M., 227
McCartney, K., 136
McCarty, C., 179, 229, 312

McCauley, C., 268
McCauley, E., 7, 311, 382, 429
McClearn, G. E., 125
McCloskey, L. A., 476
McClure, E., 66
McClure, J., 188
McCombs, H. G., 213
McConaughy, S. H., 3, 8, 388
McCrary, M., 416
McCue Horwitz, S., 392
McCullough, J. P., 456
McCullough, M. E., 259, 265
McDowell, H., 312, 335, 354, 359, 360, 361,
    368, 370, 384, 398
McEachran, A. B., 289
McEnroe, M. J., 227
McEwen, B., 19, 47, 379
McFarland, M., 429
McGee, R., 9, 12, 14, 310, 343, 476
McGirr, A., 39, 50, 61
McGonagle, K., 9, 14
McGrath, E. P., 82
McGuffin, P., 17, 19, 20, 125, 132, 133, 137,
    398, 400, 417
McGuire, S., 132, 137
McHale, J. L., 88
McIntosh, J. L., 441
McIntyre, J. S., 382
McIntyre-Smith, A., 90
McKeown, R., 299
McKnew, D., 423
McLeer, S. V., 473
McLellan, A. T., 261
McLoyd, V., 392
McMahon, R., 169
McMahon, S. D., 388
McManus, B. L., 453
McNamarra, J. J., 453
McPherson, M., 444
McWhinnie, C. M., 61, 64
McWilliams, N., 259
Mednick, S. A., 415
Medway, F. J., 88
Meehl, P. E., 46, 52, 160
Meesters, C., 157, 340
Mehta, T. G., 88
Meizitis, S., 195
Mendelsohn, S., 444
Mendelson, M., 196, 213
Menkes, D. B., 135
Mennen, F. E., 474

Merchant, M. J., 421, 426
Merikangas, K. R., 6, 15, 19
Mermelstein, R., 57, 86, 388
Merry, S., 312, 335, 354, 359, 360, 361, 368,
    370, 384, 398
Messer, S. C., 82, 84
Metalsky, G., 35, 36, 37, 38, 50, 51, 56, 64,
    82, 86, 142, 184, 311, 390, 423, 445
Metz, C., 382
Meyer, A., 289
Meyers, T., 229
Mezulis, A. H., 390, 391
Michael, S. T., 257
Midlarsky, E., 389
Miech, R., 427
Mikulincer, M., 445
Milich, R., 83
Miller, A. H., 419, 479
Miller, A. L., 447, 455, 456, 457, 458
Miller, D. N., 328, 458
Miller, E. K., 107
Miller, J. B., 319, 324
Miller, N., 49
Miller, T. L., 322
Miller, W. R., 466, 467
Mineka, S., 68
Miner, K., 273
Minor, K. L., 66
Miranda, J., 36, 63
Mirza, Y., 113
Mistry, R. S., 392
Mitchell, J., 7, 311, 382
Mittman, B. S., 382
Mock, J., 196, 213
Moerk, K. C., 153
Moffitt, C. E., 392
Moffitt, T., 9, 16, 17, 66, 153, 214, 310, 378,
    386, 392, 393, 399, 426
Moilanen, D., 183
Moilanen, I., 127
Moisan, P. A, 474
Mojica, E, 480
Moldin, S. O., 415, 419
Molnar, J., 227
Moneta, G. B., 266
Monroe, S., 20, 36, 85, 153, 183, 421, 422,
    480
Moore, A., 196, 455
Moore, G. J., 113
Moore, M., 179, 195
Moos, R., 183, 416

Moran, P. B., 388
Morano, C. D., 452
Moreau, D., 19, 131, 288, 296, 298, 384
Morgan, S, 474
Morin, A. J. S., 91
Moritz, G., 478
Morrison, M., 84
Morrow, J., 191
Mors, O., 382
Morse, J. Q., 447
Mortiz, G., 229
Moskos, M., 443
Moskowitz, D. S., 268
Moskowitz, J. T., 254, 273
Mosley, J. E., 392
Moss, H. A., 16
Moss, S., 7, 311, 382
Moye Skuban, E., 392
Mrakotsky, C., 7
Mrazek, P. J., 299, 333
Mufson, L., 17, 229, 288, 290, 296, 298, 299, 300, 303
Muller, N., 312, 354, 384, 398
Mullins, L., 183, 227, 228
Mumme, D. L., 150
Munroe-Blum, H., 230
Muraven, M., 157
Muris, P., 157, 340
Murphy, S. L., 441
Murray, C. J. L., 21
Murray, H. A, 255
Murray, K., 19, 155, 392, 417
Murray, L., 429
Murray, R., 153, 427
Mustillo, S., 9, 16, 229, 384
Myers, D. G., 268

N

Nada Raja, S., 343
Najavits, L., 180
Najman, J. M., 20
Nakamura, J., 266
Navalta, C. P., 112, 113
Navarro, A. M., 252
Nawrocki, T., 165, 423
Neale, M., 18, 20, 126, 127, 132, 139, 153, 392, 417
Nearing, G., 430
Neiderhiser, J. M., 132

Neill, J. T., 362
Nelson, B., 20
Nelson, C., 9, 14
Nelson, C. A., 105
Nelson, C. B., 9
Nelson, E. E., 66
Nelson, S., 59
Nemeroff, C. B., 116, 419, 477, 479
Nesse, R. M., 252, 277
Nestler, E. J., 19, 108, 109, 113
Neuberg, S. L., 251–252
Neuman, G., 89, 164
Newman, D. L., 9, 12, 14, 17, 153, 384, 392
Newport, D. J, 479
Nezu, A., 180
Nezu, C., 180
Ng-Mak, D. S., 480
Nichols, R. C., 419
Nisbett, R. E., 261
Nissinen, A., 254
Nitschke, J. B., 107, 160, 165, 166
Noam, G. G., 109
Nock, M. K., 448, 449
Nolan, C. L., 111
Nolan, S. A., 83, 85
Nolen-Hoeksema, S., 14, 18, 35, 36, 37, 38, 40, 41, 51, 52, 55, 56, 57, 82, 87, 90, 155, 156, 157, 191, 259, 311, 340, 377, 378, 384, 390, 391, 394, 395
Nomura, Y., 229
Norem, J., 274
Nottelmann, E., 15, 393, 421, 425
Nozik, R., 267

O

Oakes, L. M., 52
Oates, R. K., 469
Oberklaid, F., 153
O'Brien, C., 261
Obrosky, D., 7, 179, 382, 386
O'Connell, D., 214
O'Connor, T., 132, 137, 392
Offord, D. R., 3, 12, 14, 333, 424
O'Hara, M. W., 429
O'Hare, E., 89, 164
Oishi, S., 235
Oland, A. A., 168
Olfson, M., 19, 21, 131, 382, 384
Olin, S. S., 288

Olinger, L. J., 64
Olino, T. M., 162
Oliver, J. M., 64
Ollendick, T. H., 252
Olson, J., 476, 479
Olson, L., 443
Orbach, I., 445
Orlinsky, D. E., 261
Orvaschel, H., 416
Osterling, J., 165
Ostir, G. V., 254
O'Sullivan, C., 20
O'Toole, B. I., 469
Owen, M. J., 19, 20
Owens, M. J., 477

P

Paikoff, R., 229, 384, 393
Pakiz, B., 11, 14, 18, 20, 384
Palmour, R. M., 112
Panagiotides, H., 165, 420
Panak, W., 38, 41, 68, 82, 85, 183, 318, 391
Papillon, M., 388
Paradis, A. D., 9
Parducci, A., 277
Pargament, K. I., 268
Parides, M., 452
Park, N., 260, 265, 355
Parker, G., 114, 183, 385
Parker, L. E., 259
Parkhurst, J. T., 450
Parkinson, C., 38, 39, 42, 43
Parks, A. C., 269
Pastorelli, C., 390
Pattison, C., 320, 337
Patton, G., 343
Patton, K., 321, 325
Paulauskas, S. L., 14
Paulus, M. P., 299
Paus, T., 479
Pavot, W., 277
Paykel, E. S., 289
Payne, A. V. L., 39, 48, 49, 50
Payne, M. E., 109
Pedlow, R., 153
Peeke, L. A., 384
Peeke, L. G., 86, 391
Peet, M., 135

Penza, S., 169
Penza-Clyve, S., 392
Perel, J., 393
Perper, J. A., 229
Perrin, S., 15
Perrot-Sinal, T. S., 479
Perry, D. G., 85
Persons, J., 63, 180
Pesonen, A. K., 424
Petersen, A. C., 14, 83, 327, 340, 384, 395
Peterson, B. E., 268
Peterson, C., 260, 263, 265, 276
Peterson, L., 82, 183, 225, 227
Petit, J. W., 53
Petti, T. A., 213
Pettit, G. S., 386
Pettit, J. W., 7
Pevalin, D. J., 384
Pezawas, L., 13. 14, 16, 66
Pfeffer, C. R., 441, 442, 443, 451, 453, 454, 457
Pfeiffer, S. I., 328
Phelps, M. E., 420
Phillips, B. M., 392
Phillips, D. I., 127
Phillips, G., 252
Phillips, N. K., 20
Phillips, R. S. C., 227
Phillips, S. D., 21
Piacentini, J., 455
Piaget, J., 311
Pickens, J., 165, 423
Pickles, A., 8, 17, 214, 383, 389, 392–393, 399, 427
Pihl, R., 104, 107
Pike, A., 137
Pilkington, N. W., 450
Pine, D. S., 9, 16, 17, 18, 66, 160, 299, 385
Pizzagalli, D., 107, 160, 165, 166
Plancherel, B., 157
Plante, T. G., 252
Platt, R., 455
Plomin, R., 19, 125, 126, 127, 128, 131, 132, 133, 137, 417, 419
Plotsky, P. M., 116, 419, 477
Plummer, C. M., 392
Plutchik, R., 444
Podorefsky, D., 425
Poling, K, 184, 196
Pollack, S. L., 58
Pollak, S. D., 169

Pollard, J. A., 365
Pomerantz, E. M., 86
Ponton, L. E., 448
Porges, S. W., 166
Porter, C. L., 424
Porto, M., 419
Posner, M. I., 162
Pössel, P., 334, 335
Post, R. M., 480
Potthoff, J. G., 86
Potvin, P., 388
Poulin, F., 82, 343
Poulton, R., 214
Powers, B., 85
Powers, J. L., 474
Powers, T. A., 58
Poznanski, E. O., 213, 225
Prescott, C., 19, 20, 116, 392, 416, 417, 479, 480
Preskorn, S. H., 213
Presnell, K., 384
Price, J. M., 47
Price, R. H., 361
Priel, B., 44, 46, 64, 65
Prieto, S., 182
Primavera, J., 365
Prinstein, M., 38, 41, 82, 83, 84, 85, 87, 90, 91, 389, 391, 448, 449
Prior, M., 153
Proffitt, V., 197
Provost, M. A., 343
Prusoff, B. A., 19
Puig-Antich, J., 83, 84, 213, 225, 227, 229, 288, 289, 343
Purcell, S., 139
Puska, P., 254
Putnam, K., 107, 160, 165, 169

Q

Quayle, D., 320, 337, 360, 368
Quiggle, N. L., 68, 82, 318, 391
Quinlan, D. M., 388
Quitkin, F. M., 398

R

Rabin, B., 393
Rabinovich, H., 382

Racoosin, J, 219
Radke-Yarrow, M., 229, 416, 420, 421, 423, 425
Radloff, L. S., 253, 272
Rae, D. S., 9
Ragan, J., 85, 229
Raichle, M. E., 109
Raikkonen, K., 424
Rainer, K. L., 91
Raja, S. N., 9
Rajab, M. H., 452, 455
Rajkowska, G., 109
Ram, A., 480
Ramsay, J. O., 382, 383
Randall, P., 85, 229
Rao, U., 3, 20, 87
Rapaport, M. H., 299
Rapee, R., 183
Rappaport, S., 169
Rashid, T., 269, 270, 271, 272
Rasmussen, N. H., 260
Rathus, J. H., 447, 455, 456
Ray, J. S., 229
Reaven, N. M., 82, 225, 227
Rebert, C, 477
Rebgetz, M., 84
Rebok, G. W., 361
Reddy, L. A., 328
Reeder, G. D., 328
Regier, D. A., 9
Rehm, L. P., 229
Reich, T., 3
Reid, J. C., 7, 213, 451
Reinecke, M., 179, 180, 181, 182, 184, 185, 195, 198, 199, 200, 338
Reinherz, H. Z., 9, 11, 14, 18, 20, 299, 384, 385, 470
Reiss, D., 132, 133, 137, 417
Reith, D. M., 444
Reivich, K., 340
Reivich, K. J., 254, 309, 318, 319, 320, 321, 324, 337, 361, 368, 428
Reivich, K. R., 323, 324
Renaud, J., 449
Rende, R., 17–18, 133, 417
Renshaw, P. F., 109
Repetti, R. L., 82
Resch, N. L., 365
Resnick, H. S., 472
Resnick, M., 343, 444
Ressler, K. J., 419

Retzlaff, P. J., 253
Reus, V. I., 127
Reynolds, W., 195, 458
Rhodes, M. E., 379
Rholes, W. S., 51–52, 63
Rice, F., 18, 131, 132, 133, 134, 137
Rich, A. L., 450
Richards, C., 179
Richards, G. E., 362
Richards, J. M., 158
Richardson, A. S, 474
Richardson, D. T., 423
Ridder, E. M., 17
Riddle, M. A., 210
Ridley-Johnson, R., 183, 227
Rijsdijk, F., 66, 128, 133, 137
Riley, A. W., 429
Riley, B., 116
Rind, B., 390
Ringle, J. L., 452
Riniti, J., 84, 416
Riskind, J. H., 63
Rivara, F. P., 457
Roberts, B. W., 53, 153, 162
Roberts, C., 320, 337, 360, 450
Roberts, J. E., 38, 41, 48, 390
Roberts, R., 3, 7, 9, 83, 179, 382, 384, 450
Robins, C. J., 392, 447
Robins, M., 185
Robinson, J. L., 379
Robinson, N. S., 38, 41, 48, 68, 83, 476
Rochon, A., 42, 49, 94, 311, 390
Rodriguez, R. A., 474
Roeger, L., 338, 474
Roelofs, J., 157
Roesch, L., 38, 40, 41, 42, 43, 57, 86, 388
Rogers, C. R., 256, 262
Rogers, G., 180, 181
Rogosch, F. A., 311, 377, 421, 422, 430
Rohde, P., 15, 16, 20, 36, 38, 40, 41, 42, 57, 85, 86, 93, 153, 185, 196, 197, 288, 358, 385, 386
Rojas, M., 458
Rokeach, M., 256
Ronfeld, R. A., 398
Ronnestad, M. H., 261
Rosado, J., 474
Rose, A., 90, 91, 92, 380, 391, 398
Rose, D. T., 49, 57, 58, 475
Rose, G., 334
Rosenbaum, J. F., 175

Rosenberg, D. R., 113
Rosenberg, T. K., 7
Rosenthal, P. A., 442, 447, 449, 450, 451
Rosenthal, S., 442, 447, 449, 450, 451
Ross, L., 90
Ross, R. R., 474
Rosselló, J., 196, 298, 299, 303
Rossman, B. R., 228
Rosso, I. M., 109
Roth, C., 229
Roth, J. L., 354, 355, 356, 357, 358, 361
Rothbart, M. K., 55, 152, 155, 162
Rotheram-Borus, M. J., 454, 455
Rothwell, J., 455
Rouleau, M., 445
Rouse, L. W., 333
Rousseau, C., 455
Rowe, D., 133, 137, 392
Rowe, R., 383
Rowling, L., 338
Roy, A., 20
Roysamb, E., 450
Royzman, E. B., 252
Rozin, P., 252, 268
Rubenowitz, E., 450
Rubin, R. T., 379
Ruble, D. N., 228, 229, 379, 380, 381
Rudd, M. D., 55, 443, 444, 445, 448, 452, 453, 455, 456, 458
Rude, S. S., 64
Rudolph, K. D., 3, 51, 57, 67, 81, 82, 83, 84, 85, 86, 87, 89, 90, 91, 92, 94, 95, 183, 380, 388, 389, 391, 398, 480
Rueter, M. A., 116
Ruggiero, K. J., 473
Ruini, C., 257
Rumzek, H., 443
Ruscio, A. M., 7
Ruscio, J., 7, 8
Rush, A. J., 263, 340, 397, 421, 455
Rush, J., 225
Russell, B., 255
Rutter, M., 3, 8, 13, 16, 17, 18, 139, 207, 214, 339, 355, 378, 386, 390, 392–393, 399, 422, 427, 468
Ryan, J. A. M., 354
Ryan, N., 7, 20, 112, 131, 179, 210, 213, 215, 216, 289, 393
Ryan, R. M., 256
Rydell, A.-M., 167
Ryff, C. D., 252, 253, 254, 256, 260

S

Saarni, C., 163
Sabbath, J. C., 450
Sacco, W. P., 227
Sachs-Ericsson, N. J., 447
Sack, W., 15, 68
Sacks, N., 18
Sakellaropoulo, M., 44, 45, 56, 64
Salcedo, V., 257
Salomaa, V., 254
Salt, P., 338
Saltzman, H., 82
Salzinger, S., 480
Sameroff, A. J., 417, 422, 423, 424
Sanborn, K., 92, 384, 394
Sanchez, M. M., 419
Sander, J. B., 229
Sanders, M. R., 84, 429, 430
Sanders-Phillips, K, 474
Sandler, I. N., 338
Sandvik, E., 277
Sanford, M., 230
Sanson, A., 153
Santor, D. A., 382, 383
Sapolsky, R. M., 47, 477, 478
Sargeant, M., 388
Sargent, J., 343
Sargrestano, L. M., 229
Sarigiani, P. A., 14, 327, 384
Sarin, S., 38, 39, 47, 49, 50, 55
Saron, C., 420
Saunders, B. E, 472
Sayer, A. G., 399
Scales, P. C., 370
Scannell, E. D., 386
Scaramella, L., 116
Scarr, S., 136
Sceery, A., 88
Schaefer, E. S., 476
Schall, J. D., 105
Scheffler, P., 50
Schepis, T. S., 20
Scher, C. D., 63
Schkade, D., 265
Schloredt, K., 429
Schmidt, H., 340
Schmidt, K., 225
Schmidt, N. B., 456
Schmitz, S., 379
Schneider, L. S., 289

Schnoebelen, S., 227
Schoenwald, S. K., 325
Schouten, E. G., 254
Schraedley, P. K., 384, 385, 468, 470, 471, 474
Schrepferman, L., 421
Schul, Y., 361
Schulman, P., 428
Schulsinger, F., 415
Schultz, L. H., 425
Schulz, R., 277
Schulze, C. C., 290
Schwartz, B., 268, 273, 277
Schwartz, J. A., 157, 390
Schwartz, S. H., 256
Scott, K. G., 334
Scourfield, J., 19, 132, 133, 137, 417
Seeley, J., 3, 7, 8, 9, 15, 16, 20, 36, 57, 67, 68, 85, 86, 87, 153, 179, 196, 197, 288, 299, 310, 358, 382, 384, 385, 386
Seeman, M., 394
Segal, Z. V., 36, 63, 479
Segrin, C., 86
Seidlitz, L., 391
Seifer, R., 423
Seiffge-Krenke, I., 395
Seimyr, L., 424
Seiner, S. A., 430
Seligman, M. E. P., 36, 37, 38, 39, 50, 53, 58, 63, 64, 82, 142, 251, 252, 255, 258, 259, 260, 262, 263, 265, 266, 268, 269, 270, 271, 274, 276, 309, 311, 318, 319, 320, 323, 324, 337, 340, 355, 356, 360, 361, 368, 423, 428
Seligman, M. P., 154, 157
Selman, R. L., 425
Senulis, R., 420
Seroczynski, A. D., 86, 384, 391
Serrano, A. C., 326
Shadish, W. R., 252
Shaffer, D., 11, 179, 215, 217, 441, 442, 443, 449, 451, 452, 453, 454, 457, 458
Shaffery, J., 19
Shahar, G., 44, 46, 64, 65
Sham, P. C., 138
Shankman, S.A., 9
Shanley, N., 59
Shapiro, J. R., 161, 162, 450, 453
Shapiro, S. L., 262
Sharma, A. R., 370
Sharpe, K. E., 273

Shatté, A. J., 310, 319
Shaw, B. F., 225, 263, 340, 421, 455
Shaw, D. S., 168
Shaw, J. A, 474
Shea, E., 163
Shea, M. T., 159, 397
Shear, K., 378, 380, 395
Sheeber, L., 82, 83, 84, 85–86, 87, 91, 229, 230, 289, 389, 421, 425
Sheffield, J., 38, 41, 335, 336, 337, 340, 358, 361
Shekim, W. O., 213
Sheldon, K. M., 256, 265
Sherbourne, C. D., 268
Sherick, R. B., 52, 86, 227, 445
Sherman, L., 421
Sherman, T., 229, 425
Sherrill, J., 7, 382, 386
Sherrod, L. R., 355
Shields, A., 169, 480
Shih, J., 20, 67, 82, 388, 389, 390, 391
Shih, R. A., 19
Shihfen, T., 334
Shiner, R. L., 53, 55, 152
Shipman, K., 149, 169, 379, 392
Shirk, S. R., 52, 88
Shirtcliff, E. A., 378
Shneidman, E., 445
Shnit, D., 480
Shochet, I. M., 325, 334, 335, 338, 360
Shoebridge, P., 195
Shortt, J. W., 421
Shuman, D. W., 466
Shwartz, J. A. J., 36, 42, 43
Sibthrop, J., 362
Siegel, A. W., 58
Siegel, J. M., 384
Siemer, M., 154
Siever, L. J., 422
Silberg, J., 17, 18, 21, 132, 133, 137, 139, 384, 392, 393, 417
Siler, M., 38, 142
Silk, J. S., 157, 168
Silk, K. R., 169
Sills, M. R., 457
Silva, P. A., 9, 12, 14, 16, 17, 153, 310, 386, 392
Silva, S., 198
Silver, T., 309
Silverman, A. B., 11, 470, 471
Silverman, J. M., 422
Silverman, M. M., 442

Silverstein, B., 382
Simeon, J. G., 214
Simien, C., 116
Siminoff, E., 392
Simmons, R. G., 92
Simon, V. A., 82, 389
Simonds, J. F., 9, 10
Simonoff, E., 11, 15, 392–393
Simons, A., 36, 181, 338, 422
Simons, R. L., 91, 384
Simpson, J., 227, 230
Simpson, T. L, 466, 467
Sines, J. O., 19, 417
Singer, B., 252, 254, 256, 260
Sinha, R., 397
Sirota, P., 445
Skitch, S. A., 39, 41, 42, 44, 45, 48, 50, 61, 389
Skuban, E. M., 168
Skuse, D. S., 141
Slade, T., 7
Slavin, L. A., 91
Sloan, D., 255
Sloane, R. B., 289
Smailes, E. M., 472
Smailes, M., 447
Smart, J. J. C., 276
Smider, N. A., 393, 427
Smith, C. A., 470
Smith, C. L., 163
Smith, D. A., 389
Smith, K. D., 164, 169, 392
Smith, M. L., 322
Smith, N. K., 252
Smith, S., 104
Snidman, N., 424
Snyder, C. R., 257, 260
Snyder, J., 421
Sofuoglu, S., 111
Solomon, A., 8, 299
Solomon, R. L., 447
Sommerfeld, B. K., 420
Song, J., 455
Sonis, W. A., 326
Sonkowsky, M., 364
Soong, W. T., 13
Sorensen, E., 82, 83, 84, 229
Sorensen, M. J., 382
Southall, D., 38, 41, 48
Southam-Gerow, M., 166, 184
Sowell, E. R., 163

Sparkes, S., 113
Spence, S., 38, 41, 180, 181, 184, 227, 335, 337, 339, 340, 343, 358, 360, 368
Spieker, S., 420
Spinner, M., 230
Spinrad, T. L., 164, 380
Spirito, A., 446, 455
Srivastava, S., 152
Sroufe, A., 16
Sroufe, L. A., 88, 164, 389, 421
Stader, S., 289
Stahl, S. M., 210
Staley, J. E., 18
Stanger, C., 3
Stanton, A. K., 9
Stanton, W. R., 343
Stapes, F. R., 289
Stark, K., 184, 195, 225, 227, 229, 230, 243, 244, 333, 397
Starrs, C., 38, 39, 42, 43, 67
Stashwick, C. K., 9
Stattin, H., 267
Steele, R. G., 82
Steen, T. A., 252, 265
Steer, R. A., 90, 270, 445, 451, 477
Steffens, D. C., 109
Stein, M. B., 106
Steinberg, L., 15, 84, 389
Steinberg, S. J., 92
Steiner, H., 386
Steiner, M., 394
Steingard, R. J., 109, 112, 113
Steinmetz, J. L., 57
Stellrecht, N. E., 452, 454, 456
Stemmler, M., 395
Stevens, E. A., 84, 389
Stevenson, J., 132, 133, 417
Stewart, A. J, 268
Stewart, J. W., 398
Stice, E., 85, 87, 229, 384
Stifter, C. A., 164
Stinson, F. S., 20
Stockhammer, T. F., 480
Stockmeier, C. A., 112
Stolar, M., 15
Stolow, D., 38, 39, 42, 43
Stowe, Z. N., 429
Strakowski, S. M., 108, 109
Strandberg, T., 424
Strauss, C. C., 227
Stravynski, A., 450

Strazdins, L. M., 386
Strober, M., 215, 216
Stuart, S., 429
Stuewig, J, 476
Suarez, A., 447
Sudler. N., 84, 343
Sugden, K., 140
Suh, E., 277
Sullivan, C., 41, 42, 60
Sullivan, H. S., 289
Sullivan, P. F., 18, 19
Sumner, G. S., 212
Sund, A. M., 386
Suomi, S. J., 85
Susman, A., 423
Susman, E., 393
Susser, K., 68
Suveg, C., 149, 169, 392
Swanston, H., 469
Swartz, M., 7, 9, 14
Swearer, S., 225
Sweeney, L., 197
Szatmari, P., 230

T

Tackett, J. L., 117
Tageson, C., 182
Taghizadeh, P., 451
Talbot, L., 63
Tambs, K., 392
Tamres, L. K., 390
Tandon, K., 134
Tapia, M. A., 212
Tapia, M. R., 212
Taska, L., 58, 470, 474, 476
Taub, B., 384
Taxel, E., 44, 45, 56, 64
Taylor, A., 63, 426
Taylor, G., 44, 45, 48, 56, 64, 65, 90
Taylor, J. M., 263
Taylor, L., 63, 182, 416, 424
Taylor, S. E., 379, 395
Teasdale, J., 36, 423
Teasdale, J. D., 63, 142, 262, 479
Teasdale, J. E., 311
Tebbutt, J., 469, 470
Tedeschi, R. G., 273
Tellegen, A., 260, 419
Tennen, H., 273

Terman, L., 255
Terry, M., 318
Teti, D. M., 420, 422, 430
Teti, L. O., 164
Thapar, A., 17, 18, 19, 131, 132, 133, 134, 137, 400, 417
Thase, M., 180, 393, 429
Thomas, A. M., 426
Thomas, K. M., 106, 110
Thomas, L., 338
Thompson, H., 320
Thompson, M., 52
Thompson, P. M., 163
Thompson, R. A., 105, 169, 228
Thomsen, A. H., 82
Thomsen, P. H., 382
Thomson, H., 320
Thornberry, T. P., 470, 471, 472, 474, 479
Thurber, C., 197
Thurm, A. E., 388
Tierney, J. P., 365
Timbremont, B., 63
Tizard, J., 13
Tobin, R. M., 155
Todd, R. D., 109
Toga, A. W., 163
Tomarken, A. J., 116, 420
Tompson, M., 84, 230
Toth, S. L., 7, 86, 164, 168, 421, 422, 430, 466, 469, 475
Toumbourou, J., 338
Towbes, L. C., 157, 388
Trainor, G., 455
Tremaine, L. M., 398
Tromovitch, P., 390
Tronick, E. Z., 163
Troop-Gordon, W., 85
Troutman, B. R., 424
Truax, P., 200
Truglio, R., 85
Tsuang, M. T., 419
Tucker, D. M., 252, 479
Tugade, M. M., 160, 263
Tully, E. C., 416, 425, 426
Tuomilehto, J., 254
Turgeon, L., 82, 343
Turk, E., 59
Turner, J., 47, 51, 52, 55, 65, 225
Turner, L., 164
Turner, S. M., 17
Tutus, A., 111

Tversky, A., 251
Tweed, J. L., 447
Twenge, J. M., 18, 384
Tyano, S., 444

U

Udry, R. J., 379
Underwood, M., 318, 380, 392, 457, 458
Unis, A. S., 52, 445
Uno, H., 477
Usher, B., 393–394

V

Valentiner, D., 83, 476
Valeri, S., 179, 312
Valuck, R. J., 457
Van Beijsterveldt, C. E. M., 132
VandenBos, G., 149
Van den Oord, E. J., 131, 132–133
Vanderbilt, E., 42, 49, 94, 311, 390
Van der Does, A. J. W., 112
Van der Ende, J., 9, 17
Van der Valk, J. C., 132–133
Vandewater, E. A., 392
Van Dulmen, M., 480
Van Etten, M., 168
VanGeest, J., 21
Van Hulle, C. A., 379
Vanmeenen, K., 475
Van Orden, K. A., 450, 456, 458
Van Os, J., 153
Vant, J., 107
Vardi, S., 169
Vartiainen, E., 254
Vazquez, D., 107, 108, 113
Velez, C., 11, 14, 384
Verduyn, C., 184
Verheul, R., 457
Verhulst, F. C., 9, 13, 17, 131, 132–133
Véronneau-McArdle, M., 52, 64
Versage, E., 182–183, 338
Vieland, V., 457, 458
Villafuerte, S. M., 135
Villanueva, M., 253
Vinokur, A. D., 361
Vitaro, F., 82, 91, 343
Vitiello, B., 198

Vittum, J., 116
Voelz, Z. R., 53
Vohs, K. D., 251
Von Eye, A., 393
Vostanis, P., 333
Vuori, J., 361
Vythilingam, M., 478

W

Wachtel, P. L., 258
Wade, T. J., 384
Wadhwa, P. D., 419
Wadlington, S, 474
Wadsworth, M., 82, 153
Waern, M., 450
Wagner, B. M., 388
Wagner, C., 61
Wagner, E. E., 289
Waldman, I., 7, 37, 141, 142
Walker, J., 369
Walker, R. L., 53, 448
Wall, S., 88
Wallace, A. B., 262
Wallace, L. E., 116
Walsh, C, 230
Walsh, V., 362
Walsh-Allis, G., 416
Walters, C., 51–52
Walters, E. E., 7, 9, 10, 14, 20, 21, 288
Wampold, B. E., 252, 261
Wang, Z., 383
Wanner, B., 91
Ward, B., 213
Ward, C., 196, 213
Warren, M., 384, 388, 393
Wasserman, M. S., 11
Waterman, G. S., 213
Waters, E., 88, 421
Watkins, W. G, 474
Watson, D., 152, 153, 160, 162, 260, 383, 400
Watson, S. J., 135
Watts, A., 258
Weaver, G., 269
Webb, C. A., 61
Webster-Stratton, C., 421
Weersing, V., 179
Weinberg, R. A., 356
Weinberger, J., 252
Weiss, B., 7, 52, 59, 68, 157, 228–229, 325, 383

Weiss, J. M, 477
Weissman, A., 457
Weissman, M., 179
Weissman, M. M., 17–18, 19, 131, 229, 288, 289, 298, 299, 384, 441
Weissman, M. W., 416, 428, 429
Weisz, J., 179, 184, 195, 197, 198, 252, 312, 322, 325, 328
Weizman, A., 480
Weller, E., 213
Weller, R., 213
Wells, A. M., 359
Wells, J., 213
Wells, K. B., 268, 299
Wells, V., 10
Welner, A., 416
Welner, Z., 416
Welsh, J. D., 229, 423, 425
Wenzel, A., 429
Weston, D., 445, 455
Wetzler, S., 447
Wheeler, R. E., 420
Whiffen, V. E., 390, 391, 467
Whishaw, I. Q., 226
Whitaker, A., 9, 11, 14, 18
White, B. A., 384
White, G. P., 458
Whitehouse, W. G., 49
Whitman, P. B., 424
Whitmore, K., 13
Whittaker, J., 195
Whyte, I., 444
Wichstrom, L., 381, 386, 391
Wickramaratne, P., 17–18, 19, 131, 229, 290, 298, 299, 303, 384
Widstrom, A. M., 424
Wierzbicki, M., 157, 227
Wild, C. J., 335, 360
Wildes, J., 473
Wilgosh, L., 327
Wilhelm, K., 415
Wilhelmson, K., 450
Willcutt, E. G., 142
William, A., 269
Williams, B. A. O., 276
Williams, F. M., 456
Williams, G. C., 277
Williams, J. M., 479
Williams, L. M., 468, 473, 474
Williams, M., 16
Williams, R. A., 343

Williams, S., 9, 12, 14, 343
Williamson, D. E., 20, 131
Willoughby, M. T., 399
Willutzki, U., 261
Wilner, K. D., 398
Wilson, D., 255
Windle, M., 83, 85, 388, 389, 425, 426
Wingate, L. R., 447, 451, 456
Wittchen, H.-U., 9, 13, 14, 18, 20, 21
Witte, T. K., 456
Wohlfarth, T. D., 457
Wolchik, S. A., 338
Wolfe, D., 476, 479
Wolters, W. H., 446
Wonderlich, S., 159, 227
Woo, S., 84
Wood, A., 184, 196, 455
Woods, K. E., 378
Woodward, L. J., 12, 16, 18
Woody, G., 261
Worthman, C., 14, 114, 384, 393
Wostear, G., 207
Woznica, J. G., 450, 453
Wright, B. A., 252
Wright, C., 83, 184
Wright, E. J., 338
Wrzesniewski, A., 268, 269
Wu, P., 21
Wyn, J., 338

Y

Yang, H. J., 13
Yates, T., 480
Ye, W., 416
Yonkers, K. A., 397

Young, E., 19, 378, 380, 395
Young, J. E., 58, 475
Young, J. F., 288, 299, 300, 303
Young, S., 104, 112
Youngblade, L. M., 88
Yu, D. L., 320, 360
Yue, D. N., 63
Yurgelun-Todd, D., 110

Z

Zahn-Waxler, C., 164, 169, 378, 379, 384,
    385, 392, 393–394, 396, 400, 423
Zammit, S., 19, 20
Zandi, P. P., 19
Zarin, D. A., 382
Zautra, A., 53
Zax, M., 423
Zeiss, A., 299
Zeman, J., 85, 149, 168, 169, 228–229, 379,
    392
Zhao, S., 7
Ziegert, D., 42, 49, 157, 164, 390
Zimerman, B., 16
Zinbarg, J., 15
Zinbarg, R., 68
Zirinsky, L., 445, 455
Zitman, F. G., 254
Ziv, Y., 88
Zlotnick, C., 397
Zrull, J., 225
Zubernis, L. S., 319
Zung, W. W. K., 253, 270
Zupan, B., 51, 182, 424
Zuroff, D. C., 35, 36, 37, 44, 56, 58, 61, 63,
    90, 268, 383, 390

Subject Index

ABC model, 312–314
Abuse
  assessment of, 467–469
  cognitive mediation of relation of
    depression and, 474–477
  contextual factors and, 473–474
  depression in adolescents and, 470–473
  depression in children and, 469–470
  integrated psychobiological developmental
    model of depression and, 481–482
  as negative event, 390
  neurobiology of, 477–479
  overview of, 466–467, 482–483
  sexual, 472, 474
  stress sensitivity and, 479–482
  suicidal behavior and, 449–450
  type of, 473
Across Ages, 364–365, 366
ACTION treatment program
  affective education component, 234–235
  case conceptualization, 232–233
  Catch the Positive Diary (CPD), 236–237
  cognitive restructuring component, 238–243
  coping skills training component, 235–236
  goal setting, 233–234
  objectives by meeting, 231
  objectives by parent meeting, 232
  overview of, 224, 230, 232
  parent training component, 244–246
  problem-solving training component, 237–
    238
  theoretical tenets of, 224–230

Active gene–environment correlations, 136–
  137
Activity scheduling in cognitive-behavioral
  therapy, 189–190
Additive approach to vulnerability factors,
  48–49
Adoption studies
  behavioral genetic designs, 127–128
  results from, 131
Adventure programs, 362–364
Affect, linking with interpersonal events, 294
Affective education in ACTION treatment
  program, 234–235
Affective science, 149
Affective vulnerabilities, 423
Affect regulation
  cognitive-behavioral therapy and, 191
  disturbance in, 228–229
  See also Emotion regulation
Age
  of onset, studies of, 9, 14
  quantitative genetic studies and, 132–133
  symptom expression and, 7
Aggression, 386
Altruistic behavior, 259
Amitriptyline, 209
Amygdala
  primary role of, 107–108
  volume of, 109–110
"AND" rule, 8
Anger expression, 327
Anhedonia, 160

Anterior cingulate cortex and emotion
    regulation, 166
Antidepressant drugs
    classes of, 208–211
    suicidal behavior and, 457
Anxiety disorders
    comorbidity of, 15
    continuity/course and, 17–18
    emotion regulation and, 169
    sex differences and, 385
    social anxiety, 106
Assertiveness, 316–317
Assessment
    of abuse and neglect, 467–469
    challenges of, 8
    in interpersonal therapy for adolescents
        (IPT-A), 292–293
    possibility of sex bias in, 382–383
    of suicide risk, 451–453
Association studies
    findings of, 134–135
    molecular genetic designs, 130–131
Assortative mating, 127
Attachment and interpersonal vulnerability,
    88–89
Attention, reeducating, 274–275
Attributional style
    cognitive-behavioral therapy and, 182
    developmental hypothesis and, 52
    maltreatment and, 475–477
    sex differences and, 390
    as stress–diathesis model, 142
Automatic thoughts, 191–192, 226

B

Beck's cognitive theory
    developmental stage and, 51
    maltreatment and, 475
    overview of, 38, 41, 42
    parenting practices and, 58
Beck's cognitive therapy, 185–186
Behavioral disturbances, 227–228
Behavioral genetic approaches
    intermediate phenotypes and, 140–143
    molecular genetic methodology, 128–131
    overview of, 124–125
    quantitative genetic methodology, 125–128
Behavioral vulnerabilities, 423

Beliefs
    in cognitive-behavioral therapy, 181
    intermediate, 225–226
    See also Core beliefs about self
Belongingness, thwarted, 450, 452–453
beyondblue schools research initiative
    overview of, 338
    protective school environment, building,
        343–349
    rationale and content of, 339
    skills taught by year level, 341–342
    strengths, building, 340, 342
Big Brothers and Big Sisters Program, 365, 367
Biochemical disturbances, 226–227
Bioevolutionary theory, 395
Biological factors
    as correlates, 19–20
    maternal depression and, 417, 419–422
    sex differences in, 378–379, 392–394
Biological vulnerability
    emergence and onset of, 115–116
    integrative framework for, 116–118
    methodological and conceptual issues, 104–
        106
    neurochemical contributions to, 111–114
    normative neurodevelopment and
        functioning, 106–108
    overview of, 103–104
    structural imaging findings, 108–110
Black-box warning, 218–219
Borderline personality disorder
    emotion regulation and, 169
    suicidal behavior and, 447
Brain development, abnormal, 420
Brain imaging techniques
    biological vulnerability and, 104–105
    findings from, 108–110
Bupropion, 211
Burdensomeness, perceived, 450–451, 452–
    453

C

Candidate gene approach
    association studies, 130–131
    gene–environment interactions, 139–140
    molecular genetic studies, 134–135
Caregiver influences on emotion regulation,
    163–164

Catastrophic thinking, 315–316
Catch the Positive Diary (CPD), 236–237, 243
Categorical approach, 7–8
Causal factors
    neurobiological studies and, 105
    sex differences, 386–388
CBT. See Cognitive-behavioral therapy (CBT)
Child–Adolescent Suicide Potential Index, 451
Childhood Depression Rating Scale, 213
Childhood Experience of Care and Abuse
    interview, 468–469
Children's Attributional Style Questionnaire,
    52
Children's Perceptions of Parental Sadness
    Scale, 425–426
Choline, 112–113
Citalopram, 210, 216
Clinical management, 208
Clomipramine, 209
Cognitive-behavioral analysis system of
    psychotherapy, 456
Cognitive-behavioral theories, 311
Cognitive-behavioral therapy (CBT)
    activity scheduling in, 189–190
    adaptive counter-thoughts, developing, 192–
        194
    affect regulation and, 191
    automatic thoughts, cognitive distortions,
        and, 191–192
    behavioral targets of, 183
    characteristics of, 180–181
    cognitive targets of, 183
    combining with psychopharmacology, 219–
        220, 227
    effectiveness of, 194–199
    goal of, 184
    goal setting and, 188
    homework in, 188
    interventions, 186
    mood monitoring in, 188–189, 192
    overview of, 179–180, 311–312
    in practice, specific strategies, 185–187
    problem-solving skills and, 190–191
    protocols for children and adolescents, 184–
        185
    psychoeducation, 187
    recommendations for, 200–201
    relaxation training and, 194
    shortcomings and limitations of research on,
        199–200

    social interaction and, 190
    for suicidal behavior, 455–456
    taking stock, relapse prevention, and, 194
    therapeutic relationship in, 187–188
    vulnerability factors and, 181–184
    See also ACTION treatment program
Cognitive biases, 142–143
Cognitive distortions, 191–192, 225–226
Cognitive mediation of relation of abuse and
    neglect to depression, 474–477
Cognitive restructuring in ACTION treatment
    program
    negative thoughts, identifying, 241
    positive sense of self, building, 243
    rationale for, establishing, 239–240
    relationship between thoughts and moods,
        establishing, 238–239
    strategies for, 241–243
Cognitive restructuring in Penn Resiliency
    Program (PRP), 315
Cognitive styles, recognizing, 314, 476–477
Cognitive theory, Beck's
    developmental stage and, 51
    maltreatment and, 475
    overview of, 38, 41, 42
    parenting practices and, 58
Cognitive therapy, Beck's, 185–186
Cognitive vulnerability
    additive approach, 48–49
    Beck's cognitive theory and, 38, 41, 42
    developmental changes in interrelation
        among factors, 55
    developmental changes in levels of, 55–56
    developmental origins of, 56–59
    developmental stage and, 51–53
    emergence and consolidation of
        vulnerability factors, 51
    empirical status of theories, 44, 46–47
    future research on, 65–68
    hopelessness theory and, 37–38, 39–41, 46
    maternal depression and, 423–424, 425
    multiplicative approach, 48
    nomothetic versus idiographic approaches
        to analysis, 59–63
    overview of, 35–36
    personality predispositions and, 44, 45–46
    priming of factors, 63
    relationships between factors in, 47–51
    response styles theory and, 41–43
    sex differences and, 390–391

Cognitive vulnerability *(cont.)*
   specific content domains and, 63–65
   theory and evidence, 36–37
   trait-like risk factors and, 53–54
   weakest link approach, 49–51
Cognitive vulnerability–transactional stress
   theory, 67, 395–396
Combined trait/contextual model, 53, 54
Commitment to treatment statements, 453–
   454
Common cause model, 159
Communication analysis, 294
Communication skills
   in interpersonal therapy for adolescents
     (IPT-AST), 301–302
   parent–child, 244–245, 455
Community forums, 249
Community studies, 384
Comorbidity
   cognitive vulnerability and, 67–68
   concurrent and lifetime, 15–16
   maternal depression and, 416
   sex differences and, 385–386, 400
   social anxiety, 106
Competence, definition of, 355
Competence-based model, 85
Complete mental health, 253
Compliance, excessive, 392, 396–397
Complication model, 159
Concomitants model, 159
Concurrent comorbidity, 15–16
Conditional assumptions, 226
Conduct disorder
   comorbidity of, 15
   continuity/course and, 18
   suicidal behavior and, 449
Conflict resolution skills, 245
Consequences of depression
   gender and, 91
   interpersonal dysfunction as, 86–87
   overview of, 20–21
   short- and long-term, 94–95
Context of maternal depression, 426–427,
   429–430
Contextual/autoregressive model, 53, 54
Continuity/course
   heterotypic, 16, 17–18, 378, 383
   homotypic, 16–17, 378, 383
   need for research in, 22, 23
Contract for treatment, 293, 453–454
Contrasting Coaches analogy, 193

Coping skills training in ACTION treatment
   program, 235–236
Coping with Depression course, 186
Core beliefs about self
   case conceptualization and, 232–233
   dysfunctional, 225–226
   positive, building, 243
Cortisol levels
   emotion regulation and, 166
   sex differences and, 393
Counter-thoughts, 192–194
Creatine, 112–113
Crisis card, creation of, 454
Crisis hotlines, 456
Crisis intervention for suicidal behavior, 453–
   454
Culture
   as correlate, 18
   Eastern, 261–262
   Western, 261–262, 278, 380
Cytochromes, 209

D

DBT (dialectical behavior therapy), 447, 456–
   457
DEAL acronym for assertiveness, 317
Decatastrophizing, 315–316
Decision analysis, 295
Deficits, interpersonal, 297
Dependency/sociotropy
   cognitive vulnerability and, 44, 64
   interpersonal theories and, 79, 90
Depression, definitions of, 6–7, 106, 310. *See
   also* Early-onset depression; Maternal
   depression
Depression contagion model, 389
Depressive disorders, prevalence estimates of,
   9, 10–13
Desipramine, 209
Developmental assets model, 370
Developmental group psychotherapy, 455
Developmental intentionality theory, 369–370
Developmental issues
   in cognitive vulnerability to depression, 51–
     59
   in emotion regulation, 161–163
   interpersonal antecedents and consequences
     of depression, 95
   in interpersonal theories, 81

moderators of interpersonal dysfunction and depression, 95
quantitative genetic studies and, 132–133
typical sex differences, 378–381
Developmental psychopathological approach, 377–378, 399–400
Developmental timeline for emergence of sex differences in depression, 381–386
Developmental transitions and interpersonal theories, 79, 91–93
Diagnosis, confirming, 291
Diagnostic interviews, challenges of, 8
Dialectical behavior therapy (DBT), 447, 456–457
Diathesis–stress models
  attributional style and, 142
  Beck's cognitive theory and, 38, 41, 42
  cognitive-behavioral therapy and, 182, 184
  empirical status of theories, 44, 46–47
  hopelessness theory and, 37–38, 39–41
  idiographic approach to analysis of, 61–63
  nomothetic approach to analysis of, 59–63
  overview of, 35–36
  typical study examining, 60
  underlying assumptions of, 67
  See also Vulnerability–stress models
Dimensional approach, 7–8
Disinhibition, 392
Dispositional emotion regulation, 157–158
Distracting responses to symptoms of depression, 42
Dizygotic (DZ) twins, 126
Documented reports of abuse and neglect, 467
Dorsolateral prefrontal cortex, 107
"Downward arrow" technique, 232–233
Duration of depressive episode, 179
Dysthymic disorder, prevalence estimates of, 9

E

Early family disruption, 79, 87–89, 94
Early-onset depression
  as chronic disorder, 3
  cognitive-behavioral therapy and, 199–201
  continuity/course and, 17
Eastern therapeutic traditions, 261–262
Eating disorders, 386
Ecological models of mental health, 338
Ecstasy, seeking, 277

EEG (electroencephalographic) recordings
  biological vulnerabilities and, 115–116
  emotion regulation and, 165
  of frontal activation, 420
Efficacy studies
  of interpersonal therapy for adolescents (IPT-A), 298–299
  of interpersonal therapy for adolescents (IPT-AST), 303
  of Penn Resiliency Program (PRP), 318–325
  of positive youth development (PYD) programs, 356–359
  of prevention programs, 334–337, 359–361
Efficacy studies of psychopharmacological treatment
  methodological issues, 212–213
  overview of, 211–212
  of selective serotonin reuptake inhibitors (SSRIs), 214–216
  tricyclic antidepressants (TCAs), 213–214
Effortful control, 155–156
Egocentrism and cognitive vulnerability, 59
Ego control, 155
Ego resiliency, 155–156
Electrical convulsive therapy, 103
Electroencephalographic (EEG) recordings
  biological vulnerabilities and, 115–116
  emotion regulation and, 165
  of frontal activation, 420
Emotional abuse, 473, 475
Emotional development, sex differences in, 379–380
Emotional dysregulation, 446–447
Emotion regulation
  caregiver influences on, 163–164
  clarifying construct of, 150–151
  developmental models of, 161–162
  development of, 162–163
  distinctions between emotion, temperament, and, 152–156
  empirical findings regarding, 166–168
  gender differences in, 164–165
  maternal depression and, 168–169
  measurement issues in, 151–152
  neural and physiological correlates of, 165–166
  overview of, 149–150
  positive emotions, 160–161
  risk factors and, 169
  sex differences in, 392, 396–397

Emotion regulation *(cont.)*
  specific constructs linked to depression,
    155–158
  theoretical perspectives on role of in
    depression, 158–160
  See also Affect regulation; Positive emotions
Empathic listening, 245
Empathy, excessive, 392, 396–397
Endophenotypes, 140–142
The engaged life, 266–268
Environment
  family, disturbances in, 229–230
  gene–environment correlations, 136–137
  gene–environment interactions, 138–140
  invalidating, 447
  nonshared and shared factors in, 125
  social, and response styles theory, 143
Epidemiological literature, review of, 6–8
Equifinality, 422
Escape theory of suicidal behavior, 446
Ethnicity
  association studies and, 130–131
  as correlate, 18
  sex differences and, 384–385
  suicidal behavior and, 443
  treatment and, 21
Etiology
  of depression in children and adolescents,
    417–427
  integrative model of, 117–118
  need for research in, 22–23
  research on, 4
Evocative gene–environment correlations, 136, 137
Expectations, reeducating, 274–275
Expendable child, 450
Expendable Child Measure, 453
Explanatory style, pessimistic, 311
Exposure to stress. *See* Stress, exposure to
Externalizing disorders
  emotion regulation and, 169
  sex differences and, 386
  See also Conduct disorder
Extreme scoring individuals and quantitative
    genetic studies, 133–134

F

Familial factors
  as correlates, 18–19
  early family disruption, 79, 87–89, 94

emotion regulation and, 163–164
gene–environment correlations and, 137
Penn Resiliency Program (PRP) and, 326
See also Genetic influences; Maternal
    depression
Family
  environment of, disturbances in, 229–230
  gene–environment interactions and, 138–
    139
  interventions targeting, and maternal
    depression, 430–431
  relationships with, disturbances in, 83–84
  role disputes and, 296
  support of, and suicidal behavior, 450, 452–
    453, 454
Family communication and problem solving
    therapy, 455
Family studies
  behavioral genetic designs, 125–126
  results from, 131
Fathers and maternal depression, 426
Flourishing, 253
Flow, 266
Fluoxetine, 210, 214–215, 216, 227
Fluvoxamine, 210
FMRI (functional magnetic resonance
    imaging), 104, 105, 110–111
Food and Drug Administration (FDA)
    assessment of SSRIs, 218–219
Fordyce Happiness Survey, 256
Friendship quality, 83
Frontal lobe and emotion regulation, 165
The full life, 269
Functional magnetic resonance imaging
    (fMRI), 104, 105, 110–111

G

Gatekeeper training, 457
Gender
  emotion regulation and, 164–165
  hormonal influences and, 114
  interpersonal theories and, 79, 92–93
  maternal depression and, 425
  Penn Resiliency Program (PRP) and, 326–
    327
  sexual abuse and, 474
  vulnerability–stress models and, 90–91
  See also Sex differences
Gene–environment correlations, 136–137

Gene–environment interactions, 138–140
Genetic influences
    maternal depression and, 417, 419
    overview of, 18–19
    sex differences in heritability, 392–393
Girls in Transition program, 327
Glucocorticoid hypersecretion, 477
Glutamate, 112–113
Goal setting
    ACTION treatment program and, 233–
        234
    cognitive-behavioral therapy and, 188
Gray matter maturational pruning, 106–107
Grief, 296
Guided discovery, 191–192
Guided learning experiences, 242–243

H

Happiness
    components of, 263
    the engaged life, 266–268
    the full life, 269
    material possessions and, 276–277
    the meaningful life, 268–269
    the pleasant life, 263, 265
    pursuit of, 251–254
    theoretical notions of, 255–258
Heritability. See Genetic influences
Heterotypic continuity
    definition of, 16, 378
    evidence for, 17–18
    sex differences and, 383
High-risk paradigm, 415
Hippocampus
    emotion regulation and, 165–166
    maltreatment and, 477–479
    primary role of, 107–108
    stress response and, 19
    volume of, 109–110
Hispanic youth and suicidal behavior, 443
Homework assignment
    in cognitive-behavioral therapy, 181, 188
    in interpersonal therapy for adolescents
        (IPT-A), 295
Homotypic continuity
    definition of, 378
    evidence for, 16–17
    sex differences and, 383
Hope enhancement strategies, 257

Hopelessness theory
    additive approach to vulnerability factors
        and, 48–49
    attributional style and, 142
    developmental stage and, 51–52
    maltreatment and, 57–58, 475
    overview of, 37–38, 39–41
    parenting practices and, 58
    studies of, 46
    of suicide, 445
    weakest link hypothesis and, 50
Hormonal influences
    maternal depression and, 419
    sex differences and, 114, 393
Hot Seat skill, 316
Human nature, views of, 258–259
Hypothalamic–pituitary–adrenal (HPA) axis
    child abuse and neglect and, 477–479
    cortisol levels and, 166
    description of, 19–20
    hormones and, 379
    maternal depression and, 419

I

Idiographic approach to analysis, 61–63
Imaging techniques
    biological vulnerability and, 104–105
    findings from, 108–111
Imipramine, 209, 215
Inadequate parenting, 421
Indicated prevention, 333, 336–337, 359
Individualism, 268
Inhibition of emotion, 157–158
Input regulation strategies, 163
Insecure attachment, 88–89
Integrated conceptual models of sex
        differences, 394–397
Integrated psychobiological developmental
        model of child adversity and depression,
        481–482
Intentional activities, 275–276
Intentions to regulate emotions, 149–150
Interactionism, 267
Interaction of etiological mechanisms, 422
Intermediate beliefs, 225–226
Intermediate phenotypes as mediators of
        genetic and environmental risk, 140–
        143
Interpersonal factors, 182–183, 423

Interpersonal–psychological theory of suicidal
       behavior, 447–448, 450–451, 452–453,
       454
Interpersonal psychotherapy for adolescents
       (IPT-A)
   course of, 290–291
   efficacy and effectiveness research in, 298–
       299
   initial phase of, 291–293
   middle phase of, 293–297
   overview of, 289–290, 303–304
   as preventive intervention, 299–303
   termination phase of, 297–298
Interpersonal psychotherapy (IPT), 288–289
Interpersonal theories
   developmental perspective on, 81
   early family disruption and, 87–89
   overview of, 79–80, 93
   relationship disturbances and, 83–84
   research, future directions for, 93–95
   social-behavioral deficits and, 81–82
   transactions between dysfunction and
       depression, 84–87
   vulnerability–stress perspectives, 89–93
Interrelation of cognitive vulnerability factors,
       55
Interviews regarding child abuse and neglect,
       468
Invalidating environments, 447
IPT-A. See Interpersonal psychotherapy for
       adolescents (IPT-A)
IPT-AST, 299–303, 304
IPT (interpersonal psychotherapy), 288–289

K

Kindling hypothesis, 480

L

Languishing, 253
Lewinsohn's behavioral tradition, 185, 186–
       187, 189
LHPA. See Limbic–hypothalamic–pituitary–
       adrenocortical (LHPA) system
Life events, stressful, exposure to
   child abuse and neglect and, 479–482
   cognitive-behavioral therapy and, 183–184
   cognitive vulnerability and, 57

   as correlate, 20
   sex differences and, 391
Life Events and Difficulties Schedule, 480
Lifetime comorbidity, 15–16
Lifetime prevalence, 9
Limbic–hypothalamic–pituitary–adrenocortical
       (LHPA) system, 107–108, 113–114
Limbic system and trauma, 479
Limited sick role, assigning, 291–292
Linkage studies and molecular genetic designs,
       129–130
Listening, empathic, 245
Loneliness and suicide, 450

M

Major depression, prevalence of, 179
Making Hope Happen, 257
Maltreatment
   assessment of, 467–469
   cognitive mediation of relation of
       depression and, 474–477
   contextual factors and, 473–474
   depression in adolescents and, 470–473
   depression in children and, 469–470
   emotion regulation and, 169
   hopelessness theory and, 57–58
   integrated psychobiological developmental
       model of depression and, 481–482
   as negative event, 390
   neurobiology of, 477–479
   overview of, 466–467, 482–483
   sexual, 472, 474
   stress sensitivity and, 479–482
   suicidal behavior and, 449–450
   type of, 473
Manifestation of depression, potential sex
       differences in, 381–383
MAOIs (monoamine oxydase inhibitors),
       211
Marital discord, 426–427
Maternal depression
   affect regulation and, 229
   child-level interventions, 428
   core etiological mechanisms, 417–422
   empirical findings regarding, 168–169
   etiology of depression in children and
       adolescents, 417–427
   family-level interventions, 430–431
   future directions, 431

implications of, for treatment and prevention, 427–431

interacting etiological mechanisms, 422

interpersonal vulnerability and, 89

moderating variables, 424–427

mother-level interventions, 428–430

nature and extent of problem of, 415–416

pathways to depression and, 422–424

timing and course of, 427

The meaningful life, 268–269

Mediational models, 386–388, 391, 399

Meditation, 262

Memory, reeducating, 274–275

Mental pain, 446

Mentoring, 364–365

Method restriction, 456

Middle childhood and hopelessness, 51–52

Mirtazapine, 211

Modeling and maternal depression, 420–421

Modeling hypothesis and cognitive vulnerability, 58–59

Models

ABC, 312–314

combined trait/contextual, 53, 54

common cause, 159

competence-based, 85

complication, 159

concomitants, 159

contextual/autoregressive, 53, 54

depression contagion, 389

developmental assets, 370

ecological, of mental health, 338

integrated conceptual, of sex differences, 394–397

integrated psychobiological developmental, of child adversity and depression, 481–482

mediational, 386–388, 391, 399

moderational, 387–388, 399

pathoplasty, 159

predisposition, 159

titration, 37

transactional, 389, 422, 424

See also Diathesis–stress models; Vulnerability–stress models

Moderating variables, 424–427

Moderational models, 387–388, 399

Modular cognitive-behavioral therapy, 200

Molecular genetic studies

findings of, 134–136

methodology of, 128–131

Monoamine oxidase inhibitors (MAOIs), 211

Monoamines, 112, 135

Monozygotic (MZ) twins, 126

Mood monitoring in cognitive-behavioral therapy, 188–189, 192

MRI (nuclear magnetic resonance imaging), 104, 105

Muck Monster, talking back to, 242

Multifinality, 422

Multiple informants, integrating information from, 8

Multiplicative approach to vulnerability factors, 48

Multisite designs, 212–213

Multiwave longitudinal designs and cognitive vulnerability, 59–60, 61, 62

Myelination, 106–107

MZ (monozygotic) twins, 126

N

N-acetylaspartate, 112–113

Nefazodone, 211

Negative affectivity, 391–392

Negative cognitive triad, 38, 41

Negative Emotionality/Neuroticism (NE), 152–155

Negatives

dividends of focusing on, in psychotherapy, 252–253

humans as enamored with, 251–252

Negative thoughts

evaluating and replacing, 241–243

identifying, 241

Neglect. See Maltreatment

Neural activity and emotion regulation, 165–166

Neurobiology of depression, major theories of, 19–20. See also Biological vulnerability

Neurochemical disturbances, 226–227

Neurodevelopment and functioning, normative, 106–108

Neuroregulatory mechanisms, 419–420

Neurotransmitters

biological vulnerability and, 111–113

drug action and, 209

levels of, experimental manipulation of, 104

Nomothetic approach to analysis, 59–63

Nonshared environmental factors, 125

Nonsuicidal self-injury (NSSI), 448–449

Nortriptyline, 209
No-suicide contracts, 453
Nuclear magnetic resonance imaging (MRI), 104, 105
Null hypothesis significance testing, 52

O

Opponent process theory, 447
"OR" rule, 8
Overregulation of emotion, 157–158

P

Parental education, 138
Parental involvement
    in interpersonal therapy for adolescents (IPT-A), 290
    in Penn Resiliency Program (PRP), 325–326
Parental psychopathology, 19, 89. *See also* Maternal depression
Parental socialization and sex differences, 380–381
Parent–child relationships
    disturbances in, 83–84
    emotion regulation and, 163–164
    insecure, 88–89
Parenting practices
    cognitive vulnerability and, 58–59
    enhancing, 430
    maternal depression and, 420–422
Parent training in ACTION treatment program, 244–246
Paroxetine, 210, 215, 216
Passive gene–environment correlations, 136, 137
Pathoplasty model, 159
Pathways to depression, 422–424
Peers
    rejection by, 450
    relationships with, disturbances in, 83
    role disputes and, 296
Penn Resiliency Program (PRP)
    cognitive component of, 312–316
    current and future directions for, 325–328
    early adolescence, importance of, 310–311
    intervention dissemination, 324–325, 327–328

overview of, 309, 312
    research on, 318–325
    social-problem-solving component, 316–318
PE (Positive Emotionality/Extraversion), 152–155
Personality and social-cognitive style, 90
Personality predispositions, 44, 45–46
Pessimistic explanatory style, 311
PET (positron emission tomography), 104, 105
Pharmacokinetics and pharmacodynamics
    overview of, 208–209
    sex differences and, 397–398
Physical abuse. *See* Abuse
Physical appearance, perceptions of, 391
Pleasant Activities Checklist (Lewinsohn), 189
The pleasant life, 263, 265
Positive affectivity, 392
Positive Emotionality/Extraversion (PE), 152–155
Positive emotions
    building, 275
    discussing, 260–262
    the pleasant life, 263, 265
    regulation of, 160–161
    view of, 259–260
Positive psychology movement, 356
Positive Psychotherapy Inventory—Children's Version, 287
Positive psychotherapy (PPT)
    assumptions of, 258–262
    as descriptive not prescriptive, 277–278
    flexible approach of, 274
    future directions for, 279
    goal of, 272–273
    idealized session-by-session description of, 264–265
    motivation for change and, 278
    negative experiences and, 273–274
    overview of, 250–251
    potential mechanism of change, 274–277
    theoretical background of, 262–269
    therapeutic relationship in, 277
    validation studies of, 269–272
Positive reinforcement, 244
Positive youth development (PYD) programs
    Across Ages, 364–365, 366
    adventure programs, 362–364
    Big Brothers and Big Sisters Program, 365, 367

effectiveness of, 356–359, 368–370
framework of, 361
interventions, 361–368
overview of, 354, 355–356
School Transitional Environment Project, 365, 367–368, 369
theoretical framework for, 370
Positron emission tomography (PET), 104, 105
Postpartum depression, 428–429
Postpubertal-onset depression, 17
PPT. *See* Positive psychotherapy (PPT)
Predisposition model, 159
Prefrontal cortex
    emotion regulation and, 165–166
    primary role of, 107–108
    subgenual, 109
Prenatal experiences, 419
Prepubertal-onset depression, 17
Prevalence rates
    age and sex patterns of, 9, 14
    estimates of, 9, 10–13
    major depression, 179
    sex differences in, 377
    of suicidal behavior, 442–443
    in Western cultures, 3
Prevention
    definition of, 310
    of suicide, 457–458
Prevention of depression
    efficacy and effectiveness of programs for, 334–337, 359–361
    IPT-AST and, 299–303, 304
    overview of, 333
    positive psychotherapy (PPT) and, 253–254
    schools and, 328
    sex differences and, 398
    See also Penn Resiliency Program (PRP); Positive youth development (PYD) programs; School-based, universal prevention approach
Primary care settings, managing adolescent depression in, 220
Problem Solving for Life program, 335–337
Problem-solving skills
    cognitive-behavioral therapy and, 182, 190–191
    five-step approach to, 318
    ineffective, as consequence, 82

social, 316–318
    suicidal behavior and, 456
Problem-solving training in ACTION treatment program, 237–238, 245
Progress chart for school action team, 345
PRP. *See* Penn Resiliency Program (PRP)
Psychache theory of suicide, 445–446
Psychoeducation
    in ACTION treatment program, 234–235
    in cognitive-behavioral therapy, 187
    in interpersonal therapy for adolescents (IPT-A), 291–292
    in IPT-AST, 300, 301
Psychology, World War II and, 255
Psychopathology, prevention of, 253–254
Psychopharmacological treatment
    antidepressant drug classes, 208–211
    combining with psychotherapy, 219–220, 227
    efficacy studies, 211–216
    management principles, 217–218
    overview of, 207–208
    safety concerns, 218–219
    treatment-resistant depression, 218
Psychotherapy
    Beck's cognitive therapy, 185–186
    cognitive-behavioral analysis system of, 456
    combining with psychopharmacological treatment, 219–220, 227
    developmental group, 455
    dialectical behavior therapy (DBT), 447, 456–457
    dividends of focusing on negatives in, 252–253
    family communication and problem solving, 455
    interpersonal psychotherapy (IPT), 288–289
    modular cognitive-behavioral, 200
    quality of life therapy, 257
    for suicidal behavior, 454–457
    targeting happiness explicitly, 256–258
    See also Cognitive-behavioral therapy (CBT); Interpersonal psychotherapy for adolescents (IPT-A); Positive psychotherapy (PPT); Therapeutic relationship
Pubertal development and timing, 384
Putting It in Perspective skill, 315–316
PYD. *See* Positive youth development (PYD) programs

Q

Qualities of children and maternal depression, 424–425
Quality of life therapy, 257
Quantitative genetic studies
    findings of, 131–134
    methodology of, 125–128
Quantitative trait loci (QTLs), 128–129, 135–136

R

Race
    as correlate, 18
    prevalence of abuse and, 474
    treatment and, 21
Randomized clinical trials (RCT)
    of pharmacological treatment, 212, 220
    of positive psychotherapy (PPT), 269–272
Rational disputation, 192–194
Reboxetine, 211
Recurrence
    consequences of, 20
    risk for, 16–17
Relapse prevention and cognitive-behavioral
        therapy, 194
Relationships, disturbances in
    early family disruption and, 87–89
    interpersonal theories and, 79, 83–84
    long-term, 87
    as risk factor, 85–86
    short-term, 86–87
Relaxation training
    cognitive-behavioral therapy and, 194
    Penn Resiliency Program and, 317–318
Reporting bias, 382
Research
    community studies, 384
    future, directions for, 22–23
    future, on cognitive vulnerability to
        depression, 65–68
    future, on interpersonal model of
        depression, 93–95
    future, on suicidal behavior, 458–459
    overview of, 3–4
    on relation of child abuse and neglect to
        depression in adolescence, 471
    sex differences and, 399
    See also Efficacy studies; Efficacy studies of
        psychopharmacological treatment

Resourceful Adolescent Program, 325, 335
Responses to stress. See Stress, responses to
Response styles theory
    additive approach to vulnerability factors
        and, 49
    overview of, 41–43
    ruminative style, 156–157
    social environment and, 143
"Retail therapy," 277
Review of current activities for school action
        team, 346
Reviews of literature, epidemiological, 6
RIBEYE acronym, 190–191
Risk factors
    cognitive, 311
    emotion regulation and, 169
    interpersonal dysfunction, 85–86
    for suicide, 441, 443–444
Role disputes, interpersonal, 296
Role playing in interpersonal therapy for
        adolescents (IPT-A), 295
Role transitions, 297
Rumination
    as emotion regulation strategy, 155, 156–157
    Girls in Transition program and, 327
    as response to symptoms, 41–42, 94

S

Scale for Suicide Ideation, 451
Schema
    Beck's cognitive theory and, 38, 41
    cognitive-behavioral therapy and, 182, 185
School action team, 249, 343–347
School-based, universal prevention approach
    efficacy and effectiveness of, 334–338
    evaluation of, 349
    limitations of, 328
    overview of, 333–334
    pathways for care and support, building,
        347, 349
    rationale for, 343
    whole-school change process, 343–347, 348
    See also beyondblue schools research
        initiative
School Transitional Environment Project, 365,
        367–368, 369
Screening for suicidal symptoms, 458
Selected prevention, 333
Selective prevention, 359

Selective serotonin reuptake inhibitors (SSRIs)
action of, 210–211
discontinuation syndromes, 210, 218
effectiveness of, 111–112
efficacy studies of, 214–216
safety of, 218–219
selecting and monitoring, 217–218
Self, core beliefs about
case conceptualization and, 232–233
dysfunctional, 225–226
positive, building, 243
Self-actualization, 255–256
Self-consciousness and cognitive vulnerability, 59
Self-criticism/autonomy, 44, 64
Self-injury, 446–447, 448–449
Self-map, 243
Self-monitoring and Catch the Positive Diary
(CPD), 236–237, 243
Self-regulation and interpersonal dysfunction, 85
Self-reports of adversity, 467–468
Sensitivity to future stress, 479–483
Sequential comorbidity, 15
Serotonergic (5-HT) neurotransmitter system,
134–135, 139–140
Serotonin, 111–112
Sertraline, 210, 215, 216
Service utilization, factors in, 21
Severity of depression, variability in, 37
Sex differences
biological factors and, 392–394
causal explanations of, evaluating, 386–388
child abuse, maltreatment, and, 390
cognitive vulnerabilities and, 390–391
developmental psychopathological approach
to, 377–378, 399–400
developmental timeline for emergence of,
381–386
in emotion and temperament, 391–392
in heritability of depression, 133
integrated conceptual models of, 394–397
in normal development, 378–381
overview of, 398–400
in prevalence rates, 14, 377
stressors and, 388–389
in treatment and prevention, 397–398
See also Gender
Sex roles and stereotypes, 381
Sexual abuse, 472, 474
Shared environmental factors, 125
Sib-pair design, 130, 134
Signature strengths, 266–267, 273, 275–276

Similar mediating pathway, 49
Single photon emission computed tomography
(SPECT), 104, 111
Social anxiety, 106
Social-behavioral deficits
early family disruption and, 87–89
interpersonal theories and, 79, 81–82
long-term, 87
as risk factor, 85–86
short-term, 86–87
Social development, sex differences in, 380
Social interaction and cognitive-behavioral
therapy, 190
Social problem solving, 316–318
Social skills disturbances, 227–228
Socioeconomic status, as correlate, 18
Socratic stance, 192
Specific vulnerability hypothesis, 63–65
SPECT (single photon emission computed
tomography), 104, 111
SSRIs (selective serotonin reuptake inhibitors)
action of, 210–211
discontinuation syndromes, 210, 218
effectiveness of, 111–112
efficacy studies of, 214–216
safety of, 218–219
selecting and monitoring, 217–218
Strategies
cognitive-behavioral therapy (CBT), 185–187
for cognitive restructuring in ACTION
treatment program, 241–243
hope enhancement, 257
input regulation, 163
Strengths
assessment of, 260
in beyondblue schools research initiative,
340, 342
discussing, 260–262
signature, 266–267, 273, 275–276
Strengths-based program, 368–370. See also
Positive youth development (PYD)
programs
Stress
cognitive vulnerability–transactional stress
theory, 395–396
maternal depression and, 421–422
neurochemical disturbances and, 226–227
positive aspects to, 273
See also Hypothalamic–pituitary–adrenal
(HPA) axis; Stress, exposure to; Stress,
responses to; Stressors

Stress, exposure to
  cognitive-behavioral therapy and, 183–184
  as correlate, 20
  sex differences and, 388
Stress, responses to
  child abuse and neglect and, 479–482
  hippocampus and, 19
  interpersonal dysfunction and, 85
  interpersonal theories and, 82
  limbic–hypothalamic–pituitary–
    adrenocortical (LHPA) system, 113–114
  sex differences and, 388–389
  See also Diathesis–stress models;
    Vulnerability–stress models
Stress exposure hypothesis, 388
Stress generation hypothesis, 389
Stressors
  cognitive vulnerability and, 63–65
  interaction of neurobiologic forces and,
    116–117
Stress reactivity hypothesis, 388–389
Structural equation modeling, 53
Subgenual prefrontal cortex, 109
Substance use disorders, comorbidity of, 15
Suicidal behavior
  assessment of risk of, 451–453
  crisis intervention for, 453–454
  depression as predictor of, 21
  epidemiology of, 442–443
  future directions for, 458–459
  overview of, 441–442
  prevention of, 457–458
  psychotherapy for, 454–457
  risk factors for, 443–444
  SSRIs and, 218–219
  theories of, 445–451
Suicide Assessment Decision Tree, 451–452
Suppression of emotion, 157–158
Symptom expression
  age differences in, 7
  sex differences in, 381–383

T

TADS (Treatment for Adolescents with
    Depression Study) Team, 197–198, 199,
    457
TCAs (tricyclic antidepressants)
  action and side effects of, 209–210
  efficacy studies of, 213–214

"Teen Talk," 299–303
Temperament
  distinctions between emotion, emotion
    regulation, and, 152–156
  maternal depression and, 424–425
  sex differences in, 379–380, 391–392
Theory
  ACTION treatment program and, 224–230
  bioevolutionary, 395
  cognitive-behavioral, 311
  cognitive vulnerability–transactional stress,
    67, 395–396
  developmental intentionality, 369–370
  escape, of suicidal behavior, 446
  interpersonal–psychological, of suicidal
    behavior, 447–448, 450–451, 452–453,
    454
  of neurobiology of depression, 19–20
  opponent process, 447
  of positive psychotherapy (PPT), 262–269
  of positive youth development (PYD)
    programs, 370
  psychache, of suicide, 445–446
  See also Beck's cognitive theory;
    Hopelessness theory; Interpersonal
    theories; Response styles theory
Therapeutic relationship
  assumptions of, 261
  in cognitive-behavioral therapy, 187–188
  in positive psychotherapy (PPT), 277
Therapy. See Psychotherapy
Thinking styles, recognizing, 314
Thought Detective Questions, 241, 242
Thoughts
  automatic, 191–192
  catastrophic, 315–316
  counter-thoughts, 192–194
  negative, evaluating and replacing, 241–243
Threat perception, 142–143
Three Good Things exercise, 274
Titration models, 37
Trait-like risk factors, 53–54
Transactional models, 389, 422, 424
Transactions between interpersonal
    dysfunction and depression, 84–87
Trazodone, 211
Treatment
  factors in utilization of, 21
  sex differences and outcome of, 397–398
  See also Psychopharmacological treatment;
    Psychotherapy

Treatment for Adolescents with Depression
    Study Team (TADS), 197–198, 199,
    457
Treatment-resistant depression, 218
Tricyclic antidepressants (TCAs)
    action and side effects of, 209–210
    efficacy studies of, 213–214
Tryptophan, 112, 135
Twin studies
    behavioral genetic designs, 126–127
    gene–environment interactions, 139
    longitudinal, 132–133
    results from, 131
Two time point study, 53

U

Universal prevention
    description of, 333–334, 359
    studies of, 334–337, 359–361
    See also beyondblue schools research
        initiative; School-based, universal
        prevention approach

V

Vagal tone and emotion regulation, 166
Values in Action Inventory of Strengths,
    276
Venlafaxine, 211
Visualization exercise, 317
Volunteerism, 268–269
Vulnerabilities
    affective, 423
    behavioral, 423
    interpersonal, 89–93
    specific vulnerability hypothesis, 63–65
    See also Biological vulnerability; Cognitive
        vulnerability; Vulnerability–stress models
Vulnerability factors
    additive approach to, 48–49
    cognitive-behavioral therapy and, 181–184

developmental changes in interrelation
    among, 55
developmental changes in levels of, 55–56
developmental origins of, 56–59
developmental stage and, 51–53
emergence and consolidation of, 51
maternal depression and, 422–424, 428
multiplicative approach to, 48
overview of, 37
priming of, 63
relationships between, 47–51
stabilization of, into trait-like risk factors,
    53–54
weakest link approach to, 49–51
Vulnerability–stress models
    cognitive-behavioral, 311
    developmental transitions, 91–93
    gender and gender-linked processes, 90–91
    overview of, 89–90, 103
    personality and social-cognitive style, 90
    sex differences and, 394–395, 396–397
    See also Diathesis–stress models

W

Warning signs of suicidal behavior, 443, 444,
    457–458
Weakest link approach to vulnerability
    factors, 49–51
Well-being therapy, 256–257
Western culture, 261–262, 278, 380
White matter hyperintensities, 109
Whole-brain volume, 106, 108–109
Whole-school change process, 343–347, 348
Work at home in interpersonal therapy for
    adolescents (IPT-A), 295

Y

Youth development programs, 355. *See also*
    Positive youth development (PYD)
    programs